TUMORS of the SPINE
Diagnosis and Clinical Management

Edited by

NARAYAN SUNDARESAN, M.D.

Department of Neurological Surgery,
Mt. Sinai School of Medicine,
New York, New York

HENRY H. SCHMIDEK, M.D.

Vice-Chairman, Department of Neurological Surgery,
Henry Ford Hospital,
Detroit, Michigan

ALAN L. SCHILLER, M.D.

Irene Heinz Given and John LaPorte Given Professor
and Chairman, Department of Pathology,
Mt. Sinai School of Medicine,
New York, New York

DANIEL I. ROSENTHAL, M.D.

Director of Bone and Joint Radiology,
Massachusetts General Hospital;
Associate Professor of Radiology,
Department of Radiology, Harvard Medical School,
Boston, Massachusetts

And the American Association of Neurological Surgeons

1990

W.B. SAUNDERS COMPANY

Harcourt Brace Jovanovich, Inc.

Philadelphia, London, Toronto, Montreal, Sydney, Tokyo

W. B. SAUNDERS COMPANY
Harcourt Brace Jovanovich, Inc.

The Curtis Center
Independence Square West
Philadelphia, PA 19106

Library of Congress Cataloging-in-Publication Data

Tumors of the spine: diagnosis and clinical management /
Narayan Sundaresan . . . [et al.] and the American Association
of Neurological Surgeons.

    p.   cm.

1. Spine—Tumors.   I. Sundaresan, Narayan. II. American
    Association of Neurological Surgeons. [DNLM: 1. Spinal
    Neoplasms—diagnosis.   2. Spinal Neoplasms—
    therapy.   3. Spine—radiography. WE 725 T92454]

RC280.S72T87 1990   616.99'4711–dc20

ISBN 0–7216–2896–6

DNLM/DLC   89–70106

Sponsoring Editor: Martin Wonsiewicz
Developmental Editor: David H. Kilmer
Manuscript Editor: Keryn Lane
Production Manager: Frank Polizzano
Designer: Lorraine B. Kilmer
Illustration Coordinator: Joan Sinclair
Indexer: Dennis Dolan

TUMORS OF THE SPINE:
Diagnosis and Clinical Management   ISBN 0–7216–2896–6

Printed in the United States of America.

Last digit is the print number: 9   8   7   6   5   4   3   2   1

Hospital Series
POST-OPERATIVE

I come
        from the depth
        of anesthesia
Sleep the non-sleep
        of post-operative
        half life
_____

Wake up
Open my eye
        not knowing where am I
Encounter response
        in my daughter's look
She slept on the cot
        and watches
As I slowly return
        to what we call life

SIMON

Columbia Presbyterian Hospital
December 25, 1981

CONTRIBUTORS

MAX AEBI, M.D.

Associate Professor, Department of Orthopaedic Surgery, University of Bern; Chief, Spinal Surgery Service, Department of Orthopaedic Surgery, Inselspital, Bern, Switzerland

Use of the Internal Fixator in Spine Tumor Surgery

MARY AUSTIN-SEYMOUR, M.D.

Formerly of the Department of Radiation Medicine, Massachusetts General Hospital Cancer Center, Harvard Medical School, Boston, Massachusetts

The Role of Radiation Therapy

ALEX BERENSTEIN, M.D.

Professor of Radiology and Attending in Radiology, New York University Medical Center, New York, New York

Spinal Angiography and Embolization of Tumors

STEFANO BORIANI, M.D.

Orthopedic Surgeon, Rizzoli Institute, Bologna, Italy

Giant Cell Tumors of the Spine

JOHN K. BRADWAY, M.D.

Senior Resident in Orthopedics, Mayo Graduate School of Medicine, Rochester, Minnesota

Ewing's Tumor of the Spine

FRANK P. CAMMISA, JR., M.D.

Assistant Attending Orthopaedic Surgeon, The Hospital for Special Surgery, New York, New York

Benign Cartilage Tumors of the Spine; Chondrosarcoma of the Spine: Memorial Sloan-Kettering Cancer Center Experience

MARIO CAMPANACCI, M.D.

Professor of Orthopedics, University of Bologna; Chief of the First Orthopedic Clinic, Rizzoli Institute, Bologna, Italy

Giant Cell Tumors of the Spine

ROBERT C. CANTU, M.A., M.D.

Chief, Neurosurgery Service and Chairman, Department of Surgery, and Director, Service of Sports Medicine, Emerson Hospital, Concord, Massachusetts

Osseous Fusion of the Cervical, Thoracic, and Lumbar Spine with Primary and Metastatic Spine Tumors

RICHARD L. CARTER, M.D.

Senior Neurosurgery Resident, Department of Neurosurgery, University of Florida, Gainesville, Florida

Cotrel-Dubousset Instrumentation: Indications and Techniques

TED CHAGLASSIAN, M.D.

Associate Professor, Cornell University Medical College; Chief of Plastic and Reconstructive Surgery Division, Memorial Sloan-Kettering Cancer Center, New York, New York

Wound Management in Spinal Surgery

IN SUP CHOI, M.D.

Assistant Professor of Radiology, New York University Medical Center; Attending in Radiology, New York University Medical Center, New York, New York

Spinal Angiography and Embolization of Tumors

T. FORCHT DAGI, M.D.

Associate Professor of Surgery, Uniform Services of Health Sciences, Department of Clinical Neurosciences, Brown University, Providence, Rhode Island

Vascular Tumors

WALTER DICK, M.D.

Associate Professor, Department of Orthopaedic Surgery, University of Basel; Chief, Section of Adult Orthopaedic Surgery, Department of Orthopaedic Surgery, Felix-Platter-Spital, Basel, Switzerland

Use of the Internal Fixator in Spine Tumor Surgery

GEORGE V. DiGIACINTO, M.D.

Associate Attending Surgeon, St. Lukes/Roosevelt Hospital Center, New York, New York

Metastatic Tumors of the Spine; Surgical Approaches to the CervicoThoracic Junction; Complete Spondylectomy for Malignant Tumors

MAHMOUD EL-TAMER, M.D.

Fellow, Department of Surgery, Memorial Sloan-Kettering Cancer Center, New York, New York

Wound Management in Spinal Surgery

WILLIAM F. ENNEKING, M.D.

Distinguished Service Professor in Orthopaedics, University of Florida, Gainesville, Florida

Staging of Musculoskeletal Neoplasms

FRANK J. FRASSICA, M.D.

Assistant Professor of Orthopedics, Mayo Medical School; Special Fellow in Orthopedic Oncology, Mayo Graduate School of Medicine, Rochester, Minnesota

Chondrosarcoma of the Spine: Mayo Clinic Experience

DALE B. GLASSER, M.S.

Orthopaedic Research, Memorial Sloan-Kettering Cancer Center and The Hospital for Special Surgery, New York, New York

Benign Cartilage Tumors of the Spine; Chondrosarcoma of the Spine: Memorial Sloan-Kettering Cancer Center Experience

ARMANDO GIUNTI, M.D.

Professor of Orthopedics, University of Bologna; Chief of the Third Orthopedic Clinic, Rizzoli Institute, Bologna, Italy

Giant Cell Tumors of the Spine

MARK N. HADLEY, M.D., MAJOR, USAFMC

Assistant Professor, Division of Neurosurgery, Emory University, Atlanta, Georgia; Chief, Division of Neurological Surgery, David Grant USAF Medical Center, Travis Air Force Base, California

The Transoral-Transclival Approach to the Upper Cervical Spine

REGIS W. HAID, Jr., M.D.

Clinical Assistant Professor, Department of Neurosurgery, University of Florida, Gainesville, Florida; Staff Neurosurgeon, Wilford Hall Medical Center, San Antonio, Texas

Cotrel-Dubousset Instrumentation: Indications and Techniques

AKIRA HAKUBA, M.D., D.M.S.

Associate Professor of Neurosurgery, Osaka City University Medical School, Osaka, Japan

Transuncodiscal Approach to Cervical Spine Tumors

DAVID C. HARMON, M.D.

Assistant Professor of Medicine, Harvard Medical School; Assistant Physician, Massachusetts General Hospital, Boston, Massachusetts

Chemotherapy

JAMES E. O. HUGHES, M.D.

Associate Attending Surgeon, St. Lukes/Roosevelt Hospital Center, New York, New York

Metastatic Tumors of the Spine; Anterior Approaches to the Thoracic and Thoraco-Lumbar Junction; Complete Spondylectomy for Malignant Tumors

CONSTANTINE KARAKOUSIS, M.D., PH.D.

Clinical Professor of Surgery, State University of New York at Buffalo; Associate Chief, Surgical Oncology Department, and Chief, Soft Tissue–Melanoma and Bone Service, Roswell Park Memorial Institute, Buffalo, New York

Surgical Approaches to Tumors of the Pelvis Involving the Axial Skeleton

SUSAN V. KATTAPURAM, M.D.

Assistant Professor of Radiology, Harvard Medical School; Associate Radiologist, Bone and Joint Radiology, Massachusetts General Hospital, Boston, Massachusetts

Percutaneous Needle Biopsy of the Spine

SANFORD KEMPIN, M.D.

Associate Professor of Clinical Medicine, Cornell University Medical College; Associate Attending Physician and Acting Chief, Hematology Service, Memorial Sloan-Kettering Cancer Center, New York, New York

Disorders of the Spine Related to Plasma Cell Dyscrasias

GEORGE KROL, M.D.

Memorial Sloan-Kettering Cancer Center, New York, New York

Chordomas; Postradiation Sarcomas Involving the Spine; Surgical Management of Superior Sulcus Tumors; Metastatic Tumors of the Spine; Complete Spondylectomy for Malignant Tumors

JOSEPH M. LANE, M.D.

Professor, Orthopaedic Surgery, Cornell University Medical College; Chief, Orthopaedic Surgery, Memorial Sloan-Kettering Cancer Center; Chief, Metabolic Bone Disease Service, The Hospital for Special Surgery, New York, New York

Benign Cartilage Tumors of the Spine; Chondrosarcoma of the Spine: Memorial Sloan-Kettering Cancer Center Experience; Surgical Approaches to the Sacroiliac Joint

Ph. LAPRESLE, M.D.

Department of Orthopedic Surgery and Trauma, Hôpital de la Pitie, Paris, France

Treatment of Malignant Tumors of the Spine with Posterior Instrumentation

SANFORD J. LARSON, M.D., PH.D.

Professor and Chairman, Department of Neurosurgery, Medical College of Wisconsin; Attending Neurosurgeon and Director of Neurosurgery Service, Froedtert Memorial Lutheran Hospital, and Attending Neurosurgeon and Chief of Neurosurgical Service, Milwaukee County Medical Complex; Consultant, Veterans Administration Medical Center, Milwaukee, Wisconsin

Segmental Fixation of the Spine with the Luque Rod System

DAVID R. MACDONALD, M.D.

Assistant Professor (Neurology), Departments of Clinical Neurological Sciences and Oncology, The University of Western Ontario; Attending Neurologist (Active Teaching Staff), London Regional Cancer Centre, and Victoria Hospital; Consulting Neurologist, University Hospital and St. Joseph's Health Centre, London, Canada

Clinical Manifestations

RALPH C. MARCOVE, M.D.

Clinical Associate Professor of Surgery, Cornell University Medical College; Associate Attending Surgeon, Memorial Hospital, The Hospital for Special Surgery and The New York Hospital, New York, New York

The Role of Cryosurgery

C. MAZEL, M.D.

Department of Orthopedic Surgery and Trauma, Hôpital de la Pitie, Paris, France

Treatment of Malignant Tumors of the Spine with Posterior Instrumentation

R. J. McBROOM, M.D., F.R.C.S.(C)

Assistant Professor, Department of Surgery, University of Toronto; Orthopaedic Surgeon, Wellesley Hospital and St. Michael's Hospital, Toronto, Canada

Surgical Treatment for Spinal Metastases: The Posterolateral Approach

PAUL C. McCORMICK, M.D.

Assistant Professor, Department of Neurological Surgery, Columbia University College of Physicians and Surgeons, New York, New York

Surgical Considerations in Pelvic Tumors with Intraspinal Extension

DOUGLAS J. McDONALD, M.D.

Special Fellow in Orthopedic Oncology, Mayo Graduate School of Medicine, Rochester, Minnesota

Giant Cell Tumors of the Spine and Sacrum: Mayo Clinic Experience

JESSOP McDONALD, M.D.

Tacoma, Washington

Surgical Approaches to the Sacroiliac Joint

RICHARD A. McLEOD, M.D.

Professor of Radiology, Mayo Medical School; Consultant, Department of Diagnostic Radiology, Mayo Clinic and Mayo Foundation, Rochester, Minnesota

Chondrosarcoma of the Spine: Mayo Clinic Experience; Giant Cell Tumors of the Spine and Sacrum: Mayo Clinic Experience

WADE M. MUELLER, M.D.

Department of Neurosurgery, Medical College of Wisconsin, Milwaukee, Wisconsin

Segmental Fixation of the Spine with the Luque Rod System

R. G. PERRIN, M.D., M.Sc., F.A.C.S., F.R.C.S.(C)

Assistant Professor, University of Toronto; Chief of Neurosurgery, The Wellesley Hospital, Toronto, Canada

Surgical Treatment for Spinal Metastases: The Posterolateral Approach

KALMON D. POST, M.D.

Vice Chairman and Professor, Department of Neurological Surgery, Columbia University College of Physicians and Surgeons; Attending Neurosurgeon, Neurological Institute, Columbia Presbyterian Medical Center, New York, New York

Surgical Considerations in Pelvic Tumors with Intraspinal Extension

DOUGLAS J. PRITCHARD, M.D.

Professor of Orthopedics and of Oncology, Mayo Medical School; Head, Section of Orthopedic Oncology, Mayo Clinic and Foundation, Rochester, Minnesota

Ewing's Tumor of the Spine

SETTI S. RENGACHARY, M.D.

Professor and Chief, Section of Neurological Surgery, University of Missouri at Kansas City School of Medicine; Attending Neurological Surgeon, Truman Medical Center, and Trinity Lutheran Hospital, Kansas City, Missouri

Posterior and Posterolateral Surgical Approaches to the Spine

ANDREW E. ROSENBERG, M.D.

Instructor in Pathology, Harvard Medical School; Assistant in Pathology, Department of Pathology, Massachusetts General Hospital, Boston, Massachusetts

Tumorous Lesions of the Spine: An Overview

DANIEL I. ROSENTHAL, M.D.

Associate Professor of Radiology, Harvard Medical School; Director, Bone and Joint Radiology, Massachusetts General Hospital, Boston, Massachusetts

Radiology of Spine Tumors: General Considerations; Percutaneous Needle Biopsy of the Spine; An Atlas of Lesions That May Resemble Tumors on Radiographs; Osteosarcoma of the Spine; Chordomas; Postradiation Sarcomas Involving the Spine

HERBERT ROSENTHAL, M.D.

Department of Radiology, Hannover Medical School, Hannover, West Germany

An Atlas of Lesions That May Resemble Tumors on Radiographs

R. ROY-CAMILLE, M.D.

Department of Orthopedic Surgery and Trauma, Hôpital de la Pitie, Paris, France

Treatment of Malignant Tumors of the Spine with Posterior Instrumentation

VED P. SACHDEV, M.D.

Clinical Professor and Vice Chairman, Department of Neurosurgery, Mt. Sinai Hospital, New York, New York

Surgical Management of Superior Sulcus Tumors; Anterior Approaches to the Cervical Spine

G. SAILLANT, M.D.

Department of Orthopedic Surgery and Trauma, Hôpital de la Pitie, Paris, France

Treatment of Malignant Tumors of the Spine with Posterior Instrumentation

ALAN L. SCHILLER, M.D.

Chairman, Department of Pathology, Mt. Sinai Medical Center, New York, New York

Premalignant Lesions of the Osseous Spine and Classification of Primary Tumors; Tumorous Lesions of the Spine: An Overview; Osteosarcoma of the Spine; Chordomas; Postradiation Sarcomas Involving the Spine

HENRY H. SCHMIDEK, M.D.

Vice-Chairman, Department of Neurosurgery, Henry Ford Hospital, Detroit, Michigan

Premalignant Lesions of the Osseous Spine and Classification of Primary Tumors; Vascular Tumors; Tumors of the Nerve Sheath Involving the Spine; Anterior Approaches to the Thoracic and Thoraco-Lumbar Junction

JATIN P. SHAH, M.D., F.A.C.S.

Professor of Clinical Surgery, Cornell University Medical College; Attending Surgeon, Head and Neck Service, Memorial Sloan-Kettering Cancer Center, New York, New York

Transmandibular Approaches to the Upper Cervical Spine

ASHOK R. SHAHA, M.D.

Associate Professor of Surgery, SUNY Downstate Medical Center; Attending Surgeon, Downstate Medical Center and King's County Hospital, Brooklyn, New York

Transmandibular Approaches to the Upper Cervical Spine

TALI SIEGAL, M.D.

Senior Lecturer in Neurology and Oncology, Hebrew University and Hadassah Medical School; Consultant in Neurology and Neuro-Oncology, Neuro-Oncology Service, Departments of Oncology and Neurology, Hadassah Hebrew University Hospital, Jerusalem, Israel

Neurologic Compromise Due to Spinal Tumors; Surgical Intervention for Neoplastic Involvement of the Lumbar Spine

TZONY SIEGAL, M.D., D.M.D.

Director, Chosen Specialties Clinics, and Consultant, Spinal Surgery, Department of Orthopaedics, Assuta Hospital; Chief, Spinal Clinic, Meuhedet Medical Center; Consultant, Spinal Disorders, General and Leumit Sick Funds, Tel Aviv, Israel

Neurologic Compromise Due to Spinal Tumors; Surgical Intervention for Neoplastic Involvement of the Lumbar Spine

FRANKLIN H. SIM, M.D.

Professor of Orthopedics, Mayo Medical School; Consultant, Department of Orthopedics, Mayo Clinic and Mayo Foundation, Rochester, Minnesota

Chondrosarcoma of the Spine: Mayo Clinic Experience; Giant Cell Tumors of the Spine and Sacrum: Mayo Clinic Experience

DONALD A. SMITH, M.D.

Department of Surgery, University of South Florida College of Medicine, Tampa, Florida

Tumors of the Nerve Sheath Involving the Spine

VOLKER K. H. SONNTAG, M.D., F.A.C.S.

Clinical Associate Professor of Surgery (Neurosurgery), University of Arizona College of Medicine; Vice Chairman, Division of Neurological Surgery, and Chairman, Spinal Cord Injury Committee, Barrow Neurological Institute, Phoenix, Arizona

The Transoral-Transclival Approach to the Upper Cervical Spine

ROBERT F. SPETZLER, M.D.

Professor and Chairman, Division of Neurosurgery, University of Arizona College of Medicine; Director and J.N. Harber Chairman of Neurological Surgery, Barrow Neurological Institute, Phoenix, Arizona

The Transoral-Transclival Approach to the Upper Cervical Spine

BERTIL STENER, M.D., PH.D.

Professor Emeritus of Orthopaedic Surgery, Gothenburg University, Gothenburg, Sweden

Technique of High Sacral Amputation; Technique of Complete Spondylectomy in the Thoracic and Lumbar Spine

HERMAN D. SUIT, M.D.

Chairman, Department of Radiation Therapy, Harvard Medical School; Chief, Department of Radiation Medicine, Massachusetts General Hospital, Boston, Massachusetts

The Role of Radiation Therapy

GEORGE W. SYPERT, M.D., F.A.C.S.

Chairman, Southwest Florida Neurological Institute, Southwest Florida Regional Medical Center, Fort Myers, Florida

Osteoid Osteoma and Osteoblastoma of the Spine; Posterior Stabilization Using Harrington Rod Instrumentation; Spinal Orthotics

CHRISTOPHER L. TILLOTSON, M.D.

Department of Radiology, Abbott Northwestern Hospital, Minneapolis, Minnesota

Radiology of Spine Tumors: General Considerations

TADANORI TOMITA, M.D.

Associate Professor of Surgery (Neurosurgery), Northwestern University Medical School, Director of Brain Tumor Center, Children's Memorial Hospital, Chicago, Illinois

Special Considerations in Surgery of Pediatric Spine Tumors

K. KRISHNAN UNNI, M.B., B.S.

Professor of Pathology, Mayo Medical School; Consultant, Section of Surgical Pathology, Mayo Clinic and Mayo Foundation, Rochester, Minnesota

Giant Cell Tumors of the Spine and Sacrum: Mayo Clinic Experience

RAYMOND P. WARRELL, Jr., M.D.

Associate Professor, Cornell University Medical College; Associate Member, Memorial Sloan-Kettering Cancer Center, New York, New York

New Approach to Medical Management of Spinal Tumors

WALTER WICHERN, M.D.

Chief of Surgery, St. Lukes/Roosevelt Hospital, New York, New York

Surgical Management of Superior Sulcus Tumors

LESTER E. WOLD, M.D.

Associate Professor of Pathology, Mayo Medical School; Consultant, Division of Pathology, Mayo Clinic and Mayo Foundation, Rochester, Minnesota

Chondrosarcoma of the Spine: Mayo Clinic Experience

PREFACE

This textbook was originally conceived as a small monograph to provide neurosurgeons, orthopedic surgeons, and oncologists with an accurate review of the current management of spine tumors. Such a volume is useful because evaluation and management of these lesions have changed greatly within recent years.

There has been a rapid evolution of sophisticated imaging techniques, including magnetic resonance imaging, selective spinal angiography, and radioisotope studies using monoclonal antibodies. At the same time, innovations in surgical techniques and the development of sophisticated spinal instrumentation have allowed radical resection of spine tumors followed by reconstruction of the resected segments. Refinements in histologic diagnosis, progress in the interpretation of needle biopsies, and the ability to gauge the impact of medical and radiation treatment by analysis of the resected specimen have made the bone pathologist one of the most important members of the treatment team. Finally, the development of newer analogues of antineoplastic chemotherapeutic agents (such as ifosfamide and carboplatin) and the use of innovative drug delivery methods (such as intraarterial administration) have considerably expanded the possibilities for treatment by chemotherapy. To achieve the greatest benefits from all these advances requires the talents of a multidisciplinary team, and it quickly became apparent that the scope of the projected volume would have to be expanded. To bring these newer concepts to the reader, the editors have chosen experts who have distinguished themselves in the field by their research. This book has taken almost three years to produce, and we hope that our audience will accept the occasional omission or oversight of recently published material.

The editors realize that a definitive formulation of the rapidly evolving field of spinal tumor management is not possible at this time. Some of the concepts in the book may even be overshadowed by newer ideas by the time this book is published. Yet there is clearly a need for all physicians to be aware that new hope is available for successful treatment of these complex problems.

As with many multi-authored texts, some of the material is redundant, but we have decided to leave the chapters as they were written, allowing each chapter to be read by itself. In some instances, contradictory opinions expressed by different authors have been included to show the diversity of opinion in the management of these problems.

We are indebted to the American Association of Neurological Surgeons for sponsorship, and to the generous support of the Codman Shurtleff Corporation, Zimmer International Companies, Walter Wichern, M.D., and Marian Finkl. Our publisher, W.B. Saunders, and Editor, Martin Wonsiewicz, also deserve our thanks for their patience and fortitude over these years. We also acknowledge with gratitude and thanks the assistance of our wives, of our secretaries, Patience Prescott, Joan Hamilton Beachley, Elizabeth Morales, and Elizabeth Vargas, and of Michael Klein, M.D., for their devotion and help. Without them, the book would never have been completed. Finally, we owe an enormous debt to our patients, who have provided us with the necessary knowledge and experience so that others may benefit from their tribulations.

This book is dedicated to our teachers: Benjamin Castleman, M.D., Walter Putschar, M.D., Robert Gardis, M.D., Paul C. Bucy, M.D., Edir B. Siqueira, M.D., and Gwilym Lodwick, M.D.

NARAYAN SUNDARESAN, M.D.
HENRY H. SCHMIDEK, M.D.
ALAN L. SCHILLER, M.D.
DANIEL I. ROSENTHAL, M.D.

CONTENTS

SECTION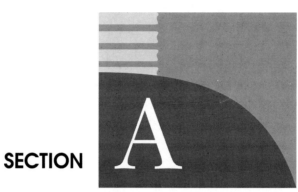

GENERAL PRINCIPLES

PREMALIGNANT LESIONS OF THE OSSEOUS SPINE AND CLASSIFICATION OF PRIMARY TUMORS

HENRY H. SCHMIDEK and ALAN L. SCHILLER

PREMALIGNANT LESIONS OF THE OSSEOUS SPINE

At a molecular level, the transition from normal to malignant cell has been shown to involve a multistep process that acts to deregulate normal cell growth and proliferation. The mechanisms underlying such deregulation of the cell have, in some cases, been shown to be related to the existence of an activated oncogene or the loss of a tumor suppressor gene. The conversion of a primary cell requires at least two separate events that act to deregulate the cell. The first stage in the process allows the cell to proliferate indefinitely in culture, but these cells are unable to produce tumors in athymic animals; at a further stage the cells demonstrate a fully malignant phenotype with deregulated proliferation, invasion of local tissues, and a propensity to metastasize. These tumors produce neoplasms where injected into athymic animals. The interaction of these "establishment" and "transformation" functions is poorly understood, as is the mechanism by which they combine to elicit the fully transformed phenotype.[2, 3, 5–11]

Based on the multistep concept of malignant transformation, the following pathologic conditions are considered to have undergone the first step in the transformation process and are then particularly susceptible to the additional changes that can result in full neoplastic transformation. In the osseous spine these lesions are clearly premalignant:

1. Von Recklinghausen's neurofibromatosis
2. Paget's disease of bone
3. Hereditary multiple osteochondromatosis
4. Enchondroma
5. Atypical osteoblastoma

Although these conditions are discussed elsewhere in this book, some features relating to their biology are discussed in this chapter. These lesions are given separate consideration because of their potential for malignant change. Patients harboring these lesions require careful lifelong follow-up. Increasing pain, change in the type of pain, onset of neurologic findings, and changing radiographic and biochemical indices reflecting bone destruction are hallmarks suggesting transformation to malignancy demanding prompt investigation and treatment.

Neurofibromatosis

Neurofibromatosis is a disorder affecting neural crest cell derivatives such as Schwann cells, melanophores, and adrenal medulla. The disease exists in two distinct forms caused by different genetic abnormalities; however, it is thought that the Schwann cell is the essential tumor-forming cell. The two forms are von Recklinghausen's neurofibromatosis (VRNF; NF1) and bilateral acoustic neurofibromatosis (BANF; NF2). The VRNF gene has been located to the long arm of chromosome 17 in the region 17q12 to 17q22, a region where the locus encoding the receptor for nerve growth factor (NGF) is also located. Using the technique of identifying restriction fragment length polymorphisms (RFLPs) among tumor samples, approximately one half of cases of bilateral acoustic tumors have a loss of heterozygosity localized to the long arm of chromosome 22. It is hypothesized that different tumor suppressor genes are located on these chromosomes, which in an as yet unknown way are important in the growth control of cells of neural crest origin. A tumor is thought to form only when a deletion or mutation occurs involving the normal copy of this gene. This occurs frequently enough to produce tumors within a predisposed patient. The acoustic neuroma associated with BANF (NF2) is invariably benign, whereas malignant tumors can and do frequently arise in association with VRNF (NF1). Both variants of this disorder have an autosomal dominant transmission and high penetrance; that is, when the genetic defect is present it is usually expressed.

Recently transgenic animals have been constructed with the *tat* gene of human T-cell lymphotropic virus I (HTLV-1) under control of its own long terminal repeat. These animals develop tumors with the morphologic and biologic properties of human neurofibromatosis.[4] These tumors are essentially benign, although in some cases malignant features are also seen. These animals develop tumors of the cranial and peripheral nerves beginning between 90 and 130 days of age, and malignant tumors develop only later in their lives.

Changes of the osseous spine occur in conjunction with bone NF1 and NF2 secondary to the effects of multiple spinal neurofibromas, spinal meningiomas arising from arachnoidal cells, neurofibromas arising from the sympathetic chain, or rarely by the invasive effects of either locally extensive neuroblastoma or of disseminated neuroblastoma. Severe nontumor-related spinal deformities, including a progressive kyphosis, result in paraplegia in about 2 per cent of patients with neurofibromatosis. In addition, when the von Recklinghausen–associated neurofibromas undergo malignant change (either spontaneously or following their irradiation), these tumors become extremely dangerous, locally destructive, and resistant to chemotherapy or radiation therapy. Often these lesions have metastasized even before the diagnosis is established, and the patient's life expectancy is short.

Paget's Disease of Bone

Characteristic inclusions have been demonstrated in the nuclei and cytoplasm of the osteoclasts in patients with Paget's disease of bone. Current evidence suggests that this disease may represent a slow virus infection, and polyclonal antibodies reveal paramyxovirus antigens, measles virus, and respiratory syncytial virus within pagetic osteoclasts. Monoclonal and monospecific polyclonal antibodies further demonstrate paramyxovirus antigens of measles virus, simian virus (SV 5), and human parainfluenza virus (PF 3). The cause and effect relationship between the presence of viral DNA in the diseased cells and Paget's disease of bone remains to be established.[1]

Paget's disease of bone is characterized by a marked increase in the osteoclastic activity of the involved bone with an intense resorption of existing bone. The affected osteoclasts often assume bizarre shapes and often harbor more than a dozen dark nuclei per cell. In the midphase of Paget's disease, waves of intense osteoclastic resorption are followed by waves of osteoblastic activity, resulting in the formation of lamellar bone; bone is thus arranged in irregular chaotic masses producing a mosaic pattern. In the late phase of this disease, massive amounts of this abnormal bone lead to structural damage with major anatomic and physiologic consequences. At this stage the degree of osteoblastic and osteoclastic activity may abate significantly, but the affected bones never return to normal structure. Malignant change of pagetic bone is a complication that occurs with an incidence of less than 1 per cent; however, in patients over the age of 40 with a sarcoma of bone, approximately 20 per cent have an underlying associated Paget's disease.

Three cell types are involved in the pagetic process—osteoblast, osteoclast, and fibroblast—and the malignancies are predominantly either osteosarcomas or fibrosarcomas. Rarely, patients develop benign, hyperplastic, or low grade neoplasms of osteoclastic origin, the so-called giant cell lesion of Paget's disease.

The radiographic hallmarks of Paget's disease of bone in the spine are as follows: the vertebrae are larger than normal and possess lucent and osteoblastic foci; in addition, there is thickening and coarseness of the bone's trabeculae. In advanced cases, the spinal canal is diminished in caliber owing to enlargement of the bodies and the vertebral arches, producing spinal cord and/or nerve root compression. The spinal cord is the most frequently compressed in the upper thoracic spine. Characteristically, when spinal cord compression is present, three to five adjacent vertebrae are involved by this disease; when the lumbar spine is associated with neural compression, the pagetic process is usually restricted to a single vertebra. Malignant degeneration of pagetic vertebrae can result in osteogenic sarcoma or chondrosarcoma, although this is quite rare.[12–14]

Hereditary Multiple Osteochondromatosis

Multiple osteocartilaginous exostosis is a disease of unclear etiology, inherited by a single autosomal dominant gene, and characterized by multiple cartilage-capped bony protrusions from the surface of bones. These growths originate adjacent to the cortex or near the zone of endochondral growth, the epiphyseal growth plate. The pathogenetic mechanism most widely accepted maintains that the disease results from the defective development of the periosteal ring surrounding the epiphysis. Endochondral ossification in this region permits a cartilaginous mass to grow into the neighboring soft tissue, producing a cartilage-capped exostosis without an underlying cortex. Initially, the bone and the cartilage are histologically normal. At the site where these lesions develop, the cortex is not formed and the exostosis joins underlying spongy bone. Continued stimulation of the cartilaginous rests of cells results in newly directed endochondral growth, which usually ceases when the overall epiphyseal growth stops. Residual microfoci of cartilage almost always remain into adulthood. Malignant transformation in the form of chondrosarcoma may arise from the cells of the cartilaginous cap or the internal rests of cartilage. The overall incidence of secondary chondrosarcomatous degeneration in these patients is rare, and we have never seen such a case involving the spine.

Endochondroma

Endochondromas compose up to 20 per cent of benign bone tumors and 3 per cent of all bone tumors. These tumors represent a benign cartilaginous mass occurring within the medulla of the bone,

TABLE 1–1. CLASSIFICATION OF PRIMARY TUMORS OF THE OSSEOUS SPINE

TISSUE OF ORIGIN	BENIGN TUMOR	MALIGNANT TUMOR
Fibrous tissue	Fibroma Fibrous dysplasia	Fibrosarcoma Malignant fibrous histiocytoma
Cartilage	Chondroblastoma Osteochondroma Enchondroma Chondromyxoid fibroma	Chondrosarcoma
Bone	Osteoid osteoma Osteoblastoma	Osteosarcoma Osteosarcoma associated with Paget's disease and previous radiation
Hematopoietic elements		Plasma cell myeloma Lymphoma
Fat cells	Lipoma	Liposarcoma

Vascular system
  Blood vessels
  Lymphatics
	Hemangioma
	
	Lymphangioma
		Angiosarcoma
		Hemangiopericytoma
		Lymphangiosarcoma

Nerve	Schwannoma (neurilemmoma) Neurofibromatosis Pigmented nerve sheath tumors Ganglioneuroma	Malignant nerve sheath tumor
Notochord		Chordoma
Unknown		Giant cell tumor Ewing's sarcoma

which arises during growth and becomes symptomatic in the third and fourth decades. While most often occurring in the bones of the hand and in long bones, approximately a dozen cases have been reported in the spine. In multiple enchondromatosis (Ollier's disease) or in Maffucci's syndrome (multiple enchondromas and hemangiomas), the process also occurs in long bones and in the bones of the hand. Cases involving the vertebrae have been reported. Chondrosarcomatous change in multiple enchondromatosis is well known, with an incidence of this complication exceeding 50 per cent, and even higher in Maffucci's syndrome.

Atypical Osteoblastoma (Epithelioid Osteoblastoma)

Osteoblastoma, although histologically similar to osteoid osteoma, is a progressively growing lesion usually of a larger size than the osteoid osteoma at the time of diagnosis. Osteoblastomas occur predominantly among males before the age of 30. Over 30 per cent of cases occur in the spine. These tumors are premalignant lesions with features that include large, plump osteoblasts with atypical nuclei. These tumors are aggressive and will almost always recur following treatment by curettage. In some cases the recurrences are difficult to distinguish from osteosarcoma; in other cases these tumors will eventually metastasize. We therefore believe this subset of osteoblastoma should be treated aggressively.

CLASSIFICATION OF PRIMARY TUMORS OF THE OSSEOUS SPINE

There is no universally accepted classification of primary bone tumors. The proposed classification is one that is simple and based on histologic origin and

will be used in this book. The tissue of origin is either fibrous, cartilaginous, bone-forming, hematopoietic, fat, vascular, neural, notochordal, or unknown (see Table 1–1).

REFERENCES

1. Basic MF, Rebel A, Fournier JG, et al: On the trail of paramyxoviruses in Paget's disease of bone. Clin Orthop 217:9–15, 1987.
2. Friend SM, Berbards RM, Rigekhu S, et al: A human DNA segment with properties of the gene that predisposes to retinoblastoma and osteosarcoma. Nature 323:643–646, 1986.
3. Hanahan D: Heritable formation of pancreatic beta-cell tumors in transgenic mice expressing recombinant insul/simian virus 40 oncogenes. Nature 315:115–122, 1985.
4. Hinrichs SH, Nirenberg M, Reynolds RK, et al: A transgenic mouse model for human neurofibromatosis. Science 237:1340–1343, 1987.
5. Land H, Parada L, Weinberg R: Cellular oncogenes and multistep carcinogenesis. Science 222:771–778, 1983.
6. Land H, Parada L, Weinberg R: Tumorigenic conversion of primary embryo fibroblasts requires at least two cooperating oncogenes. Nature 305:596–602, 1983.
7. Land H, Chen A, Morgenstern J, et al: Behavior of myc and ras oncogenes in transformation of rat embryo fibroblasts. Cell Biol 6:1917–1925, 1986.
8. Newbold RF, Overell RW: Fibroblast immortality is a prerequisite for transformation by EJ and H-ras oncogene. Nature 304:648–651, 1983.
9. Parada LF, Land H, Weinberg RA, et al: Cooperation between gene encoding p53 tumor antigen and ras in cellular transformation. Nature 312:649–651, 1984.
10. Ruley H: Adenovirus early region 1A enables viral and cellular transforming genes to transform primary cells in culture. Nature 304:602–606, 1983.
11. Ruley HE: Analysis of malignant phenotypes by oncogene complementation. Adv Viral Oncol 6:1–20, 1987.
12. Schmidek HH: Neurologic and neurosurgical sequelae of Paget's disease of bone. Clin Orthop 127:70–77, 1977.
13. Schmidek HH: The molecular genetics of nervous system tumor. J Neurosurg 67:1–16, 1987.
14. Singer FR, Mills BG: Critical evaluation of viral antigen data in Paget's disease of bone. Clin Orthop 217:16–25, 1987.

CLINICAL MANIFESTATIONS

DAVID R. MACDONALD

INTRODUCTION

The physician has a difficult task when a patient presents with symptoms or signs of a spinal problem. Benign spinal conditions are very common; up to 5 per cent of the population will have back pain each year, and the lifetime prevalence of back pain is 60 to 90 per cent.[11, 24, 62] Almost all spinal conditions are benign, do not require extensive investigations, and are either self-limiting or treatable with routine symptomatic measures. Tumors of the spine are uncommon in the general population; primary tumors are very rare, although metastases to the spine from systemic cancer are more common. Up to 70 per cent of persons dying with systemic cancer will have spinal metastases at careful postmortem examination.[26, 43, 75] A similar percentage will have spinal metastases detected by bone scintigraphy (isotope bone scanning),[54, 69, 81] although only half of these patients will have been symptomatic during life. A delay in diagnosis of a primary or metastatic spinal tumor subjects the patient to unnecessary pain and possibly preventable disability. Five to 10 per cent of patients with advanced systemic cancer will develop signs and symptoms of spinal cord compression in whom early diagnosis and appropriate treatment may effectively treat symptoms and prevent neurologic deficits, but late diagnosis and treatment may result in permanent paralysis.[6, 9, 29, 33, 66, 67]

The physician is thus faced with the dilemma of either overinvestigating many patients with benign back pain—resulting in unnecessary anxiety, expense, and discomfort—or delaying investigations and risking missing early, treatable disease. This chapter will discuss the clinical manifestations of spinal tumors, including primary and metastatic tumors, the investigation of patients with suspected spinal tumors, and the clinical aspects of three major clinical problems in cancer patients—epidural metastases, brachial or lumbosacral plexopathy, and leptomeningeal metastases. A detailed discussion of specific tumors, radiologic investigations, and treatment is beyond the scope of this chapter but can be found in other chapters of this book.

SYMPTOMS AND SIGNS

Tumors of the spine typically present with any combination of pain, neurologic dysfunction, mass lesion, or spinal deformity (Tables 2–1 and 2–2). The incidental discovery of an asymptomatic spinal tumor is uncommon; most asymptomatic tumors, found during the investigation for other medical problems, are benign tumors such as hemangiomas.[16, 71]

Pain

Pain is *the* cardinal symptom of spinal tumors. Pain is the presenting symptom, and often the only symptom, at time of diagnosis in 80 to 100 per cent of all primary spinal tumors.[8, 20, 89]

Bone metastases are frequently asymptomatic initially; only half the patients with bone metastases found by bone scintigraphy (isotope bone scans) may be symptomatic during life.[39] In patients with painful systemic cancer, however, bone metastases are the most common cause of the pain.[20] Epidural spinal cord compression develops in 5 to 10 per cent of all patients with systemic cancer and is heralded by pain in over 95 per cent of cases.[29, 33, 88] Primary intraspinal tumors may also present with pain. Patients with spinal schwannomas and neurofibromas frequently

TABLE 2–1. PRESENTING SIGNS AND SYMPTOMS OF PRIMARY SPINAL TUMORS

Sign/Symptom	At Presentation (%)
Pain	85–100
Weakness	40–75
Reflex change	35–45
Autonomic dysfunction	5–20
Sensory loss	30–50
Mass	15–60
Scoliosis	10–70

References: 10, 36, 44, 55, 89.

Supported in part by grant SRC-5-P50-NS20023 from the National Institutes of Health.

TABLE 2–2. PRESENTING SIGNS AND SYMPTOMS OF METASTATIC EPIDURAL SPINAL CORD COMPRESSION

SIGN/SYMPTOM	FIRST SYMPTOMS (%)	SYMPTOMS AT DIAGNOSIS (%)	SIGNS AT DIAGNOSIS (%)
Pain (tenderness)	96	96	63
Weakness	6	76	87
Reflex change	—	—	65
Autonomic dysfunction	0	57	57
Sensory loss	1	51	78
Ataxia	2	5	7
Herpes zoster	0	2	2

References: 29, 33.

have pain for months or years prior to diagnosis. Only two thirds of patients with intramedullary spinal cord tumors (astrocytoma, metastases) present with pain, perhaps because other signs and symptoms of neurologic dysfunction occur earlier in these patients.[27, 34, 36, 65, 73]

Pain may precede the diagnosis of a spinal tumor by months to years. The duration of pain tends to be longer in benign spinal tumors, such as chondromas, osteoblastomas, or osteoid osteomas, and in benign intraspinal tumors, such as neurofibromas or schwannomas, than in malignant spinal tumors, such as osteogenic sarcomas, Ewing's sarcomas, or bone metastases.[23, 29, 37, 55, 60, 82, 91] In Weinstein and McLain's series of patients with primary tumors of the spine, the mean interval from onset of symptoms to diagnosis was 10.4 months in patients with malignant lesions and 19.3 months in those with benign lesions.[89] Even in patients with malignant lesions, the duration of pain before a diagnosis is made can be variable and may be more than one year. Pain precedes the diagnosis of epidural spinal cord compression from metastatic cancer an average of one to two months but may be present for as long as two years.[29, 33]

The pathogenesis of pain in patients with spinal tumors includes infiltration and destruction of bone (especially distention of the periosteum); compression or pathologic fracture of bone; spinal instability; compression or infiltration of spinal cord, nerve root, or plexus; and pain due to cancer therapy (surgery, radiation therapy, chemotherapy).[8, 20, 21, 42, 46, 49, 80] Patients with tumor infiltration or destruction of bone generally complain of a dull, constant, aching pain that is localized to the area of vertebral involvement. The pain is usually gradual in onset, progressively increasing in severity and analgesic requirements. Sudden movements may exacerbate the pain. There is often percussion tenderness over the involved vertebra. The pain may occasionally begin or increase after trivial trauma.

Compression or pathologic fracture of the tumor-damaged vertebral body may occur spontaneously (i.e., during a transfer from bed to chair), following a minor trauma, or after a fall. Severe localized and/or radiating pain develops, which is exacerbated by any movement and is somewhat relieved by rest. There may be new onset of neurologic disturbance (myelopathy or radiculopathy) if fragments of bone

or tumor are displaced into the spinal canal or intervertebral foramina. Spinal instability is suggested by the persistence of incident pain (pain with movement) longer than pain from benign compression fractures should last.

Tumor compression of the spinal cord is suggested by the development of progressive severe back pain that is increased by coughing, sneezing, straining, and other Valsalva maneuvers that increase intraspinal pressure. The pain of spinal cord compression, unlike that of disc herniation, is frequently exacerbated by bed rest and is partly relieved by standing or activity. Nocturnal pain is common.

Pain typically precedes the development of a myelopathy by days to weeks and sometimes by many months.[29, 33] Tumor compression or infiltration of nerve roots or plexus (brachial or lumbosacral) produces a neuralgia that is often described as a severe constant burning, sometimes with painful paresthesias or with sharp lancinating pains superimposed, radiating along the course of the nerve, with weakness or numbness in the distribution of the involved nerve root or plexus. The skin in the involved dermatomes may be tender to the touch.

The pain of spinal tumors may be localized to the back (over the involved vertebral body), may be referred to a site distant from the site of local pathology (but not in the usual dermatomal distribution of a nerve root), and may be associated with tenderness of subcutaneous tissues or muscles at the site of referral. The pain may be radicular (along the course of the involved nerve root, in its cutaneous—dermatomal—or muscular—myotomal—distribution) or funicular (in the distribution of compressed long tracts of the spinal cord—often described as a cold, tight unpleasant sensation in the extremity). Spinal tumors may cause local muscle pain due to reflex spasm of adjacent paraspinal muscles, usually described as a deep aching pain felt lateral to the midline accompanied by paravertebral neck or back muscle spasm and tenderness.[62]

Several well-characterized pain syndromes are recognized. Tumor involvement of the odontoid process of the axis can produce severe neck pain radiating over the occiput to the vertex which is exacerbated by movement, especially flexion of the neck.[76] Flexion may induce sharp electric-like paresthesias that radiate into the arms or down the back (Lhermitte's sign) or weakness or numbness beginning in the arms and progressing to the legs. Tumor involvement of the C7-T1 vertebral bodies may produce pain that radiates across the posterior aspect of one or both shoulders and down the medial aspect of the arms to the elbows or ulnar aspect of the hands. Numbness in the fourth and fifth fingers, weakness, and wasting of intrinsic hand muscles, wrist and finger extensors and triceps may occur. Horner's syndrome suggests paraspinal involvement of sympathetic fibers. Pancoast's syndrome, from infiltration of the inferior brachial plexus by a primary or secondary tumor in the superior pulmonary sulcus, may mimic tumor involvement of the C7-T1 vertebrae.[46]

Tumor involvement of midthoracic vertebrae can

produce pain that radiates around the chest, is often described as a tight band, and may sometimes be confused with anginal pain of cardiac origin. Similarly, involvement of lower thoracic or upper lumbar vertebrae may produce pain that radiates to the anterior abdominal wall and can sometimes be mistaken for the pain of cholecystitis, appendicitis, diverticulitis, or bowel obstruction, especially if autonomic involvement has produced a paralytic ileus. Pain from tumor involvement of the L1 vertebral body may radiate to the sacroiliac region, superior iliac crest, or inguinal regions on one or both sides. Loss of bowel, bladder, or sexual function, with leg weakness or numbness and extensor plantar reflexes, may indicate compression of the conus medullaris.

Tumor involvement of mid to low lumbar vertebral bodies may produce typical sciatica-like pain and neurologic disturbance, mimicking lumbar disc herniation, although the pain is often increased rather than relieved by bed rest. Sacral involvement by tumor produces pain in the low back or coccygeal region which may radiate into the perineum or perianal region. Early loss of bowel, bladder, or sexual function may occur before perianal or perineal sensory loss develops. The pain from tumor involvement in the lumbosacral spine is often exacerbated by sitting or lying and is reduced by standing. Traction signs (i.e., pain increased by straight leg raising or reverse straight leg raising), radiation of pain into the legs or buttocks, and development of weakness or numbness in the legs indicate compression or infiltration of the cauda equina, nerve roots, or lumbosacral plexus.

Neurologic Dysfunction

Neurologic dysfunction develops when spinal tumors compress or infiltrate the spinal cord, nerve roots, or paraspinal nerve plexuses. Neurologic dysfunction is usually a late manifestation of spinal tumors, preceded by days, weeks, or months of local back pain or radicular pain. Once neurologic dysfunction develops, treatment of the tumor may prevent further progression of disability but often does not reverse the neurologic deficit. Compression of neurologic structures of mild degree or short duration may produce local demyelination or edema, which may be reversible once the compression is relieved. More severe or prolonged compression, especially if rapid in onset, may produce axonal damage, possibly by ischemia.[48, 86] If compression is relieved, some recovery is possible in damaged nerve roots or plexuses by axonal sprouting and regeneration, although recovery is often limited and very slow. Regeneration of central nervous system (i.e., spinal cord) axonal damage is minimal. Early diagnosis and treatment, ideally before the development of abnormal neurologic signs, are important if neurologic dysfunction is to be avoided. Once the neurologic examination is abnormal, urgent investigation and therapy are crucial if permanent neurologic disability is to be prevented. Compression of very

gradual onset, such as from spinal meningiomas, is tolerated much better. The spinal cord may be able to adapt to severe degrees of compression and deformity without axonal loss if sufficiently slow in development; subsequent decompression, even when patients are severely disabled, often produces complete recovery from neurologic dysfunction.

Primary or metastatic tumors of the spine seldom present with the signs or symptoms of only neurologic dysfunction, although neurologic dysfunction is more common at time of diagnosis. Primary tumors of the spine present with symptoms of motor weakness in up to 40 per cent of patients; sensory loss is less common and autonomic dysfunction is rare (except sacral tumors). By the time of diagnosis, over 55 per cent of patients with malignant primary spinal tumors have objective signs of neurologic dysfunction, while only 35 per cent of patients with benign primary spinal tumors have such findings.[89]

Metastatic epidural cord compression initially presents with symptoms of motor weakness in only 5 per cent of cases and with sensory loss or autonomic dysfunction in fewer still. By the time of diagnosis, however, up to 75 per cent will have evidence of motor weakness, 50 per cent will have sensory loss, and almost 60 per cent will have autonomic dysfunction.[29, 33] Ataxia, due to posterior column damage with severe proprioceptive loss or due to damage to the spinocerebellar pathways, is an uncommon presenting complaint. Spinal cord signs are usually symmetric, whereas root or plexus signs or symptoms are often asymmetric. Herpes zoster occasionally develops at the level of epidural spinal cord compression, presumably due to activation of a latent virus by tumor involvement of the dorsal root ganglion.[6, 29, 58]

Compression of the spinal cord produces a myelopathy: weakness, sensory loss, and spasticity below the level of the lesion, often with autonomic dysfunction (loss of bowel, bladder, or sexual function). Initial symptoms or signs may be asymmetric, but bilateral abnormalities are usually found on careful neurologic examination. The sensory loss may be patchy or may involve some sensory modalities more than others, depending upon which pathway is affected most (pain and temperature loss contralateral to lateral spinothalamic tract damage; vibration and proprioceptive loss ipsilateral to posterior column damage). The upper level of sensory loss may exhibit a narrow band of intense dysesthetic painful sensitivity, possibly due to nerve root irritation at that level. Spasticity (increased motor tone, deep tendon reflexes, and extensor plantar reflexes) is the hallmark of a myelopathy but may not initially be present if the myelopathy is rapid in onset (so-called spinal shock) or if the reflexes are suppressed due to prior chemotherapy (vincristine or cisplatin) or peripheral neuropathy.

Compression or infiltration of nerve roots or a plexus produces radicular signs and symptoms (pain, weakness, muscle wasting, sensory loss, reflex loss, and sometimes autonomic loss) in the distribution of the affected nerve roots or plexus. Muscle wasting and fasciculations are late findings, indicative of denervation. Compression of the nerve roots in the cauda equina may produce early autonomic dysfunction before other signs or symptoms of radiculopathy develop.

Mass and Deformity

A palpable mass on the neck or back or a deformity of the spine may indicate the presence of an underlying spinal tumor. The frequency of such findings depends upon the type of tumor. Benign, slow-growing primary spinal tumors such as osteoblastoma, osteochondroma, or aneurysmal bone cysts may present as a painful or painless mass.[52, 55, 82] A palpable, often tender mass may be indicative of malignant primary spinal tumors such as osteogenic sarcoma or Ewing's sarcoma. Ewing's sarcoma often presents as a painful, warm, tender mass, sometimes with fever, mimicking an abscess.[91]

Metastatic spinal tumors seldom present with a mass as the initial finding, but a palpable, sometimes asymmetric mass may be present at diagnosis. Intraspinal tumors such as dermoids or epidermoids frequently have an overlying subcutaneous mass or skin dimple, especially in the lumbar or sacral region. The presence of multiple café au lait spots or subcutaneous masses along nerve roots indicates von Recklinghausen's neurofibromatosis and may be accompanied by spinal neurofibromas, schwannomas, or meningiomas.

Spinal deformities such as scoliosis or kyphosis are common with some types of spinal tumors. Osteoid osteomas and osteoblastomas may have an associated scoliosis of the spine in up to 70 per cent of cases; the tumor is usually located on the concave side.[37, 44, 55] Scoliosis may also be caused by intraspinal tumors, especially in children.[10, 36, 65] Spinal metastases from systemic cancer may produce spinal deformities, usually as a result of bone destruction with collapse of vertebral bodies. Widespread vertebral involvement in breast cancer, prostate cancer, or multiple myeloma may occasionally produce a striking kyphosis or kyphoscoliosis. Marked collapse of a single or several adjacent vertebral bodies may result in a sharp kyphotic angulation of the spine (gibbus deformity). Severe spinal deformity may produce sufficient compression or distortion of the spinal cord to cause a myelopathy. Spinal deformities may also compress nerve roots in the intervertebral foramina to produce a radiculopathy.

INVESTIGATIONS

History and Physical Examination

Every patient with presumed or possible spinal tumor (or back pain) should have a thorough history and complete physical examination. A detailed description of the pain should be obtained, including nature of the pain (sharp, dull, aching, burning, lancinating); location of the pain; patterns of radiation or referral of pain (into arms, around chest, into legs, and so forth); precipitating and relieving factors (effects of coughing, sneezing, straining, moving, standing, sitting, lying, or bed rest); behavior over time (stable, increasing, decreasing, intermittent); associated neurologic problems (weakness, sensory loss, bowel/bladder/sexual dysfunction); previous history of similar or other pain; and response to analgesics or other treatments. Patients with spinal tumors, especially if there is spinal cord or nerve root compression, typically have a dull, aching pain that progressively increases in severity and is localized to the back over the involved vertebral body and/or radiates into the arm, around the chest or abdomen as a tight band, or down the leg. This pain is increased by coughing, sneezing, straining, and movement (especially flexion) of the back, is not relieved by bed rest, is often associated with progressive neurologic deficits, and requires increasing analgesics over time.

A detailed inquiry should be made of the patient's current and past health. The following may indicate the development of a primary or metastatic tumor that can involve the spine: Weight loss unexplained by dieting; history of smoking or excessive alcohol use; change in cough or sputum production; change in bowel habits (especially constipation or melena); change in urinary function (slowness, retention, incontinence, hematuria); change in appearance or texture of the breasts or breast masses; unexplained fever or night sweats; change in appearance of pigmented skin lesions (enlargement, bleeding, or color change); presence of lymph node or other masses. The presence of café au lait spots or other "birthmarks" should be sought, as neurofibromatosis and other neurocutaneous syndromes may be accompanied by spinal tumors. A past history of cancer or removal of any growths, cysts, or other lesions may indicate a metastatic cancer to the spine. The possibility of the acquired immunodeficiency syndrome (AIDS) should be considered in patients belonging to high-risk groups (male homosexuals, intravenous drug users, and so forth) or in those with unusual opportunistic infections. The incidence of some tumors (especially non-Hodgkin's lymphomas) is increased in patients with AIDS, and these tumors may involve the spine or spinal cord.

A history of childhood cancer (leukemia or lymphoma) or prior treatment with radiotherapy or chemotherapy (especially alkylating agents) increases the risk of developing second malignancies (especially leukemia or lymphoma, but also sarcomas and other solid tumors), which may not appear until years later. Studies have shown that the relative risk for all second cancers after treatment for Hodgkin's disease is over 5 times that in the general populaton, while the relative risk of developing a bone sarcoma after treatment of childhood cancer with radiotherapy or chemotherapy is over 100 times, and the 20-year cumulative risk is almost 3 per cent.[84, 85]

Patients known or suspected to have a spinal tumor should be asked directly regarding the presence of any neurologic symptoms. The typical pain pattern from spinal tumors has already been discussed. Weakness and/or sensory loss, especially if in a radicular or myelopathic pattern, gait disturbances, or autonomic dysfunction may indicate the early development of spinal cord or nerve root compression.

A complete physical and neurologic examination is required in all patients with known or suspected spinal tumors. The clues to the presence of a systemic malignancy should be carefully sought: lymphadenopathy, pigmented skin lesions, subcutaneous masses, hepatic or splenic enlargement, ascites, other intraabdominal masses, pleural effusion, apical lung dullness, oral lesions, breast masses, skin or nail changes (such as clubbing of fingers), testicular masses, and so forth. All patients require a rectal examination, and most women should have a gynecologic examination as well. The spine must be examined, looking for masses or deformity, and must be percussed, looking for local tenderness indicating vertebral involvement by tumor. The range of neck and spine movements, including straight leg and reverse straight leg raising, should be checked.

A careful neurologic examination is required including speech, mental status, and cranial nerves (to help exclude coexisting intracranial tumor involvement) as well as motor, sensory, coordination, and reflex testing of the limbs and trunk. Neurologic deficits should be particularly sought in patients with any neurologic symptoms; the neurologic examination is frequently abnormal in these patients and may give clues to the location, level, and extent of neurologic involvement by a spinal tumor.

Laboratory Tests

A wide range of hematologic and biochemical laboratory tests are available which may be useful in the investigation of patients with spinal tumors. A complete blood count (CBC) should be done on all patients. In patients who have not had extensive prior or recent chemotherapy or radiotherapy, the presence of leukopenia, anemia, or thrombocytopenia (especially if accompanied by the presence of immature white blood cells or red blood cells) indicates possible bone marrow involvement by metastatic or primary tumors. Anemia alone can be due to blood loss from gastrointestinal (stomach, colon, rectal) carcinomas or renal cancers or from reduced red blood cell production seen in many cancers. Leukocytosis, especially of immature blast cells, may indicate leukemia or a leukemoid reaction secondary to systemic cancer.· The white blood cell differential may separate benign leukocytosis (such as from infections) from malignant causes. Thrombocytosis can also be seen in response to systemic malignancies. The erythrocyte sedimentation rate (ESR) is often increased as a nonspecific finding in patients with primary or metastatic spinal tumors. Primary spinal cord tumors, benign intraspinal tumors, and benign vertebral body tumors seldom affect the CBC or ESR.

The prothrombin time (PT) should be checked in patients with metastatic tumor or if there is any history or evidence of bleeding or easy bruising. An elevated PT suggests liver involvement by tumor with underproduction of vitamin K–dependent clotting factors and may make any invasive diagnostic test (such as myelography or needle biopsy) hazardous until corrected.

Many biochemical tests are available to aid the investigation of patients with spinal tumor. Serum total protein and albumin should be checked. If the total protein is elevated or the globulin fraction is increased, myeloma should be suspected, and serum protein electrophoresis, serum immunoglobulins, serum immunoelectrophoresis, and urinary proteins (such as Bence Jones protein) should be obtained. Marked elevation of serum proteins, especially if accompanied by any elevation of serum urea (BUN) or creatinine to suggest renal insufficiency, makes the use of intravenous contrast radiography (such as intravenous pyelography [IVP] or contrast-enhanced computed tomography) hazardous, as acute renal failure may be precipitated. An elevated serum calcium may indicate widespread bone metastases and may require urgent therapy. Hyperuricemia may be seen in hematologic malignancies. Hypoglycemia may occasionally be found in widespread systemic malignancies, such as sarcomas, or from liver metastases. Liver metastases may cause elevated serum bilirubin (early in obstructive jaundice, late from hepatic destruction) and elevated liver enzymes, such as alkaline phosphatase, gamma glutamyltransferase (GGT), 5'-nucleotidase, aspartate aminotransferase (AST, SGOT), or alanine aminotransferase (ALT, SGPT). Elevated liver enzymes raise the suspicion of hepatic involvement by malignancy but are not diagnostic alone, as many processes in addition to malignancy may cause elevation of these enzymes. Alkaline phosphatase can also be increased by bone destruction from primary or metastatic tumors. Isoenzyme determination can separate liver from bone production. Serum electrolytes are seldom directly affected by spinal tumors.

A variety of tumor markers may be useful in the diagnosis or follow-up of malignancy. Prostate cancer, especially if metastatic, is often accompanied by elevation of serum acid phosphatase or prostatic specific antigen. Elevated serum carcinoembryonic antigen (CEA) is typically associated with carcinoma of the colon but can also be found in a variety of other solid tumors, such as breast cancer. Its greatest clinical value is in the follow-up of patients rather than in initial diagnosis. Elevated serum beta human chorionic gonadotropin (beta-HCG) or alpha fetoprotein (AFP) may be found in testicular or ovarian carcinomas. Neuronal specific enolase (NSE) has been reported increased in some patients with small cell carcinomas of the lung or neuroblastomas. Elevated serum or urinary catecholamines, vanilmandelic acid (VMA) or homovanillic acid (HVA) may be found in many patients with neuroblastoma or pheochromocytoma.

These tumor markers may also be present in cerebrospinal fluid (CSF) in leptomeningeal or sometimes cerebral involvement by metastatic cancer.

Epidural spinal cord compression may produce elevation of the CSF protein (sometimes to very high levels) and occasionally a mild CSF leukocytosis (typically all lymphocytes) below the level of a spinal block. Low CSF glucose and/or marked CSF leukocytosis is suggestive of direct leptomeningeal metastases by tumor (or infective—bacterial or fungal—meningitis). The CSF cytology is usually positive for malignant cells in leptomeningeal metastases, but several lumbar punctures may be required.[87]

Radiology

A thorough radiologic investigation of patients with suspected or known spinal tumors is required in order to delineate the site and extent of tumor involvement of the spine, to determine the presence or absence of intraspinal extension of tumor and thus the degree and extent of spinal cord or nerve root compression, to distinguish benign primary spinal tumors from malignant primary tumors and spinal metastases, to exclude benign (i.e., nontumor related) lesions of the spine, to determine the degree of bone destruction and spinal stability, and to determine the extent of paraspinal involvement by tumor. Such information is important for diagnosing spinal tumors and helps guide treatment decisions concerning surgery, radiotherapy, and chemotherapy.

The radiologic investigation also plays an important part in the search for occult primary tumors that may have spread to the spine and in the determination of the extent of systemic involvement by primary spinal tumors.

Plain Films

All patients with spinal tumors should have plain anteroposterior and lateral radiographs of the complete spine. Oblique films of the cervical and lumbar spine occasionally increase the diagnostic yield, and special films of the odontoid (open mouth) or cervicothoracic junction (swimmer's view) may be required. Patients with known systemic cancer who have back pain or neurologic deficit, patients without known spinal tumors who have progressive or persistent back pain or neurologic deficit, all children with back pain (especially in the presence of a painful scoliosis), and elderly patients with the sudden onset of back pain suggestive of a pathologic fracture should also have plain spinal radiography. Plain film changes of spinal involvement by tumor include focal or multifocal areas of sclerosis or blastic change (especially metastatic carcinomas of prostate or breast and some primary spinal tumors, such as osteoid osteoma or osteoblastoma); focal or multifocal areas of bone lysis or reduced density (myeloma, metastatic lung, breast, or renal carcinoma, primary malignant bone tumors); mixed blastic and lytic lesions; diffuse rarefaction of bone simulating osteoporosis (most common in myeloma but also seen with diffuse bone marrow involvement by leukemia, lymphoma, or metastatic solid cancers); expansion of bone with new bone formation (especially primary benign and malignant bone tumors); vertebral body collapse; and paraspinal soft tissue masses. Unfortunately, plain films may also be normal despite extensive involvement of the spine by tumor. It is estimated that in the absence of a blastic or sclerotic reaction to tumor at least 30 to 50 per cent of the bone will be destroyed before plain radiographs will be abnormal.[39, 43] The clinician should review the radiographs with the radiologist to ensure that the symptomatic areas were adequately visualized and that subtle abnormalities were not overlooked.

The clinical features and plain film findings are used to guide further investigations. In patients with cancer, the presence of back pain and a myelopathy or radiculopathy is highly suggestive of epidural metastasis; almost all of these patients have abnormal plain spine radiographs and should be further investigated. Two thirds of patients with localized back pain and a normal neurologic examination but abnormal plain films had epidural metastasis on myelography in one series.[66, 67] Graus and colleagues[32] correlated the degree of plain spinal radiographic abnormality with the likelihood of epidural disease. In patients with cancer and local back pain alone, epidural metastasis was found in 87 per cent of patients with a major (> 50 per cent) vertebral collapse, in 31 per cent of those with pedicle erosion, and in only 7 per cent with metastasis restricted to the vertebral body without collapse. In patients with radiculopathy, epidural metastasis was found in 75 per cent of patients with a destroyed pedicle and in 42 per cent of those with metastasis restricted to the vertebral body without collapse. In patients with negative plain spine films, epidural metastasis was found on myelography in only 3 per cent of patients with localized back pain and a normal neurologic examination, in 9 per cent of patients with radicular pain, and in 29 per cent of patients with a paraspinal tumor mass.

Plain film tomography can increase the sensitivity of plain radiography and may better differentiate benign from malignant spinal lesions but has generally been supplanted by computed tomography (CT) or magnetic resonance imaging (MRI) of the spine.

Computed Tomography (CT Scan)

Computed tomography of the spine is more sensitive and more specific than plain spinal radiography in the detection and delineation of spinal tumors. CT scanning is effective in differentiating benign (i.e., degenerative or discogenic) spinal disease from neoplastic disease, in determining the extent of bone destruction, and in demonstrating the extent of paraspinal tumor involvement. CT scanning is not an effective screening test for spinal tumors; visualization of the entire spine is a time-consuming and inefficient use of CT. Areas of interest should first be localized by clinical examination and by either plain spinal radiography, isotope bone scanning, or myelography, then studied by CT scanning (Fig. 2–1). In patients with systemic cancer and new lesions identified on isotope bone scanning but with normal neurologic examinations and plain spine radiographs, 67 to 80 per cent had metastases identified by CT scanning; the remainder had benign discogenic or degenerative disease.[57, 64]

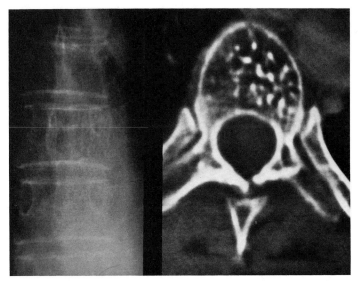

FIGURE 2–1. A 70-year-old woman with back pain, normal neurologic examination. Left, plain spine radiograph, antero-posterior film, faint vertically oriented sclerosis in vertebral body. Right, CT scan (bone window), characteristic speckled pattern in vertebral body of hemangioma.

Although CT scanning may demonstrate intraspinal extension of tumor (and thus spinal cord or nerve root compression), the spinal canal is often not well visualized due to the presence of artifacts from surrounding bone, and the accurate visualization of the spinal cord, thecal sac, and epidural space may be difficult without the presence of an intrathecal contrast agent (CT-myelography). CT-myelography cannot be performed in patients allergic to intrathecal contrast agents or in whom a lumbar puncture for instillation of contrast cannot be safely done (those with coagulopathies, intracranial mass lesions, and so forth). In a series of 60 patients with cancer, new isotope bone scan lesions, and normal neurologic examinations reported by O'Rourke[57] and Redmond,[63] 72 per cent had spinal metastases on plain spine CT scanning, and 47 per cent of these (33 per cent of entire group) had epidural spinal cord compression on CT-myelography.

CT scanning after conventional myelography may demonstrate the upper end of a complete spinal block not visualized by lumbar myelography, may show the degree of bone destruction and extent of paraspinal tumor spread, but may miss other skip epidural lesions remote from the site of myelographic blockage[18, 32, 61] (Fig. 2–2).

The CT characteristics of spinal tumors include cortical bone destruction, focal medullary trabecular loss, focal medullary sclerosis unassociated with discogenic disease or other pathology, and soft tissue mass with bone destruction.[64] The CT demonstration of cortical bone disruption around the spinal canal is highly suggestive of intraspinal extension by tumor and epidural spinal cord compression. In one series, 78 per cent of patients with such findings had epidural spinal cord compression[90]; and in another series, 100 per cent of patients with cord compression on CT-myelography had adjacent contiguous destruction of the posterior vertebral cortex by tumor.[57, 63]

Myelography

Myelography is the current gold standard for the demonstration of epidural extension of tumor. My-

elography is indicated in the evaluation of almost all patients with suspected epidural spinal cord compression in order to confirm the diagnosis, to determine the rostral-caudal extent of tumor (to guide radiotherapy or surgical decompression), and to diagnose coexistent leptomeningeal (by direct visualization or CSF analysis) or intramedullary tumor.

Although the clinical examination and plain spinal radiographs may suggest the diagnosis and localization of spinal cord compression, false-positive (such as radiation myelopathy) and false-negative cases occur, which can be excluded by myelography. Rodichok reported a series of patients in whom plain spinal radiographs correctly predicted the myelographic results in only 80 per cent. A radiotherapy portal, based on the plain spinal radiographic findings, encompassed all epidural disease found at myelography in only 79 per cent and could not be designed due to widespread vertebral involvement in 19 per cent.[67] In over 60 per cent of patients with epidural spinal cord compression from lymphoma, the plain spinal radiographs may be normal.[34a] Myelography is indicated in patients with myelopathy or radiculopathy in whom plain spinal films, spinal CT scanning, or clinical examination suggest a paraspinal tumor mass (such as Pancoast's syndrome).[46] Paravertebral tumors may gain access to the spinal canal through the intervertebral foramina and produce epidural spinal cord compression without producing vertebral body destruction.[62]

Myelography may discover silent epidural disease distant from the symptomatic lesion in up to 10 per cent of patients with multiple vertebral lesions.[32, 61] Furthermore, the degree of myelographic block alters prognosis[5] and influences the urgency of treatment.[33, 61, 62]

Myelography, however, is an invasive procedure that is difficult to perform if the patient is in considerable pain or is unstable medically or neurologically. As many as 14 per cent of patients with spinal cord compression may deteriorate neurologically after lumbar myelography.[40] It is contraindicated in patients with a coagulopathy, increased pressure from intracranial mass lesions or obstructive hydrocepha-

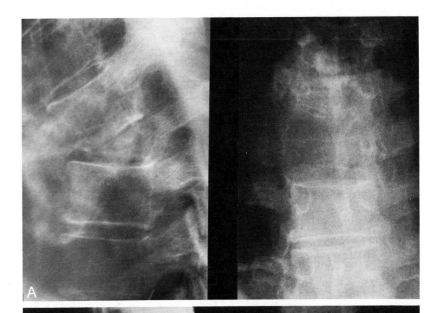

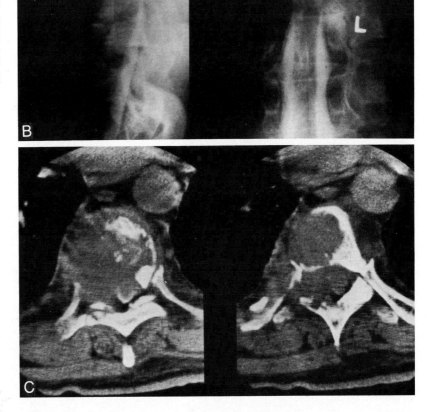

FIGURE 2–2. A, Plain spine radiographs in a 53-year-old man with metastatic renal carcinoma, midthoracic back pain, and normal neurologic examination. Left, lateral film, marked collapse of vertebral body, angulation. Right, anteroposterior film, loss of right pedicle, right paravertebral mass. B, Myelogram (metrizamide). Left, lateral film, complete extradural block. Right, anteroposterior film, complete extradural block from right side at level of missing pedicle. C, CT scan, postmyelogram. Left, destruction of vertebral body by tumor mass, paravertebral tumor and extradural tumor on right; thecal sac, outlined by metrizamide, pushed to left. Right, higher level than slice on left, right pedicle destroyed; no contrast in thecal sac.

lus, or an allergy to intrathecal contrast agents. Oil-based myelographic agents can be left in the thecal sac for repeat myelography at a future date but may produce an arachnoiditis. Water-soluble nonionic agents produce better visualization of nerve roots, allow CT-myelography, and do not have to be removed, but may produce a transient encephalopathy in some patients and seizures in patients with epilepsy. If a complete myelographic block is found after a lumbar injection, a lateral C1-2 puncture should be done to introduce contrast from above to determine the upper border of the block and exclude other lesions. Myelography alone cannot determine the degree of vertebral destruction, evaluate spinal stability, or visualize paravertebral extension of tumor; CT or MR scanning may be a useful adjunct to myelography in these areas. Spinal angiography is sometimes advised to assess the degree of vascularity of epidural metastases discovered at myelography and for embolization of highly vascular tumors (such as metastases from renal carcinoma) prior to surgery.[77]

Magnetic Resonance Imaging

Magnetic resonance imaging is a new imaging modality that offers considerable promise in the visualization of spinal tumors. On MRI, T1-weighted images demonstrate good anatomic visualization, including the vertebral bodies (bone marrow in vertebral bodies) and the spinal cord; whereas the intervertebral discs and subarachnoid space are well-demonstrated on T2-weighted images. Compared with normal bone marrow, most tumors demonstrate decreased signal intensity on T1-weighted images and increased signal intensity on T2-weighted images. A combination of T1- and T2-weighted images

can usually reliably detect tumor involvement of the spine and accurately visualize intraspinal and paravertebral extension of tumor. MR imaging can reliably differentiate tumor masses (low signal intensity on T1-weighted images) from acute hematomas or fat tissue (increased signal intensity).

Magnetic resonance imaging has several potential advantages over conventional imaging techniques, including: lack of exposure to ionizing radiation; no degradation of image quality by bone artifacts; superior soft tissue contrast resolution; good intraspinal resolution (spinal cord, thecal sac) without requiring intrathecal contrast agents (i.e., noninvasive); direct multiplanar visualization capacity (axial, coronal, sagittal) allowing visualization of spinal, intraspinal, and paravertebral tissues; and capacity to visualize the entire spine (thus able to demonstrate lesions at several different levels). MR imaging is superior to plain radiography and isotope bone scanning in the early detection of vertebral metastases by demonstrating altered signal characteristics of bone marrow involved by tumor[14, 31, 70, 72, 93] (Figs. 2–3 and 2–4).

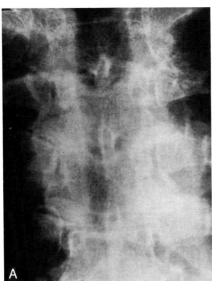

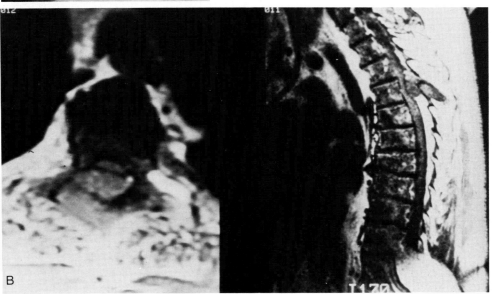

FIGURE 2–3. A 60-year-old man with prior melanoma, back pain, and myelopathy. *A,* Plain spine radiograph: AP film, questionable lucency of right pedicle. *B,* MRI scan, T1-weighted. Left, axial image, tumor (high signal) compressing spinal cord from posterior. Right, sagittal image, tumor in spinous process and epidural space compressing spinal cord.

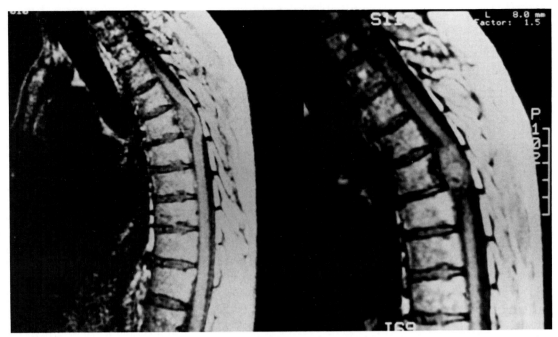

FIGURE 2–4. A 45-year-old man with a two-year history of back pain, recent myelopathy, and radiculopathy (left intercostal nerve). MRI scan, T1-weighted sagittal images: tumor compressing spinal cord from left and anterior. Sclerosis (low signal intensity) in vertebral body adjacent to tumor indicates long-standing process and spinal neurofibroma.

Using a combination of T1-weighted and T2-weighted images, Sze and coworkers[79] were able to reliably detect all epidural lesions in patients with metastatic cancer previously demonstrated by myelography or CT-myelography. Smoker and colleagues[72] reported that MR imaging was judged diagnostic in 60 of 64 examinations (94 per cent) in patients with suspected epidural metastases. In 22 patients, myelography, CT-myelography, and MR imaging were performed. Myelography was diagnostic in 16 of 22 cases (73 per cent); in 4 cases the upper end of a spinal block was not visualized. MR imaging provided the same diagnosis as myelography in 19 of the 22 studies (in no case did myelography provide more information about a clinically significant epidural lesion) and provided additional information not seen at myelography in 13 of 22 patients (59 per cent). This additional information included visualization of both the upper and lower end of cord compressions and demonstration of significant paraspinal muscle involvement, additional areas of cord compression, and additional areas of osseous spinal metastatic disease. Similar findings have been reported in other studies.[4, 14, 31, 47, 70] Hagenau and coworkers,[35] however, reported that in patients with systemic cancer being investigated for back pain or myelopathy, small clinically significant extradural lesions were identified in 9 of 19 patients by myelography and not MRI. Technical factors and the completeness of the MRI study may have accounted for some of the discrepancies among these studies.

Magnetic resonance imaging does have several potential disadvantages, including: relative inaccessibility to quality MRI (this problem is being corrected with the increased availability of MRI units); relative expense of MRI (high resolution requires an expen-

sive, superconducting, high magnetic strength unit); long duration of image acquisition required to produce complete images in multiple planes of the entire spine (often 60 to 90 minutes or more); relative inability to visualize small intrathecal lesions such as leptomeningeal metastases; lumbar puncture still required to obtain CSF for analysis; and technical problems associated with MRI such as artifacts from movement or metallic clips, difficulty visualizing patients with spinal deformities (scoliosis or kyphosis), difficulty studying patients with critical illness requiring close monitoring or ventilatory support, and claustrophobia in patients confined in small bore MRI units for prolonged studies.

Optimal MR imaging of the spine should include both sagittal T1- and T2-weighted images as well as axial T1-weighted images, with additional images as required to produce adequate visualization of clinically suspicious areas. The use of a superconducting, high magnetic field strength magnet and cardiac gating may improve image quality. The use of intravenous paramagnetic contrast agents such as gadolinium-DTPA (gadopentetate dimeglumine) may improve the delineation and characterization of epidural metastases and may allow the visualization of intradural extramedullary metastases not detectable by conventional noncontrast MR imaging.[78, 79]

Radionuclide Bone Scan

The radionuclide bone scan (isotope bone scan, bone scintigraphy) is widely used in the initial diagnosis and follow-up of bone tumors. Bone scintigraphy has a relatively limited role in the initial diagnosis of most primary bone lesions, as these lesions are usually evident on plain radiographs when the patient first presents with local symptoms. Bone scans are useful to determine the local extent and whether a lesion is solitary or multifocal in expression.[69, 83] Some primary bone tumors, such as osteoid osteoma, may be detected earlier on isotope bone scans than on plain radiographs as a well-localized area of intensely increased isotope uptake, before the plain x-ray film shows the typical bull's-eye appearance of a lucent nidus with a surrounding area of sclerosis.

Bone scintigraphy is very useful in the initial assessment and follow-up of systemic neoplasms that typically metastasize to bone. The presence or absence of bone metastases at initial diagnosis can influence the treatment of the primary tumor and obviously the prognosis of the patient. In breast cancer, radionuclide evidence of bone metastases is found in 2 to 3 per cent of patients with presumed Stage I disease, in 5 to 7 per cent with Stage II disease, and in up to 25 per cent with Stage III disease. At initial diagnosis, at least 35 per cent of patients with prostate cancer have radionuclide evidence of bone metastases.[38, 39, 54]

In patients with bone metastases, the isotope bone scan may be positive while the plain radiographs are negative in up to 36 per cent of patients, and the plain x-rays may lag 3 to 18 months behind bone scan positivity.[7, 19, 25] Radionuclide bone scanning detects changes in bone metabolism (especially new bone formation by osteoblasts) and in blood flow. Radionuclide imaging, using technetium-99m (Tc-99m)–labeled phosphate compounds, can detect as little as a 5 to 15 per cent alteration in local bone turnover; whereas a minimum size of 1 cm and a 50 per cent decrease in bone density are required for plain radiographs to detect a lytic lesion, and a 30 per cent increase in bone density is required to detect sclerotic lesions. Radionuclide bone imaging is thus 50 to 80 per cent more sensitive in detecting early skeletal metastases.[69]

Radionuclide bone imaging, however, is less specific than plain radiographs or CT scanning, as many different pathologic processes (trauma, infection, degenerative disorders, and so on) or physiologic processes (normal growth in children) may produce focal areas of increased isotope uptake ("hot spots"). Multiple areas of increased isotope uptake in patients with known malignancies that commonly spread to bone are likely to be metastases, but other benign processes must be considered, especially if a lesion is solitary, the clinical history is atypical, or the pattern of distribution of lesions is unusual for metastatic disease. Radiologic confirmation may be needed.

Neoplastic processes that produce intense bone destruction without concomitant new bone deposition (i.e., pure lytic lesions) may produce a "cold spot" or a negative bone scan. Multiple myeloma and thyroid cancer are the tumors most likely to produce cold spots or a negative bone scan despite lytic lesions detected on plain x-rays, but metastases from other solid tumors, including breast and lung cancer, can also occasionally produce cold lesions.[45] Prior radiotherapy may make an entire area cold, despite active

bone metastases in the area. In general, the false-negative rate of radionuclide scans (i.e., bone scan negative when plain radiographs are positive) is very low, probably less than 2 to 3 per cent.

Biopsy

The surgical treatment of suspected spinal tumors has several goals, including: biopsy (to establish the histologic nature of the tumor and guide further therapy); exclusion of other nonneoplastic disorders (infection, hemorrhage, and so forth); decompression of neural structures (spinal cord, cauda equina, nerve roots); stabilization of the spine; and removal of tumor. Biopsy of spinal tumors can be done by an open or closed (needle) approach. Almost all areas of the spine are accessible to needle biopsy, although x-ray fluoroscopic or CT guidance may be required, especially for small or deep lesions and lesions near the spinal canal. Prior to biopsy the local and systemic extent of the tumor should be determined (as a widely disseminated tumor may require only a needle biopsy or more limited open resection than a solitary lesion in which complete resection may be a goal), the presence or absence of spinal epidural extension should be determined (a more aggressive approach may be appropriate if neural structures are potentially at risk), and the general medical condition of the patient should be assessed. Coagulopathies and the possibility of renal carcinoma should be excluded as the inadvertent biopsy of lesions in these patients may result in excessive bleeding.[77, 89]

CLINICAL PROBLEMS

Several clinical problems may produce symptoms or signs that may mimic the presence of a spinal tumor or may confuse or complicate its investigation or treatment. These problems include epidural metastases, brachial or lumbosacral plexopathy, and leptomeningeal metastases.

Epidural Metastases

The development of epidural metastases, possibly leading to spinal cord, cauda equina, or nerve root compression, is a serious complication of spinal tumors which requires early detection and urgent investigation and treatment if serious neurologic disability is to be avoided. Epidural extension may complicate primary or metastatic spinal tumors. In patients with primary spinal tumors, the risk of epidural extension is highest in those with malignant histology. Epidural metastases, estimated to complicate 5 to 10 per cent of all patients with systemic cancer,[6] are most common in patients with carcinomas of breast, lung, prostate, and kidney, as well as in those with sarcomas, melanoma, and lymphoma. The mechanism of metastasis is most commonly hematogenous spread to the vertebral body or pedicle with extension into the spinal epidural space (85 per cent). Direct extension along spinal nerve roots into the epidural space, without vertebral body involvement, may occur in retroperitoneal or paravertebral tumors such as lymphoma or neuroblastoma. Direct metastases to the epidural space or drop metastases from intracranial tumors are very uncommon (< 5 per cent). The incidence of epidural metastases is likely to increase as cancer patients survive longer with more advanced disease and as detection methods improve.

The signs and symptoms of epidural metastases are summarized in Table 2–2. Back pain, either midline spinal pain or radicular pain, is the initial symptom in over 95 per cent of patients. The pain is usually described as a severe dull constant aching discomfort that is exacerbated by coughing, sneezing, straining, or bending and that is not relieved by bed rest. Radicular pain may be dull, constant, and aching or sharp, burning, and lancinating. At diagnosis, over 95 per cent of patients have severe pain, three quarters complain of weakness, and over one half complain of sensory loss and autonomic (bowel, bladder, or sexual) disturbance. Abnormalities on neurologic examination are more common than the corresponding symptoms.

Patients with signs or symptoms suggestive of epidural spinal cord compression (or cauda equina compression) require urgent investigation and treatment. Admission to hospital is usually needed. Posner,[62] Portenoy,[61] Rodichok,[66] O'Rourke,[57] and others have suggested algorithms for the investigation and treatment of patients (usually cancer patients) with back pain and/or suspected epidural spinal cord compression. Plain spine radiographs followed by myelography are recommended to localize the sites of vertebral involvement, to determine the site, degree, and extent of epidural or leptomeningeal involvement, as well as to provide a sample of CSF for analysis. CT or CT-myelography may provide additional information. MRI is gradually replacing myelography as the definitive investigation of epidural metastases. The advantages and disadvantages of CT, MRI, and myelography were discussed in the section on "Investigations" earlier.

Patients with back pain or radicular pain, without clinical evidence of a myelopathy, still require investigation. Plain spine radiography and/or radionuclide bone scanning are used to search for evidence of metastases. Posner,[62] Portenoy,[61] and Rodichok[67] support the early use of myelography to exclude epidural metastases in cancer patients with back pain and plain film or isotope bone scan abnormalities. O'Rourke[57] and Redmond[63, 64] suggest that spinal CT or CT-myelography can accurately determine the presence of epidural metastases. Colman,[14] Godersky,[31] Karnaze,[47] Sarpel,[70] and Smoker[72] report that MR imaging is equal or superior to CT scanning and/ or myelography in detecting and determining the degree and extent of epidural metastases, although Hagenau[35] found that conventional myelography was superior to MRI in 47 per cent of cases with small epidural lesions. The use of paramagnetic contrast

agents (gadolinium-DTPA) for MRI may improve the delineation and characterization of some extradural lesions[79] and may allow the detection of leptomeningeal metastases.[78] The early diagnosis and treatment of epidural metastases are important, as the major factor determining the outcome of treatment is the patient's neurologic status at the time of diagnosis: ambulatory patients do well, nonambulatory patients do very poorly, and paraplegic patients almost never regain useful function.[15, 29, 33]

Brachial and Lumbosacral Plexopathy

By compressing one or multiple nerve roots, spinal tumors may mimic a brachial or lumbosacral plexopathy. Brachial or lumbosacral plexopathy, from either benign or neoplastic causes, may mimic the signs and symptoms of a spinal tumor. Spinal tumors and plexus lesions may also coexist. Any of the above situations may confuse or complicate investigation and treatment and may lead to errors in diagnosis and treatment.

Neoplastic brachial plexopathy may occur owing to direct invasion of the plexus by carcinomas of the lung (especially apical squamous carcinomas arising in the superior pulmonary sulcus—Pancoast's tumor), compression and/or invasion from lymphatic metastases from carcinomas of the breast or head and neck, or hematogenous metastases from distant sites. Sarcomas and peripheral nerve sheath tumors (neurofibroma, neurofibrosarcoma, and so forth) are important but less common causes. Prior radiotherapy may produce a brachial plexopathy that must be distinguished from neoplastic involvement of the plexus.

The signs and symptoms that help differentiate neoplastic from radiation plexopathies are summarized in Table 2–3. In neoplastic brachial plexopathy,

TABLE 2–3. PLEXOPATHY: TUMOR VERSUS RADIATION

	TUMOR	RADIATION
Clinical		
Pain	Early, severe (>95%)	Late, mild (35%)
Level of involvement		
Brachial	Lower	Upper
Lumbosacral	Unilateral	Bilateral
Edema	Mild	Severe
Interval	Anytime	Usually > 1 year
Radiotherapy dose	Any dose	> 6000 cGy
Course	Progressive	Late stabilization
Horner's syndrome	Common (50%)	Uncommon
Myelopathy	Epidural tumor (50%)	Rare
Investigations		
CT scan		
Brachial	Mass (>80%); Fibrosis (10%)	Fibrosis (80%)
Lumbosacral	Mass (74%)	Normal; fibrosis
EMG	Denervation (>90%)	Myokymia (60%)

References: 13, 41, 46, 49, 80.

pain is an early and severe symptom in over 95 per cent of patients. The lower plexus is preferentially involved. Edema is mild. The course is relentlessly progressive unless effective tumor therapy can be given. Up to 50 per cent of patients may have epidural metastases and/or Horner's syndrome, although few present with a myelopathy.[46] The CT scan shows a discrete mass in over 80 per cent of patients. Patients who have a Horner's syndrome, CT evidence of paraspinal tumor, bilateral arm symptoms, or a myelopathy require either a myelogram or MRI scan to exclude epidural spinal cord compression. Electromyogram reveals denervation in over 90 per cent of patients; myokymic discharges are rare.

In radiation brachial plexopathy, pain is a late and relatively mild feature, occurring in 35 per cent of patients. Numbness, tingling, and paresthesias occur early and are followed later by weakness and reflex loss. The upper plexus is involved more than the lower plexus. Lymphedema of the arm may be severe. The course is usually slowly progressive with late stabilization. Relatively high radiation doses, usually over 6000 cGy, are required to produce radiation plexopathy. Local skin changes and induration may be severe. The interval from treatment to onset is usually over one year, unless the radiation dose has been excessively high. Most patients do not show a myelopathy. The CT scan shows diffuse fibrosis and loss of tissue planes in over 80 per cent of patients. Electromyogram studies reveal myokymia (spontaneous rapid semirhythmic bursts of potentials) in up to 60 per cent of patients.[1, 13, 49, 74]

Surgical exploration of the plexus is helpful if tumor is found, but the absence of tumor (and presence of fibrosis) on biopsy does not exclude tumor infiltration of the plexus. Stabilization of the clinical course and failure to develop metastatic disease after a prolonged observation period (over five years) is suggestive of radiation fibrosis. Development of a painful mass and progressive neurologic dysfunction many years after radiotherapy (up to 40 years, median > 15 years) is suggestive of a radiation-induced sarcoma or peripheral nerve sheath tumor.[17, 22]

Lumbosacral plexopathy may complicate gynecologic malignancy (cervix, endometrium, ovary), urologic malignancy (kidney, bladder, prostate, testis), colon carcinoma, lymphoma, or sarcoma. Radiotherapy to the pelvis may produce a radiation lumbosacral plexopathy as well. Radiation lumbosacral plexopathy is typically bilateral although asymmetric. CT scans are often normal or show only diffuse fibrosis and loss of tissue planes. Neoplastic lumbosacral plexopathy is usually unilateral, painful, and progressive. The CT scan shows a discrete tumor mass in three quarters of patients. Electromyogram shows similar changes as for brachial plexopathy.[42, 80] Epidural involvement is common. Myelography or MRI should be done, especially in patients with proximal, paravertebral plexus involvement on CT scan, spinal/vertebral involvement on plain films, isotope bone scan, or CT scan, or bilateral symptoms without prior radiotherapy.

Benign causes of brachial or lumbosacral plexopathy, such as diabetes mellitus, neuralgia amyotrophy, polyarteritis nodosa, trauma, and many others, must be considered but usually pose little diagnostic difficulty.

Leptomeningeal Metastases

Leptomeningeal metastases (carcinomatous meningitis) are a rare complication of primary benign or malignant spinal tumors, but may develop in up to 5 per cent of all patients with solid tumors (especially carcinomas of breast and lung, and melanoma); in up to 40 per cent of patients with relapsed small cell carcinoma of lung; in up to 30 per cent of patients with lymphoma (especially patients with high grade tumors, diffuse histology, and advanced—Stage IV—disease); occasionally in patients with primary brain tumors (especially medulloblastoma and ependymoma, but also anaplastic gliomas); and still occurs in patients with leukemia despite CNS prophylaxis.[2, 12, 51, 87, 92] Leptomeningeal metastases may present with signs and/or symptoms of cerebral, cranial nerve, or spinal dysfunction. As leptomeningeal metastases are often a late complication of disseminated cancer, many patients may have coexisting spinal bony metastases. The symptoms and signs of leptomeningeal metastases thus could be mistaken for more localized disease, leading to inappropriate treatment. At diagnosis, cerebral symptoms (headache, mental change, nausea, etc.) or signs (mental change, seizures, papilledema, etc.) are present in 50 per cent of patients with leptomeningeal metastases from solid tumors. Cranial nerve symptoms (diplopia, hearing loss, visual loss, etc.) or signs (ocular muscle paresis, facial weakness, deafness, etc.) are present in 56 per cent of patients. Spinal symptoms (weakness, numbness, radicular pain, back pain, and bowel/bladder dysfunction) or signs (reflex loss, lower motor neuron weakness, sensory loss, meningeal irritation, etc.) are present in 82 per cent of patients.[87] A careful neurologic examination often discloses more cranial nerve or spinal signs than the patient's symptoms had initially suggested. While spinal symptoms or signs are found in over 80 per cent of patients with leptomeningeal metastases, and thus could possibly be attributed to spinal bony metastases, epidural metastases, or plexopathies, cerebral and/or cranial nerve symptoms or signs are also found in over 50 per cent of these patients. A careful history and neurologic examination may reveal the more extensive findings that would suggest leptomeningeal metastases. In patients with spinal dysfunction the presence of multifocal radicular symptoms or signs (radicular pain, reflex loss, radicular weakness, or sensory loss) or prominent signs of meningeal irritation (nuchal rigidity, positive straight leg raising) should suggest possible leptomeningeal metastases.

The single most important diagnostic test for leptomeningeal metastases is the examination of the CSF. According to Wasserstrom,[87] leptomeningeal metastases from solid tumors may produce CSF leukocytosis (> 5 × 10⁶/l in 72 per cent), increased CSF protein (> 500 mg/l in 89 per cent), reduced CSF glucose (< 2.2 mmol/l or < 40 mg/dl in 41 per cent), or increased CSF pressure (> 160 mm Hg in 71 per cent). The CSF cytology is positive for malignant cells in 54 per cent of patients on the initial lumbar puncture, in 84 per cent after two lumbar punctures, and in over 90 per cent after subsequent lumbar punctures. A positive CSF cytology for malignant cells almost always indicates leptomeningeal metastases.[30] Elevated CSF levels of biochemical markers of metastatic disease (beta-glucuronidase, CEA, or lactic dehydrogenase isoenzymes [LDH-5]) may be found in over 80 per cent of patients with leptomeningeal metastases from carcinomas of the breast or lung. In leukemia or lymphoma, the CSF beta$_2$-microglobulin level is often elevated in patients with meningeal involvement.[53] Immunocytochemistry analysis, sometimes using a fluorescent-activated cell sorter, looking for a monoclonal population of abnormal lymphocytes may assist the diagnosis of leptomeningeal leukemia or lyumphoma.

Myelography may be abnormal (leptomeningeal nodules, thickened or matted nerve roots) in 25 to 50 per cent of patients with leptomeningeal metastases, may be abnormal in some patients with negative CSF cytology, and helps to exclude coexisting epidural metastases.[59, 87] Spinal CT scanning is usually negative, but cranial CT scanning is frequently abnormal (hydrocephalus, obliteration of basal cisterns or cortical sulci, enhancement of cortical gyri, meningeal or subependymal enhancement, enhancing superficial nodules), showing specific or nonspecific abnormalities in 50 to 75 per cent of patients.[3, 41, 87] MR imaging is usually negative, although the paramagnetic contrast agent gadolinium-DTPA may allow visualization of enhanced nodules over 2 to 3 mm in size and thickened nerve roots in up to 90 per cent of patients with leptomeningeal metastases.[78]

It is important to differentiate leptomeningeal metastases from more localized processes producing spinal dysfunction, as the treatment is different and prognosis often worse in patients with leptomeningeal metastases.

CONCLUSIONS

Spinal tumors may present with a wide variety of clinical manifestations: pain is an early and often severe symptom; neurologic dysfunction, mass, or deformity develop later. A high degree of suspicion must be maintained as benign back pain is very common and spinal tumors are relatively uncommon. A delay in diagnosis, however, may result in the development of neurologic disability that may be permanent despite appropriate treatment. The symptoms, signs, and investigation of spinal tumors have been discussed, with emphasis on early diagnosis, differentiation from benign spinal disorders, and the manifestations of epidural metastases, plexopathies, and leptomeningeal metastases.

ACKNOWLEDGMENT: Secretarial assistance of Maggi Stawarski and Michelle Chui is gratefully appreciated.

REFERENCES

1. Albers JW, Allen AA, Bastron JA, Daube JR: Limb myokymia. Muscle Nerve 4:494–504, 1981.
2. Aroney RS, Dalley DN, Chan WK, et al: Meningeal carcinomatosis in small cell carcinoma of lung. Am J Med 71:26–32, 1981.
3. Ascherl GF, Hilal SK, Brisman R: Computed tomography of disseminated meningeal and ependymal malignant neoplasms. Neurology 31:567–574, 1981.
4. Bale JF, Bell WE, Dunn V, et al: Magnetic resonance imaging of the spine in children. Arch Neurol 43:1253–1256, 1986.
5. Barcena A, Lobato RD, Rivas JJ, et al: Spinal metastatic disease: Analysis of factors determining functional prognosis and choice of treatment. Neurosurgery 15:820–827, 1984.
6. Barron KD, Hirano A, Arakis S, Terry RD: Experiences with metastatic neoplasms involving the spinal cord. Neurology 9:91–106, 1959.
7. Belliveau RE, Spencer RP: Incidence and sites of bone lesions detected by 99m-Tc-polyphosphate scans in patients with tumors. Cancer 36:359–363, 1975.
8. Benedetti C, Bonica JJ: Cancer pain: Basic considerations. *In* Benedetti C, et al (eds): Advances in Pain Research and Therapy, Vol 7. New York, Raven Press, 1984, pp 529–555.
9. Black P: Spinal metastasis: Current status and recommended guidelines for management. Neurosurgery 5:726–746, 1979.
10. Boggan JE, Hoff JT, Wara WM, Boldrey EB: Intraspinal tumors in children. West J Med 133:108–114, 1980.
11. Bonica JJ: Historical, socioeconomic and diagnostic aspects of the problem. 1. The nature of the problem. *In* Carron H, McLaughlin RE (eds): Management of Low Back Pain. Bristol, The Stonebridge Press, 1982, pp 1–15.
12. Bunn PA, Schein PS, Banks PM, DeVita VT: Central nervous system complications in patients with diffuse histiocytic and undifferentiated lymphoma: Leukemia revisited. Blood 47:3–10, 1976.
13. Cascino TL, Kori S, Krol G, Foley KM: CT of the brachial plexus in patients with cancer. Neurology 33:1553–1557, 1983.
14. Colman LK, Porter BA, Redmond J, et al: Early diagnosis of spinal metastases by CT and MR studies. J Comput Assist Tomogr 12:423–426, 1988.
15. Constans JP, de Divitiis E, Donzelli R, et al: Spinal metastases with neurological manifestations. Review of 600 cases. J Neurosurg 59:111–118, 1983.
16. Dahlin DC, Unni KK: Bone Tumors. General Aspects and Data on 8,542 Cases. 4th Ed. Springfield, IL, Charles C Thomas, 1983.
17. Ducatman BS, Scheithauer BW: Postirradiation neurofibrosarcoma. Cancer 51:1028–1033, 1983.
18. Fink IJ, Garra BS, Zabell A, et al: Computed tomography with metrizamide myelography to define the extent of spinal canal block due to tumor. J Comput Assist Tomogr 8:1072–1075, 1984.
19. Fletcher JW, Solaric-George E, Henry RE, et al: Radioisotope detection of osseous metastases. Arch Intern Med 135:553–557, 1975.
20. Foley KM: Pain syndromes in patients with cancer. *In* Bonica JJ, Ventrafridda V (eds): Advances in Pain Research and Therapy. Vol 2. New York, Raven Press, 1979, pp 59–75.
21. Foley KM: Pain syndromes in patients with cancer. Med Clin North Am 71:169–184, 1987.
22. Foley KM, Woodruff JM, Ellis FT, Posner JB: Radiation-induced malignant and atypical peripheral nerve sheath tumors. Ann Neurol 7:311–318, 1980.
23. Friedlauder GE, Southwick WO: Tumors of the spine. *In* Rothman RH, Simeone FA (eds): The Spine. 2nd ed, Vol 2. Philadelphia, WB Saunders Co, 1982.

24. Frymoyer JW: Back pain and sciatica. N Engl J Med 318:291–300, 1988.

25. Galasko CSB: The significance of occult skeletal metastases, detected by skeletal scintigraphy, in patients with otherwise apparently "early" mammary carcinoma. Br J Surg 62:694–696, 1975.

26. Galasko CSB: The anatomy and pathways of skeletal metastases. *In* Weiss L, Gilbert HA (eds): Bone Metastasis. Boston, GK Hall & Co, 1981, pp 49–63.

27. Garcia DM: Primary spinal cord tumors treated with surgery and postoperative irradiation. Int J Radiat Oncol Biol Phys 11:1933–1939, 1985.

28. Gilbert HA, Kagan AR: Metastases: Incidence, detection, and evaluation without histologic confirmation. *In* Weiss L (ed): Fundamentals of Metastasis. Amsterdam, North Holland Publishing Company, 1976.

29. Gilbert RW, Kim JH, Posner JB: Epidural spinal cord compression from metastatic tumor: Diagnosis and treatment. Ann Neurol 3:40–51, 1978.

30. Glass JP, Melamed M, Chernik NL, Posner JB: Malignant cells in cerebrospinal fluid (CSF): The meaning of a positive CSF cytology. Neurology 29:1369–1375, 1979.

31. Godersky JC, Smoker WRK, Knutzon R: Use of magnetic resonance imaging in the evaluation of metastatic spinal disease. Neurosurgery 21:676–680, 1987.

32. Graus F, Krol G, Foley KM: Early diagnosis of spinal epidural metastasis (SEM): Correlation with clinical and radiological findings. Proc Am Soc Clin Oncol 4:269, 1985.

33. Greenberg HS, Kim JH, Posner JB: Epidural spinal cord compression from metastatic tumor: Results with a new treatment protocol. Ann Neurol 8:361–366, 1980.

34. Grem JL, Burgess J, Trump DL: Clinical features and natural history of intramedullary spinal cord metastasis. Cancer 56:2305–2314, 1985.

34a. Haddad P, Thaell JF, Kiely JM, et al: Lymphoma of the spinal extradural space. Cancer 38:1862–1866, 1976.

35. Hagenau C, Grosh W, Currie M, Wiley RG: Comparison of spinal magnetic resonance imaging and myelography in cancer patients. J Clin Oncol 5:1663–1669, 1987.

36. Hahn YS, McLone DG: Pain in children with spinal cord tumors. Child's Brain 11:36–46, 1984.

37. Haibach H, Farrell C, Gaines RW: Osteoid osteoma of the spine: Surgically correctable cause of painful scoliosis. Can Med Assoc J 135:895–899, 1986.

38. Harbert JC: Efficacy of bone and liver scanning in malignant disease: Facts and opinions. *In* Freeman LM, Weissmann HS (eds): Nuclear Medicine Annual. New York, Raven Press, 1982.

39. Harrington KD: Orthopaedic Management of Metastatic Bone Disease. St. Louis, CV Mosby, 1988.

40. Hollis PH, Malis LI, Zappulla RA: Neurological deterioration after lumbar puncture below complete spinal subarachnoid block. J Neurosurg 64:253–256, 1986.

41. Jaeckle KA, Krol G, Posner JB: Evolution of computed tomographic abnormalities in leptomeningeal metastases. Ann Neurol 17:85–89, 1985.

42. Jaeckle KA, Young DF, Foley KM: The natural history of lumbosacral plexopathy in cancer. Neurology 35:8–15, 1985.

43. Jaffe WL: Tumors and Tumorous Conditions of the Bones and Joints. Philadelphia, Lea & Febiger, 1958.

44. Janin Y, Epstein JA, Carras R, et al: Osteoid osteomas and osteoblastomas of the spine. Neurosurgery 8:31–38, 1981.

45. Kagan AR, Stekel RJ, Bassett LW: Lytic spine lesion and cold bone scan. AJR 136:129–131, 1981.

46. Kanner RM, Martini N, Foley KM: Incidence of pain and other clinical manifestations of superior pulmonary sulcus (Pancoast) tumors. *In* Bonica JJ, et al (eds): Advances in Pain Research and Therapy. Vol 4. New York, Raven Press, 1982, pp 27–39.

47. Karnaze MG, Gado MH, Sartor KJ, Hodges FJ: Comparison of MR and CT myelography in imaging the cervical and thoracic spine. Am J Radiol 150:397–403, 1988.

48. Kato A, Ushio Y, Hayakawa T, et al: Circulatory disturbance of the spinal cord with epidural neoplasm in rats. J Neurosurg 63:260–265, 1985.

49. Kori SH, Foley KM, Posner JB: Brachial plexus lesions in patients with cancer: 100 cases. Neurology 31:45–50, 1981.

50. Low JC: The radionuclide scan in bone metastasis. *In* Weiss L, Gilbert HA (eds): Bone Metastasis. Boston, GK Hall & Co, 1981, pp 231–244.

51. MacKintosh FR, Colby TV, Podolsky WJ, et al: Central nervous system involvement in non-Hodgkin's lymphoma: An analysis of 105 cases. Cancer 49:586–595, 1982.

52. Martinez V, Sissons HA: Aneurysmal bone cyst. A review of 123 cases including primary lesions and those secondary to other bone pathology. Cancer 61:2291–2304, 1988.

53. Mavligit GM, Stuckey SE, Cabanillas FF, et al: Diagnosis of leukemia or lymphoma in the central nervous system by beta₂-microglobulin determination. N Engl J Med 303:718–722, 1980.

54. McNeil BJ: Rationale for the use of bone scans in selected metastatic primary bone tumors. Semin Nucl Med 8:336–345, 1978.

55. Myles ST, MacRae ME: Benign osteoblastoma of the spine in childhood. J Neurosurg 68:884–888, 1988.

56. Olsen ME, Chernik NL, Posner JB: Infiltration of the leptomeninges by systemic cancer. A clinical and pathologic study. Arch Neurol 30:122–137, 1974.

57. O'Rourke T, George CB, Redmond J, et al: Spinal computed tomography and computed tomographic metrizamide myelography in the early diagnosis of metastatic disease. J Clin Oncol 4:576–583, 1986.

58. Patchell R, Posner JB: Neurologic complications of systemic cancer. Neurol Clin 3:729–750, 1985.

59. Pedersen AG, Paulson OB, Gyldensted C: Metrizamide myelography in patients with small cell carcinoma of the lung suspected of meningeal carcinomatosis. J Neuro-Oncol 3:85–89, 1985.

60. Pilepich MV, Vietti TJ, Nesbit ME, et al: Ewing's sarcoma of the vertebral column. Int J Radiat Oncol Biol Phys 7:27–31, 1981.

61. Portenoy RK, Lipton RB, Foley KM: Back pain in the cancer patient: An algorithm for evaluation and management. Neurology 37:134–138, 1987.

62. Posner JB: Back pain and epidural spinal cord compression. Med Clin North Am 71:185–205, 1987.

63. Redmond J, Friedl KE, Cornett P, et al: Clinical usefulness of an algorithm for the early diagnosis of spinal metastatic disease. J Clin Oncol 6:154–157, 1988.

64. Redmond J, Spring DB, Munderloh SH, et al: Spinal computed tomography scanning in the evaluation of metastatic disease. Cancer 54:253–258, 1984.

65. Reimer R, Onofrio BM: Astrocytomas of the spinal cord in children and adolescents. J Neurosurg 63:669–675, 1985.

66. Rodichok LD, Harper GR, Ruckdeschel JC, et al: Early diagnosis of spinal epidural metastases. Am J Med 70:1181–1188, 1981.

67. Rodichok LD, Ruckdeschel JC, Harper GR, et al: Early detection and treatment of spinal epidural metastases: The role of myelography. Ann Neurol 20:696–702, 1986.

68. Rogers LR, Weinstein MA: Magnetic resonance imaging in the detection of metastatic epidural spinal cord or nerve root compression. Neurology 37(Suppl 1):337, 1987.

69. Rosenthall L, Lisbona R: Skeletal Imaging. Norwalk, CT, Appleton-Century-Crofts, 1984.

70. Sarpel S, Sarpel G, Yu E, et al: Early diagnosis of spinal-epidural metastasis by magnetic resonance imaging. Cancer 59:1112–1116, 1987.

71. Sim FH, Unni KK, Wold LE, McLeod RA: Benign tumors. *In* Sim FH (ed): Diagnosis and Treatment of Bone Tumors: A Team Approach (A Mayo Clinic Monograph). Thorofare, NJ, Slack Inc, 1983, pp 107–151.

72. Smoker WRK, Godersky JC, Knutzon RK, et al: The role of MR imaging in evaluating metastatic spinal disease. Am J Radiol 149:1241–1248, 1987.

73. Stein BM: Spinal intradural tumors. *In* Wilkins RH, Rengarchary SS (eds): Neurosurgery. New York, McGraw-Hill, 1984, pp 1048–1061.

74. Stohr M: Special types of spontaneous electrical activity in radiogenic nerve injuries. Muscle Nerve 5:S78–S83, 1982.

75. Stoll BA: Natural history, prognosis and staging of bone metastases. *In* Stoll BA, Parbhoo S (eds): Bone Metastasis: Monitoring and Treatment. New York, Raven Press, 1983, pp 1–20.

76. Sundaresan N, Galicich JH, Lane J: Treatment of odontoid fractures in cancer patients. J Neurosurg 54:468–472, 1981.

77. Sundaresan N, Scher H, DiGiacinto GV, et al: Surgical treatment of spinal cord compression in kidney cancer. J Clin Oncol 4:1851–1856, 1986.

78. Sze G, Abramson A, Krol G, et al: Gadolinium-DTPA in the evaluation of intradural extramedullary spinal disease. Am J Radiol 150:911–921, 1988.

79. Sze G, Krol G, Zimmerman RD, Deck MDF: Malignant extradural spinal tumors: MR imaging with Gd-DTPA. Radiology 167:217–223, 1988.

80. Thomas JE, Cascino TL, Earle JD: Differential diagnosis between radiation and tumor plexopathy of the pelvis. Neurology 35:1–7, 1985.

81. Tofe A, Francis MD, Harvey WJ: Correlation of neoplasms with incidence and localization of skeletal metastases: An analysis of 1355 diphosphonate bone scans. J Nucl Med 16:986–989, 1975.

82. Torma T: Benign osteogenic and chondrogenic tumours of the spine. *In* Vinken PJ, Bruyn GW (eds): Tumors of the Spine and Spinal Cord, Part 1. Handbook of Clinical Neurology. Vol 19. New York, North-Holland, 1975, pp 293–312.

83. Treves ST, Kirkpatrick JA: Bone. *In* Treves ST (ed): Pediatric Nuclear Medicine. New York, Springer-Verlag, 1985.

84. Tucker MA, Coleman CN, Cox RS, et al: Risk of second cancers after treatment for Hodgkin's disease. N Engl J Med 318:76–81, 1988.

85. Tucker MA, D'Angio GJ, Boice JD, et al: Bone sarcomas linked to radiotherapy and chemotherapy in children. N Engl J Med 317:588–593, 1987.

86. Ushio Y, Posner R, Posner JB, Shapiro WR: Experimental spinal cord compression by epidural neoplasms. Neurology 27:422–429, 1977.

87. Wasserstrom WR, Glass JP, Posner JB: Diagnosis and treatment of leptomeningeal metastases from solid tumors: Experience with 90 patients. Cancer 49:759–772, 1982.

88. Weidner A: Extradural tumors of the spine. Adv Neurosurg 14:10–15, 1986.

89. Weinstein JN, McLain RF: Primary tumors of the spine. Spine 9:843–851, 1987.

90. Weissman DE, Gilbert M, Wang H, Grossman SA: The use of computed tomography of the spine to identify patients at high risk for epidural metastases. J Clin Oncol 3:1541–1544, 1985.

91. Wilkins RM, Pritchard DJ, Burgert EO, Unni KK: Ewing's sarcoma of bone. Experience with 140 patients. Cancer 58:2551–2555, 1986.

92. Yung WA, Horten BC, Shapiro WR: Meningeal gliomatosis: A review of 12 cases. Ann Neurol 8:605–608, 1980.

93. Zimmer WD, Berquist TH, McLeod RA, et al: Bone tumors: Magnetic resonance imaging versus computed tomography. Radiology 155:709–718, 1985.

3

STAGING OF MUSCULOSKELETAL NEOPLASMS

WILLIAM F. ENNEKING

INTRODUCTION

The purposes of a staging system for musculoskeletal neoplasms are to: (1) incorporate the significant prognostic factors into a system that describes progressive degrees of risk of local recurrence and distant metastases to which a patient is subject, (2) stratify the stages so that they have specific implications for surgical management, and (3) provide guidelines for adjunctive therapies.

Over a number of years, staging systems for various classes of malignant tumors have been developed under the auspices of the American Joint Committee for Cancer Staging and End Results Reporting (AJC). The systems vary among cancers related to the natural course of a particular type of cancer. In 1980, a system for the surgical staging of musculoskeletal sarcoma was proposed, studied, and adopted by the Musculoskeletal Tumor Society[3] and was subsequently adopted by the AJC.

In this review, the natural evolution of benign and malignant lesions of connective tissue derivation which led to the staging system, the system for both benign and malignant lesions, its articulation with surgical treatment, and early experience with its use will be described.

NATURAL EVOLUTION

The natural course in progression from the most benign to the most malignant connective tissue tumor is the same, lesion for lesion, whether the tumor arises in bone or in somatic soft tissue. A fibrosarcoma behaves as a fibrosarcoma whether it arises in soft tissues and invades bone or vice versa. Aggressive benign fibrous lesions in soft tissue (fibromatosis) behave the same as their counterparts arising in bone (desmoplastic fibroma). Therefore, a common staging system, as opposed to separate systems, was devised for bone and soft tissue lesions. The system, as befits the natural history, applies only to lesions of connective tissue histogenesis and not to primary

lesions of round cell origin (leukemias, lymphomas, myeloma, Ewing's sarcoma) or metastatic lesions.

The significant progressive changes in the biologic behavior of musculoskeletal lesions are: (1) localized, latent or static, inactive, benign; (2) localized, active, benign; (3) aggressive, invasive, but still benign; (4) indolent, invasive, malignant, low risk of regional lymphatic or distant metastases; (5) rapidly destructive, malignant, high risk of local, regional, and distant metastases; and (6) regional and/or distant metastases. Each of these progressions has distinctive clinical, radiographic, and histologic features that form the basis for the staging system and will be presented in some detail. The radiographic features that express these evolutionary changes in skeletal lesions have been previously studied and classified by their probability of occurrence by Lodwick and colleagues.[11]

Inactive Benign Lesions

Inactive benign lesions are usually asymptomatic, discovered incidentally, and seldom related to pathologic fracture or mechanical dysfunction. They may slowly attain large size but eventually reach a steady state in which they no longer grow. These lesions appear quite responsive to contact inhibition and remain completely encapsulated. They remain intracompartmental and seldom deform the compartmental boundaries of cortical bone, articular cartilage, or dense fascial septae. When palpable in soft tissue, inactive benign lesions are often small, movable, nontender, with little or no significant enlargement on subsequent clinical observation. Radiographic studies show lesions that are well marginated by a mature shell of cortical-like reactive bone, without deformation or expansion of the encasing bone (Lodwick IA). Angiographic staging studies show little or no increase in isotope uptake and no intralesional neoangiogenesis or significant reactive neoangiogenesis about the lesion. Computed tomographic (CT) scanning shows a homogeneous, well-marginated density, with no cortical broaching or cross-fascial extension.

The histologic characteristics of the lesion are: (1) low cell-to-matrix ratio; (2) mature, well-differentiated matrices; (3) benign cytologic characteristics (no hyperchromasia, anaplasia, or pleomorphism); (4) encapsulation by mature fibrous tissue or cortical bone; and (5) little or no reactive mesenchymal proliferation, inflammatory infiltrate, or neoangiogenesis about the lesion.

Active Benign Lesions

Active benign lesions are mildly symptomatic, discovered because of discomfort, and are occasionally associated with pathologic fracture or mechanical dysfunction. They grow steadily and continue to enlarge during observation. These lesions appear responsive to contact inhibition but not at normal levels, as they can expand by deformation of overlying cortical bone, articular cartilage, or fascial septae. They remain encapsulated and have only a thin layer of filmy areolar tissue forming the reactive zone between the lesion and surrounding normal tissue. When palpable in soft tissue, they are usually small, movable, moderately tender, and grow slowly during clinical observation. Radiographic characteristics of active lesions in bone are irregular but well-marginated defects. The margin is a mature cancellous ring rather than a cortical shell, and the inner aspect is often irregular or corrugated, giving a septated appearance. Expansion, bulging, or deformation of the combination of overlying cortex/reactive bone (Lodwick IB) is frequently observed.

Staging studies show increased isotope uptake that conforms closely to the limits of the radiographic defect and reactive changes. A thin but discernible rim of reactive neoangiogenesis about the lesion is often observed, but seldom any significant intralesional neoplastic neoangiogenesis. CT scanning shows a homogeneous density, irregular but intact reactive bone, expansion of the overlying cortex, and intracompartmental containment by bone or fascia. The histologic characteristics of active benign lesions are: (1) a relatively balanced cell-to-matrix ratio with homogeneous distribution of the matrix; (2) well-differentiated matrices; (3) benign cytologic characteristics; (4) an intact capsule of mature fibrous tissue and/or cancellous bone; (5) a narrow zone of mesenchymal, inflammatory, and vascular reactive tissue between the capsule and the surrounding normal tissue; and (6) resorption of preexisting bone by osteoclasts rather than by neoplastic cells as the mechanism of expansion. Intermittent areas of resorption often produce an irregular, serrated, sometimes corrugated interface between the capsule and the adjacent reactive bone.

Aggressive Benign Lesions

Aggressive benign lesions are often symptomatic, discovered because of discomfort and/or a growing mass, and when in a stress-bearing bone, associated with a pathologic fracture. When palpable in soft tissues, they grow rapidly, sometimes alarmingly. These lesions are frequently tender and may have an inflammatory appearance. They are little affected by contact inhibition and readily penetrate or permeate the natural barriers to tumor growth: cortical bone, fascial septae, and in some cases, articular cartilage or joint capsules. They penetrate the capsule with finger-like extensions protruding directly into the surrounding zone. The reactive zone is thick, edematous, and often inflammatory. These aggressive lesions invade by destroying or resorbing the restraining bone or fascia and permeating into adjacent tissues or compartments, rather than by expanding through concomitant endosteal resorption and subperiosteal apposition.

When aggressive benign lesions involve unrestrained areas (medullary canal, cancellous bone, adventitial intermuscular planes within muscle bellies, periarticular tissues), they extend rapidly although usually preceded by a pseudocapsule of reactive tissue.

Aggressive soft tissue lesions are usually firm, fixed, and tender and have a rapid growth history. The radiographic features of aggressive benign lesions are a ragged permeative interface with adjacent bone, incomplete attempts at containment by reactive bone, cortical destruction, endosteal buttresses and periosteal Codman's triangles, and rapid soft tissue extension (Lodwick IC). Staging studies often reflect the aggressive nature and behavior of these lesions. Isotope scans show increased uptake in both the early vascular phase and the late bone phase. The extent of the increased uptake is often well beyond the apparent radiographic limits. Angiograms show a distinct reactive zone of neovasculature on the early arterial phase and an intralesional hypervascular blush on the late venous phase of the study. CT scans show nonhomogeneous mottled densities with defects in attempts at reactive containment, early extracompartmental extension from bone, and indistinct margins in soft tissues. Otherwise, occult involvement of major neurovascular bundles is often shown by either angiography or CT scans in aggressive soft tissue lesions.

Histologic features of aggressive lesions are: (1) high cell-to-matrix ratio; (2) clearly differentiated matrices of varying maturity; (3) predominantly benign cytologic characteristics without anaplasia or pleomorphism, but with frequent hyperchromatic nuclei. Mitoses are occasionally encountered. Vascular invasion within the lesion may also be found; (4) finger-like projections of tumor extending through gaps in the capsule and growing into the surrounding reactive zone. These extensions usually maintain continuity with the main mass, although occasional apparently isolated satellites are seen; and (5) a thick, succulent zone of reactive tissue interposed between the penetrated capsule and the more peripheral normal tissue. This zone or pseudocapsule encircles but does not inhibit growth of an aggressive tumor. The reactive zone prevents tumor nodules from extending directly into normal tissue. Destruction of surrounding bone is by reactive osteoclasts rather than by tumor cells, although fingers of tumor grow rapidly into the reactive bone.

Despite the benign cytologic characteristics, the invasive behavior of these lesions is more like that of a low grade malignancy than of an active benign process. The reliability of the benign cytologic features is occasionally challenged by the occurrence of distant, usually pulmonary, metastases. These metastases look histologically as benign as the primary tumor and have a much better prognosis than the metastases of frankly malignant lesions.

Low Grade Sarcomas

Low grade sarcomas have all the invasive growth mechanisms of local malignancy but have a low risk of distant metastases and an indolent rate of evolution. With time and particularly with repeated cycles of unsuccessful excisions and recurrences, the risk of dedifferentiating into high grade and distant metastases is increased.

Low grade sarcomas often present as slow-growing, painless masses with an indolent but steady growth rate. They are seldom symptomatic. They stimulate generous amounts of reactive bone or fibrous tissue that often impart a false impression of encapsulation. These lesions are not inhibited by the natural barriers to tumor growth, but their extension through them is one of gradual erosion rather than rapid destruction. Their relentless progression often produces extraosseous or extracompartmental extension and neovascular bundle involvement. They seldom traverse articular cartilage or joint capsule to extend intraarticularly. They may, however, stimulate reactive synovitis and effusion when adjacent to joints in either bone or soft tissue. Similarly, they do not extend through tendon sheath, nerve sheath, or the outer adventitial layer of major arteries but tend to push these structures aside. Tendons, nerves, and vessels, however, are often involved by the reactive zone about the lesion.

When low grade sarcomas arise in the soft tissue, they are apt to be small, superficial, fixed, nontender, and without inflammatory signs from the reactive zone. The radiographic features of low grade skeletal sarcomas are similarly apt to be less ominous than many aggressive benign lesions (Lodwick II). They often have a generous reactive rim of cancellous bone admixed with defects of extracapsular and/or soft tissue extension. Buttressing in the medullary canal, Codman's triangles externally, and especially endosteal scalloping are features of these lesions. Staging studies again accurately reflect the behavior of these lesions. Isotope scans in both bone and soft tissue show increased early and late uptake that is more extensive than the radiographic limits would suggest. The angiographic findings show little or no reactive neovasculature or intralesional neoangiogenesis and often appear deceptively benign. CT findings show nonhomogeneous density, a thick perforated

ring of reactive bone, and occult soft tissue or intraosseous extension.

The histologic features of locally invasive low grade malignancies are: (1) a relatively even proportion of cells to matrix; (2) well-differentiated and usually mature matrices; (3) malignant cytologic characteristics—anaplasia, pleomorphism, and hyperchromasia—with a modest number of mitoses. These features are consistent with Broders' Grades 1 and occasionally 2 in other malignancies[2]; (4) varying amounts of necrosis, hemorrhage, and vascular invasion found in these lesions which are seldom seen in benign lesions; and (5) numerous interruptions in the continuity of the capsule where the tumor extends directly into the reactive zone which, in turn, forms a pseudocapsule about the lesion. In the reactive zone, nodules of isolated tumor-forming satellites are almost universally found. Skip lesions in normal tissue beyond the reactive zone are rarely if ever seen about low grade lesions.

Due to the indolent growth rate of low grade, locally invasive sarcomas, they remain contained by the natural barriers to tumor growth within their compartments of origin for long periods. With their ability to destroy or pervade normal tissue, however, they eventually extend through their barriers to involve adjacent extracompartmental tissues. Metastasis to regional lymph nodes is unusual. Distant pulmonary metastases occur late in the course and are often solitary.

High Grade Sarcomas

High grade sarcomas usually appear as destructive symptomatic masses that are often associated with pathologic fractures when they involve bone. They stimulate generous amounts of reactive tissue but overgrow it so rapidly that they appear to have little or no pseudoencapsulation. They are uninhibited by the natural barriers to tumor growth and rapidly extend into adjacent tissues by destruction of cortical bone, fascial septae, articular cartilage, or joint capsules. They quickly extend extracompartmentally, involve adjacent neurovascular bundles, and extend proximally along ill-defined extracompartmental fascial plane and spaces. They often cross epiphyseal growth plates and, although they respect articular cartilage, will extend intraarticularly at sites of capsular or ligamentous attachment.

High grade sarcomas of soft tissue origin are usually deep, large, fixed, and tender and stimulate a soft, edematous, succulent, inflammatory-like reaction about them. The radiographic features of high grade sarcomas arising in bone are quite predictive of their behavior (Lodwick III). The reactive response is so rapidly destroyed that the interface between the lesion and the surrounding bone is poorly marginated with a diffuse permeative border. Patchy cortical destruction, early occult soft tissue extension, obliteration of periosteal reaction with only small Codman's triangles remaining, and ill-defined intramedullary extension beyond the extent suggested by the periosteal reaction are all features of high grade primary skeletal sarcomas.

Staging studies are usually accurate in suggesting the high grade nature of these lesions. Isotope scans show increased uptake both early and late which extends beyond the radiographic limits of the lesion. Increased isotope uptake in radiographically normal bone adjacent to high grade soft tissue sarcomas may be the only clue of occult reaction to the soft tissue lesion. They may also be the first hint of a "skip" metastasis. Angiograms show a vigorous zone of reactive neovasculature about the lesion on the early arterial phase and often a hypervascular intralesional "blush" on the late venous phase. The extent of involvement of neurovascular bundles is often best shown on angiography; CT scans show occult intraosseous extension, skip lesions in the medullary canal, occult soft tissue extension, and extracompartmental extension through cortical bone and across fascial septae.

The histologic features of high grade sarcomas are: (1) high cell-to-matrix rate; (2) poor differentiations of immature matrices; (3) all the cytologic characteristics of high grade malignancy. Mitoses are abundant. Vascular invasion, necrosis, hemorrhage, and direct destruction of normal tissue by tumor cells are part of this picure. These findings are those of Broders' Grade 2, 3, or 4 lesion[2]; (4) little or no encapsulation is apparent, and isolated satellites are found in the pseudocapsule of reactive tissue about the lesion; (5) skip metastases—isolated nodules of tumor in the normal tissue well beyond the reactive zone—are found in a significant proportion (approximately 25 per cent) in both bone and soft tissue sarcomas.[4] In bone, they are either in the medullary canal or occasionally transarticularly in an adjacent metaphysis. In soft tissue, they may occur more proximally in either the ill-defined extracompartmental spaces and planes or within skeletal muscle.

For the spine, skip lesions are exceptionally rare. Lesions do not "skip" from one vertebral body to another nor from the body anteriorly to the posterior elements. High grade primary sarcomas involving more than one vertebra do so by direct extension through the disc or are considered to be of multicentric origin. The one common exception to the foregoing generalization is the chordoma that extends into the neural canal. Once within the canal, the

TABLE 3–1. STAGES OF MUSCULOSKELETAL LESIONS

Benign
  1. Latent
  2. Active
  3. Aggressive

Malignant
  I. Low grade without metastases
    A. Intracompartmental
    B. Extracompartmental
  II. High grade without metastases
    A. Intracompartmental
    B. Extracompartmental
  III. Low/high grade with metastases
    A. Intracompartmental
    B. Extracompartmental

From Enneking WF: A system of staging musculoskeletal neoplasms. Clin Orthop 204:9–24, 1986.

lesion often skips along the extradural space, producing intermittent droplets of tumor proximal to the primary level of involvement.

High grade sarcomas quickly cross barriers to tumor extension, and a relatively small proportion (approximately 10 per cent) are still intracompartmental at the time of presentation. The majority extend extracompartmentally: an occasional lesion, usually of soft tissue origin, will develop with regional lymphatic metastasis; and a significant proportion (approximately 10 per cent) will present with distant (usually pulmonary) metastases.

These behavioral changes (latent, active, aggressive, invasive, destructive, and metastatic) that form the basis of the staging system together with their clinical, radiographic, and staging studies are summarized in Tables 3–1 (summary), 3–2 (benign), and 3–3 (malignant).

THE STAGING SYSTEM

The system is based on the interrelationship of three factors: grade (G), site (T), and metastases (M). Each of these in turn is stratified by components that influence both prognosis and response to treatment.

Grade

The grade is an assessment of the biologic aggressiveness of the lesion. It is not a purely histologic

TABLE 3–2. STAGES OF BENIGN MUSCULOSKELETAL LESIONS

	1	2	3
Grade	G_0	G_0	G_0
Site	T_0	T_0	T_{1-2}
Metastasis	M_0	M_0	M_{0-1}
Clinical course	Latent, static, self-healing	Active, progressing, expands bone or fascia	Aggressive, invasive, breaches bone or fascia
Radiographic grade	IA	IB	IC
Isotope scan	Background uptake	Increased uptake in lesion	Increased uptake beyond lesion
Angiogram	No neovascular reaction	Modest neovascular reaction	Moderate neovascular reaction
CT scan	Crisp, intact margin; well-defined, homogeneous	Intact margin; "expansile"—thin capsule, homogeneous	Indistinct broached margin, extracapsular and/or extracompartmental extension; nonhomogeneous

From Enneking WF: A system of staging musculoskeletal neoplasms. Clin Orthop 204:9–24, 1986.

TABLE 3–3. STAGES OF MALIGNANT MUSCULOSKELETAL LESIONS

	IA	IB	IIA	IIB	IIIA	IIIB
Grade	G_1	G_1	G_2	G_2	G_{1-2}	G_{1-2}
Site	T_1	T_2	T_1	T_2	T_1	T_2
Metastasis	M_0	M_0	M_0	M_0	M_1	M_1
Clinical course	Symptomatic indolent growth	Symptomatic mass, indolent growth	Symptomatic rapid growth	Symptomatic rapid growth, fixed mass, pathologic fracture	Systemic symptoms, palpable nodes, pulmonary symptoms	
Isotope scan	Increased uptake	Increased uptake	Increased uptake, beyond radiographic limits	Increased uptake, beyond radiographic limits	Pulmonary lesions, no increased uptake	
Radiographic grade	II	II	III	III	III	
Angiogram	Modest neovascular reaction, involvement of neurovascular bundle	Modest neovascular reaction, involvement of neurovascular bundle	Marked neovascular reaction—no invovement of neurovascular bundle	Marked neovascular reaction—involvement of neurovascular bundle	Hypervascular lymph nodes	
CT scan	Irregular or broached capsule—intracompartmental	Extracompartmental extension or location	Broached (pseudo) capsule—intracompartmental	Broached (pseudo) capsule—extracompartmental	Pulmonary lesions or enlarged nodes	

From Enneking WF: A system of staging musculoskeletal neoplasms. Clin Orthop 204:9–24, 1986.

assessment (as in Broders' 1, 2, 3, 4 grading of malignancies),[2] a purely radiographic assessment (as in Lodwick's IA, IB, IC, II, and III radiographic classification of probabilities),[11] or a purely clinical reflection of growth rate, doubling time, size, temperature, tissue pressure, or biochemical markers. It is a blending of all of these into patterns. The three stratifications of grade are G_0, G_1, and G_2. Their identifying characteristics are:

1. G_0 (benign). *Histologic*—benign cytology, clearly differentiated, low to moderate cell-to-matrix ratio. *Radiographic*—Lodwick IA, IB, or IC ranging from clearly marginated to those with capsular broaching and soft tissue extensions. *Clinical*—distinct capsule, no satellites, no skips, rare metastases, variable growth rate, predominantly in adolescents and young adults.

2. G_1 (low grade malignant). *Histologic*—Broders' Grades 1 and some 2. Few mitoses, moderate differentiation, distinct matrix. *Radiographic*—Lodwick II with indolent invasive features. *Clinical*—indolent growth, extracapsular satellites in the reactive zone, no skips, and only occasional distant metastases.

3. G_2 (High grade malignant). *Histologic*—Broders' Grades 2, 3, and 4. Frequent mitoses, poorly differentiated, sparse and immature matrix. High grade cytologic features: anaplasia, pleomorphic, and hyperchromatic. *Radiographic*—Lodwick III: destructive, invasive. *Clinical*—rapid growth, symptomatic, both satellites and skips, occasional regional and frequent distant metastases.

The behavior of G_0 benign lesions may be latent, active, or aggressive. Their histologic features are often poor indicators of their behavior, and within this spectrum G_0 lesions are often better predicted by their radiographic, staging, and clinical features (see Table 3–2). The histologic characteristics of G_1

low grade sarcomas make their distinction from G_2 high grade lesions on histologic grounds predictably accurate, and their radiographic staging and clinical features are supportive and confirmatory of the histologic distinction. However, it may be difficult to distinguish G_0 from G_1 lesions on purely histologic features, and in many instances the radiographic and particularly the staging studies may be of more value than the histologic findings (Table 3–3).

A promising new method of assessing grade is the determination of the nuclear DNA concentration (ploidy) by flow cytometry. Individual cell nuclei are stained with a specific fluorescent DNA dye, and the concentration is assessed rapidly by fluorometric assay of the cells as they pass through a focused laser beam. Normal cells are euploid and so are most G_0 lesions. G_1 lesions have increased numbers of cells in normal replicative activity (tetraploidy). G_2 lesions have abnormal numbers of cells in tetraploidy and also may show an abnormal cell line (aneuploid) quite distinctive for high grade neoplasms. These correlations between ploidy and prognosis have been shown to be valid for other classes of neoplasia—particularly myelomas and lymphomas—and preliminary results suggest that this technique may be quite helpful in connective tissue lesions.[10]

Spinal lesions are graded by the same clinical, radiographic, and histologic criteria as other lesions. Chordoma largely presents as a low grade G_1 lesion but accelerates to a high grade G_2 lesion, particularly after several recurrences have been observed.

In summary, surgical grading into G_0, G_1, G_2 requires histologic, radiographic, and clinical correlation to achieve accuracy and reliability. Although certain histogenic types of sarcomas may have a preponderance of their lesions graded G_1 or G_2 (Table 3–4), each lesion must be assessed on its own characteristics before a grade is assigned. For exam-

TABLE 3–4. SURGICAL GRADE (G)

Low (G_1)	High (G_2)
Parosteal osteosarcoma	Classic osteosarcoma, radiation sarcoma, Paget's sarcoma
Endosteal osteosarcoma	
Secondary chondrosarcoma	Primary chondrosarcoma
Fibrosarcoma, Kaposi's sarcoma, atypical malignant fibrous histiocytoma	Fibrosarcoma, malignant, fibrous histiocytoma, undifferentiated primary sarcoma
Giant cell sarcoma of bone	Giant cell sarcoma of bone
Hemangioendothelioma, hemangiopericytoma	Angiosarcoma, hemangiopericytoma
Myxoid liposarcoma	Pleomorphic liposarcoma, neurofibrosarcoma (schwannoma)
	Rhabdomyosarcoma
	Synovioma
Clear cell sarcoma, tendon sheath epithelioid sarcoma	
Chordoma	
Adamantinoma	
Alveolar cell sarcoma	Alveolar cell sarcoma
Other and undifferentiated	Other and undifferentiated

From Enneking WF: A system of staging musculoskeletal neoplasms. Clin Orthop 204:9–24, 1986.

ple, most parosteal osteosarcomas are G_1, but a few dedifferentiate into G_2 lesions and accordingly have a much more ominous prognosis. Conversely, although most classic osteosarcomas are G_2, occasionally one will be G_1 with a much more favorable prognosis.

Site

The anatomic setting of the lesion has a direct relationship to the prognosis and the choice of surgical procedure. The three strata of anatomic settings are T_0, T_1, and T_2. These are determined primarily by clinical and radiographic techniques. Staging studies (isotope scanning, angiography, CT, and magnetic resonance imaging [MRI], ultrasonography, myelography, and so forth) can make valuable contributions in preoperatively assessing the anatomic setting. The identifying characteristics are:

1. T_0. The lesion remains confined within the capsule and does not extend beyond the borders of its compartment of origin. While the boundaries of the capsule and/or the compartment of origin may be distorted or deformed, they both remain intact.

2. T_1. The lesion has extracapsular extensions, either by continuity or isolated satellites, into the reactive zone, but both the lesion and the reactive zone about it are contained within an anatomic compartment bounded by the natural barriers to tumor extension: cortical bone, articular cartilage, joint capsule, or the dense fibrous tissue of fascial septa, ligaments, or tendon (sheath). To be classified as T_1, both the lesion and its (pseudo)capsule must be within the compartment. If the reactive zone extends outside the compartment while the tumor remains within, the lesion is classified as extracompartmental. The anatomic compartments of both bone and soft tissue are shown in Table 3–5.

Three particular points about compartmentalization require elaboration. The skin and subcutaneous tissue are classified as a compartment, even though there are no longitudinal boundaries. In the transverse dimension, however, the deep fascia forms an effective barrier between the subcutaneous and deeper tissues. The paraosseous compartment is a potential compartment between cortical bone and overlying muscles. Lesions on the surface of bone that have not invaded either the underlying cortical bone or the overlying muscle but have pushed them apart are defined as intracompartmental. Lesions within muscular compartments that contain more than one muscle (e.g., the volar compartment of the forearm) are considered intracompartmental despite involving more than one muscle.

3. T_2. Lesions extending beyond compartmental barriers into the loosely bounded fascial planes and spaces that have no longitudinal boundaries are extracompartmental or T_2. Extracompartmental involvement may occur by virtue of extension of a previously intracompartmental lesion, by arising de novo in the extracompartmental tissues, or by inadvertent transmission by trauma or surgical excision. The various sites that are extracompartmental are shown in Table 3–5. Almost without exception, lesions (or their reactive zones) that abut or involve major neurovascular bundles are extracompartmental by virtue of the extracompartmental location of these structures.

For the spine, site is classified as in the extremities. Well-encapsulated benign lesions within bone or the paravertebral soft tissues are T_0. Extracapsular lesions within the vertebral bodies or posterior elements are intracompartmental T_1. Lesions extending from bone into the paravertebral soft tissues (or vice versa) are extracompartmental or T_2. Lesions arising within the paravertebral soft tissues are extracompartmental (T_2), since these muscles and fascia have no longitudinal barriers to tumor extension. Lesions arising within bone which encroach on the neural canal and remain extradural are intracompartmental

TABLE 3–5. SURGICAL SITES (T)

Intracompartmental (T_1)	Extracompartmental (T_2)
Intraosseous	Soft tissue extension
Intraarticular	Soft tissue extension
Superficial to deep fascia	Deep fascial extension
Paraosseous	Intraosseous or extrafascial
Intrafascial compartments	Extrafascial planes or spaces
Ray of hand or foot	Mid- and hindfoot
Posterior calf	Popliteal space
Anterolateral leg	Groin-femoral triangle
Anterior thigh	
Middle thigh	Intrapelvic
Posterior thigh	Midhand
Buttocks	Antecubital fossa
Volar forearm	Axilla
Dorsal forearm	Periclavicular
Anterior forearm	Paraspinal
Posterior arm	Head and neck
Periscapular	

From Enneking WF: A system of staging musculoskeletal neoplasms. Clin Orthop 204:9–24, 1986.

(T_1), despite broaching the bone, because the dura is an excellent tumor barrier. Lesions that broach the dura are T_2. Lesions that penetrate the subchondral plate and involve the intravertebral disc remain T_1, as long as the lesion does not penetrate the annular or longitudinal ligaments.

Metastasis

In most staging systems for carcinomas, metastases are stratified by virtue of being regional (N for nodes) or distant (M), since the prognosis and treatment are significantly different for these two sites of metastasis.

For sarcomas, metastatic involvement of either regional lymph nodes or distant organs has the same ominous prognosis, and both are designated by M. There are only two strata of metastasis—M_0 and M_1. M_0 indicates no evidence of regional or distant metastases, while M_1 signifies either regional or distant metastases.

These three factors—G, T, and M—are combined to form the criteria for the progressive stages of benign and malignant lesions (see Table 3–1).

Benign lesions are designated by Arabic numerals 1, 2, or 3 that are synonymous with latent, active, or aggressive. The characteristics of Stage 1 latent, Stage 2 active, and Stage 3 aggressive lesions are shown in Table 3–2 and were described in detail as the latent, active, and aggressive progressions in the preceding section on evolution. As indicated, Stages 1, 2, and 3 correspond closely to the Lodwick classification of radiographic features as IA, IB, and IC.

Malignant lesions are designated by the Roman numerals I, II, or III that are synonymous with low grade, high grade, and metastatic. These three stages of sarcomas are further stratified into A or B depending on whether the lesion is anatomically intracompartmental (A) or extracompartmental (B). The characteristics of these malignant lesions are shown in Table 3–3 and were described in detail as low grade invasive and high grade destructive lesions in the evolution of connective tissue lesions. Their radiographic characteristics correspond closely to Stages II and III in the Lodwick classification. Only after each lesion has been studied clinically and radiographically and biopsied for histogenic typing and cytologic grading can it be staged according to its characteristics. Although particular lesions tend to cluster in particular stages (i.e., more than 90 per cent of classic osteosarcomas present as Stage IIB), others tend to be more evenly distributed (e.g., of giant cell tumors of bone, approximately 10 per cent are Stage 1, 75 per cent are Stage 2, and 15 per cent are Stage 3).

Clearly a particular lesion may undergo transition from one stage to another. Benign lesions that are Stage 2 active or even Stage 3 aggressive during adolescence frequently undergo involution into Stage 1 latent lesions after growth has ceased. On the other hand, certain benign lesions of any stage may undergo transformation into Stage I, II, or even III sarcomas. Obviously, high grade Stage II and occa-

sionally low grade Stage I lesions become Stage III lesions after presentation by virtue of either regional or distant metastases. Certain factors have been implicated directly or by inference in the upstaging of benign or malignant lesions. Radiation has been held responsible for transition of giant cell tumor, chondroblastoma, and other benign lesions to sarcomas. Repeated inadequate surgical interventions have been implicated in the evolution of low grade fibrous lesions into high grade fibrosarcomas and in the dedifferentiation of Stage I parosteal osteosarcoma into Stage II or III high grade osteosarcoma.

ARTICULATION WITH SURGICAL TREATMENT

Articulating the staging system with the surgical treatment of connective tissue tumors requires precise definitions of the procedures as well as the stages. The traditional terms of incisional biopsy, excisional biopsy, resection, and amputation are difficult to define in either biologic, anatomic, or physical terms. After a number of physical and surgical criteria were postulated, a method of definition was devised based on the margin that the procedure obtained in relation to the lesion and the barriers to its extension.

The four oncologic surgical margins, the plane of dissection that achieves them, and the microscopic appearance of the tissue at the margin of the wound are shown in Table 3–6. The four margins are described in surgical terms (intracapsular, marginal, wide, and radical), and they reflect the progressive barriers to tumor extension in their natural evolution—for example, the (pseudo)capsule, reactive zone, intracompartmental normal tissue, and compartmental boundaries. Although marginal, wide, and radical margins may all be tumor-free, the residual reactive tissue at a marginal margin often contains extensions or satellites, and the residual normal intracompartmental tissue beyond a wide margin occasionally contains skip lesions. For high grade sarcomas only a radical margin with an intact barrier of normal tissue between the margin and the reactive zone consistently and reliably can be called tumor-free.

Determinations of margins may be estimated by inspection of the cut surface of either bone or soft tissue. Tetracycline-labeling may be quite helpful in visually identifying the type of osseous margin as it

TABLE 3–6. SURGICAL MARGINS

Type	Plane of Dissection	Microscopic Appearance
Intracapsular	Within lesion	Tumor at margin
Marginal	Within reactive zone—extracapsular	Reactive tissue, ± microsatellites tumor
Wide	Beyond reactive zone through normal tissue	Normal tissue, ± skips
Radical	Normal tissue extracompartmental	Normal tissue

From Enneking WF: A system of staging musculoskeletal neoplasms. Clin Orthop 204:9–24, 1986.

TABLE 3–7. MUSCULOSKELETAL ONCOLOGIC SURGICAL PROCEDURES

| | How Margin Achieved | |
MARGIN	Limb Salvage	Amputation
Intracapsular	Intracapsular piecemeal excision	Intracapsular amputation
Marginal	Marginal en bloc excision	Marginal amputation
Wide	Wide en bloc excision	Wide through-bone amputation
Radical	Radical en bloc resection	Radical exarticulation

From Enneking WF: A system of staging musculoskeletal neoplasms. Clin Orthop 204:9–24, 1986.

distinguishes reactive from normal bone. Often specimens will have to be taken for histologic study from questionable areas to verify whether nonneoplastic tissue at a margin is reactive or normal. The microscopic appearance of wide and radical margins are histologically identical (i.e., normal), and the distinction as to the type of margin obtained is made by identifying whether or not the margin is beyond a compartmental barrier. This is usually accomplished by gross inspection or radiographic examination of the specimen. As shown in Table 3–7, each of the four margins can be achieved by a local or limb-salvaging procedure or an amputation making eight possible oncologic procedures.

The four types of limb-salvaging procedures are: (1) *intracapsular excision,* that is, debulking, cytoreductive excision, and so forth, done piecemeal within the (pseudo)capsule; (2) *marginal (local) excision,* that is, en bloc excisional biopsy, shell-out, and so forth, done en bloc extracapsularly within the reactive zone; (3) *wide (local) excision,* that is, en bloc excision done through normal tissue beyond the reactive zone, but within the compartment of origin leaving in situ some portion of that compartment; or (4) *radical (local) resection,* that is, en bloc excision of the lesion and the entire compartment of origin leaving no remnant of the compartment of origin.

Due to the anatomic constraints of the spine, radical resection is not technically feasible without sacrifice of the contents of the neural canal. Excising an entire vertebra piecemeal to preserve neurologic function is not the same as resecting en bloc the entire femur. The contamination attending a piecemeal vertebral excision, despite the magnitude of the procedure, obtains at best a contaminated marginal or wide margin depending on whether the wound margins are composed of reactive or normal tissue. Aggressive surgical resections of vertebral bodies and

adjacent soft tissues which leave residual tumor that extends posteriorly into the pedicles achieve intracapsular margins. Peeling the dura off of underlying lesions achieves either an intracapsular or marginal margin depending on whether the lesion was isolated by the dissection. To achieve a wide margin under such circumstances, the intact dura must be removed en bloc with the lesion. If the lesion has penetrated the subchondral plate into the disc, the entire disc must be removed en bloc by osteotomy through an adjacent body to achieve a wide margin.

The terms excision and resection are coupled with wide and radical to emphasize the biologic differences between the two procedures. Wide excision and radical resection are correct; by definition wide resection or radical excision become incompatible terms. This is important conceptually, if not semantically, because in Europe the term "radical" in terms of margin is synonymous with tumor-free and can be either marginal, wide, or radical. Therefore, in the European literature, excision and resection are used interchangeably with radical, taken to mean any local procedure with a tumor-free margin.

The other four types of oncologic procedures are amputations that achieve various margins: (1) an intracapsular amputation in which the level passes within the (pseudo)capsule; (2) a marginal amputation through the reactive zone; (3) a wide amputation through normal tissue proximal to the reactive zone, but with the compartment of involvement (usually a through-bone); and (4) a radical amputation proximal to the involved compartment, usually a disarticulation (the entire compartment at risk is removed).

In terms of these definitions, articulation of the stages with the surgical margins and procedures can be done with anatomic and biologic meaning rather than in less significant physical dimensions. The articulation for benign lesions is shown in Table 3–8, and the articulation for malignant lesions is summarized in Table 3–9.

Benign Lesions

Stage 1 latent lesions have a negligible recurrence rate following intracapsular excision (i.e., curettage, piecemeal removal) as their natural history is to heal spontaneously. Examples would be ganglion, nonossifying fibroma, solitary eosinophilic granuloma, simple cyst, giant cell tumor of tendon sheath, and so forth, in which the lesion's behavior is latent. While desirable for insurance, en bloc marginal or even wide excision, if feasible without additional morbidity

TABLE 3–8. ARTICULATION OF BENIGN STAGES WITH SURGICAL MARGINS

STAGE	GRADE	SITE	METASTASIS	MARGIN FOR CONTROL
1	G_0	T_0	M_0	
2	G_0	T_0	M_0	
3	G_0	T_{1-2}	M_{0-1}	Wide or ? Marginal plus effective adjuvant

From Enneking WF: A system of staging musculoskeletal neoplasms. Clin Orthop 204:9–24, 1986.

TABLE 3–9. ARTICULATION OF MALIGNANT STAGES WITH SURGICAL MARGINS

STAGE	GRADE	SITE	METASTASIS	MARGIN FOR CONTROL
IA	G_1	T_1	M_0	Wide—usually excision
IB	G_1	T_1	M_0	Wide—consider amputation vs. joint or neurovascular deficit
IIA	G_2	T_1	M_0	Radical—usually resection or wide excision plus effective adjuvant
IIB	G_2	T_2	M_0	Radical—consider exarticulation or wide excision or amputation plus effective adjuvant
IIIA	G_{1-2}	T_1	M_1	Thoracotomy—radical resection or palliative
IIIB	G_{1-2}	T_2	M_1	Thoracotomy—radical exarticulation or palliative

From Enneking WF: A system of staging musculoskeletal neoplasms. Clin Orthop 204:9–24, 1986.

or disability, is unnecessary to achieve a low-risk margin for Stage 1 lesions.

Stage 2 active lesions have a significant recurrence rate after intracapsular procedures and negligible recurrence rates after marginal en bloc excision. Since active lesions are by definition intracapsular (T_0), dissection through the extracapsular reactive zone carries little risk of leaving residual neoplastic tissue with a marginal margin. Whereas obtaining a marginal margin by an en bloc excision carries a significant risk of morbidity or disability, then either these risks or the risks of recurrence after an intra-capsular procedure must be assumed or considera-tion must be given to extending the margin of an intracapsular procedure to the equivalent of a mar-ginal (or better) margin by the use of nonsurgical adjuvants. Since both chemotherapy and radiation therapy are effective by virtue of their effect on mitotically active cells, their effectiveness on benign G_0 lesions is limited, and the side effects make their use inappropriate. Physical adjuvants such as phenol, hypertonic saline, Merthiolate, methylmethacrylate, and repeated freezing and thawing (cryosurgery) all have had trials and advocates. Only cementation with thermal (and perhaps chemotoxic necrosis) and cryo-surgery producing cell rupture have been docu-mented to produce significant extensions of surgical margins.[6, 7] Both have been shown to produce milli-meters of necrosis and, when used appropriately and judiciously, can reliably extend an intracapsular mar-gin to become the equivalent of a marginal margin with significant reduction in recurrence rates for active Stage 2 benign lesions.

Stage 3 aggressive benign lesions with their extra-capsular extensions (T_1 or even T_2) have high recur-rence rates after either intracapsular or marginal procedures. Wide surgical margins beyond the exten-sions in the reactive zone are the least that provide a low-risk procedure for these aggressive lesions. Mar-ginal procedures coupled with effective adjuvants may be clinically prudent when location makes wide surgical procedures impractical. Thermotherapy has been ineffective, albeit largely untried; but radiation therapy, when coupled with marginal excision, has considerably reduced the risk of recurrence. Sur-gically inaccessible lesions such as aggressive fibro-matosis, aggressive recurrent aneurysmal bone cysts, and aggressive giant cell tumors are in this category. The effectiveness of physical adjuvant for Stage 3 lesions has not been as extensively investigated as for

Stage 2 lesions, but may be rational in lieu of disabling wide procedures. Despite their appeal, to date no combination of adjuvant/marginal surgery has been as effective as wide surgery. When prior recurrences after inadequate excisions have occurred, the pattern of local dissemination is often so diffuse that only amputation offers a practical method for achieving a low-risk wide margin.

Articulation of benign lesions with surgical margins has the same connotation in the spine as in any other anatomic setting. Intracapsular margins for Stage 2 lesions carry the same risk for recurrence in the spine as in the extremities. The generally higher incidence of recurrence in the spine as opposed to the extrem-ities speaks to the oncologic compromise preservation of neurologic function or mechanical stability often entails. This difficulty becomes magnified by compli-cations produced by the use of physical adjuvants about the spine. Whereas in the limbs, intracapsular or marginal margins may often be extended by the use of cryosurgery or cementation, proximity to the spinal cord may make these useful oncologic adju-vants too risky for clinical use.

Malignant Lesions

Stage IA

Low grade G_1 locally invasive tumors with predi-lection for occult extracapsular satellites in the en-veloping reactive zone have high recurrence rates after either intracapsular or marginal procedures. Wide procedures are low risk, and because of their intracompartmental location, Stage IA lesions are usually excellent candidates for excision rather than amputation. Marginal excision plus an effective ad-juvant is less risky than marginal excision alone, but identification of an effective adjuvant is difficult. Adjuvant radiation therapy has been effective in reducing the incidence of recurrence after marginal excision in soft tissue lesions but is of limited value in skeletal lesions. Chemotherapy has been ineffective in G_1 sarcomas. Physical adjuvants are largely un-tested, but as their effectiveness is difficult to predict and is usually measured in millimeters, they would not seem rational for G_1 sarcomas that have a low incidence of recurrence after wide procedures.

Stage IB

Extracompartmental G_1 lesions require the same margins as their intracompartmental counterparts. The extracompartmental location often makes a wide margin unattainable by anything short of amputation or wide excision with sacrifice of significant neurovascular or articular stuctures. Marginal surgery coupled with an adjuvant is no more effective in IB than in IA lesions. When the extracompartmental status has occurred as a result of recurrences after prior inadequate excision, achieving a wide margin in the face of widely disseminated occult disease by limb-salvaging excision becomes less and less practical, and amputation more and more a serious consideration.

Stage IIA

High grade, high risk destructive lesions are seldom intracompartmental and have a significant incidence of skips. Low-risk control is offered by either radical resection (frequently practical in the unusual circumstance of intracompartmental confinement), radical amputation, or the combination of a wide margin and an effective adjuvant(s). Soft tissue sarcomas are more often intracompartmental, and radiation therapy is an effective adjuvant for local control of the majority of the various histogenic types of soft tissue sarcomas. (Exception: chemotherapy is more effective in rhabdomyosarcoma.) Chemotherapy may be effective in assisting local control in some skeletal lesions (e.g., osteosarcoma and perhaps malignant fibrous histiocytoma), while it has little benefit in others (e.g., chondrosarcoma and fibrosarcoma). It is quite clear, however, that all combinations of wide surgery with adjuvant therapy carry significantly greater risk of local recurrence than radical procedures (approximately 25 per cent versus less than 5 per cent), whether achieved by limb salvage or amputation.

Stage IIB

Radical margins are the most effective way of assuring local control and, in IIB lesions, are often attainable only by disarticulation. Wide margins, coupled with adjuvant therapy, have significant risks of recurrence in their own right and often achieve only marginal margins because of the proclivity of these lesions to have occult proximal microextensions along the major neurovascular bundles. The risk of local recurrence in Stage IIB sarcomas treated by wide excision without adjuvant therapy is 40 to 60 per cent, and with adjuvant therapy in responsive lesions it is 20 per cent. When the wide margin is achieved by through-bone amputation, the risk of recurrence with effective adjuvant is less than with wide excision—approximately 10 per cent rather than 20 per cent.

For the spine and adjacent soft tissues, obtaining wide or radical en bloc margins, while oncologically optimal for Stage I and II lesions, often requires extensive sacrifice of neurologic function. In making this assessment, it is well to consider that if the oncologic margin is compromised and recurrence ensues, the subsequent neurologic loss produced by the recurrence(s) will often produce some amount of neurologic dysfunction without the oncologic benefit of an appropriate margin. With a diffuse paraspinal recurrence, local control of the lesion becomes surgically impractical. In all of the above reasons, successful surgical management of malignancies about the spine often requires effective adjuvant management combined with an aggressive surgical procedure to produce an oncologically adequate margin.

Stage III

Control of the disease requires the appropriate surgical management of the primary as well as of the pulmonary or other distant metastases. When the appropriate wide or radical procedure entails significant morbidity or disability, a lesser palliative procedure may be rational unless control of the metastasis can be reasonably anticipated. Both preliminary aggressive chemotherapy (with decision as to subsequent thoracotomy) and definitive surgical treatment of the primary tumor—based on the response of the metastases to the chemotherapy or, alternatively, aggressive thoracotomy and definitive radical surgery followed by postoperative adjuvant chemotherapy in the clinically tumor-free state—are recommended by some authors, although long-term results are not yet known. Either procedure appears preferable to palliation alone, as each has significant salvage rates at five years.

DISCUSSION

In its preliminary trials by the Musculoskeletal Tumor Society, this staging system was shown to be practical, reproducible, and of significant prognostic value for sarcomas of both bone and soft tissue origin.[3] Subsequent reports have shown its value in surgical planning and treatment evaluation.[1, 5, 8, 9, 12]

Since the original presentation of the definitions of surgical margins and procedures in 1980, some misperceptions need clarification. The common ones are how to describe the margins (and procedures) about superficial lesions, extracompartmental lesions, and lesions that are inadvertently entered but subsequently reexcised. A superficial lesion in the skin and/or subcutaneous tissue that has not penetrated the deep fascia is intracompartmental. En bloc removal with a plane of dissection deep to the deep fascia and through normal tissue well around the lesion obtains an extracompartmental radical margin in depth (on the other side of the deep fascia—a natural barrier). However, it obtains only a wide margin circumferentially (there are no natural barriers within skin and subcutaneous tissue, and so an extracompartmental radical margin in the defined sense is not possible). This ambiguity has been resolved by arbitrarily calling a margin that is less than 5 cm about the reactive zone, wide, and a margin that is more than 5 cm, radical. This dimension was chosen in conformity with the melanoma experience. Thus, a superficial IA lesion excised en bloc deep to the deep fascia with a surrounding margin of 2 cm has been widely excised, while the same lesion with a 6-cm margin about it has been radically resected. Whether or not these physical dimensions are appropriate for the articulation of margin and stage remains to be seen.

By definition, extracompartmental "B" lesions—whether by extension or origin—cannot be radically resected since the extracompartmental spaces and planes have no longitudinal barriers. For such lesions, a local procedure that removes en bloc a lesion with a margin of normal tissue is a wide excision for an en bloc procedure. Resection of an extracompartmental lesion that is beyond natural barriers in the transverse plane, but by definition cannot be radical in the longitudinal sense, is arbitrarily defined as a radical resection when the longitudinal margin is at the same level as the origin or insertion of the adjacent muscles. For example, a lesion in the subsartorial canal abutting the femoral neurovascular bundle which was removed en bloc (including the bundle with a plane of dissection beyond the fascial boundaries of the canal [i.e., radical transversely], but with a proximal and distal margin less than the musculotendinous junctions of the sartorius) would have been widely excised. The same procedure with the proximal and distal margins at or beyond the musculotendinous junctions of sartorius would be a radical resection. If the lesion were removed en bloc by dissection within the canal sacrificing the bundle, the procedure would be a marginal excision. If the lesion were dissected away from the bundle thereby preserving the bundle, the procedure would be designated as either an intracapsular or marginal excision, depending on whether the dissection was within the (pseudo)capsule or the extracapsular reactive zone.

If a lesion involves two compartments, that is, a lesion arising in bone extending into the adjacent soft tissues, then to achieve a radical margin both compartments would have to be removed en bloc in toto. For example, a radical resection of a lesion of the distal femoral metaphysis extending into the posterior thigh would require removal of the entire femur, hamstrings, and sciatic nerve en bloc. From the above discussion, it is evident that in certain instances the only practical way of achieving a radical margin is by amputation. This may be particularly true in certain anatomic sites (i.e., popliteal fossae, femoral triangle, axillae, antecubital fossae, flexor canal of the forearm) where a radical margin can be obtained by resection; but the virtually functionless salvaged limb hinders rather than aids rehabilitation.

When lesions are entered, the wound is contaminated and all the exposed tissues are at risk for recurrence. If these at-risk tissues are not removed, the margin is intracapsular. If the tissues are removed, the margin becomes what the subsequent removal achieves in relation to the lesion as if the exposure had not happened. The procedure is said to be a contaminated procedure. For example, if a lesion in the quadriceps were inadvertently entered exposing the rectus femoris muscle, and if the lesion were subsequently widely excised with a cuff of normal tissue, then the procedure would be designated a contaminated wide excision since some of the exposed, more proximal, rectus femoris would remain in the wound.

If, under the same circumstance, the entire quadriceps compartment were removed en bloc by extracompartmental dissection, then the procedure would be an (uncontaminated) radical resection. This means that after incisional biopsy, the entire tract at risk must be appropriately excised en bloc with the lesion and tissues to achieve wide or radical margins. It also means that if the (pseudo)capsule is inadvertently entered during attempted excisional biopsy, a great deal more tissue will have to be removed to achieve an uncontaminated wide or radical margin than if such contamination had not occurred. In certain instances, contamination may take place in such a way that the only way of achieving an uncontaminated wide or radical margin is by amputation (previously unnecessary to achieve an uncontaminated wide or radical margin); in other circumstances (e.g., the pelvis), inadvertent contamination may make obtaining an uncontaminated margin of any kind impossible.

It is evident that continuous refinement and classification of these terms, definitions, and concepts are needed for them to be of optimal value.

A serious consideration of stratification of Stage III is also in order. It is becoming clearer that the prognosis of a patient who develops a solitary pulmonary metastasis from a G_0 or G_1 primary tumor some years following local control is significantly different than that of a patient with multiple metastases from a G_2 lesion at the time of presentation or shortly after apparent local control of the primary lesion.[12] It may well be that meaningful stratifications will offer guidelines for the management of these lesions.

The final objective of this staging system—development of guidelines for adjunctive therapy—has yet to be realized. The effectiveness of adjuvant therapy continues to be judged by survival rates of various histogenic types of sarcomas, largely ignoring the influence of the stage, surgical margin, or adequacy of the surgical procedure on survival rates. This lamentable state is exemplified by the fact that one decade after the enthusiastic widespread adoption of prophylactic chemotherapy, serious doubt continues whether the increase in survival rates during this period is the result of adjuvant chemotherapy or of improvement in staging techniques with resultant improvements in surgical control of the primary tumor. In light of this, it would seem obvious that data concerning staging, surgical margins, and surgical procedures must be gathered to establish significant variables in the assessment of the current explosive proliferation of protocols for adjunctive management of musculoskeletal lesions.

REFERENCES

1. Boriani S, Bacchini P, Bertoni F, Campanacci M: Periosteal chondroma. J Bone Joint Surg 65A:205, 1983.
2. Broders AC, Hargrave R, Meyerding HW: Pathological features of soft tissue fibrosarcoma. Surg Gynecol Obstet 69:267, 1939.

3. Enneking WF, Kagan A: "Skip" metastases in osteosarcoma. Cancer 36:2192, 1975.
4. Enneking WF, Spanier SS, Goodman MA: A system for the surgical staging of musculo-skeletal sarcoma. Clin Orthop 153:106, 1980.
5. Eriksson AI, Schiller A, Mankin HJ: The management of chondrosarcoma of bone. Clin Orthop 153:44, 1980.
6. Feith R: Side effects of acrylic cement implanted into bone. Acta Orthop Scand (Suppl) 161:1, 1975.
7. Gage AA, Greene GW, Jr, Neiders ME, Emmings FG: Freezing bone without excision—An experimental study of bone cell destruction and manner of regrowth in dogs. JAMA 196:770, 1966.
8. Gherlinzoni F, Rock M, Picci P: Chondromyxofibroma. J Bone Joint Surg 65A:198, 1983.
9. Gitelis S, Bertoni F, Picci P, Campanacci M: Chondrosarcoma of bone. J Bone Joint Surg 63A:1248, 1981.
10. Kreicbergs A, Boquist L, Borssén B, Larsson SE: Prognostic factors in chondrosarcoma. Cancer 50:577, 1982.
11. Lodwick GS, Wilson AJ, Farrell C, et al: Determining growth rates of focal lesions of bone from radiographs. Radiology 134:577, 1980.
12. Sim FJ: Diagnosis and treatment of bone tumors—A teaching approach. *In* Sim FJ (ed): Principles of Surgical Treatment. Thorofare, NJ, Slack, 1983, pp 164–168.

4

RADIOLOGY OF SPINE TUMORS:
General Considerations

CHRISTOPHER L. TILLOTSON and DANIEL I. ROSENTHAL

INTRODUCTION

There has been extraordinary progress in medical imaging with the development of many new modalities. Although conventional radiography remains a mainstay in the diagnosis, management, and follow-up of primary bone neoplasms, it is necessary to integrate the information from a variety of imaging studies. The techniques of plain tomography, radionuclide imaging, computed tomography (CT) and magnetic resonance imaging (MRI) serve to complement, rather than supplant, plain film interpretation. After eliciting the patient history, performing a physical examination, and obtaining the appropriate radiographic studies, the clinician will have several questions for the radiologist:

1. Is there an abnormality present? Conversely, what degree of bony alteration can be seen; what may escape detection?

2. If conventional films are adequate and unremarkable, yet clinical suspicion remains high, what additional studies might be helpful?

3. If an abnormality is detected, are other regions of the skeleton affected, or is the lesion solitary?

4. What are the diagnostic possibilities? Characteristics of the lesion such as location, margin, matrix and size, must be systematically examined in order to arrive at a coherent differential diagnosis.

5. What is the extent of local and distant involvement?

QUESTION #1: Detection

Proper radiographic evaluation requires technically adequate images. Attention to radiographic technique (kV, mAS) is needed, especially in the cervicothoracic junction and in the thoracolumbar junction, where there are large changes in radiographic density. At least two orthogonal views should be obtained of the region in question. A multitude of special views exist which complement the standard anteroposterior and lateral views. However, for tumors these are generally supplanted by more complex imaging studies.

Most, but not all, skeletal neoplasms arise from the medullary space of the bone. This compartment is composed of varying proportions of trabecular bone, fat, and marrow elements depending on the age, nutrition, and clinical status of a patient. The cortex is predominantly composed of crystalline hydroxyapatite with little in the way of soft tissue elements. The vertebral body is composed of approximately 95 per cent trabecular bone and 5 per cent cortical bone. The posterior elements are largely cortical so that the overall distribution is 65 per cent trabecular and 35 per cent cortical.[23]

Subtle differences in medullary density can be exceedingly difficult to detect. To quantitate the minimum detectable destruction, Ardran[2] removed progressively larger amounts of medullary bone from an isolated vertebra. Specimen radiographs revealed that at least 30 per cent must be removed before a radiographic change is discernible. Edelstyn and colleagues, experimenting with a whole lumbar spine complete with local soft tissues, demonstrated that 50 to 75 per cent of the medullary space must be replaced before a radiographic change can be noted.[12] This decrease in sensitivity as compared with Ardran's work is attributed to the superimposed soft tissues that degrade the bony detail seen in the isolated vertebra (Fig. 4–1). In the setting of osteopenia, even greater trabecular replacement is necessary in order to result in an identifiable abnormality. The degree of radiographic detail seen in the extremities is thus not obtainable in the spine, a fact that is also significant in the identification of tumor matrix and margins.

Ancillary radiographic findings may facilitate localization of subtle bony lesions. For instance, painful lesions may result in a scoliosis concave to the side of the tumor[16, 20] owing to paravertebral muscle spasm (Fig. 4–2). Similarly, a soft tissue mass may result in distortion of surrounding soft tissue planes.

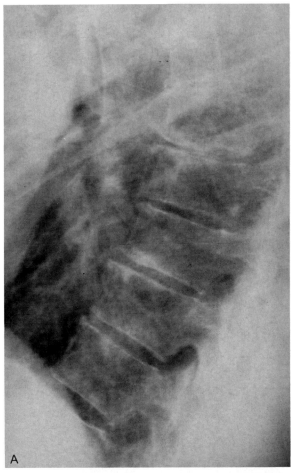

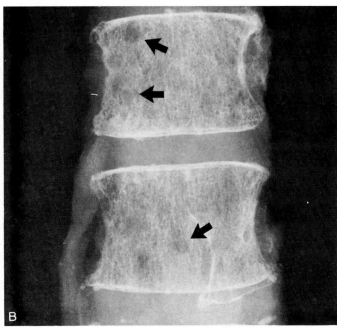

FIGURE 4–1. Multiple myeloma. *A,* Lateral plain film of the thoracic spine demonstrates no focal abnormality, although generalized osteopenia is present. This is one of several typical radiographic presentations of myeloma. *B,* A postmortem specimen radiograph reveals multiple well-circumscribed, lytic foci due to myelomatous involvement of bone (*arrows*). This abnormality was not visible in vivo due to overlying bone and soft tissue.

FIGURE 4–2. Osteoid osteoma of L4. *A,* Anteroposterior (AP) plain film of the lumbar spine shows a scoliosis concave to the left, centered at the L3/L4 level. There is a sclerotic abnormality involving the left lamina at L4 (*arrowheads*). Painful neoplasms typically result in a scoliosis concave to the side of the lesion. *B,* AP tomogram at the level of the posterior elements of L4 shows a lucent lesion in the left lamina measuring roughly one centimeter (*arrows*). Note the small focus of ossification of the nidus (*asterisk*).

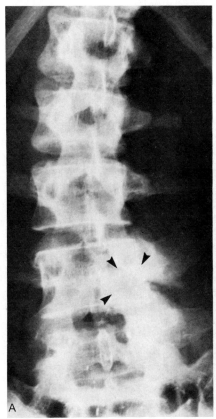

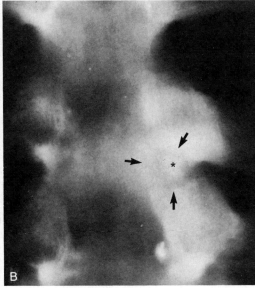

QUESTION #2: Additional Studies

Radionuclide bone scanning with technetium-labeled phosphate analogues provides a significant improvement in sensitivity over conventional radiography for most types of lesions. In a study of metastatic lesions, Pistenma and coworkers have demonstrated false-negative rates for radionuclide scanning and conventional radiography of 1.6 per cent and 17 per cent, respectively.[27] Exceptions to these observations include multiple myeloma,[34] histiocytosis X,[24, 28] and certain highly anaplastic metastatic neoplasms to bone, such as neuroblastoma.[15] These lesions are more likely than others to result in a false-negative bone scan. In those patients with multiple myeloma and positive bone scan, roughly one third are attributable to superimposed pathologic fracture.[34] Furthermore, in a review of children with histiocytosis X, Parker and colleagues demonstrated that only 35 per cent of individual lesions detected on radiographs were seen on radionuclide bone scan.[24]

If both plain films and radionuclide scans are negative, it is possible that the lesion may go undetected. Film tomography, an old and less frequently utilized technique, may still be helpful in such cases (Fig. 4–3). Both CT and MRI may also be useful in revealing lesions not detected otherwise (Fig. 4–4). Solomon and coworkers have demonstrated occult lytic foci within the spine in 66 per cent of patients with multiple myeloma and normal plain films using CT.[30] In addition, they showed that CT may more accurately describe the number and extent of vertebral lesions in those patients who do have plain film findings of multiple myeloma.

Detection of paraspinal soft tissue lesions and of the soft tissue component of bone lesions is difficult on plain radiographs. Displacement of fat planes can be recognized in the cervical spine, and displacement of the pleura may be seen at thoracic levels. Generally, there are no findings when the lesion is confined to the lumbar spine or the posterior elements. In such cases, magnetic resonance or computed tomography must be used.[2, 5–7, 10, 13, 33]

QUESTION #3: Primary Bone Neoplasm Versus Metastasis

Metastatic disease of the skeleton is far more common than primary neoplasia. Bone metastases from cancer of the breast, lung, and prostate are encoun-

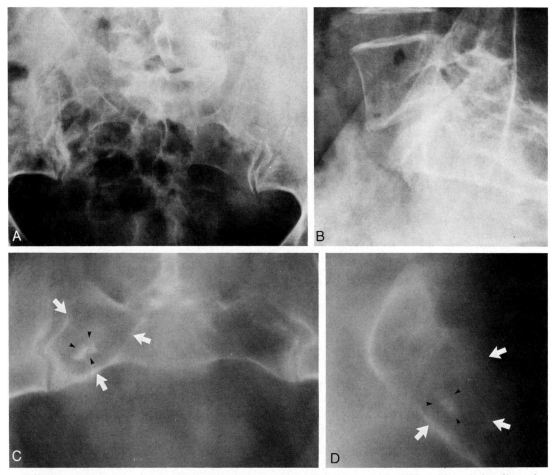

FIGURE 4–3. Chondrosarcoma of the right sacral ala. *A* and *B*, Anteroposterior (AP) and lateral plain films of the sacrum reveal no abnormality, although bony detail is partially obscured by overlying bowel gas. *C* and *D*, AP and lateral tomograms of the sacrum show a lytic, slightly expansile lesion of the right ala (*arrows*). Contained within this tumor is a dense focus of flocculent calcification suggesting a neoplasm of cartilaginous origin (*arrowheads*).

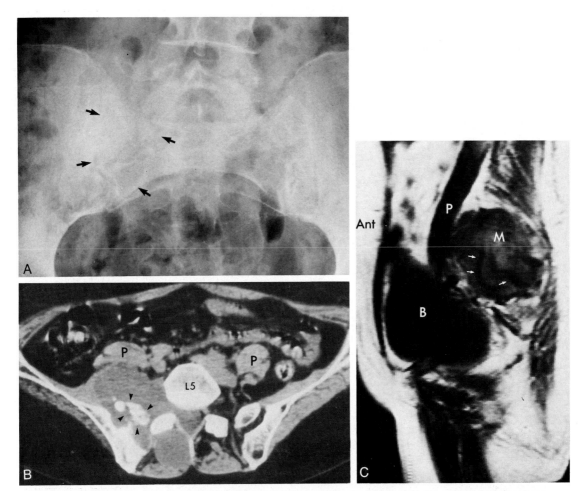

FIGURE 4—4. Chondrosarcoma of the right sacral ala. *A,* Anteroposterior plain film of the sacrum. Close scrutiny reveals a faintly detectable pattern of mixed lytic and blastic change in the right sacral wing (*arrows*). *B,* CT scan reveals an extensive, destructive lesion arising in the right sacral ala with extension into the ilium and retroperitoneal soft tissues. Note the anterior displacement of the psoas (P). The noncalcified portions of the tumor are of low density and exhibit a lobular configuration, typical of cartilage tumors. Flocculent calcification is also consistent with a chondroid tumor (*arrowheads*). *C,* Right parasagittal MR scan (T1 weighted) confirms the presence of a large mass (M) posterior to the psoas (P). Regions of decreased signal represent calcification seen on CT (*arrows*). B = bladder.

tered most often and are disseminated via the hematogenous route. Because of greater vascularity, the parts of the skeleton containing red marrow, such as the spine, are preferentially affected. Wilson and Calhoun have demonstrated that in patients with extraosseous primaries complicated by bone metastases, the vertebral column is affected in 26 per cent of cases.[32]

Most primary bone tumors, with the exception of multiple myeloma, are unifocal. Metastatic lesions are usually multifocal, although bone metastases may be solitary in 10 to 15 per cent of patients.[32] There is usually a known primary malignancy elsewhere, but bone pain from metastatic disease may be the patient's initial complaint in some cases. The likelihood that bone lesions will be symptomatic appears to depend upon the type of primary lesion. In our experience, lung cancer metastases are usually symptomatic; breast and prostate lesions may be clinically silent.

Since metastatic lesions greatly outnumber primary

tumors, a radionuclide bone scan is probably indicated whenever an unknown spinal lesion is encountered. Occasionally, a radionuclide scan will be done to assess the degree of activity of a known lesion. However, since most destructive lesions of bone cause increased uptake of the radiopharmaceutical, the primary use of scanning is to evaluate the skeleton for additional lesions. As noted previously, multiple myeloma, histiocytosis X, and certain highly anaplastic metastatic neoplasms may show decreased uptake or appear normal; if these lesions are known or suspected, a radiographic metastatic survey is required.

QUESTION #4: Differential Diagnosis
Location

Location is important in differential diagnosis. Features of location include both the spinal level and the portion of the vertebra which is affected. The sacrum is the most common site for primary neoplasms, and certain tumors have a distinct propensity to arise there. Dahlin reports that in patients with Ewing's sarcoma, giant cell tumor, chordoma, or fibrosarcoma of the spine, the sacrum is affected in roughly two thirds of the cases[8] (Fig. 4–5). Conversely, osteoid osteomas (see Fig. 4–2) and osteoblastomas tend to be more evenly distributed throughout the spine, with lumbar and thoracic involvement being more common.[8]

The portion of the vertebra from which the lesion arose is also important. Although this delineation is difficult in the sacrum, it can be made in the more rostral portions of the spine in most cases. Osteoblastomas, osteoid osteomas (Fig. 4–2), and aneurysmal bone cysts (Fig. 4–6) are most prevalent in the posterior elements. Metastatic lesions usually affect pedicles or the junction of pedicles and body. Conversely, osteosarcoma[3, 25] chondrosarcoma,[14] heman-

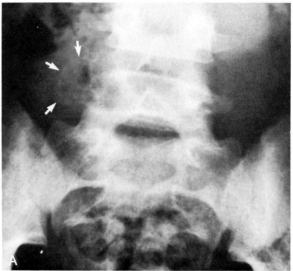

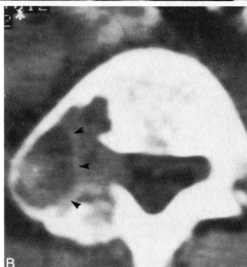

FIGURE 4–6. Aneurysmal bone cyst of L5. *A,* Anteroposterior plain film demonstrates an expanded right pedicle and transverse process of L5. There is a thin shell of periosteal new bone surrounding the lesion (*arrows*). *B,* CT scan reveals an expansile, lytic lesion with a thin, but intact, shell of periosteal new bone surrounding the lesion. Low density regions are present (*arrowheads*) corresponding to cystic areas within the mass.

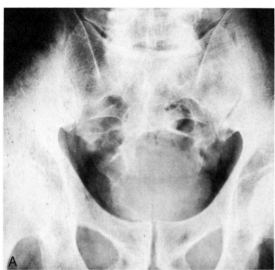

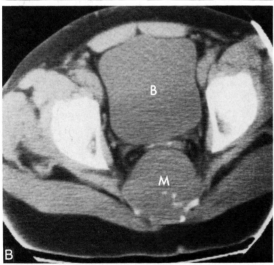

FIGURE 4–5. Chordoma of the sacrum. *A,* Anteroposterior plain film of the sacrum demonstrates a large, destructive mass centered in the third sacral segment on the left. No calcifications are noted. *B,* CT scan through the lower sacrum and coccyx shows extensive destruction of the sacrum with a soft tissue mass (M) extending anteriorly behind the bladder (B). Although the surrounding fat and muscle planes are preserved, microscopic invasion cannot be excluded.

gioma (Fig. 4–7), giant cell tumor, and lymphoma often involve the vertebral body, although varying degrees of extension into the pedicles may be present. Multiple myeloma, which arises within the medullary space, is also predominant in the vertebral body.[17, 30]

Margins

The margin between bone and tumor is a dynamic interface at both the microscopic and gross level. The radiographic appearance of this margin may reflect both destructive (osteoclastic) and reparative (osteoblastic) changes. Different neoplastic entities, owing to their inherent growth characteristics, may demonstrate a characteristic radiographic margin that is

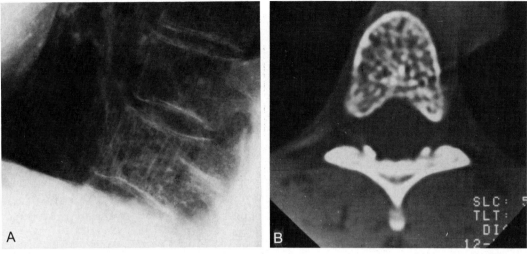

FIGURE 4–7. Hemangioma of T12. *A,* Lateral plain film of the lower thoracic spine demonstrates a prominent vertical trabecular pattern in the body of T12, characteristic of a hemangioma. Bony replacement by tumor results in coarsening of the vertical, weight-bearing trabeculae. *B,* CT scan through the body of T12 shows the thickened, vertical trabeculae imaged in cross-section. No soft tissue mass is seen, although one may occasionally be noted, especially in younger patients.

a reflection of the "balance" between these forces. The relation between radiographic margin and growth or biologic activity was described by Lodwick and colleagues [18, 19] and was recently summarized by Madewell and coworkers.[21] The margin grading system developed by these authors is an accepted standard. Margin analysis helps to understand the local aggressiveness of the lesion but does not invariably correlate with metastatic potential.

A static lesion or one with indolent growth characteristics results in a well-demarcated interface with normal bone. About this interface, a shell of reactive new bone may form, resulting in the sclerotic rim of type IA lesions. Such margins are typical of simple cysts (Fig. 4–8), nonossifying fibroma, and chondromyxoid fibroma (lesions not generally seen in the spine), as well as enchondroma, chondroblastoma, and sometimes plasmacytoma and osteoblastoma.

In tumors with a slightly faster growth rate, this reactive bony shell may not have sufficient time to form. This results in a geographic margin without sclerosis, or a "punched-out" appearance. This type IB pattern may be seen typically in giant cell tumor and multiple myeloma (see Fig. 4–1*B*).

Type IC lesions demonstrate greater local infiltration at the boundary with normal bone than lesions in the IA or IB category. Although the overall appearance is geographic, this infiltrative tendency results in a margin that is comparatively ragged and indistinct. Complete penetration of the cortex is also a characteristic of tumors in this category. Neoplasms that typically display this margin include giant cell tumors (Fig. 4–9) and low grade sarcomas.

The type II margin is characterized by numerous discrete areas of bony rarefaction with intervening residual bone. Individual lucencies have indistinct

FIGURE 4–8. Subchondral cyst of C5. Anteroposterior *(A)* and lateral *(B)* tomograms of the cervical spine reveal a well-circumscribed, round lesion in the right aspect of the vertebral body *(arrowheads).* There is a thin, sclerotic rim of reactive new bone bordering the cyst indicating a type IA margin. Degeneration of the adjacent uncovertebral joint is present.

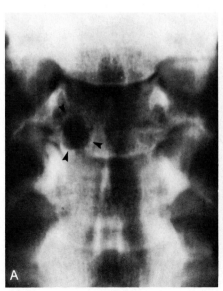
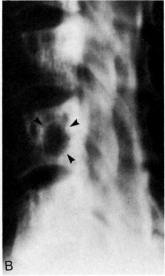

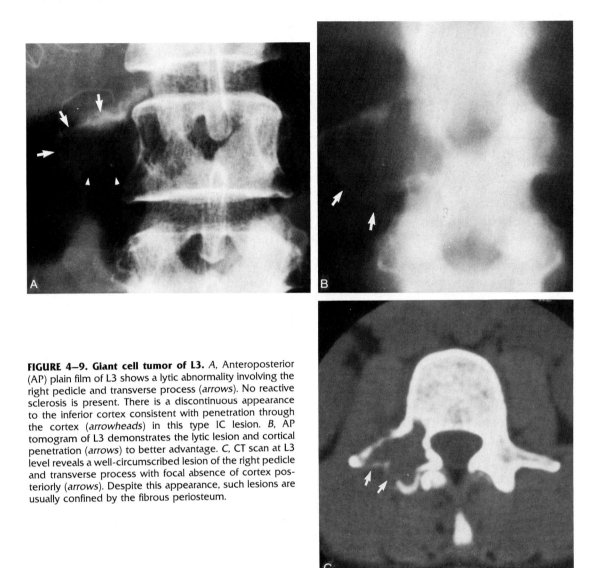

FIGURE 4–9. Giant cell tumor of L3. *A*, Anteroposterior (AP) plain film of L3 shows a lytic abnormality involving the right pedicle and transverse process (*arrows*). No reactive sclerosis is present. There is a discontinuous appearance to the inferior cortex consistent with penetration through the cortex (*arrowheads*) in this type IC lesion. *B*, AP tomogram of L3 demonstrates the lytic lesion and cortical penetration (*arrows*) to better advantage. *C*, CT scan at L3 level reveals a well-circumscribed lesion of the right pedicle and transverse process with focal absence of cortex posteriorly (*arrows*). Despite this appearance, such lesions are usually confined by the fibrous periosteum.

margins and coalesce in varying degrees around the center of the lesion. The term moth-eaten is often used to describe the appearance of these lesions. Type II neoplasms are more aggressive than type I lesions. Osteosarcoma, fibrosarcoma, and chondrosarcoma were the histologies most often encountered in this group by Lodwick and colleagues.[18] Although less common, Ewing's sarcoma and lymphoma must also be considered.

Neoplasms that display a permeated or type III margin represent the most aggressive end of the growth rate spectrum. The appearance of a permeative lesion is that of innumerable, minuscule lucencies with a rounded or slit-like quality. As a result of the marked infiltrative nature of these tumors, no discrete margin is detected. Instead, the lesion fades imperceptibly into the surrounding normal bone. Osteosarcoma and round cell tumors such as Ewing's sarcoma (Fig. 4–10) and lymphoma (Fig. 4–11) are most frequent, although other high grade sarcomas are also seen. In general, it is difficult to distinguish between type II and III margins especially in the

spine. Fortunately, the clinical significance of this distinction is minimal. Metastatic lesions may demonstrate any of the above patterns except (generally) for type IA.

This system of grading margins was primarily developed for lesions of the extremities and is most applicable to them. In the spine it is often difficult to characterize margins adequately by plain films alone. The type of cortical penetration as demonstrated by CT scan has been shown to correlate with tumor type and grade and may be used to complement margin analysis.[7] Figure 4–12 summarizes the margin patterns of common spine neoplasms.

Matrix

The term matrix refers to the intercellular substance produced by mesenchymal cells.[31] Some tumors demonstrate characteristic forms of matrix mineralization which can be appreciated radiographically. These patterns are useful in narrowing diag-

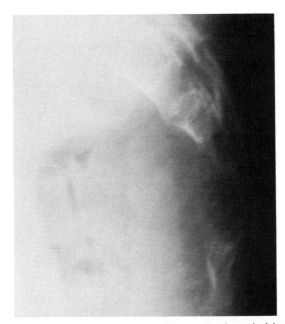

FIGURE 4–10. Ewing's sarcoma of the sacrum. Lateral plain film of the sacrum reveals a lytic lesion of the midsacrum. The margins are difficult to identify due to the highly infiltrative nature of this type III neoplasm.

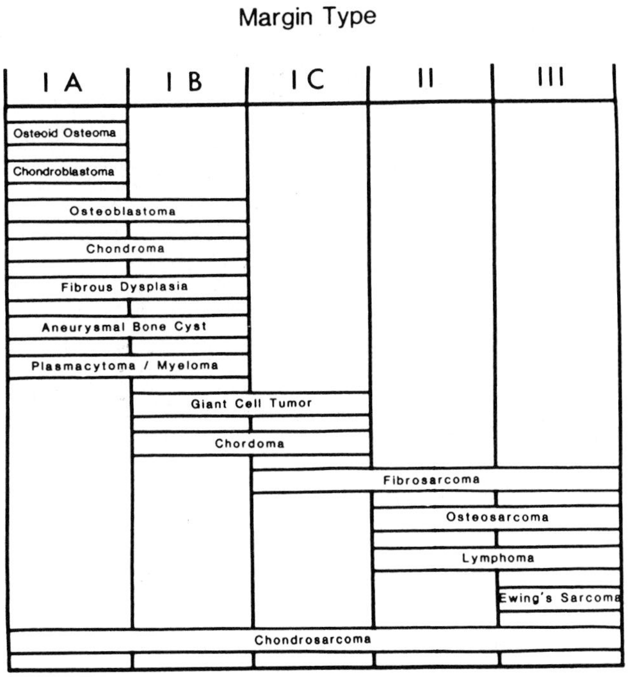

Margin Type

	I A	I B	I C	II	III
Osteoid Osteoma	■	■			
Chondroblastoma	■	■			
Osteoblastoma	■	■	■		
Chondroma	■	■	■		
Fibrous Dysplasia	■	■	■		
Aneurysmal Bone Cyst	■	■	■		
Plasmacytoma / Myeloma	■	■	■		
Giant Cell Tumor		■	■		
Chordoma		■	■		
Fibrosarcoma				■	■
Osteosarcoma				■	■
Lymphoma				■	■
Ewing's Sarcoma					■
Chondrosarcoma	■	■	■	■	■

FIGURE 4–12. Margin patterns of common bone neoplasms.

nostic considerations, but it must be emphasized that not all bone neoplasms produce matrix. For example, lymphoma, myeloma, and giant cell tumor are purely cellular neoplasms. Even lesions that characteristically produce matrix, such as osteosarcoma and chondrosarcoma, may be too poorly differentiated to produce recognizable matrix.

Bone matrix generally assumes a puffy or hazy appearance. When it is exuberant, a diffuse increase in density or ivory-like appearance is noted (Fig. 4–13).[31] In contrast, cartilage is often lobular in configuration. These lobules may vary in size and degree

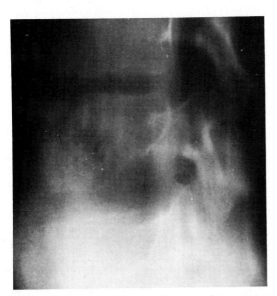

FIGURE 4–11. Primary lymphoma of L4. Lateral tomogram of L4 shows an ill-defined lytic process involving the vertebral body. This high-grade tumor/bone interface could be classified as either a type II or type III lesion.

of maturation. Calcification of the cartilage and ossification of the surface of the lobules result in the characteristic stippled or arcuate pattern of mineralization often noted in these tumors (Fig. 4–14).[31]

Age

Age is an important factor in formulating a differential diagnosis of bone lesions. Malignant neoplasms such as osteosarcoma and Ewing's sarcoma occur most commonly between the first and third decades of life. Benign entities such as chondroblastoma, osteoblastoma, osteoid osteoma, and bone cysts are also encountered at this age. Conversely, other malignancies primarily affect the older population. These include chondrosarcoma and multiple myeloma, which are seen after the fourth decade and beyond. In the middle ground between these two periods, other neoplasms are commonly diagnosed and include fibrosarcoma, lymphoma, giant cell tumor, and enchondroma (Fig. 4–15).

Predisposing Factors

Some preexisting conditions are known to predispose to skeletal malignancy. The association between bilateral retinoblastoma and subsequent development of osteosarcoma is a case in point.[11] Disorders such as Paget's disease have a known association with osteosarcoma and fibrosarcoma.[8] Solitary enchondromas or those of multiple enchondromatosis may undergo malignant degeneration into chondrosarcoma.[8] The relationship between radiation therapy and subsequent development of bone sarcomas was

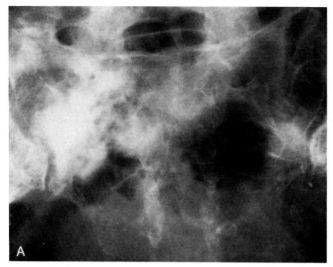

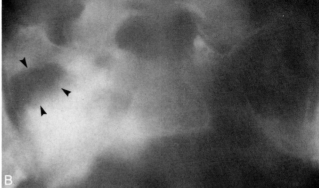

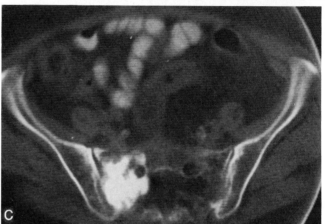

FIGURE 4–13. Osteosarcoma of the sacrum. *A,* Anteroposterior (AP) plain film of the sacrum demonstrates a region of mixed lysis and mineralization in the right ala. This matrix ossification has a cloud-like or hazy appearance indicative of a bone-forming neoplasm. *B,* AP tomogram of the sacrum more clearly demonstrates the mixed lytic (*arrowheads*) and blastic changes present on the plain films. *C,* CT scan shows the uniformly dense, ivory-like quality of neoplastic bone in this osteosarcoma.

first described in 1922 by Beck.[4] Several large reviews have demonstrated that 2 to 4 per cent of osteosarcomas may be secondary to previous irradiation.[9, 22] In general, any condition resulting in an accelerated rate of bone growth, repair, or remodeling appears capable of malignant change.

QUESTION #5: Involvement
Local Extent

The staging system of musculoskeletal neoplasms is discussed in Chapter 3. Accurate staging depends upon localization of the lesion to one or more anatomic compartments. For lesions that are clearly confined to bone, plain radiographs and tomography are probably sufficient to make this determination.

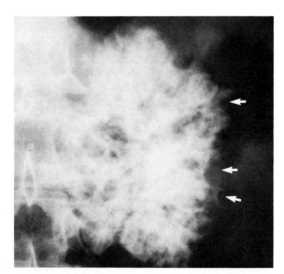

FIGURE 4–14. Osteochondroma of L1. Anteroposterior plain film displays a large, exophytic mass arising from the left transverse process of L1. The lobular nature of cartilaginous growth can be recognized by the arcuate pattern of mineralization. This represents "framing" of the neoplastic cartilage lobules by enchondral ossification (*arrows*).

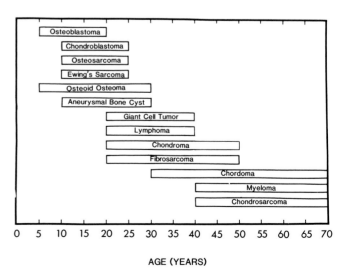

FIGURE 4–15. Common age distribution of selected bone neoplasms.

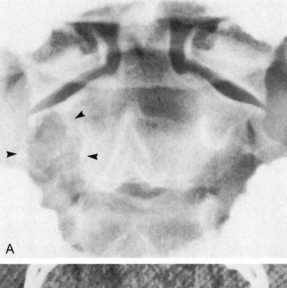

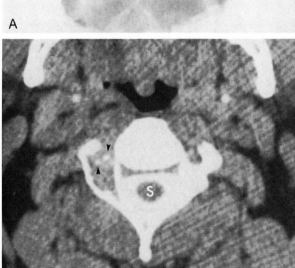

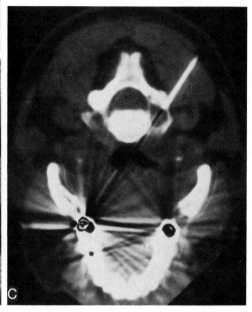

FIGURE 4–16. Chondrosarcoma of C2. *A,* Anteroposterior odontoid view reveals a well-circumscribed, lytic lesion of the right lateral mass of C2 (*arrowheads*). No matrix mineralization is identifiable. *B,* CT myelogram through the body of C2 confirms the presence of a geographic lesion with cortical disruption. In addition, punctate matrix calcification is noted, indicative of a cartilage-forming neoplasm (*arrowheads*). S = spinal cord. *C,* The patient was placed in the prone position within the scanner and a CT-guided needle biopsy was performed. Linear streak artifacts are due to the metallic needle and dental work.

Radionuclide bone scan techniques may overestimate the degree of bony involvement especially for hypervascular lesions.[29] As stated before, the utility of radionuclide scanning rests on the exclusion of additional foci of involvement.

Computed tomography is an important adjunct to plain radiography in the further delineation of bone neoplasms. CT may help to identify soft tissue features of the lesion which are not apparent on plain films, leading to more accurate diagnosis and staging [7, 10, 13, 33] (Fig. 4–16).

Several recent comparisons of MRI with CT have defined a key role for MRI in the evaluation of bone neoplasms.[1, 6] MR imaging is capable of producing exquisite soft tissue discrimination. It is often superior to CT in delineating the intramedullary and extraosseous extent of bone lesions. In addition, the multiplanar capability of MRI is helpful in evaluating the relationship with adjacent structures. However, as a result of the relatively immobile nature of protons within bone and mineralized matrix, MRI is inferior to CT in the determination of cortical integrity and matrix mineralization patterns. Calcified tissues appear as regions of decreased signal with relatively poor spatial resolution as compared with more cellular areas. In the spine, MRI has a demonstrable advantage over CT in the assessment of marrow space involvement, canal invasion, and paravertebral extension.[5] When myelographic contrast is administered, the two modalities are roughly equivalent for evaluation of intrathecal structures (Fig. 4–17).

In tumor staging, CT is preferred when the compartmental boundary in question is composed of bone, since MR images have relatively poor sensitivity for thin bone interfaces. MRI is preferred when compartmental boundaries are composed of soft tissues or fascia and when it is necessary to evaluate a longitudinally oriented structure such as the spinal canal.

Detection of pulmonary metastases is an important part of staging. A combination of chest radiography and CT is necessary to detect pulmonary metastases when they are fewest in number and smallest in size, thus affording the best chance of curative resection. In particular, chest CT is superior in detecting metastatic lesions and most accurately depicts their number and location.[26] MRI is not useful in this instance due to motion artifact from transmitted cardiac pulsation. Also, due to the relative paucity of mobile

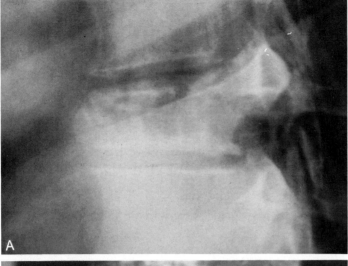

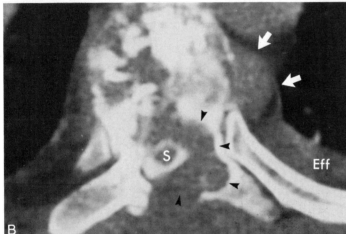

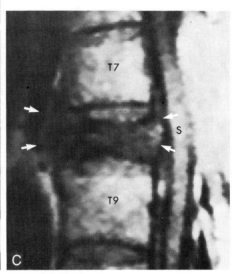

FIGURE 4–17. Giant cell tumor of T8. *A,* Lateral plain film demonstrates a mixed lytic/blastic process involving the body of T8 with pathologic compression fracture. *B,* CT/myelogram at the level of the T8 body shows extensive bony replacement by tumor with soft tissue extension into the spinal canal (*arrowheads*) and left paravertebral region (*arrows*). An associated left pleural effusion is also noted (Eff). Previous decompressive laminectomy has been performed. S = spinal cord. *C,* Midsagittal MR scan (T1 weighted) demonstrates a diffuse, low signal abnormality of the body of T8 indicative of neoplastic replacement. Tumor extends both anteriorly and posteriorly (*arrows*) with resultant deformation of the thecal sac. The spinal cord (S) is bowed posteriorly.

protons within air-filled lungs, information density is low.

REFERENCES

1. Aisen AM, Martel W, Braunstein EM, et al: MRI and CT evaluation of primary bone and soft tissue tumors. AJR 146:749–756, 1986.
2. Ardran GM: Bone destruction not demonstrable by radiography. Br J Radiol 24:107–109, 1951.
3. Barwick KW, Huvos AG, Smith J: Primary osteogenic sarcoma of the vertebral column. Cancer 46:595–604, 1980.
4. Beck A: Zuir Frage des Rontgensarkomas zugleich ein Beitrag zur Pathogenese des Sarkoms. Muench Med Wochenschr 69:623–625, 1922.
5. Beltran J, Noto AM, Chakeres DW, Christoforidis AJ: Tumors of the osseous spine: Staging with MR versus CT. Radiology 162:565–569, 1987.
6. Bohndorf K, Reiser M, Lochner B, et al: Magnetic resonance imaging of primary tumors and tumor-like conditions of bone. Skel Radiol 15:511–517, 1986.
7. Brown KT, Kattapuram SV, Rosenthal DI: Computed tomography analysis of bone tumors: Patterns of cortical destruction and soft tissue extension. Skel Radiol 15:448–451, 1986.
8. Dahlin DC: Bone Tumors. 3rd ed. Springfield, IL, Charles C Thomas, 1978, pp 99–115, 274–287, 315–343.
9. Dahlin DC, Coventry MB: Osteogenic sarcoma: A study of 600 cases. J Bone Joint Surg 49A:101–110, 1967.
10. deSantos LA, Goldstein HM, Murray JA, Wallace S: Computed tomography in the evaluation of musculoskeletal neoplasms. Radiology 128:89–94, 1978.
11. Draper GJ, Sanders BM, Kingston JE: Second primary neoplasms in patients with retinoblastoma. Br J Cancer 53:661–671, 1986.
12. Edelstyn GA, Gillespie PJ, Grebbell FS: The radiological demonstration of osseous metastases: Experimental observations. Clin Radiol 18:158–162, 1967.
13. Heelan RT, Watson RC, Smith J: Computed tomography of lower extremity tumors. AJR 132:933–937, 1979.
14. Hermann G, Sacher M, Lanzieri CF, et al: Chondrosarcoma of the spine: An unusual radiographic presentation. Skel Radiol 14:178–183, 1985.
15. Kaufman RA, Thrall JH, Keyes JW, et al: False negative bone scans in neuroblastoma metastatic to the ends of long bones. AJR 130:131–135, 1978.
16. Keim HA, Reina EG: Osteoid osteoma as a cause of scoliosis. J Bone Joint Surg 57A:159–163, 1975.
17. Kyle RA: Multiple myeloma: Review of 869 cases. Mayo Clin Proc 50:29–40, 1975
18. Lodwick GS, Wilson AJ, Farrell C, et al: Determining growth rates of focal lesions of bone from radiographs. Radiology 134:577–583, 1980.
19. Lodwick GS, Wilson AJ, Farrell C, et al: Estimating rate of growth in bone lesions: Observer performance and error. Radiology 134:585–590, 1980.
20. Maclellan DI, Wilson FC: Osteoid osteoma of the spine. J Bone Joint Surg 49A:111–121, 1967.
21. Madewell JE, Ragsdale BD, Sweet DE: Radiologic and pathologic analysis of solitary bone lesions. Part One. Internal margins. Radiol Clin North Am 19(4):715–748, 1981.

22. McKenna RJ, Schwinn CP, Soong KY, Higinbotham NL: Sarcomata of the osteogenic series (osteosarcoma, fibrosarcoma, chondrosarcoma, parosteal osteogenic sarcoma, and sarcomata arising in abnormal bone): An analysis of 552 cases. J Bone Joint Surg 48A:1–26, 1966.

23. Ott SM, Chesnut CH III, Hanson JA, et al: Comparison of bone mass measurements using different diagnostic techniques in patients with postmenopausal osteoporosis. Proceedings of the Copenhagen International Symposium on Osteoporosis. *In* Christiansen C, Arnaud CD, Nordin BEC, et al (eds): Osteoporosis. Glostrup, Denmark, Aalborg Stiftsbogtrykkeri.

24. Parker BR, Pinckney L, Etcubanas E: Relative efficacy of radiographic and radionuclide bone surveys in the detection of the skeletal lesions of histiocytosis X. Radiology 134:377–380, 1980.

25. Patel DV, Hammer RA, Levin B, Fisher MA: Primary osteogenic sarcoma of the spine. Skel Radiol 12:276–279, 1984.

26. Peuchot M, Libshitz HI: Pulmonary metastatic disease: Radiologic-surgical correlation. Radiology 164:719–722, 1987.

27. Pistenma DA, McDougall IR, Kriss JP: Screening for bone metastases—Are only scans ncessary? JAMA 231(1):46–50, 1975.

28. Siddiqui AR, Tashjian JH, Lazarus K, et al: Nuclear medicine studies in the evaluation of skeletal lesions in children with histiocytosis X. Radiology 140:787–789, 1981.

29. Simon, MA, Kirchner PT: Scintigraphic evaluation of primary bone tumors. J Bone Joint Surg 62A(5):758–764, 1980.

30. Soloman A, Rahamani R, Seligsohn U, Ben-Artzi F: Multiple myeloma: Early vertebral involvement assessed by computerized tomography. Skel Radiol 11:258–261, 1984.

31. Sweet DE, Madewell JE, Ragsdale BD: Radiologic and pathologic analysis of solitary bone neoplasms. Part Three. Matrix patterns. Radiol Clin North Am 19(4):785–814, 1981.

32. Wilson MA, Calhoun FW: The distribution of skeletal metastases in breast and pulmonary cancer: Concise communication. J Nucl Med 22:594–597, 1981.

33. Wilson JS, Korobkin M, Genant HK, Borill EG: Computed tomography of musculoskeletal disorders. AJR 131:55–61, 1978.

34. Woolfenden JM, Pitt MJ, Durie BGM, Moon TE: Comparison of bone scintigraphy and radiology in multiple myeloma. Radiology 134:723–728, 1980.

5

PERCUTANEOUS NEEDLE BIOPSY OF THE SPINE

SUSAN V. KATTAPURAM and DANIEL I. ROSENTHAL

Needle biopsy of the spine is a procedure that intimidates many patients and some physicians. The technical difficulty of the technique and fear of complications have prevented this valuable procedure from being used as fully as its merits indicate. These fears are partly an outgrowth of the early development of percutaneous techniques. Initially, less sophisticated biopsy implements and imaging devices were available, leading to suggestions that the procedure be limited to the lumbar and lower thoracic spine.[69] However, recent advances in imaging modalities and in cytologic and histologic techniques have greatly enhanced its safety and have extended its application to previously inaccessible or invisible lesions. When performed under local anesthesia, needle biopsy can spare the patient a major operation.

HISTORY

Percutaneous biopsy of the skeleton is well described in the literature. The earliest bone biopsies consisted of bone marrow aspirates for hematologic evaluation.[4, 70] A blind approach was used, since the sites (iliac crest and sternum) were palpable. Percutaneous biopsy of individual skeletal lesions was first discussed by Martin and Ellis in 1930,[47] and then by Coley and colleagues,[10] Hoffman,[38] and Martin.[48] Biopsy of spine lesions was first reported by Ball in 1934.[7] In 1935 Robertson and Ball[61] reported 15 cases in which needle aspiration was used to diagnose various spinal conditions. The authors warned of the danger of injury to the cord and the difficulties in obtaining cartilaginous or fibrous tissue by their method.

A breakthrough came in 1943 when Turkel and Bethell[68] introduced the first trephine biopsy needle. The set contains a 10-gauge outer sheath, through which a toothed cutting needle can be introduced. This needle is capable of cutting through thick cortices and blastic lesions. In 1947, Ellis[19] introduced the drill biopsy method. In 1948, Valls and Ottolenghi[69] presented an ingenious device for making an accurate needle approach to the vertebral

bodies at a measured angle of 35 degrees. Their device consisted of two needles and a guide. A long thin stylet was used for exploration. A shorter aspiration needle performed the biopsy. Valls and Ottolenghi described techniques for approaching all spinal levels, including the pharyngeal path for the upper three cervical bodies, but advised against reaching above the ninth thoracic vertebra due to the possibility of injury to the azygos and hemiazygos systems. In 1949, Sieffert and Arkin[63] modified Valls' technique by introducing a bevelled, serrated, toothed needle. Mazet and Cozen[49] in 1952 and Ray[59] in 1953 modified Valls' technique to biopsy cervical and lumbar vertebral bodies. Later, Ottolenghi,[55] Schajowicz,[63] Ackermann,[1] and Craig[12] contributed significantly by describing in detail the instrumentation and techniques of spinal biopsy. Ackermann added the option of a smaller caliber needle to the basic Turkel needle design.[2] Craig[12] introduced a needle with a handle attached to the back of the cutting cannula.

The initial spine biopsies were done blindly. Later Snyder and Coley[64] elaborated the technique described by Martin and Ellis in 1934 and mentioned the use of radiographic and fluoroscopic guidance for their biopsies. The development of image intensifier fluoroscopy further simplified the procedure.[42, 43, 56] Since that time, further refinements include the application of more advanced imaging modalities (especially computed tomography [CT]), allowing safer access to difficult locations,[8, 11, 29, 35, 39, 44, 72] and various reports of extensive experience detailing techniques and complications.[3, 5, 6, 9, 13–18, 20–23, 25–29, 31–34, 36, 37, 41, 45, 50, 51, 53, 57, 60, 67, 71]

BIOPSY PROCEDURE AND TECHNIQUE

Preliminary Studies

Our biopsies are performed by the radiologist in the Radiology Department. However, close cooperation between the orthopedist, radiologist, and pathologist is of utmost importance. The pathologist must be experienced with bone lesions and should be aware of the clinical, roentgenographic, and laboratory findings. The cytologist also plays an important role by providing "on the spot" diagnosis or by confirming that adequate tissue is available. Consultation with the surgeon is important, since it may sometimes be desirable to excise the needle path if the lesion proves to be malignant.

A detailed prebiopsy radiographic evaluation is indicated in all spine biopsies. The precise localization of the lesion to be biopsied is important to the success of the procedure. Thus all available studies, including radiographs, tomograms, and CT scans, are reviewed to determine the exact site of the lesion, the choice of needle, and a safe route of approach. A radionuclide scan should be available to ascertain if the lesion is solitary. A spine biopsy should not be done if there are other more easily approachable lesions. We routinely perform blood counts and clotting studies if the lesion is in a location where hemostasis might be difficult to achieve by external pressure. A careful history of any bleeding tendency or ingestion of nonsteroidal anti-inflammatory drugs is obtained. This is important because aspirin and certain similar products can prolong the bleeding time, an effect that may persist for up to two weeks after use is terminated.[46]

Needles

A variety of needles are commercially available. The instruments developed by Craig (Becton-Dickinson, Rutherford, NJ) and Turkel (Turkel Instruments Inc., Southfield, MI) continue to be commercially available. The Ackermann needle is no longer commercially available. Other commonly used needles include the Jamshidi needle (Kormed Co., Minneapolis, MN), TruCut (for soft tissues) (Travenol Laboratories Inc., Deerfield, IL), Vim Silverman (Becton-Dickinson, Rutherford, NJ), and Chiba needles (for fine needle aspirations) (Cook Co., Bloomington, IN). All of these are cutting needles, except the Jamshidi needle, which combines the features of the cutting and trephine needles. The Jamshidi needle is available in two calibers (11 and 12 gauge) and in two lengths. Spinal needles, ranging in gauge from 16 to 22, are also used in most procedures as guides for the introduction of the larger needle and for performing local anesthesia. They can also be used for aspiration of purely lytic lesions or fluid collections.

The choice of the needle depends on the type of lesion (osteoblastic, osteolytic, or mixed), location (bony or soft tissue), the critical areas around it, and the amount of tissue needed by the pathologist. We prefer a trephine needle (Turkel) if an intact cortex has to be penetrated or if the lesion is blastic. Occasionally, a hand drill may be needed if the cortex is hard to penetrate[40] (Fig. 5–1). For medullary lesions surrounded by an intact or thickened cortex, a trephine needle is used to create a window through which a TruCut or other soft tissue needle can be passed to obtain a sample of marrow. When the

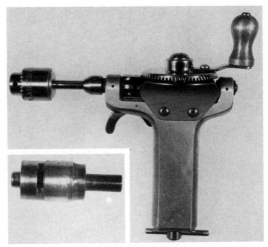

FIGURE 5–1. A manual hand-held drill is useful for obtaining samples of cortical bone and for penetrating intact cortex to sample intraosseous tissues. An adapter consisting of a Luer-Lok fitting welded to a solid metal post is used to connect the drill to the trephine needle. (From Kattapuram SV, Rosenthal DI, Phillips WF: Trephine biopsy of the skeleton with the aid of a hand drill. Radiology 152:231, 1984.)

cortex is destroyed or when there is a soft tissue mass, a TruCut needle provides an excellent specimen. These needles are rather large; for lytic metastatic lesions or for lesions located in difficult anatomic sites, aspiration using a fine needle is preferred.

Imaging Systems

Biopsy using fluoroscopic guidance is faster and easier to perform than CT-directed biopsy and is probably less costly. Fluoroscopic guidance is usually adequate for lumbar vertebral lesions. Cervical and thoracic levels are more difficult, and CT guidance offers a greater margin of safety for surrounding structures such as blood vessels or viscera. In addition, small or poorly visible lesions may require CT guidance.

Technique

Almost all of our biopsies are done under local anesthesia. An alert and cooperative patient can warn the examiner if the needle approaches a spinal sensory nerve. The use of local anesthesia allows most biopsies to be done as outpatient procedures.

For biopsy of the thoracic and lumbar spine, a posterior oblique approach is employed. The patient may be positioned in either the prone, oblique, or decubitus position. For lumbar biopsy the needle is introduced into the skin approximately 7 to 8 cm from the spinous process and directed obliquely toward the posterior lateral aspect of the vertebral body (Fig. 5–2). For biopsy of the thoracic spine, a more medial site is selected to avoid the pleura (Fig. 5–3).

For purposes of biopsy, the cervical spine can be

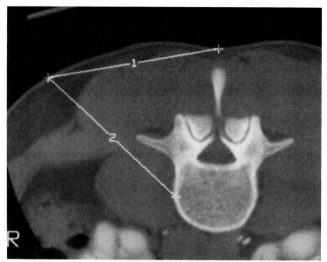

FIGURE 5–2. For lumbar vertebral biopsy a point is selected approximately 8 cm from the midline (line 1). The needle is introduced at approximately 45 degrees from the vertical (line 2). The needle is advanced until it encounters the posterolateral aspect of the vertebral body. Such an approach avoids both the abdomen and the spinal canal.

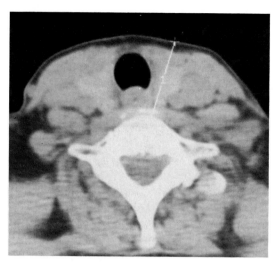

FIGURE 5–4. An anterior approach to the cervical vertebral bodies can be performed by advancing the needle through the thyroid gland (line 1). If necessary, the structures of the carotid sheath can be manually retracted for ease of access.

divided into two different areas: (1) the upper cervical spine (C1–C3) and (2) the lower cervical vertebrae and the first thoracic level. Three different approaches are described: anterior or pharyngeal, lateral, and posterior. An anterior approach is used for the first three cervical vertebral bodies. These vertebrae are deeply situated and are surrounded laterally by vital organs that pass from head to neck and vice versa. Needle puncture of any of these structures could cause serious damage, and thus a lateral approach is contraindicated. An anterior approach through the thyroid gland can be done safely, manually retracting the carotid sheath to the side (Fig. 5–4).

For the lower cervical bodies and discs a lateral or posterolateral approach is preferable. For a lateral approach the needle is introduced at the posterior

edge of the sternocleidomastoid muscle. At the lowest cervical levels it is possible to manually retract the carotid sheath.

A posterior approach is used for biopsy of posterior elements. The risk of injury to vertebral artery is minimized by careful CT control[39] (Fig. 5–5).

A small radiopaque marker is used to identify the point of entry on the skin. The skin is prepared with antiseptics and is draped. A small caliber (20 or 22 gauge) spinal needle is introduced by increments, infiltrating the subcutaneous and deep tissue with 1 per cent xylocaine as the needle is advanced. A generous amount of local anesthetic is deposited within and around the periosteum. The needle position is checked frequently using fluoroscopy or CT. It is best to use rather thick (1 cm) CT scans for this

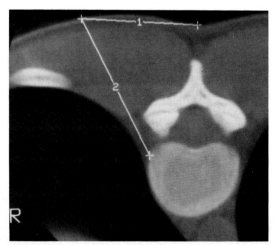

FIGURE 5–3. For biopsy of the thoracic spine a point is selected approximately 5 cm from the midline (line 1). A more steeply vertical approach toward the posterior corner of the vertebral body is selected to avoid the pleura and the intraspinal structures (line 2).

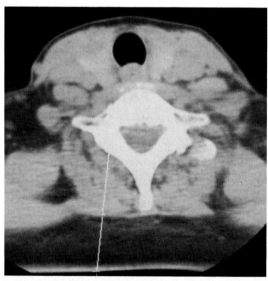

FIGURE 5–5. Biopsy of the posterior elements of the cervical vertebrae can be easily accomplished (line 1). Care must be taken to prevent the needle from violating the spinal canal or entering the soft tissues anterior to the transverse processes.

purpose, except when very small lesions are being biopsied. If radicular symptoms are produced, the needle is redirected slightly. In general, pain is mild to moderate and adequately controlled by xylocaine infiltration. This is especially true in destructive bone lesions. Although the bone itself cannot be anesthetized, destructive lesions seem to impair sensation such that relatively little pain is produced with adequate soft tissue anesthesia. Occasionally, we supplement xylocaine anesthesia with intravenous morphine.

When the tip of the needle encounters the bone and satisfactory local anesthesia has been established, the definitive biopsy needle is introduced as closely as possible along the same path through a small skin incision. The location of the biopsy needle is confirmed by radiographs or scans. A twisting or drilling movement is used to advance the needle (except for Tru-Cut needles), delivering a core of the desired length. Before the core is removed, a second radiograph or scan is done to verify the exact position of the needle in relation to the lesion. We usually take two or three core biopsies, although one core may be adequate. The spinal needle used for anesthesia and guidance can also be used to obtain an aspiration specimen. A bloody aspirate should be heparinized.

Specimen

Aspirated material is used to make smears on frosted glass slides and is fixed immediately in 90 per cent alcohol. Paper clips are used on alternate slides to prevent them from sticking to each other. The rest of the aspirate is sent to cytology and/or bacteriology. The tissue cores are immediately placed in normal saline and are hand delivered to the Pathology Department. On occasion, when the lesion is in a critical location, the cytologist is called in to see whether a diagnostic sample has been obtained or a frozen section is performed.

Indications

Percutaneous needle biopsy is a safe, simple, and fast technique with significant advantages over open biopsy for surgically difficult areas such as the spine.[6, 8, 16, 18, 26, 39, 44, 53, 55, 61, 67, 71] It is also useful when an open biopsy may weaken the bone to such an extent as to impair its mechanical stability or risk pathologic fracture. When the ultimate treatment is not surgical, percutaneous biopsy may save the patient from an open surgical procedure.

Metastatic disease has been and continues to be the most common indication for percutaneous needle biopsy. Spinal osteomyelitis is another major indication. Needle biopsy can provide a histologic diagnosis, but in addition the organisms can be cultured, leading to the appropriate therapy.

The value of percutaneous needle biopsy of the spine in cases of primary bone tumors has been much less understood and accepted. Pathologists have been reluctant to make these diagnoses on small tissue samples. In addition, most primary tumors need surgical intervention as part of their treatment. However, with improvements in technology and with skillful skeletal pathologists, percutaneous biopsy is used increasingly in suspected primary bone neoplasms.

Percutaneous needle biopsy is especially useful in the following groups of patients with primary bone tumors:

1. Patients with suspected round cell tumors (e.g., Ewing's sarcoma, myeloma, lymphoma) or with tumors for which the definitive treatment may be radiation or chemotherapy.

2. Patients with primary tumors that require reconstructive surgery, including suspected giant cell tumors, osteoblastomas, aneurysmal bone cysts, and so forth. A needle biopsy can confirm the clinical impression, allowing the surgeon to plan the reconstruction with confidence in the diagnosis and with no biopsy scar.

3. Patients with conditions such as eosinophilic granuloma for whom the biopsy may be adequate treatment.

4. Patients with recurrent tumors or changes from previous radiation therapy.

Contraindications

There are a few relative contraindications. Needle biopsy of the spine should be avoided in patients who are at high risk for hemorrhage. Platelet counts below 40,000 to 50,000 are not considered safe. In general, cartilaginous and fibrous lesions are not well suited to needle biopsy because of difficulty obtaining representative tissue. Parosteal osteosarcomas are difficult to diagnose for similar reasons. If these lesions are to be biopsied, an attempt should be made to select an area that appears most aggressive on the radiographs.

RESULTS

The recent results of percutaneous needle biopsy of the spine have been encouraging, although early reports suggested a low success rate. In 1932, Robertson and Ball correctly diagnosed only 6 of 15 patients with various diseases of the spine without using radiographic guidance. Ackermann's series yielded only 20 per cent success. This is probably because the majority of biopsies were done for suspected neoplastic involvement of the spine, not necessarily with radiographic confirmation.

Later, Valls and coworkers reported an accuracy rate of 80 per cent. This was followed by 71 per cent by Ray, 59 per cent by Frankel, and 67 per cent by Kendall. In 1964, Ottolenghi had a 79 per cent success rate in his 34 cervical spine biopsies. In the same year Cramer reported 71 per cent accuracy in 31 spinal lesions. In 1969, Ottolenghi achieved an accuracy rate of 92 per cent in a series of 1078 vertebral punctures: 78 in the cervical spine, 28 in the thoracic region, and 972 in the thoracolumbar spine.[21] Since then variable accuracy rates ranging from 68 per cent to 90 per cent have been reported.[5, 8, 39, 44] At our institution, out of 75 spine biopsies performed for a variety of reasons, we have an accuracy rate of 90.7 per cent.

COMPLICATIONS

A number of complications associated with percutaneous spinal biopsy have been reported in the literature. The reported incidence varies from 0 to 10 per cent. These range from mild discomfort to severe neurologic damage, including a few occurrences of paraplegia.[5, 8, 11, 28, 34, 51, 52, 58, 62, 65, 66, 71]

Pain and mild discomfort are the most common complications. They may be caused by introduction of the needle, penetration of an intact cortex, or negative pressure in the medullary cavity when suction is applied to retrieve the tissue sample.

Bleeding and infection are other potential complications. However, their incidence is quite low. Ottolenghi has reported a deep hematoma following a lumbar spine biopsy (1 out of 204 cases). A large hematoma requiring transfusion followed a bone marrow biopsy in a leukemic patient.[24] A soft tissue tuberculous abscess[5] and pneumonia[5, 28] have also been reported.

The incidence of pneumothorax following thoracic spine biopsy varies from 0 to 6.6 per cent. In Armstrong's series of percutaneous biopsy of 19 spinal infections, one patient developed a pneumothorax that led to pneumonia. The danger of pneumothorax can be significantly reduced by proper precautions and prompt remedial action. The use of CT guidance should greatly lessen the incidence of this problem since the medial aspect of the pleura is easily seen and avoided. In our experience with thoracic spine cases, there has been only one case of pneumothorax.

The possibility of tumor spread along the needle track is often mentioned.[21] However, this complication has not been reported in spinal or, for that matter, bone biopsies.

Neurologic damage is the most serious complication reported from percutaneous spinal biopsies. There have been scattered individual case reports of transient paresis,[11, 22, 45] transient spinal anesthesia,[28] foot drop,[52] paraplegia,[51, 52, 66] paraplegia and death,[30] and meningitis and death.[58]

The most frequent adverse outcome of percutaneous needle biopsy is inadequate tissue for diagnosis. There are several reasons for failure to obtain adequate tissue. The location of the lesion may be such that multiple needle passes may be dangerous. The choice of needle used could affect the tissue obtained. Also, certain dense tumors by their texture may present great difficulty in aspiration. Cystic, necrotic, or highly vascular lesions may yield bloody material with insufficient cells for diagnosis. Densely blastic lesions may be difficult to penetrate and may yield a macerated specimen. In such cases, the radiologist should biopsy the least sclerotic part of the blastic lesion.

CONCLUSION

Percutaneous biopsy of the spine is a safe, effective, and reliable method for diagnosis of skeletal lesions. Fear of complications is the major deterrent to the widespread acceptance of this procedure. This is especially true in cases of cervical and thoracic spine biopsies. Although relatively safe, the procedure requires expertise. An experienced individual skilled in the technique and familiar with the potential complications is essential. The need for cooperation from an experienced skeletal pathologist cannot be overemphasized. Recent technical advances have made the procedure safer. Even when guided by CT, needle biopsy is less expensive than an open procedure and can signficantly decrease the length of hospital stays. The cost-effectiveness of the procedure, its safety, and its accuracy have made it an important diagnostic tool.

REFERENCES

1. Ackermann W: Vertebral trephine biopsy. Ann Surg 143:373–385, 1956.
2. Ackermann W: Application of the trephine for bone biopsy. Results of 635 cases. JAMA 184:11–17, 1963.
3. Adler O, Rosenberger A: Fine needle aspiration biopsy of osteolytic metastatic lesions. AJR 133:15–18, 1979.
4. Arinkin M: Die intravitale untersuchungs methodik des knochenmarks. Folia Hematol 38:233, 1929.
5. Armstrong P, Chalmers AH, Green G, Irving FD: Needle aspiration/biopsy of the spine in suspected disc space infection. Br J Radiol 51:333–337, 1978.
6. Ayala AG, Zornosa J: Primary bone tumors: Pathologic study of 222 biopsies. Radiology 149:675–679, 1983.
7. Ball RP: Needle (aspiration) biopsy. J Tenn State Med Assn XXVII:203, 1934.
8. Bender CE, Berquist TH: Imaging assisted percutaneous biopsy of the thoracic spine. Mayo Clin Proc 61:942–950, 1986.
9. Bernardino ME: Percutaneous biopsy. AJR 142:41–45, 1984.
10. Coley BL, Sharp GS, Ellis EB: Diagnosis of bone tumors by aspiration. Am J Surg 13:215–224, 1931.
11. Collins JD, Bassett L, Main GD, Kagan C: Percutaneous biopsy following bone scans. Radiology 132:439–442, 1979.
12. Craig FS: Vertebral body biopsy. J Bone Joint Surg 38A:93–102, 1956.
13. Cramer LE, Khun C III, Stein AH Jr: Needle biopsy of bone. Surg Gynecol Obstet 118:1253–1256, 1964.
14. de Santos LA, Lukeman JM, Wallace S, et al: Percutaneous needle biopsy of bone in cancer patient. AJR 130:641–649, 1978.
15. DeSantos LA, Murray JA, Ayala AG: The value of percutaneous needle biopsy in the management of primary bone tumors. Cancer 43:735–744, 1979.
16. de Santos LA, Zornosa J: Bone and soft tissue. In Zornosa J (ed): Percutaneous Needle Biopsy. Baltimore, Williams and Wilkins, 1981.
17. Debnam JW, Staple TW: Trephine bone biopsy by radiologists. Radiology 116:607–609, 1975.
18. Debnam JW, Staple TW: Needle biopsy of bone. Rad Clin North Am XIII:157–164, 1975.
19. Ellis F: Needle biopsy in the clinical diagnosis of tumors. Br J Surg 34:240–261, 1947.

20. Ellis LO, Jensen WN, Westerman MP: Needle biopsy of bone and marrow. An experience with 1445 biopsies. Arch Intern Med 114:213–221, 1964.
21. Engzell U, Esposti PL, Rubio C, et al: Investigation of tumor spread in connection with aspiration biopsy. Acta Radiol Ther Phys 10:385–398, 1971.
22. Evarts CM: Diagnostic techniques: Closed biopsy of bone. Clin Orthop 107:100–111, 1975.
23. Fang HSY, Ong GB: Direct anterior approach to the upper cervical spine. J Bone Joint Surg 44A:1588–1604, 1962.
24. Fisher WB: Hazard in bone marrow biopsy. N Engl J Med 285:804, 1971.
25. Fornasier VL, Cameron HU: Techniques of closed bone biopsy. Crit Rev Lab Sci 6:145–155, 1975.
26. Frankel CJ: Aspiration biopsy of the spine. J Bone Joint Surg 36A:69–74, 1954.
27. Fyfe IS, Henry APJ, Mulholland RC: Closed vertebral biopsy. J Bone Joint Surg 65B:140–143, 1983.
28. Gladstein MO, Grantham SA: Closed skeletal biopsy. Clin Orthop 103:75–79, 1974.
29. Haaga JR: New techniques for CT-guided biopsies. AJR 133:633–641, 1979.
30. Haaga JR, Lipuma JP, Bryan PJ, et al: Clinical comparison of small and large caliber cutting needles for biopsy. Radiology 146:665–667, 1983.
31. Hajdu SI: Aspiration biopsy of primary malignant bone tumors. Radiat Ther Oncol 10:73–81, 1975.
32. Hajdu SI, Melamed MR: Needle biopsy of primary malignant bone tumors. Surg Gynecol Obstet 133:829–832, 1971.
33. Hajdu SI, Melamed MR: The diagnostic value of aspiration smears. Am J Clin Pathol 59:350–356, 1973.
34. Hanafee WN, Tobin PL: Closed bone biopsy by a radiologist. Radiology 92:605–606, 1969.
35. Hardy DC, Murphy WA, Gilula LA: Computed tomography in planning percutaneous bone biopsy. Radiology 134:447–450, 1980.
36. Hartman JT, Phalen GS: Needle biopsy of bone. Report of three representative cases. JAMA 200:113–115, 1967.
37. Hewes RC, Vigorita VJ, Freiberger RH: Percutaneous bone biopsy. The importance of aspirated osseous blood. Radiology 148:69–72, 1983.
38. Hoffman WJ: Punch biopsy in tumor diagnosis. Surg Gynecol Obstet LVI:829, 1933.
39. Kattapuram SV, Rosenthal DI: Percutaneous biopsy of the cervical spine using CT guidance. AJR 149:539–541, 1987.
40. Kattapuram SV, Rosenthal DI, Phillips WJ: Trephine biopsy of the skeleton with the aid of a hand drill. Radiology 152:231, 1984.
41. Kendall PH: Needle biopsy of the vertebral bodies. Ann Phys Med 5:236–242, 1960.
42. Lalli AF: Roentgen-guided aspiration biopsies of skeletal lesions. J Can Assoc Radiol 21:71–73, 1970.
43. Lalli AF: The direct fluoroscopically guided approach to renal, thoracic and skeletal lesions. Curr Prob Radiol 2:30–41, 1972.
44. Laredo JD, Bard M: Thoracic spine: Percutaneous trephine biopsy. Radiology 160:485–489, 1986.
45. Legge D, Ennis JT, Dempsey J: Percutaneous needle biopsy in the management of solitary lesions of bone. Clin Radiol 29:497–500, 1978.
46. Lind S: Prolonged bleeding timer. Am J Med 77:305–312, 1984.
47. Martin HE, Ellis EB: Biopsy by needle puncture and aspiration. Ann Surg 92:169–181, 1930.
48. Martin HE, Ellis EB: Aspiration biopsy. Surg Gynecol Obstet 59:578–589, 1934.
49. Mazet R, Cozen L: The diagnostic value of vertebral body needle biopsy. Ann Surg 135:245–252, 1952.
50. McCollister EC: Diagnostic techniques. Closed biopsy of bone. Clin Orthop 107:100–111, 1975.
51. McLaughlin RE, Miller WR, Miller CW: Quadriparesis after needle aspiration of the cervical spine. Report of a case. J Bone Joint Surg 58A:1167–1168, 1976.
52. Moore TM, Meyers MH, Patzakis MJ, et al: Closed biopsy of musculoskeletal lesions. J Bone Joint Surg 61A:375–380, 1979.
53. Murphy WA, Destouet JM, Gilula LA: Percutaneous skeletal biopsy 1981: A procedure for radiologists—Results, review and recommendations. Radiology 139:545–549, 1981.
54. Nagel DA, Albright JA, Keggi KJ, Southwick WO: Closer look at spinal lesions: Open biopsy of vertebral lesions. JAMA 191:103–106, 1965.
55. Ottolenghi CE: Diagnosis of orthopaedic lesions by aspiration biopsy. Results of 1061 punctures. J Bone Joint Surg 37A:443–464, 1955.
56. Ottolenghi CE: Aspiration biopsy of the spine. Technique for the thoracic spine and results of twenty-eight biopsies in the region and overall results of 1050 biopsies of other spinal segments. J Bone Joint Surg 51A:1531–1544, 1969.
57. Ottolenghi CE, Schajowicz F, DeSchant FA: Aspiration biopsy of the cervical spine. Technique and results in thirty-four cases. J Bone Joint Surg 46A:715–733, 1964.
58. Ramgopal V, Geller M: Iatrogenic Klebsiella meningitis following closed needle biopsy of the lumbar spine: Report of a case and review of literature. Wis Med J 76:41–42, 1977.
59. Ray RD: Needle biopsy of the lumbar vertebral bodies. A modification of the Valls technique. J Bone Joint Surg 35A:760–762, 1953.
60. Rix RR, Brooks SM: Needle biopsy in bone lesions. N Engl J Med 246:373–375, 1952.
61. Robertson RC, Ball RP: Destructive spine lesions. Diagnosis by needle biopsy. J Bone Joint Surg 17:749–758, 1935.
62. Schajowicz F: Aspiration biopsy in bone lesions. J Bone Joint Surg 37A:465–471, 1955.
63. Sieffert RS, Arkin AM: Trephine biopsy of bone with special reference to the lumbar vertebral bodies. J Bone Joint Surg 31A:146–149, 1949.
64. Snyder RE, Coley BL: Further studies on the diagnosis of bone tumors by aspiration biopsy. Surg Gynecol Obstet 80:517–522, 1945.
65. Southwick WO, Robinson RD: Surgical approaches to the vertebral bodies in the cervical and lumbar regions. J Bone Joint Surg 39A:631–644, 1957.
66. Stahl DC, Jacobs B: Diagnosis of obscure lesions of the skeleton: Evaluation of biopsy methods. JAMA 201:229–231, 1967.
67. Tehranzadeh J, Freiberger RH, Ghelman A: Closed skeletal needle biopsy. AJR 140:113–115, 1983.
68. Turkel H, Bethell FH: Biopsy of bone marrow performed by a new and simple instrument. J Lab Clin Med 28:1246–1251, 1943.
69. Valls J, Ottolenghi CE, Schajowicz F: Aspiration biopsy in diagnosis of lesions of vertebral bodies. JAMA 136:376–382, 1948.
70. Ward GR: Bedside Haematology. An Introduction to the Clinical Study of the So-Called Blood Disease and of Allied Disorders. Philadelphia, WB Saunders Co, 1914, p 129.
71. Zornosa J: Percutaneous Needle Biopsy. Baltimore, Williams and Wilkins, 1981.
72. Zornosa J, Bernardino ME, Ordonez NG, et al: Percutaneous needle biopsy of soft tissue tumors guided by ultrasound and computed tomography. Skel Radiol 9:33–36, 1982.

6

SPINAL ANGIOGRAPHY AND EMBOLIZATION OF TUMORS

IN SUP CHOI and ALEX BERENSTEIN

INTRODUCTION

Selective angiography of the spinal cord and spine was first described by Djindjian and DiChiro in 1964. Since then a number of publications have outlined angiographic anatomy of the spinal medullary arteries and vascular supply to the spinal column.[8, 11, 14] However, previous clinical applications of spinal angiography have largely been limited to the diagnosis of intramedullary vascular lesions.

With recent developments resulting in a more aggressive and curative approach toward tumors of the spinal column, including metastasis,[22, 35, 42] the indications and scope of spinal angiography have broadened. Prior to surgical intervention, it is important not only to know the vascularity of the tumor in order to avoid unexpected excessive bleeding but also to identify the presence of any radiculomedullary arteries to avoid clipping of unrecognized spinal arteries at the time of operation.

With the first description of transfemoral embolizations by Djindjian in 1971, a new era of endovascular treatment has developed. Techniques of superselective catheterizations have rapidly improved, and new catheter systems and embolic materials[4, 5, 12, 44] have been introduced in the last 15 years. The value of endovascular embolization is increasingly recognized, and it has become a valuable tool for preoperative or palliative treatment of vascular neoplasms involving all organ systems. By devascularizing the tumor, surgical resection is now feasible in otherwise inoperable cases.[39, 43] In some instances, unresectable lesions become resectable by decreasing the actual size of a tumor mass. For widespread metastatic lesions, embolization provides symptomatic relief of agonizing pain, resulting in patients becoming less dependent on strong analgesics.[37, 41, 45]

In this chapter, we present our experience of spinal angiography and embolization of spinal tumors from the last 12 years.

VASCULAR ANATOMY OF THE SPINE

Since the introduction of selective catheterizations of the intercostal and lumbar arteries, a number of articles have described angiographic anatomy of the spinal arteries and radiculomedullary branches. Less attention has been paid to the vascular supply of the vertebral bodies. In 1979, Chiras and colleagues[8] described angiographic and anatomic studies of the intercostal and lumbar arteries, including blood supply to the vertebral body and appendages as well as to the muscular branches. In this section, the discussion is focused upon the vascular supply of the spinal column.

Each vertebra is developed from a metamere that gives rise to its own segment of nervous, vascular, musculoskeletal, and cutaneous system. Therefore, the basic vascular supply to each vertebra is essentially the same regardless of its level. However, due to different embryonic development, the arrangement of each pedicle becomes different depending upon the levels of the spinal column. Rather than discussing individual arterial supplies at different levels of the spinal column, we will discuss them by territorial approach.

Arterial supply of the spine can be divided simply into four territories (Fig. 6–1): (1) anterolateral supply, (2) anterior spinal canal supply, (3) posterior spinal canal supply, and (4) posterior supply.

Anterolateral Supply

These are fine perforating branches that enter the anterior and lateral surfaces and supply the anterolateral portion of the vertebral body. In the cervical region, the vertebral and ascending cervical arteries give branches to the corresponding vertebral bodies. In the thoracolumbar region, several osseous branches originate directly from the intercostal or

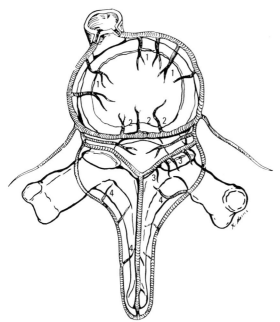

FIGURE 6–1. Vascular supply of the spine: anterolateral supply (1), Anterior spinal canal supply (2), Posterior spinal canal supply (3), Posterior supply (4).

lumbar arteries, which then traverse the vertebral body from the aorta to its lateral surface. Consequently, the right-sided arteries contribute more perforating branches than the left-sided arteries. In the lower lumbar and sacral spines, the midsacral artery is the counterpart of the intercostal or lumbar arteries.

Anterior Spinal Canal Supply

This arterial arcade supplies the posterior surface of the vertebral body. A branch of the dorsal spinal artery enters the spinal canal and then lies underneath the posterior longitudinal ligament. A few perforating branches enter at the posterior surface of the body. In the cervical region, branches originate directly from the vertebral artery and give rise to ascending and descending branches that form a longitudinal anastomosis with corresponding branches of the adjacent levels. Its terminal branches anastomose with the contralateral anterior spinal canal branches. These anastomoses result in a classic ladder pattern or H-shaped arterial arcade on the posterior surface of the vertebral body. In the thoracolumbar region, branches originate from the posterior spinal branch (dorsospinal artery) of the intercostal or lumbar artery. These may originate as a common trunk with the intermediate spinal artery (radiculomedullary artery). A similar vascular pattern can be seen in the lower lumbar and sacral region from the iliolumbar arteries.

Posterior Spinal Canal Supply

These arteries enter the spinal canal posterior to the nerve root, then run through the posterior

epidural space and anastomose with their contralateral counterparts in the midline. The laminae of the spine obtain their blood supply as these arteries enter the spinal canal. There is a somewhat prominent midline branch that penetrates the spinous process from the base and runs posteriorly to the tip of the process. In the cervical region, there are small-caliber posterior spinal canal branches originating from the vertebral artery. In the thoracolumbar region, these arteries originate from the trunk of the dorsispinal artery. As they enter the spinal canal, a descending branch passes along the medial surface of the apophyseal joint and forms a longitudinal anastomosis.

Posterior Supply

The main trunk of the dorsispinal artery passes posteriorly along the outer surface of the lamina and then forms an "open meshed plexus" close to the spinous process. Many fine arteries penetrate the lamina and spinous process from the outer surface. Near the base of the spinous process there is a longitudinal anastomosis with the ipsilateral branch. In the cervical region, the ascending and deep cervical arteries and descending anastomotic branch of the occipital artery provide branches to the posterior element. In the lower lumbar and sacral area, the iliolumbar and lateral sacral arteries represent the corresponding vascular supply.

Anterior Longitudinal Anastomosis

As mentioned above there are many anastomotic channels between the adjacent vertebrae in and out of the spinal canal (Fig. 6–2). However, there are anastomotic branches between the proximal portion of the two intercostal arteries. Chiras and colleagues[8] described two types of anastomosis. One lies on the lateral surface of the vertebral bodies formed by the ascending and descending branches prior to bifurcation of the intercostal arteries. The second type lies in the posterolateral border of the vertebral body. These are seen only in the upper thoracic and lumbar regions. We have seen the anterior longitudinal anastomosis in 10 per cent of the cases in the lower thoracic levels.

SPINAL ANGIOGRAPHY

Indications

Spinal angiography in most instances is performed as a preoperative or prebiopsy evaluation. In other instances, spinal angiography is requested after an unsuccessful attempt to remove the tumor has been aborted because of excessive bleeding. Even though noninvasive diagnostic imaging methods using state-of-the-art equipment in computed tomography (CT)

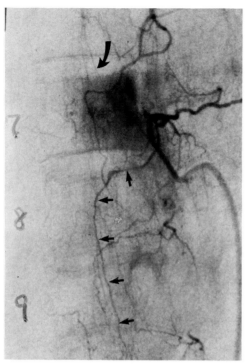

FIGURE 6–2. Normal angiographic appearance of vertebral body in anteroposterior view. Note that a square-shaped hemivertebra is opacified homogeneously. Branches of T8 and T9 intercostal arteries are also opacified by several collaterals from the T7 intercostal artery injection. Small arrows indicate long anastomotic channels. A posterior spinal artery (*curved arrow*) originates from the same pedicle as the anterior spinal canal supply.

and magnetic resonance imaging (MRI) provide extensive information, accurate determination of the vascularity of tumors is still difficult. Indications for spinal angiography largely depend on the nature and extent of the lesion and on the proposed surgical approach.[20, 42] Based on our experience of the last 12 years, we believe the following lesions should be evaluated by spinal angiography:

1. Tumors that are to be removed by a transthoracic or transabdominal approach in order to localize the spinal arteries.

2. Tumors of the cervical and lower thoracic upper lumbar spine where the anterior spinal artery frequently originates.

3. Tumors with moderate to high enhancement on the contrast-enhanced CT scan.

4. Tumors with signal void areas on MRI which are suggestive of high blood flow.

5. Tumors of known vascular origin.

6. Tumors to be treated by embolization or chemoembolization.

Angiographic Protocol

We suggest the following angiographic protocol for thorough evaluation of the lesions. As indicated in the section on vascular anatomy, different levels of the spinal column have different vascular arrangements. The origins and names are different, especially in the cervical and lower lumbosacral regions. For practical purposes we have divided the spinal column into five regions. The following list includes all possible arterial supplies to a given tumor in the corresponding region. Is it necessary to do the selective catheterization of individual arteries? We believe that once a decision is made to study a vascular lesion by angiography, all possible information should be obtained. Global injection of the aorta or subclavian artery will provide an answer as to whether or not a tumor is highly vascular. Certain tumors with a low or moderate vascularity may not be recognized as vascular, and dangerous anastomosis may be unrecognized by a global study. We therefore insist that all arteries be studied by selective catheterization. In addition, the spine is a midline structure. Therefore, all the angiograms should include bilateral studies.

The arteries to be evaluated are:

1. Upper cervical region (C1–C4) (Fig. 6–3)
   Vertebral artery
   Occipital artery
   Ascending pharyngeal artery
   Thyrocervical trunk (ascending cervical artery)
   Costocervical trunk (deep cervical artery)

2. Lower cervical region (C5–C7)
   Vertebral artery
   Thyrocervical trunk (ascending cervical artery)
   Costocervical trunk (deep cervical artery)
   Supreme intercostal artery

3. Upper thoracic region (T1–T4) (Fig. 6–4)
   Supreme intercostal artery
   Thyrocervical trunk (superior intercostal artery)
   Costocervical trunk

4. Thoracic and upper lumbar region (T5–L3) (Fig. 6–5)
   Intercostal or lumbar arteries of involved level
   Intercostal arteries two levels above and two levels below the involved segment

5. Lower lumbar and sacral regions (L4–sacrum)
   Lower lumbar arteries (L3 and L4)
   Iliolumbar artery
   Lateral sacral artery
   Median sacral artery

Many symptomatic vertebral tumors are not confined to the spine itself. For example, even benign hemangiomas often have extraspinal components that are seen at the time of surgery.[19] As the tumor grows into the adjacent vertebra or extends into the paraspinal space, new vascular supplies are recruited.[21] By a systemic study outlined in the above protocol, all possible arterial supplies can be thoroughly evaluated and the presence of a spinal artery can be documented. In addition, if embolization is attempted, it is important to know the anastomosis surrounding the lesion in order to prevent inadvertent embolization of a spinal artery (see Fig. 6–4C).

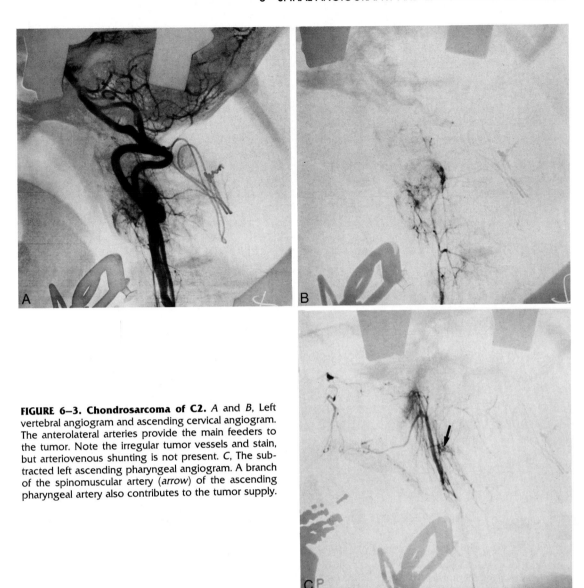

FIGURE 6–3. Chondrosarcoma of C2. *A* and *B*, Left vertebral angiogram and ascending cervical angiogram. The anterolateral arteries provide the main feeders to the tumor. Note the irregular tumor vessels and stain, but arteriovenous shunting is not present. *C*, The subtracted left ascending pharyngeal angiogram. A branch of the spinomuscular artery (*arrow*) of the ascending pharyngeal artery also contributes to the tumor supply.

Technique

Since each institution has different approaches, and individual preferences for catheters and techniques vary, it is difficult to standardize angiographic techniques. However, we would like to describe our own techniques and catheter systems.

The patient is routinely sedated by neuroleptic analgesia or anesthesia with Phentanyl and droperidol. These analgesics are least likely to interfere with the somatosensory evoked potential monitoring, which will be discussed below.

Our standard approach is the femoral route unless selective catheterizations of the feeders had previously failed, in which case an axillary approach is chosen. An introducer sheath (7 French) is used for easy catheter exchanges.[4] Several preshaped spinal catheters in different sizes are commercially available, but some angiographers shape their own curves depending upon difficulty of selective catheterizations

of the intercostal or lumbar arteries. Several types of catheters may be necessary to complete the angiography, since the angulation of the origin of the artery from the aorta changes gradually from the supreme intercostal to the lower lumbar artery. Further, the diameter of the aorta varies from thoracic to abdominal levels. We frequently use H1H, HS1, HS2 catheters (5.7, 6.5, or 7 French, Cook) and Cobra 1 (7 French, USCI) and/or Mikaelsson catheter (7 French).

Angiography can be recorded by the digital subtraction angiogram (DSA) technique or by the film-screen combination technique. DSA is especially useful for embolization procedures since it eliminates all bony densities during the injections of the embolic material. If the patient has undergone surgical intervention previously, metallic devices for stabilization of the spine may obscure the spinal arteries. In these situations, oblique or lateral views are necessary to visualize any intradural vessels.

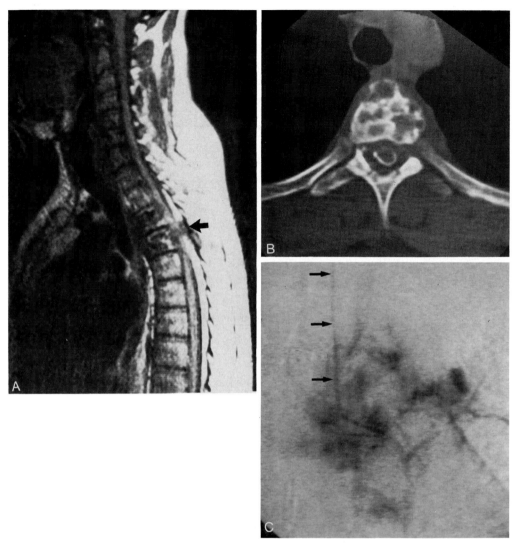

FIGURE 6–4. Hemangioma of T4 and T5 with unusual radiographic findings. *A,* Magnetic resonance T1-weighted image. Destruction of T4 and T5 (low signal) with epidural compression is seen. The posterior element of T5 (*arrow*) is also destroyed. *B,* Myelogram/CT scan at T5 level. Incomplete block by the extraspinal component is clearly seen. Note atypical large areas of destruction. *C,* Digital subtraction angiogram of left T4 intercostal artery. Irregular tumor stain is seen, which is different from that in Figure 6–5*B* and *C.* The histologic diagnosis is ordinary hemangioma. Small arrows point to the anterior spinal artery. Therefore, this pedicle could not be embolized.

Spinal Cord Monitoring

Somatosensory evoked potentials (SEPs) have been proven effective in functional monitoring of the spinal cord in cases of spinal cord injury as well as with orthopedic or neurosurgical procedures of the spine or spinal cord. We use SEP monitoring during spinal angiography and endovascular embolization to minimize the complication rate, which has previously been reported as high as 10–15 per cent.[16] With the use of SEPs our complication rate has been lowered to less than 1 per cent. This technique has proven to be very sensitive and effective in recognizing spinal arteries, especially the anterior spinal artery.[2, 25, 47] When contrast material is injected into the anterior spinal artery, the SEPs immediately decrease in amplitude, and at times this is associated with an increase in latency. Since the SEP is monitoring the posterior columns that are primarily supplied by the posterior spinal artery, there are several possible explanations for this SEP change. One is an increased potassium ion level in the extracellular space induced by ischemia or cellular toxicity of the contrast material. However, the exact neurophysiologic changes have not yet been proved, and further studies may be necessary to understand SEP changes and their significance. Our clinical experience suggests that the presence of the anterior spinal artery can be recognized by SEP changes in over 80 per cent of cases prior to angiographic confirmation.

SEPs are also useful to monitor the actual embolizations. Even though SEPs fluctuate due to different factors and conditions (depth of anesthesia, anesthetic agent, level of consciousness, and so forth),

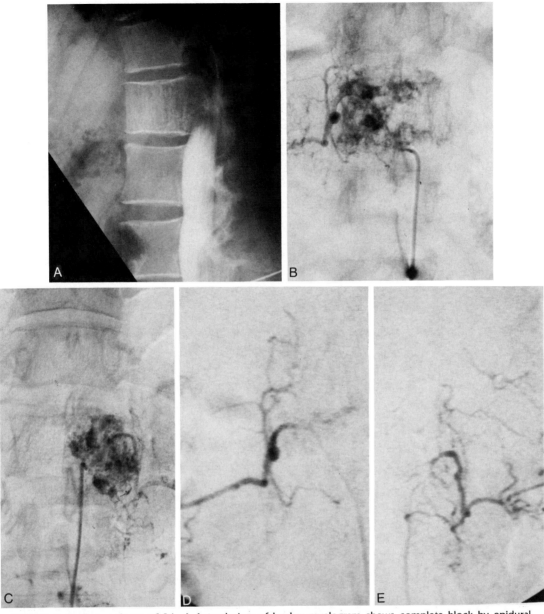

FIGURE 6–5. Hemangioma of L1. *A,* Lateral view of lumbar myelogram shows complete block by epidural extension of the tumor. Note the typical plain radiographic appearance of the vertebral hemangioma. *B* and *C,* Digital subtraction angiograms of the right and left L1 lumbar arteries; punctate contrast pools of various sizes without enlargement of feeding artery and arteriovenous shunting are the typical angiographic findings of hemangioma. *D* and *E,* Postembolization (PE) digital subtraction angiograms of the right and left L1 lumbar arteries. All tumor feeders were embolized with polyvinyl alcohol foam particles (149 to 250 microns). The T12 and L2 branches are also opacified through collaterals without further supply to the tumor. If the proximal trunk of the lumbar artery were embolized, these collaterals would take over supply to the tumor immediately.

they provide important warning signals during injection of embolic material. In cases in which there is decrease of amplitude of SEPs, embolization is stopped until the SEPs return to baseline. SEPs are also excellent physiologic indicators for provocative tests to be discussed later. The basic technique and findings have been discussed in a previous report.[2]

Provocative Test

In many instances, the anterior or posterior spinal artery can be readily recognized in conventional or digital subtraction angiography. Occasionally it may not be possible to document the presence of the spinal artery due to patient motion, subtraction artifacts, or confusion with other long anastomotic vessels. If there is any doubt, we perform a provocative test with Amytal Sodium (amobarbital sodium). This short-acting barbiturate is used to determine the dominance of the cerebral hemispheres prior to neurosurgical procedures (Wada test). We have applied this principle to evaluate the territory to be embolized, especially for intracerebral or intraspinal arteriovenous malformations. Fifty to 70 mg of Amytal Sodium (25 mg/cc dilution) is injected in the artery

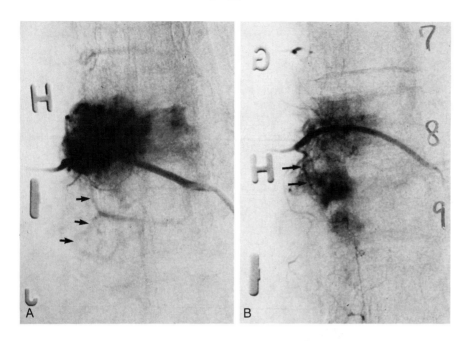

FIGURE 6–6. Plasmocytoma of T9. *A,* Right T9 angiogram demonstrates dense irregular tumor stain with arteriovenous shunting. Note extension of tumor stain to the left hemivertebra, which is often seen in malignant lesions. Small arrows indicate draining veins. *B,* Right T8 angiogram shows parasitic supply *(arrows)* due to extension of tumor into the paraspinal and intervertebral spaces.

to be embolized, and neurologic status is monitored clinically and electrophysiologically. If this test is positive, embolization is aborted. There may be false-negative tests with arteriovenous malformations due to high flow and "sump effect." We have not experienced any false-negative tests in cases of spinal tumors. Injection of xylocaine has been proposed for similar purposes in the spinal cord, but we have no experience with it.

Angiographic Findings

In general, the angiographic findings of spinal tumors are not pathognomonic, except for a few benign lesions such as vertebral hemangiomas and osteoid osteomas. Voegeli and Fuchs[46] have stated that arteriography in bone tumors increases the accuracy of the histologic diagnosis by 20 per cent. As illustrated in Figures 6–6 and 6–7, two lesions can have similar vascular patterns; however, these are two different malignant tumors. One is a plasmacytoma, the other is a Ewing's sarcoma. Therefore, analysis of the angiography should emphasize the differentiation between benign and malignant neoplasms, the extent of tumor, and recognition of spinal arteries (see Fig. 6–4C). The identification of typical vascular patterns may help to differentiate certain benign tumors.

Benign Tumors

HEMANGIOMA (see Figs. 6–4 and 6–5)

Hemangioma is the most common benign vascular tumor in the spine. On conventional radiography, the typical findings include a striated appearance of the vertebral body with thick trabeculations (Fig. 6–5A). Hemangiomas are often found incidentally. The usual presenting symptoms are backache, segmental

pain, and/or progressive paraparesis. Sudden paraplegia may occur due to compression fractures of the affected vertebra.[23] The angiographic appearances are well recognized.[1, 14, 19] In general, the caliber of the corresponding intercostal artery is not enlarged. There is irregular opacification of the vertebral body with a small pocket of contrast pooling. These pools of contrast are of various size, without arteriovenous (AV) shunting, and persist in the late venous phase (Fig. 6–5). The draining veins are not dilated. Occasionally, atypical irregular vascular pools and stains may be seen which suggest a malignant lesion (Fig. 6–4). However, the lack of AV shunting and a normal caliber filling artery suggests a nonmalignant tumor. In its early stages, the tumor is confined to the vertebral body. However, most symptomatic lesions have paraspinal or epidural extension that is easily

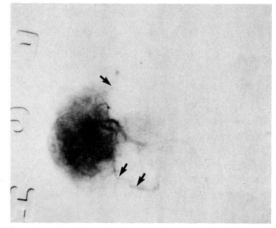

FIGURE 6–7. Ewing's sarcoma of T9. Right T9 angiogram demonstrates irregular neovascularity with dense tumor stain. Early draining veins *(arrows)* are clearly seen. Compared with Figure 6–6A there is no specific angiographic feature. For malignant spinal tumors, angiographic differentiation is difficult.

recognized on CT scan[19] (Fig. 6–4*B*). There may be multiple hemangiomas in the spine, or they may be associated with hemangiomas elsewhere in the body.

ANEURYSMAL BONE CYST

A ballooned-out distention of subperiosteal shell of bone with eccentric destruction of underlying cortex and cancellous bone is the typical radiographic appearance.[32] Paraspinal extension is common. The angiographic pictures are similar to the lesions of long bones.[31] The feeding arteries are usually dilated, and the cystic area is often opacified by contrast in the late arterial phase. The tumor stain is often patchy and remains to the venous phase. Lindbom and colleagues suggest that patchy opacification could be due to wash-out by unopacified blood through the cystic areas. There may be some degree of AV shunting but not as intense as is seen in malignant tumors.

GIANT CELL TUMORS

Giant cell tumors, classically described by Jaffe and colleagues, are now regarded as benign aggressive or occasionally malignant neoplasms. In the spinal column, the sacrum is most commonly involved, and cervical and thoracic spines are rarely affected.[13] Since the angiographic findings for giant cell tumors are similar to those for aneurysmal bone cysts, they are described in this section for comparison.

These tumors are highly vascular and the feeding arteries are dilated. Multiple dilated feeders can be seen on the surface which then enter the tumor. Dense irregular tumor stains are common. The center of the tumor may show lack of stain. Arteriovenous shunting and early venous return are part of the usual picture. The differentiation from aneurysmal bone cysts or hypervascular malignant tumors may be difficult.

OTHER VASCULAR BENIGN TUMORS

Spinal angiography for other benign tumors is not commonly performed, since conventional radiology and the CT scan are more useful for specific diagnosis.

Malignant Tumors

Because we believe that the differential diagnosis among malignant tumors is not practical, only the general angiographic findings of malignancy will be discussed.

1. The feeding arteries are usually dilated and small osseous branches are recognizable. There may be an increased number of these vessels, with caliber being somewhat irregular, and abrupt angulations may be seen.

2. Vascularity may vary from lesion to lesion. Compared with benign lesions, tumor stains are seen earlier, and irregular vascular lakes are often present. The tumor vessels are irregular in caliber and have a distorted course with abrupt angulations within the tumor.

3. Venous drainage often shows AV shunting.

Early filling of the epidural or paravertebral venous plexuses is common. The draining veins may or may not be dilated.

As discussed previously, malignant lesions often extend to the adjacent vertebrae and recruit a parasitic supply (Fig. 6–6). To recognize the extent of the lesion, the boundary of the tumor must be identified by studying *all* possible collateral circulations.

EMBOLIZATION

Since the introduction of selective spinal angiography followed by the development of selective endovascular embolization,[15] many reports have been published on the value of embolization of vascular tumors of the spine.[1, 7, 19, 45] Repeatedly it has been proven that embolization can reduce mass effect, relieve spinal block,[24] and eventually reduce symptoms.[37, 41] Embolization is not a curative treatment for spinal tumors, but it can palliate immediate symptoms, mainly intolerable pain, and can possibly retard tumor growth.[45] When surgical intervention is indicated, preoperative embolization sometimes allows the tumor to be totally resected.[43] Moreover, tumors that are considered unresectable may become resectable after embolization. As a preoperative or palliative measure, embolization is now an accepted mode of treatment for many benign or malignant vascular tumors of the spine.[7]

In the last 15 years, techniques of embolization have progressed rapidly in conjunction with new developments of catheter systems and embolic materials. In order to maximize the effects of embolization, several factors have to be considered.

1. The anatomy and flow characteristics in a given tumor.

2. The size and physical characteristics of the catheter system to be used.

3. The position of the catheter tip.

4. The physical, chemical, and biologic characteristics of the embolic material.

5. The goal of the embolization: preoperative, prebiopsy, or palliative.

6. The type of lesion: benign or malignant.

These factors will help to determine proper selection of the embolic agent so that the best and safest results can be obtained. Various embolic materials are available as shown in Table 6–1. The following are commonly used.

Gelfoam. Gelfoam is available in powder form with particle sizes of 40 to 60 microns. These penetrate into the tumor beds, producing perivascular necrosis. However, these particles are smaller than the caliber of the dangerous anastomosis and of certain AV shunts. We have not had satisfactory results in using Gelfoam powder for spinal tumors. Strips or large particles have been used by other authors.[23] However, these do not penetrate into the tumor bed, which therefore will be resupplied by collateral vessels.

Polyvinyl alcohol foam (PVA).[3, 44] PVA is a non-

TABLE 6–1. EMBOLIC AGENTS

Absorbable solid particles
Autologous blood clot
Gelatin sponge and/or powder (Gelfoam)
Oxidized cellulose (Oxycel)
Microfibrillar collagen (Avitene, Angiostat)
Glutaraldehyde cross-linked collagen (GAX)
Nonabsorbable solids
Lyophilized dura (Lyodura)
Polyvinyl alcohol foam (PVA, Ivalon)
Silastic beads
Steel coils
Fluids
Low-viscosity silicone rubber
Isobutyl-2-cyanoacrylate (IBCA)
N-butyl-cyanoacrylate (NBCA)
95% ethanol
Ethanol in various concentrations
Opacificants
Tantalum dust (1–2 microns)
Tantalum oxide (1–2 microns)
Retardants
Iophendylate (Pantopaque)
Acetic acid

absorbable biocompatible sponge material. A particulate form is used on most occasions. Particulate PVA varies in size from 149 to 1000 microns (149–250, 250–590, or 590–1000 microns). It is prepared in sterile water and is then autoclaved.[3] These particles can be easily injected through conventional or coaxial catheter systems, and they penetrate into the vascular bed (Fig. 6–5D and E). Various concentrations of PVA suspensions can be used depending upon flow rate and vascularity of a given tumor. If there are any dangerous anastomoses, particles larger than the caliber of anastomotic vessels are needed to prevent inadvertent embolization. Consequently, PVA is an excellent embolic agent for preoperative devascularization of tumors.

Stainless steel coils. Metallic Gianturco coils are small, short pieces of guidewire to which a Dacron thread is attached to promote thrombosis. The coil occludes the artery at the point of exit from the catheter tip. If it is used alone, it gives the same effect as surgical ligation of the feeding intercostal artery. It can be used in conjunction with particle embolization. Following injection of particles (PVA or Gelfoam), stainless steel coils can occlude the trunk of the feeding artery and maximize the effect of particle embolization.

Isobutyl-2-cyanoacrylate (IBCA).[12] IBCA is a low viscosity liquid that polymerizes quickly when in contact with ions or changes in pH. It has tissue adhesive properties and causes an inflammatory reaction of the vascular walls. It is useful for recurrent or unresectable tumors as well as for tumors with fast AV shunting. Polymerization time can be delayed by adding pantopaque so that the distal tumor bed can be reached. It is not commonly used for tumors because it is difficult to handle and a great deal of experience is needed for proper use. Furthermore, there is controversy related to the carcinogenicity of IBCA. It is not obtainable at the present time.

Ethyl alcohol. Ellman and colleagues[18] and Eke-

lund and coworkers[17] have reported the value of absolute alcohol as an embolic agent. When ethyl alcohol is injected intravascularly, it causes intimal damage and sludging of blood cellular elements, which then produce mechanical emboli. Latchaw and colleagues[29] have reported the long-term effect of intraarterial ethanol infusion. For up to 91 days, there was complete vascular occlusion and permanent infarction without evidence of recanalization. Its flow characteristics, availability, and effectiveness as a long-term occlusive agent make ethanol the best embolic agent for vascular tumors. However, if inadvertently perfused into normal tissue, serious complications can occur. During renal artery embolization, bowel infarction due to reflux into the aorta has been reported.[10, 34] It can also cause extensive skin necrosis if it enters cutaneous branches. Therefore, we limit the use of ethanol to embolization of malignant tumors.

Ninety-five per cent ethyl alcohol is opacified by metrizamide powder, which enables it to be seen under fluoroscopy. It is used *only* when superselective catheterization of the tumor-feeding pedicle can be accomplished. Two to 3 cc of opacified ethanol is injected slowly each time. Because of low viscosity, it can easily reflux to the normal territory. Therefore, at the end stage of embolization, small quantities (0.5 to 1 cc) should be injected at a slower rate. For larger and highly vascular lesions, ethanol can be mixed with PVA particles. The PVA provides mechanical occlusion and increases stasis of alcohol in the neovascular region. As illustrated in Figure 6–8, significant tumor necrosis can be achieved by alcohol embolization.

Several other embolic materials have been used clinically. Bovine dura mater in particulate form is commonly used in Europe. It is not available in the United States. Silicone fluid was first introduced as an embolic agent in 1978 by Hilal and coworkers.[27] It can penetrate into the smaller feeders and forms a complete cast of the major tumor supply.[36] The disadvantages of silicone fluid are that it is difficult to handle and it requires catheters with larger lumens due to high viscosity. Since it does not have adhesive properties, it can easily pass into the venous circulation if fast AV shunting is present.

Direct retrograde injection of methyl methacrylate into a hemangioma of vertebral body was reported recently by Nicola and Lins.[38] Following transarterial embolizations, laminectomy was performed and methyl methacrylate was injected through a cannula positioned in the vascular pedicles. Authors claimed that polymerized acrylate supports a weakened vertebral body so that no further stabilizations are necessary. Its long-term effects have not been reported.

CHEMOEMBOLIZATION

The term chemoembolization was first introduced by Kato and Nemoto in 1978.[28] In order to increase the topical release of an active anticancerous agent in high concentrations, they prepared mitomycin-C

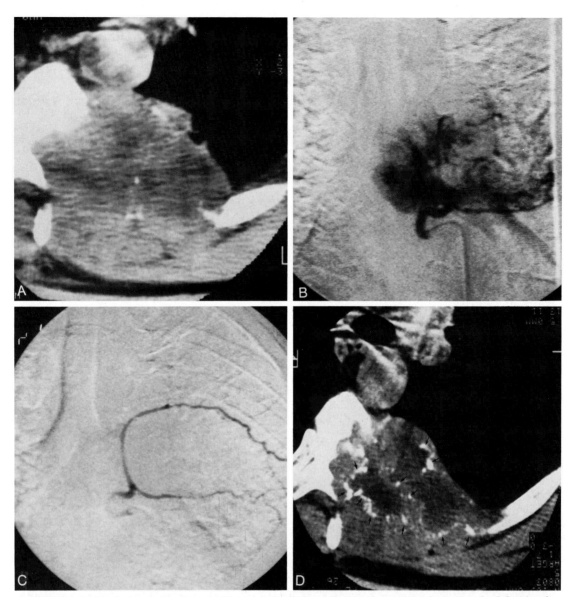

FIGURE 6–8. Alcohol embolization. *A*, CT scan at the T5 level shows a large mass destroying the left side of T5 including the posterior elements and the proximal portion of the rib. *B*, Selective digital subtraction angiogram of left T5 intercostal artery. Despite large volume injection (10 cc), only a portion of the tumor is opacified. *C*, Postembolization control angiogram of left T5. The tumor was embolized with 95 per cent ethanol for a total of 25 cc in the first procedure. Further embolization was performed two days later. Thirty cc more of ethanol mixed with PVA particles (149 to 250 microns) was then injected. Complete obliteration of the tumor stain was accomplished. *D*, Follow-up CT scan after one month at the same level. Note marked reduction of mass effect. The hypodense areas within the tumor are believed to be necrosis. Small increased densities at the periphery are PVA particles in the tumor vessels (*small arrows*).

microcapsules with particle size of 224.6 ± 45.9 microns and injected these particles through the angiographic catheter to the target organ. The microcapsules produced local ischemia, and the sustained release of mitomycin-C from the capsule increased the duration of contact between the drug and target cells.

Courtheoux and colleagues reported their experience of chemoembolization of spine metastases in 1985.[8] Mitomycin-C microcapsules or Adriamycin mixed with dura mater was used. Improvement of clinical symptoms, pain, and neurologic deficits was noticed in 58 months of follow-up.

Early results of chemoembolization indicate that it can be an excellent palliative treatment for unresectable metastases. Further clinical and pharmacologic studies are needed in conjunction with comparative studies with other cytotoxic embolic agents such as ethyl alcohol.

REFERENCES

1. Benati A, Da Pian R, Mazza C, et al: Preoperative embolisation of a vertebral haemangioma compressing the spinal cord. Neuroradiology 7:181–183, 1974.
2. Berenstein A, Young W, Ransohoff J, et al: Somatosensory

evoked potentials during spinal angiography and therapeutic transvascular embolization. J Neurosurg 60:777–785, 1984.

3. Berenstein A, Graeb D: Convenient preparation of ready to use particles in polyvinyl alcohol foam suspensions for embolization. Radiology 145:38–46, 1982.

4. Berenstein A, Kricheff II: Catheters and material selections for transarterial embolization: Technical considerations. I. Catheters. Radiology 132:619–631, 1979.

5. Berenstein A, Kricheff II: Catheter and material selections for transarterial embolization: Technical considerations. II. Materials. Radiology 132:631–641, 1979.

6. Blaylock R, Kempe L: Chondrosarcoma of the cervical spine. J Neurosurg 44:500–503, 1976.

7. Bowers T, Murray J, Charnsangavej C, et al: Bone metastases from renal carcinoma. J Bone Joint Surg 64A:749–754, 1982.

8. Chiras J, Morvan G, Merland JJ: The angiographic appearances of the normal intercostal and lumbar arteries. Analysis and the anatomic correlation of the lateral branches. J Neuroradiol 6:169–196, 1979.

9. Courtheoux P, Alachkar F, Casasco A, et al: Chimioembolisation des metastases du rachis lombaire. J Neuroradiol 12:151–162, 1985.

10. Cox GG, Lee KR, Price HI, et al: Colonic infarctions following ethanol embolizations of renal-cell carcinoma. Radiology 145:343–345, 1982.

11. Crock HV, Yoshizaua H: Origins of arteries supplying the vertebral column. *In* Crock HV, Yoshizaua H (eds): The Blood Supply of the Vertebral Column and Spinal Cord in Man. New York, Springer-Verlag, 1977, pp 1–21.

12. Cromwell KD, Kerber CW: Modification of cyanoacrylate for therapeutic embolization: Preliminary experience. AJR 132:779–801, 1979.

13. Dahlin D: Giant-cell tumor of vertebrae above the sacrum. Cancer 39:1350–1356, 1977.

14. Djindjian R, Merland JJ: Angiography of Spinal Column and Spinal Cord Tumors. Stuttgart, Georg Thiem Verlag, 1981.

15. Djindjian R, Cophignon J, Rey A, et al: Superselective arteriographic embolizations by the femoral route in neuroradiology, study of 50 cases: Embolizations in vertebro medullary pathology. Neuroradiology 6:132–142, 1973.

16. Doppman JL, DiChiro G: Risks and complications. *In* Doppman JL, DiChiro G, and Ommaya AK (eds): Selective Angiography of the Spinal Cord. St. Louis, Warren H Green, Inc., 1969, pp 51–58.

17. Ekelund L, Jonsson N, Trengut H: Transcatheter obliterations of the renal artery by ethanol injection: Experimental results. Cardiovasc Intervent Radiol 4:1–7, 1981.

18. Ellman B, Green CE, Eigenbradt E, et al: Renal infarction with absolute ethanol. Int Rad 15:318–322, 1980.

19. Esparza J, Castro S, Portillo J, et al: Vertebral hemangiomas: Spinal angiography and preoperative embolization. Surg Neurol 10:171–173, 1978.

20. Fielding W, Pyle R, Fietti V: Anterior cervical vertebral body resection and bone-grafting for benign and malignant tumors. J Bone Joint Surg 61A:251–253, 1979.

21. Folkman J: The vascularization of tumors. Sci Am 234:59–70, 1976.

22. Gilbert R, Kim J, Posner J: Epidural spinal cord compression from metastatic tumor: Diagnosis and treatment. Ann Neurol 3:40–51, 1978.

23. Graham J, Yang W: Vertebral hemangioma with compression fracture and paraparesis treated with preoperative embolization and vertebral resection. Spine 9:97–101, 1984.

24. Gross C, Hodge C, Binet E, et al: Relief of spinal block during embolization of a vertebral body hemangioma. J Neurosurg 45:327–330, 1976.

25. Hacke W: Neuromonitoring. Neurology 232:125–133, 1985.

26. Hastings D, Macnab I, Lawson V: Neoplasms of the atlas and axis. Can J Surg 11:290–296, 1968.

27. Hilal SK, Sane P, MiChilson WJ: The embolization of vascular malformations of spinal cord with low viscosity silicone rubber. Neuroradiology 16:430–433, 1978.

28. Kato T, Nemoto R: Microencapsulation of mitomycin C for intra-arterial infusion chemotherapy. Proc Japan Acad 54B:413–417, 1978.

29. Latshaw RF, Pearlman RL, Schaitkin BM, et al: Intraarterial ethanol as a long-term occlusive agent in renal hepatic and gastrosplenic arteries of pigs. Cardiovasc Intervent Radiol 8:24–30, 1985.

30. Laurin S: Angiography in giant cell tumors. Radiologe 17:118–123, 1977.

31. Lindbom A, Soderberg G, Spjut H, et al: Angiography of aneurysmal bone cyst. Acta Radiol 55:12–16, 1961.

32. MacCarty C, Dahlin D, Doyle J, et al: Aneurysmal bone cysts of the neural axis. J Neurosurg 18:671–677, 1981.

33. Maclellan D, Wilson F: Osteoid osteoma of the spine. J Bone Joint Surg 49A:111–121, 1967.

34. Malligan BD, Espimosa GA: Bowel infarctions: Complications of ethanol ablation of a renal tumor. Cardiovasc Intervent Radiol 6:55–57, 1983.

35. Marshall L, Langfitt T: Combined therapy for metastatic extradural tumors of the spine. Cancer 40:2067–2070, 1977.

36. Muraszko K, Antunes L, Hilal S, et al: Hemangiopericytomas of the spine. Neurosurgery 10:473–479, 1982.

37. Nickolisen R, Fallon B: Locally recurrent hypernephroma treated by radiation therapy and embolization. Cancer 56:1049–1051, 1985.

38. Nicola N, Lins E: Vertebral hemangioma: Retrograde embolization-stabilization with methyl methacrylate. Surg Neurol 27:481–486, 1987.

39. Roy-Camille R, Chiras J, Gagna G, et al: L'interet de l'arteriographie dans la chirurgie rachidienne. Chirurgie 112:567–570, 1986.

40. Slatkin N, Posner J: Management of spinal epidural metastases. Clin Neurosurg 30:698–716, 1984.

41. Soo C, Wallace S, Chuang V, et al: Lumbar artery embolization in cancer patients. Radiology 145:655–659, 1982.

42. Sundaresan N, Galicich J, Lane J, et al: Treatment of neoplastic epidural cord compression by vertebral body resection and stabilization. J Neurosurg 63:676–684, 1985.

43. Sundaresan N, Scher H, DiGiacinto G, et al: Surgical treatment of spinal cord compression in kidney cancer. J Clin Oncol 4:1851–1856, 1986.

44. Tadavarthy SM, Moller JH: Polyvinyl alcohol (Ivalon): A new embolic material. AJR 125:609–616, 1974.

45. Treves R, Legoff J, Doyon D, et al: L'embolisation therapeutique ou embolisation palliative à visée antalgigue des metastases osseuses d'origine renale. Rev Rhum 51:1–5, 1984.

46. Voegeli E, Fuchs W: Arteriography in bone tumours. Br J Radiol 49:407–415, 1976.

47. Young W, Berenstein A: Somatosensory evoked potential monitoring of intraoperable procedures. *In* Schramm J, Jones SJ (eds): Spinal Cord Monitoring. Heidelberg, Springer-Verlag, 1985, pp 197–203.

AN ATLAS OF LESIONS THAT MAY RESEMBLE TUMORS ON RADIOGRAPHS

HERBERT ROSENTHAL and DANIEL I. ROSENTHAL

The following illustrations show conditions such as genetic defects that may cause confusion during the process of diagnosis by their resemblance to malignant neoplasms. The correct diagnoses are given along with a succinct discussion of the particular condition.

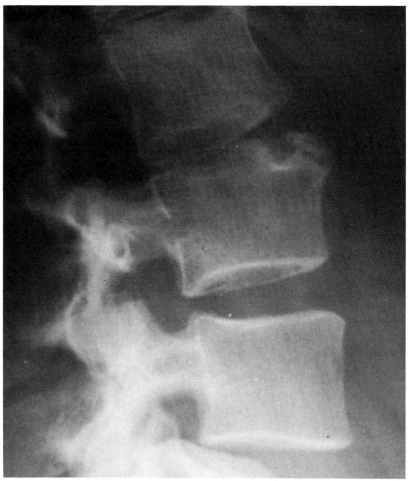

FIGURE 7–1. A 33-year-old female.

Description: A lateral plain film shows a deformity of the anterior margin of the upper end plate of L3. A 1-cm diameter triangular bony fragment is separated from the vertebral body. The opposing margins are sclerotic.

Diagnosis: Limbus vertebra.

Discussion: The limbus vertebra results from herniation of disc material during childhood. This herniation separates a part of the ring apophysis that continues to ossify as a triangular-shaped isolated bony fragment.[8] The anterosuperior corner of a single vertebral body in the midlumbar spine is most frequently affected.

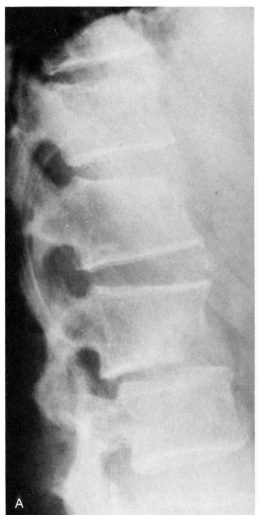

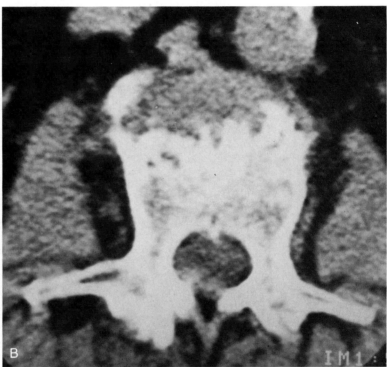

FIGURE 7–2. A 73-year-old male.

Description: A lateral plain film (A) of the thoracolumbar junction shows an osteolytic defect of L2. There is a complete absence of the inferior corner of the vertebral body, surrounded by a faint zone of sclerosis. The adjacent superior end plate of L3 seems intact. Significant narrowing of the intervertebral disc and retrolisthesis of the vertebral segment T12 and L1 are noted. The CT (B) at the level of destruction shows no paravertebral soft tissue mass. There is irregular but sclerotic margin of destruction.

Diagnosis: Intravertebral disc herniation.

Discussion: This is an uncommon presentation of a common disorder. Although the amount of bone destruction is usually less extensive, other diagnoses are even less likely. The disc space narrowing is not generally associated with tumors, although intravertebral disc herniations into areas of metastatic bone destruction have been described.[20] An infection with this amount of bone destruction should have affected the adjacent vertebral body. Small Schmorl's nodes at T12 and L1 increase the level of confidence.[24]

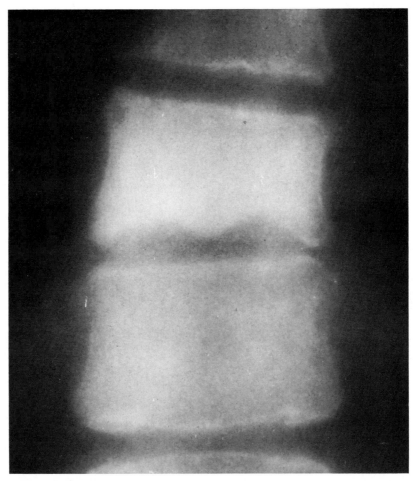

FIGURE 7–3. A 13-year-old male.

Description: An anteroposterior tomogram of T11 shows a slight sclerosis of the whole vertebral body with loss of height and irregular inferior end plate.

Diagnosis: Juvenile kyphosis (Scheuermann's disease) with intravertebral disc herniation.

Discussion: Juvenile kyphosis is a common disorder characterized by irregular end plates due to multiple intravertebral disc herniations. It is predominantly seen in the low thoracic and upper lumbar spine. Exaggerated kyphosis and anterior wedging of the affected vertebral bodies may or may not be associated with clinical symptoms. Sclerotic changes are uncommon.[23]

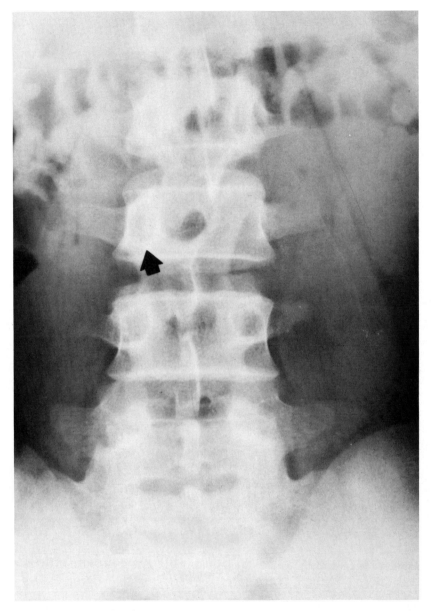

FIGURE 7–4. A 24-year-old male.

Diagnosis: Congenitally absent pedicle.

Discussion: Congenital absence of a pedicle is a rare developmental anomaly.[29] It has to be differentiated from osteolytic destruction due to tumors. The hyperplasia of the contralateral side offers a valuable clue in the differential diagnosis. Radionuclide scan may reveal increased uptake in the sclerotic pedicle.[16] This variable degree of hypertrophy may also be found opposite hypoplastic pedicles.[2]

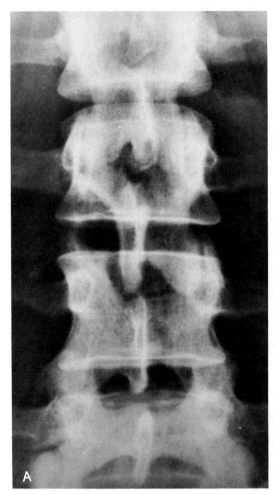
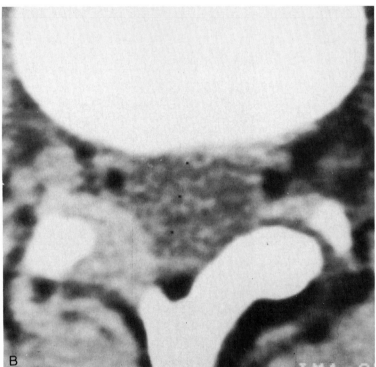

FIGURE 7–5. A 23-year-old female.

Description: Anteroposterior plain film (*A*) of the midlumbar spine shows a defect of the posterior elements at L3/L4 with absent apophyseal joint on the right side. An axial CT scan (*B*) reveals replacement of the right posterior lamina at this level with soft tissue density.

Diagnosis: Spinal anomaly with defect of posterior elements.

Discussion: Developmental defects of the posterior elements of the spine may be variable and may include the apophyseal joints.[13] The extent of the defect is best demonstrated on CT scans.[29] Recognition of the anomaly is important to prevent unnecessary surgery.

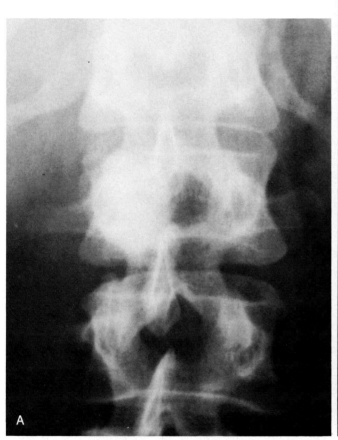

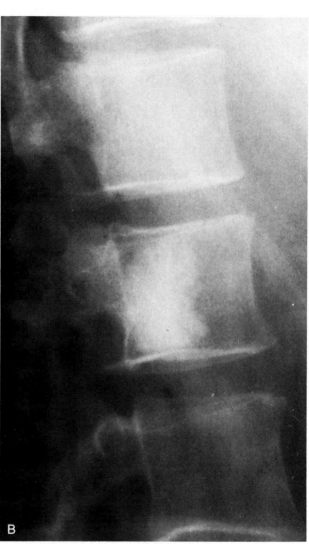

FIGURE 7–6. A 46-year-old female.

Description: The anteroposterior and lateral plain films of L1 reveal a 3-cm area of dense sclerosis in the right posterior part of the vertebral body. No osteolytic changes are detectable. The lesion has sharp borders, and there is no evidence of cortical destruction.

Diagnosis: Bone island.

Discussion: Bone islands are areas of mature bone producing a dense sclerosis within normal trabecular bone. They are asymptomatic.[19] Although usually located in the pelvis or proximal femur and measuring up to 1 cm in size, they can occur in all parts of the body. So-called giant bone islands are rare.[26] The films are useful in distinguishing them from other significant pathologic processes such as osteoblastic metastases. Bone islands may be static for many years but can either grow slowly or regress.[14]

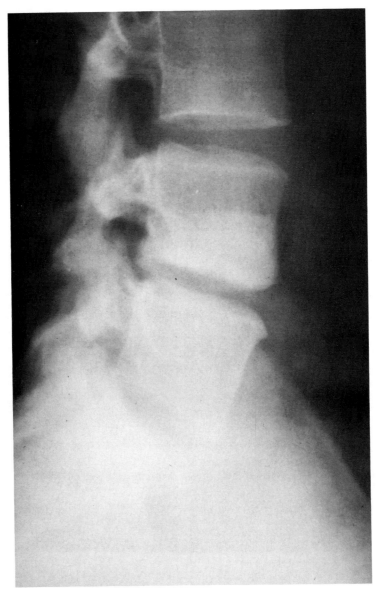

FIGURE 7–7. A 45-year-old male.

Description: A lateral plain film of the lower lumbar spine demonstrates an area of sclerosis of L4 adjacent to the inferior end plate with involvement of the lower half of the vertebral body. No osteolytic destructions are noticed. There is significant loss of disc height at the affected level.

Diagnosis: Discogenic sclerosis.

Discussion: Sclerotic changes of vertebral bodies are common findings in degenerative disc disease.[18] In some cases these sclerotic changes may be the predominant finding, involving large parts of the trabecular bone. Sclerosis may take several forms, often involving the anteroinferior aspect of the vertebral bodies and having a hemispherical shape. Disc space narrowing may be minimal, and degenerative spurs are usually absent.[12]

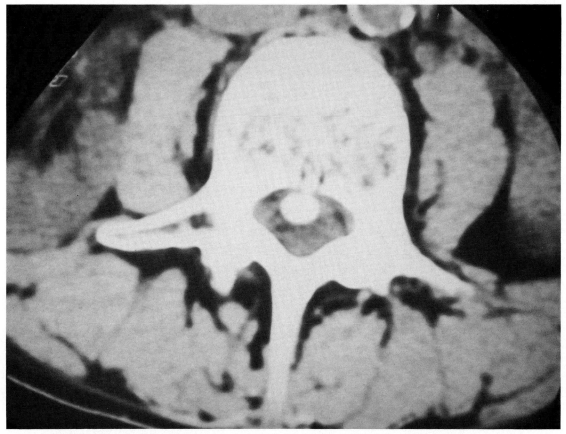

FIGURE 7–8. A 62-year-old male.

Description: The axial CT scan through a lumbar vertebral body shows a calcification in the spinal canal midline and attached to the posterior margin of the vertebral body.

Diagnosis: Calcification of the posterior longitudinal ligament.

Discussion: Calcification in the posterior longitudinal ligament is less conspicuous than calcification in the anterior longitudinal ligament on plain films.[10] This can occur with or without associated disc herniation and is an uncommon cause of spinal cord compression especially in the cervical spine.[15]

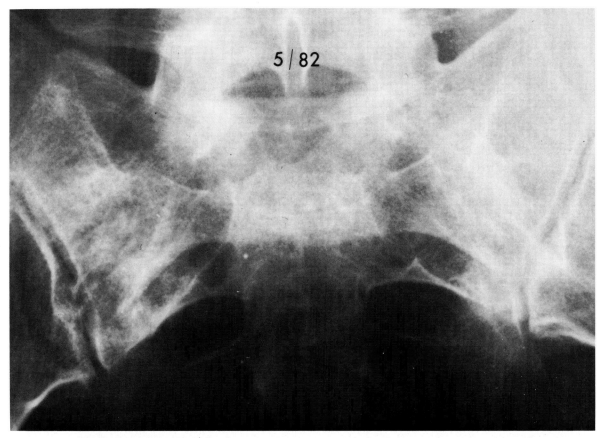

FIGURE 7–9. A 65-year-old female.

Description: An anteroposterior plain film of the sacrum shows a diffuse osteopenia and irregular densities in the sacral wings. These findings correspond to an area of increased uptake on bone scan. The patient had prior radiation.

Diagnosis: Radiation osteitis with insufficiency fracture.

Discussion: Radiation osteitis is a well-known complication of high dose irradiation of bone. The incidence is less than 1 per cent in recent series using megavoltage radiation.[4, 11] Among the complications of radiation is insufficiency fracture. These fractures can be overlooked or confused with metastatic disease. Osteoporosis is another important predisposing factor for insufficiency fractures in the sacrum.[5]

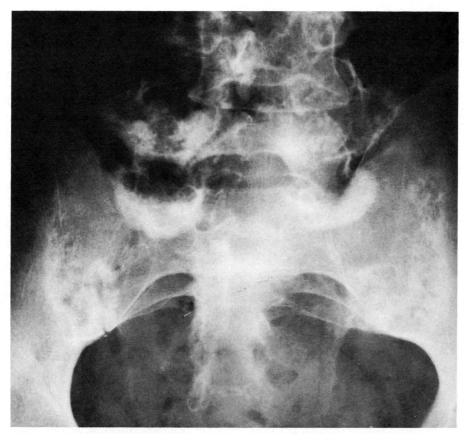

FIGURE 7–10. A 25-year-old male.

Description: An anteroposterior plain film of the sacrum and fifth lumbar vertebra reveals dense calcifications projecting over the sacroiliac joints and the apophyseal joints. Erosive changes of the sacroiliac joints are also demonstrated.

Diagnosis: Gout.

Discussion: Arthritis of the axial skeleton including the sacroiliac joints is a rare manifestation of gout.[1] When present there is usually also involvement of peripheral sites, as in this case. In the absence of peripheral tophi, confident diagnosis of tophaceous gout of the spine probably requires biopsy.[28] The radiographic findings vary considerably from degenerative osteochondrosis to erosive changes, and tophi with or without calcifications.

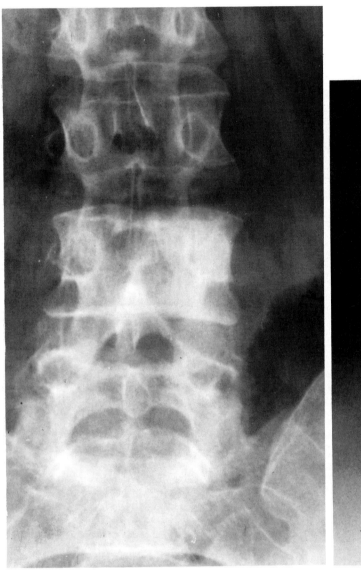

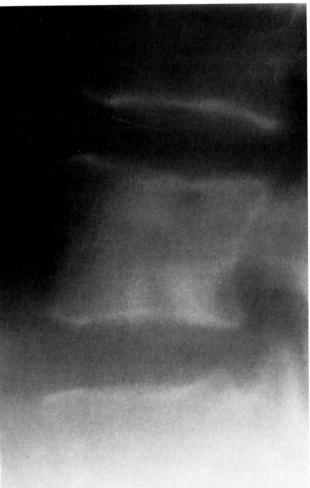

FIGURE 7–11. A 43-year-old female.

Description: Anteroposterior plain film and lateral tomogram. There is sclerosis of the left part of the fourth vertebral body in this patient with a one-year history of low back pain. The area of sclerosis is ill defined and two small lytic foci of about 1 cm in diameter are detected on a lateral tomogram near the end plates. The intervertebral disc space seems unremarkable on either side of the affected vertebra.

Diagnosis: Osteomyelitis (*Staphylococcus aureus*).

Discussion: Pyogenic infection of the spine usually produces acute clinical symptoms and rapidly progressive destruction of the vertebral end plates. Involvement of the disc space is considered a radiographic hallmark of infection. Despite this, insidious onset of symptoms and less aggressive findings on x-rays are part of the spectrum of the disease.[9]

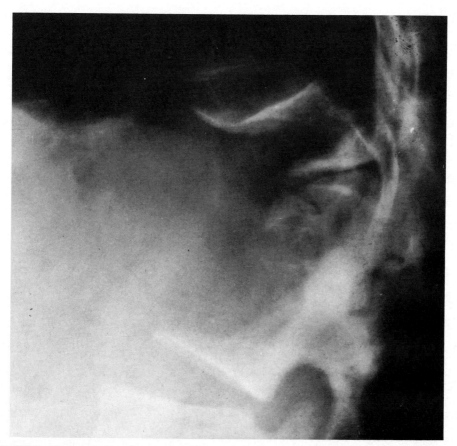

FIGURE 7–12. An elderly male.

Description: A lateral plain film of the thoracolumbar junction reveals a large area of bone destruction involving the anterior parts of several vertebral bodies with resulting angular kyphosis.

Diagnosis: Aortic aneurysm with bone erosion.

Discussion: Erosions of the spine due to aneurysms of the aorta are uncommon. They are most often seen in the thoracic spine. This case is an extreme example of erosion due to an abdominal aortic aneurysm. Erosions of the posterior elements may be caused by tortuous vertebral arteries.[3]

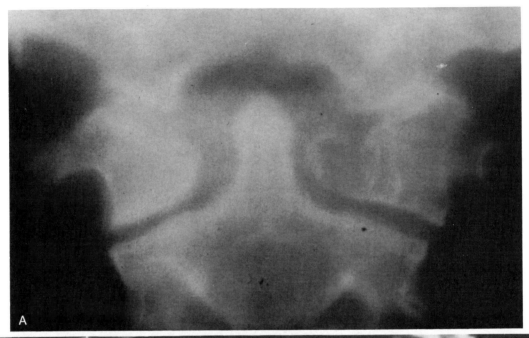

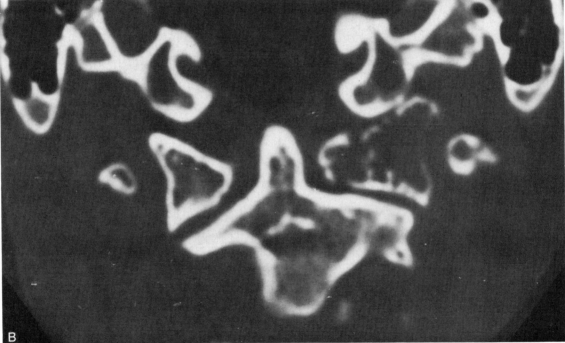

FIGURE 7–13. A 19-year-old male.

Description: Anteroposterior tomogram (*A*) and coronal CT scan (*B*) of the occipitocervical junction. There is osteolysis of the left lateral mass of C1 and slight enlargement of the affected segment. No calcified matrix is seen within the lesion.

Diagnosis: Fibrous dysplasia of C1.

Discussion: This disease of unknown etiology presents in two major clinical forms: monostotic or polyostotic. Spinal involvement is unusual in either form.[7, 17] In the early bone-replacing phase of fibrous dysplasia, the lesions are lucent as in this case. Weakening of the vertebra may lead to compression fracture.

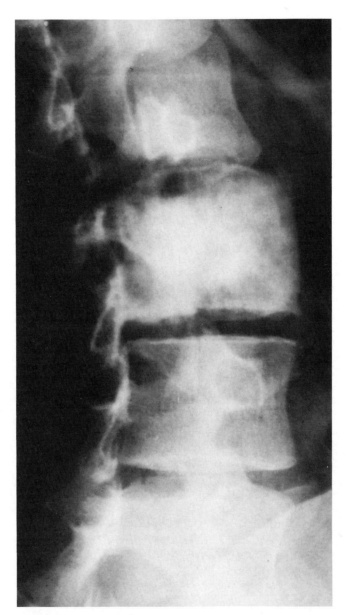

FIGURE 7–14. A 24-year-old female.

Description: An oblique plain film of the midlumbar spine shows a predominantly dense L3 vertebral body with considerable enlargement. Small osteolytic foci are seen within the lesion. The anterolateral margin is convex compared with the normal concavity seen at L2 and L4.

Diagnosis: Fibrous dysplasia.

Discussion: Another example of spinal involvement with fibrous dysplasia illustrates the bone-forming phase.[21] The osteoid produced by the lesion mineralizes within the medullary cavity. The mineralization is not always homogeneous enough to give the typical "ground-glass" appearance.

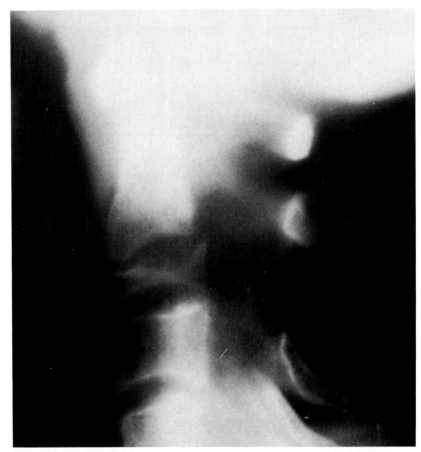

FIGURE 7–15. A 52-year-old female.

Description: A lateral tomogram of the cervical spine shows a compression fracture of C3. The underlying osteolytic destruction involves the posterior elements.

Diagnosis: Paget's disease (osteolytic).

Discussion: Paget's disease is a common disorder in elderly persons of Western European origin. Spinal involvement is also common, with a decreasing incidence from the sacrum to the cervical spine. In the development of the disease, sclerotic changes are preceded by a lytic phase. This leads to osteoporosis circumscripta of the skull and a V-shaped or flame-shaped resorption in the tibia or other long bones.[6] A purely lytic phase in the spine with compression factor is a rare event.[22] Involvement of the posterior elements narrows the differential diagnosis and favors Paget's disease over metastatic destruction.

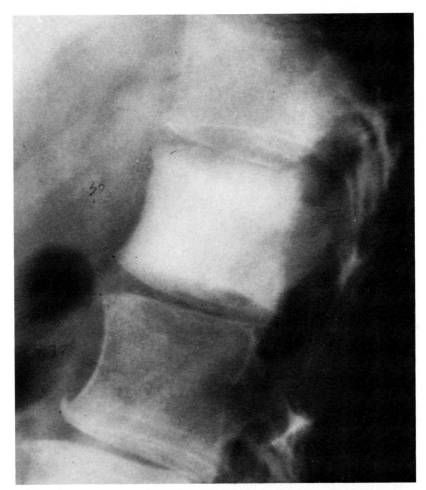

FIGURE 7–16. A 60-year-old asymptomatic female, with normal alkaline phosphatase levels.

Description: A lateral coned-down plain film of the first lumbar vertebra shows a homogeneous sclerosis of the body and the posterior elements. Enlargement of the affected bone is not obvious.

Diagnosis: Paget's disease (osteoblastic).

Discussion: In the osteoblastic phase of Paget's disease the vertebral bodies may become homogeneously dense as in the presented case. The involvement of the posterior elements is again helpful in establishing the diagnosis.[27] The blastic phase is relatively inactive, and with small areas of skeletal involvement the alkaline phosphatase activity may be normal.

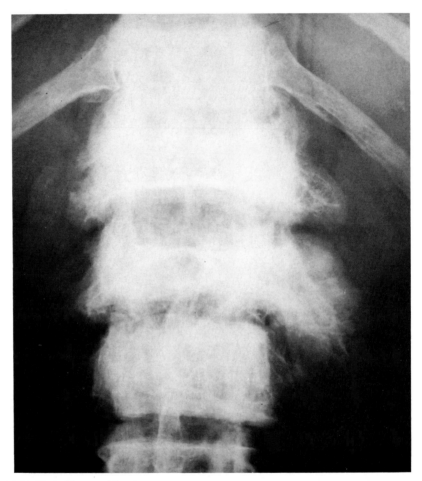

FIGURE 7–17. A 49-year-old male.

Description: Anteroposterior plain film of the upper lumbar spine. All vertebral bodies show a structural change with coarsening of the trabecular pattern, sclerosis, and severe enlargement.

Diagnosis: Paget's disease.

Discussion: In this extensive case no other differential diagnosis has to be considered. Due to the bony overgrowth, cord compression may occur.[25] CT allows the direct visualization of the narrowing of the spinal canal.[30] Extramedullary hematopoiesis can occur as paravertebral masses in these severe cases.

REFERENCES

1. Alarcon GS, Reveille JD: Gouty arthritis of the axial skeleton including the sacroiliac joints. Arch Intern Med 147:2018, 1987.
2. Bardsley JL, Hanelin LG: The unilateral hypoplastic pedicle. Radiology 101:315, 1971.
3. Brooks BS, El Gammal T, Beveridge WD: Erosions of vertebral pedicles by unusual vascular causes. Neuroradiology 23:107, 1982.
4. Brown KT, Rosenthal DI, Rosenberg A: Case report 247. Postradiation osteitis of the sacrum. Skeletal Radiol 10:269, 1983.
5. Cooper KL, Beabout JW, Swee RG: Insufficiency fractures of the sacrum. Radiology 156:15, 1985.
6. Frame B, Marel GM: Paget disease: A review of current knowledge. Radiology 141:21, 1981.
7. Garfin SR, Rothman RH: Case report 346. Fibrous dysplasia (polyostotic). Skeletal Radiol 15:72, 1986.
8. Ghelman B, Freiberger RH: The limbus vertebra: An anterior disc herniation demonstrated by discography. AJR 127:854, 1976.
9. Griffith HED, Jones DM: Pyogenic infection of the spine. A review of twenty-eight cases. J Bone Joint Surg 53B:383, 1971.
10. Hiramatsu Y, Nobechi T: Calcification of the posterior longitudinal ligament of the spine among Japanese. Radiology 100:307, 1971.
11. Howland WJ, Loeffler RK, Starchman RK, Johnson RG: Postirradiation atrophic changes of bone and related complications. Radiology 117:677, 1975.
12. Katz ME, Teitelbaum SL, Gilula LA, et al: Invest Radiol 23:447, 1988.
13. Klinghoffer R, Murdock MG, Hermel MB: Congenital absence of lumbar articular facets. Clin Orthop 106:151, 1975.
14. Onitsuka H: Roentgenologic aspects of bone islands. Radiology 123:607, 1977.
15. Palacios E, Brackett CE, Leary DJ: Ossification of the posterior longitudinal ligament with a herniated intervertebral disk. Radiology 100:313, 1971.
16. Papanicolaou N, Wilkinson RH, Emans JB, et al: Bone scintigraphy and radiography in young athletes with low back pain. AJR 145:1039, 1985.
17. Resnik CS, Lininger JR: Monostotic fibrous dysplasia of the cervical spine: Case report. Radiology 151:49, 1984.
18. Resnick D: Degenerative diseases of the vertebral column. Radiology 156:3, 1985.
19. Resnick D, Nemcek AA Jr, Haghighi P: Spinal enostosis (bone islands). Radiology 147:373, 1983.
20. Resnick D, Niwayama G: Intervertebral disk herniations: Cartilaginous (Schmorl's) nodes. Radiology 126:57, 1978.
21. Rosendahl-Jensen SV: Fibrous dysplasia of the vertebral column. Acta Chir Scand 111:490, 1956.
22. Rosenthal DI, Raymond K: Case report 148. Paget disease (osteoporosis circumscripta) of C3. Skeletal Radiol 6:205, 1981.
23. Scheuermann H: Kyphosis dorsalis juvenilis. Ugeskr Laeger 82:384, 1920.
24. Schmorl G, Junghanns H: The Human Spine in Health and Disease. 2nd ed. New York, Grune & Stratton, 1971.
25. Schwarz G, Reback S: Compression of the spinal cord in osteitis deformans (Paget's disease) of the vertebrae. AJR 42:345, 1939.
26. Smith J: Giant bone islands. Radiology 107:35, 1973.
27. Steinbach HL: Some roentgen features of Paget's disease. AJR 86:95, 1961.
28. Varga J, Giampaolo C, Goldenberg DL: Tophaceous gout of the spine in a patient with no peripheral tophi: Case report and review of literature. Arthritis Rheum 28:1312, 1985.
29. Wortzmann G, Steinhardt MI: Congenitally absent lumbar pedicle: A reappraisal. Radiology 152:713, 1984.
30. Zlatzkin MB, Lander PH, Hadjipavlou AG, Levine JS: Paget disease of the spine: CT with clinical correlation. Radiology 160:155, 1986.

8

TUMOROUS LESIONS OF THE SPINE:

An Overview

ANDREW E. ROSENBERG and ALAN L. SCHILLER

The human spine has a complex embryology and anatomy. It functionally integrates 33 vertebrae, more than 97 diarthroses and amphiarthroses, and numerous collagenous and elastic ligaments. A large array of nerves and blood vessels course throughout its compartments, and tendons insert into its surface. Unlike the remainder of the skeleton, its embryologic origins are from both the mesoderm and ectoderm (notochord). Its complexity is also reflected by the diverse cell and tissue types that compose or are associated with its structures: bone, hyaline and fibrocartilage, notochord, tendon, ligament, elastic tissue, peripheral and central nervous tissue, fat, hematopoietic elements, smooth muscle, skeletal muscle, blood vessels, and synovium. Benign and malignant tumors may potentially arise from any of these components, and furthermore the vertebral column serves as a common reservoir for metastases. The heterogeneity of possible neoplasms predisposes to diagnostic difficulty, and the restrictions imposed by the anatomy of the spine limit its accessibility to diagnostic and therapeutic procedures.

GENERAL OVERVIEW

Primary neoplasms of the spine are uncommon, with the exception of myeloma. Similar to other portions of the skeleton, the type of tumors that affect the spine and their anatomic localization tend to be restricted. We have not encountered any primary tumors of the intervertebral disc or ligamentum flavum.

BENIGN TUMORS

The common benign tumors of the spine include hemangioma, osteoid osteoma, osteoblastoma, giant cell tumor, and aneurysmal bone cyst. Fibrous, cartilaginous, neural, myogenic, and fatty tumors are unusual.

Hemangioma is the most common benign tumor of the spine. Hemangiomas occur throughout the skeleton; however, the spine is the most common site of origin. Hemangiomas of the spine are usually asymptomatic and are typically detected as an incidental finding.[6] In Schmorl's large autopsy study they were present in 10.7 per cent of examined spines.[6] The most frequent location was the thoracic spine, followed by the lumbar, cervical, and sacral regions. Most hemangiomas are limited to the vertebral body, but larger tumors can extend into the pedicles and spinal processes.

Osteoid osteoma and osteoblastoma are benign bone-forming tumors. They typically affect the posterior vertebral elements in adolescents and young adults.[2] Osteoid osteoma is a known cause of painful scoliosis in teenagers. Osteoid osteoma tends to induce more abundant reactive bone than osteoblastoma. Although both lesions are usually easily diagnosed, the aggressive variant of osteoblastoma may be difficult to distinguish from an osteosarcoma on a limited biopsy sample.

Giant cell tumors of bone are locally aggressive benign tumors. A very small percentage may metastasize following pathologic fracture or repeated incomplete surgery, since these procedures increase the tumor's access to blood vessels. They usually involve the vertebral body and can cause extensive destruction with soft tissue masses.[3] Approximately 10 per cent of giant cell tumors arise in the spine, and the sacrum is most frequently involved.[3] Giant cell tumors of bone should be distinguished from other tumors rich in giant cells, such as brown tumor of hyperparathyroidism, pigmented villonodular synovitis, chondroblastoma, and aneurysmal bone cyst.

Aneurysmal bone cyst is a diagnosis of exclusion. Primary bone lesions may undergo massive cystic degeneration and hemorrhage and may mimic an aneurysmal bone cyst. Such lesions include osteosarcoma, giant cell tumor, osteoblastoma, chondroblastoma, and fibrous dysplasia. The spine is a common location for aneurysmal bone cysts, and the lumbar region is most frequently affected.[1] It typically involves the posterior elements and, unlike most other primary benign bone tumors, may extend into adjacent bones.[1]

MALIGNANT TUMORS

In contrast to the rest of the skeleton, the spine is *more* commonly affected by malignant tumors than benign neoplasms. Metastatic disease and myeloma occur magnitudes more frequently than do primary tumors such as osteosarcoma, chondrosarcoma, Ewing's sarcoma, and chordoma.

Metastases greatly outnumber primary tumors of the spine by a ratio of at least 5 to 1. Approximately 70 per cent of all tumors of the vertebral column are metastatic. In Schmorl's review of 1000 spines obtained at autopsy from patients with cancer, 17.6 per cent had metastases.[6] The most common sites of origin are carcinoma of the breast, prostate, and lung. Metastases most frequently localize to the lumbar region followed by the thoracic and cervical segments.[6] Most spinal metastases are multifocal, and in about two thirds of the cases the thoracic and lumbar vertebrae are affected concurrently. Most metastases involve the vertebral bodies; however, the transverse processes and neural arches may be affected by continuous spread or as independent sites.[6]

Myeloma refers to a solid malignant proliferation of plasma cells. It may appear as a solitary focus, called plasmacytoma, or may diffusely involve the marrow, for which the term multiple myeloma applies. The proliferation of plasma cells in myeloma usually arises in the hematopoietic marrow but may also occur in extraskeletal sites. Myeloma may involve both the vertebral bodies and posterior elements. It can present as diffuse osteoporosis, single or multiple punched-out lytic defects, and uncommonly as osteosclerotic lesions. Expansile tumors may cause cord compression and neurologic deficits.[4]

Osteosarcoma is the most common primary malignant (nonhematopoietic) tumor of the skeleton. However, osteosarcoma of the spine is unusual. Only 1 to 3 per cent of osteosarcomas arise in the vertebral column, and osteosarcoma accounts for approximately 5 per cent of all primary malignant tumors of the spine.[7] Osteosarcoma of the spine occurs in an older patient population than that which is afflicted by standard osteosarcoma of the extremities. Some cases arise in the setting of Paget's disease or in sites of previous radiation (i.e., sacrum irradiated during treatment for uterine carcinoma).[7]

Chordoma is a rare malignant tumor that arises from the notochord. It occurs exclusively in the midline of the axial skeleton along the anatomic pathway of the notochord. Approximately 85 per cent of cases arise in the sacrococcygeal or sphenocipital region. For unknown reasons, spinal chordomas arise in the vertebral bodies rather than in the intervertebral disc. The lumbar and cervical vertebrae are affected more frequently than the thoracic vertebrae. Chordomas are slow growing, locally invasive, and may metastasize.[5]

Other malignant tumors such as Ewing's sarcoma and chondrosarcoma are rare, and the reader is referred to Chapters 16, 17, and 24.

THE PATHOLOGIST'S ROLE

The pathologist has a vital role in diagnosing tumors of the spine and should be an active member of the multidisciplinary team that cares for affected patients. It is imperative that the pathologist review the x-rays with the radiologist, since the x-rays represent the gross pathology. The pathologist should discuss with the surgeons the location of the biopsy and the allotment of tissue needed. Furthermore, the pathologist should explore the ramifications of the diagnosis with the surgeon, radiation therapist, and oncologist.

Tissue Diagnosis

Central to the pathologist's task is the receipt of representative tissue that permits an accurate diagnosis. To ensure that the biopsy specimen is adequate, a frozen section should be performed. This requires that the tissue be given to the pathologist in the fresh state. Depending upon the results of the frozen section various steps can be initiated to further secure the diagnosis: (1) request additional tissue because of a sampling problem; (2) suggest that cultures be taken; (3) place tissue in certain fixatives (e.g., 95 per cent alcohol for glycogen preservation, glutaraldehyde for electron microscopy, B-5 fixative for nuclear preservation, formalin for standard H & E preparation); (4) keep tissue frozen for immunohistochemistry; (5) submit tissue for cell surface marker analysis for suspected lymphomas; (6) submit fresh tissue for flow cytometry; (7) submit fresh tissue for genetic analysis. In cases in which special studies are needed, then a minimum of three needle cores of tissue should be obtained: a core for frozen section, which can be kept for immunohistochemistry; a core for standard processing; and a core for electron microscopy. Open biopsies usually provide abundant tissue. Fine needle aspirates can be done to confirm metastatic disease or a recurrent tumor.

Electron microscopy in many situations is crucial, since identifying specific ultrastructural features will lead to a definitive diagnosis. Electron microscopy is important in distinguishing the round cell tumors, including small cell carcinoma, lymphoma, Ewing's sarcoma, rhabdomyosarcoma, histiocytosis, and neuroblastoma. Ultrastructural analysis can also delineate the spindle cell tumors such as fibrosarcoma, malignant schwannoma, malignant fibrous histiocytoma, leiomyosarcoma, sarcoma-like carcinomas, and spindle melanomas.

Immunohistochemistry utilizes monoclonal and polyclonal antibodies directed against specific antigens. The most useful antibodies are those that distinguish among lymphoma, carcinoma, and sarcoma, including the small round cell tumors. Many of the anti-

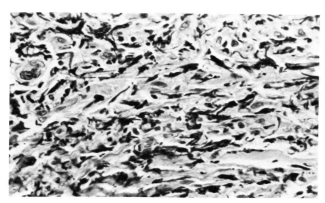

FIGURE 8–1. Malignant lymphoma with extensive squeeze artifact, which prevents accurate diagnosis (H & E ×500).

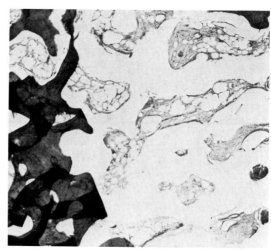

FIGURE 8–3. Trabecular bone has become folded with the spaces mimicking a vascular tumor (H & E ×31).

bodies that are utilized in this regard are directed against the intermediate filaments that form the cytoskeleton of cells. Because the sensitivity of these antibodies is greatest on fresh frozen tissue, the biopsy specimens have to be handled properly.

Flow cytometry is a recently developed method that measures cell cycle and the quantity of DNA within a cell. It is based on the premise that benign tumors tend to have few cells in the replicative stages and a normal complement of DNA. However, in malignant tumors the cells cycle more frequently and have abnormal amounts of DNA. Furthermore, the more primitive or malignant the tumor, the more replicative activity occurs and the more abnormal the quantity of DNA. FLow cytometry has been used with some success in distinguishing benign from malignant bone tumors. It has also added valuable prognostic information concerning the degree of aggressive behavior of malignant tumors and their responsiveness to chemotherapy. Flow cytometry can be performed on both fresh and formalin-fixed paraffin wax embedded tissue. Since there are nuclear alterations caused by decalcification, flow cytometry analysis should be done on nondecalcified tissue.

Genetic analysis usually requires fresh sterile tissue to grow tumor cells in cell culture. Recently, genetic studies on bone tumors have centered on identifying patient populations predisposed to developing neo-

plasms (i.e., retinoblastoma and osteosarcoma). Specific chromosomal abnormalities have been used to subclassify or elucidate the histogenesis of tumors (e.g., many Ewing's sarcomas are now considered primitive neuroectodermal malignancies).

PITFALLS AND TRAPS IN DIAGNOSING NEOPLASMS OF THE SPINE

The pitfalls and traps in diagnosing spinal neoplasms may result from (1) tissue artifact, (2) not recognizing normal structures, (3) confusing degenerative and reactive changes with neoplasms, and (4) mistaking lymphoma or myeloma with infection.

Tissue artifact can be introduced during any step from the time of biopsy to staining of the tissue. Inappropriate pressure applied to the tissue during the surgical procedure or in the pathology laboratory can produce "squeeze" or smear artifact (Figs. 8–1 and 8–2). The distortion of the cells prevents their identification. Cells most susceptible to squeeze artifact are those that have very few cytoskeletal filaments such as the small round cell tumors (Ewing's sarcoma, lymphoma, neuroblastoma, small cell carcinoma), inflammatory cells, and hematopoietic elements.

Cells that are not fixed promptly or adequately may lose nuclear and cytoplasmic detail which can prevent a diagnosis from being rendered. Bone needs to be well fixed before it is exposed to decalcifying agents. If not, the gas bubbles (usually carbon dioxide) produced by decalcification solutions such as 5 per cent nitric acid may greatly distort cells by causing marked vacuolization. The vacuoles compress and push the nucleus aside and cause confusion with signet ring cell adenocarcinoma or fatty tumors. If bony specimens are not adequately decalcified, then the bony trabeculae may shatter or be pushed out of the paraffin block during sectioning. The empty spaces left behind can simulate vascular tumors (Fig. 8–3). Furthermore, too much decalcification can digest cells and simulate conditions with necrosis.

The major components of the vertebral body are

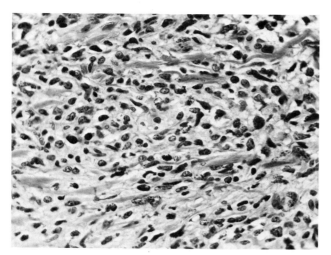

FIGURE 8–2. Different part of same tumor in Figure 8–1 with better preserved areas (H & E ×500).

bone, hyaline cartilage of the end plates and articulating facets, fibrocartilage of the annulus fibrosus, and notochord tissue of the nucleus pulposus. In biopsy specimens fragmentation of tissue usually occurs, and the normal hyaline cartilage may be mistaken for a cartilage tumor. Similarly, notochord may be misdiagnosed as chordoma and the annulus fibrosus as some sort of fibrous lesion.

Compression fractures and herniations of the intervertebral disc into the vertebral body (Putschar-Schmorl's nodule) can clinically and pathologically simulate neoplasms. In both of these conditions the associated reactive bone, cartilage, and fibrous tissue (callus) can be features that may lead to a misdiagnosis of malignant tumor (Fig. 8–4).

In cases of vertebral chronic osteomyelitis, lymphocytes or plasma cells may predominate. In these situations a diagnosis of lymphoma or myeloma can be avoided by careful clinical pathologic correlation, utilization of cell markers, and the appreciation of a

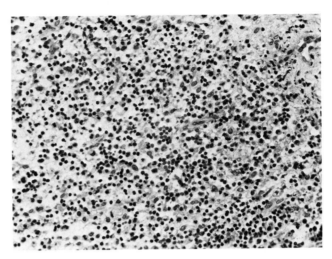

FIGURE 8–5. Chronic osteomyelitis with a predominance of lymphocytes simulating malignant lymphoma (H & E ×313).

heterogeneous population of inflammatory cells (Fig. 8–5). In contrast, some lymphomas may have reactive lymphocytes intermixed with neoplastic cells. This admixture of cell types may simulate infection.

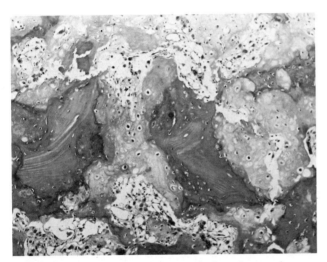

FIGURE 8–4. Fracture callus composed of cartilage and woven bone surrounding necrotic fragments of trabecular bone. This can simulate either osteosarcoma or chondrosarcoma (H & E ×125).

REFERENCES

1. Capanna R, Albisinni V, Picci P, et al: Aneurysmal bone cyst of the spine. J Bone Joint Surg 67(A):527–531, 1985.
2. Keim HA, Reina E: Osteoid osteoma as a cause of scoliosis. J Bone Joint Surg 57(A)159–163, 1975.
3. McDonald DJ, Sim F, McLeod RA, Dahlin DC: Giant cell tumor of bone. J Bone Joint Surg 68(A):235–242, 1986.
4. Resnick D, Niwayama G: Diagnosis of Bone and Joint Disorders. 2nd ed. Philadelphia, WB Saunders Co, 1988.
5. Rich TA, Schiller A, Suit HD, Mankin H: Clinical and pathologic review of 48 cases of chordoma. Cancer 56:182–187, 1985.
6. Schmorl G, Junghanns H: The Human Spine in Health and Disease. New York, Grune and Stratton, 1975.
7. Shives TC, Dahlin DC, Sim F, et al: Osteosarcoma of the spine. J Bone Joint Surg 68(A):660–668, 1986.

THE ROLE OF
RADIATION THERAPY

HERMAN D. SUIT and MARY AUSTIN-SEYMOUR

The general principles that govern the outcome of treatment of patients with malignant tumors of the spine are the same as those for tumors of any other site. First, for a patient to be considered cured all tumor cells at the primary, regional, and distant sites must be inactivated or removed. Second, the determinants of probability of success are the anatomic site and size of tumor and the histopathologic type and grade of tumor. Malignant lesions of the spine are often nonresectable with secure margins because of the constraints imposed by the proximity of the spinal cord and nerve roots, major vessels (especially along the thoracic column), and organs (e.g., esophagus, which lies anterior to the lower cervical spine). An intact spine is critical to an individual's anatomic integrity. The role of radiation treatment for malignant tumors of the spine is often severely limited by the necessity to include the spinal cord in the high dose region because tumor abuts on the dura and/or cord.

The rationale for combining radiation with surgery in the treatment of malignant lesions is that the volume of grossly normal tissue that must be removed in order to resect all of the microscopic extensions around the tumor often demands a prohibitively high price in function and/or cosmesis. Radiation in moderate doses can inactivate, at an important clinical probability, those subclinical extensions into grossly normal tissues. That is, the net result of combining radiation and surgery should be tumor control probability equivalent to that achieved by the radical ablative surgical procedure, but with reduced morbidity and/or functional decrement. Thus, in those situations where resection of grossly normal but microscopically involved tissue is unattractive, the combined approach should be considered. In the case of tumors of the spine, resection may not be grossly complete, and hence the radiation dose would have to be high. Even so, the likelihood of success of treatment of mesenchymal tumors could be modest for conventional x-ray therapy. We present data from our study of high dose proton beam therapy for incompletely resected chordomas and chondrosarcomas.

Radiation is the treatment of choice for several tumor types that are relatively readily controlled by radiation, namely, Ewing's sarcoma, primary lymphoma of bone, solitary plasmacytoma. The mesenchymal tumors—for example, chordomas, chondrosarcomas, osteosarcoma, fibrosarcoma—are best managed by surgery alone or where achievement of negative margins is difficult by the combination of the two modalities. Radiation alone offers good prospect of control of giant cell tumor, and the need to push for complete resection is not compelling when the procedure would constitute a *major* morbidity for the patient.

The likelihood of success of surgical treatment of sarcomas is set by the actual anatomic site and size of the individual lesion. For example, a 4-cm sarcoma arising in the pedicle of C2 probably could not be resected with good margins; a similar size lesion arising in S4 could in most circumstances be readily resected. The probability of development of distant metastasis is a function of histologic type and grade and tumor size in patients who have achieved local control of their tumor. Although data on this point are not known to the authors for bone sarcoma, we do show related data for sarcomas of soft tissue in Table 9–1.[17] Distant metastasis is quite uncommon from Grade 1 sarcomas at any size, but the incidence

TABLE 9–1. FIVE-YEAR ACTUARIAL DISTANT METASTASIS PROBABILITY AS A FUNCTION OF TUMOR SIZE AND GRADE IN PATIENTS WITH LOCAL CONTROL OF SARCOMA

SIZE (mm)	GRADE 1		GRADES 2 AND 3	
	No. Pts.	DM (%)	No. Pts.	DM (%)
<25	5	0	23	5
26–50	11	0	39	14
51–100	17	6	78	42
101–150	5	0	27	52
151–200	4	25	14	70
>200	3	0	6	83
Total	45	6	187	37

DM = Distant metastasis.
From Suit HD, Mankin HJ, Wood WC, et al: Treatment of the patient with Stage M$_0$ sarcoma of soft tissue. J Clin Oncol 6:854–862, 1988.

This investigation was supported by PHS grant number CA21239 awarded by the National Cancer Institute, DHHS.

increases very steeply with size for tumors of Grade 2 and 3. This dependence of probability of distant metastasis on grade and size might well be shown to be specific for each histologic type. At present, the data are pooled for all histologic types. In an analysis of 130 patients with primary chondrosarcoma treated at Mayo Clinic by radical surgical resection, Pritchard and colleagues showed that there was a steep decrease in disease-free survival at 10 years with increasing grade. Further, patients who failed locally experienced a much less satisfactory 10- and 20-year survival than patients who had achieved local control.[14] The same dependency of metastasis on histologic grade was shown in the analysis by Gitelis and colleagues[7] and Kreicbergs and coworkers.[12] In the latter investigation, DNA ploidy was determined in 44 patients with chondrosarcoma; they reported a higher local recurrence and a higher death rate among patients whose lesions were hyperdiploid. This finding is supported by the work of Alho and coworkers, who found a progressively smaller proportion of diploid cells in benign, low grade, and high grade cartilaginous tumors.[1] The same behavioral characteristics are likely to apply to fibrosarcoma, malignant fibrohistiocytoma, and osteosarcoma. Data on this point are not currently available.

HISTOPATHOLOGIC TYPES OF BENIGN AND MALIGNANT SPINAL TUMORS

The histopathologic types of tumors arising in the vertebrae and sacrum from two large series—the Mayo Clinic and the Netherlands Committee on Bone Tumors (NCBT)[5, 15]—are presented in Table 9–2.

TABLE 9–2. HISTOLOGIC TYPES OF TUMORS OF BONE

	VERTEBRAL Mayo*/NCBT†	SACRAL Mayo/NCBT
Benign		
Osteochondroma	11/–	1/–
Chondroma	3/1	–/–
Chondroblastoma	1/–	–/–
Osteoid osteoma	3/2	–/–
Osteoblastoma	9/5	2/1
Giant cell tumor	3/5	14/2
Other	9/1	1/–
Total	39/14	18/3
Vertebral and sacral/Total skeleton	Mayo 57/956 = 5.9% NCBT 17/361 = 4.7%	
Malignant		
Chordoma	20/2	62/9
Chondrosarcoma	25/0	7/6
Primary lymphoma	19/0	8/0
Osteosarcoma	10/1	4/1
Fibrosarcoma	4/1	7/0
Ewing's sarcoma	7/1	9/0
Other	3/0	1/0
Total	88/5	98/16
Vertebral and sacral/Total skeleton	Mayo 186/953 = 19.5% NCBT 21/626 = 3.3%	

*Mayo Clinic, see ref. 5.
†Netherlands Committee on Bone Tumors, see ref. 15.

There is a substantial difference in the relative importance of the vertebral/sacral sarcomas among all skeletal tumors in these two series. This may reflect the large geographic area from which patients with unusual malignant tumors of bone were referred to the Mayo Clinic as distinct from the population-based origin of the patients seen by the NCBT. Namely, of patients with malignant bone tumors seen at Mayo Clinic, 19.5 per cent of the tumors were located in the vertebrae and/or sacrum as compared with only 3.3 per cent in the NCBT series. Nonetheless, of the vertebral/sacral malignant tumors, apparently half were chordomas. In the United States there are approximately 2000 new malignant tumors of bone arising every year.[16] Accordingly, we may estimate that there would be 80 to 400 newly diagnosed sarcomas of the spine every year in the United States. Thus, the opportunity at a single institution to develop a detailed understanding of the natural history and response to therapies for any one histologic type of tumor of bone originating in the spine would be very limited.

TUMORS TREATED BY RADIATION ALONE

Ewing's Sarcoma

Ewing's sarcoma is an uncommon malignant tumor of bone primarily involving adolescents. These tumors comprise approximately 20 per cent of all primary malignant tumors of bone, and of Ewing's tumors approximately 10 per cent arise in the spine.[11, 19] The treatment of Ewing's tumor arising in the vertebrae or sacrum will in most instances involve intensive multidrug, multicycle chemotherapy combined with radiation. After several cycles of chemotherapy, radiation is commenced. Following radiation, the drug therapy is continued, usually for about one year. The total radiation dose in most protocols is about 50 Gy if given at 1.8 to 2.0 Gy per fraction, 5 fractions per week. For lesions in the upper lumbar (L1-L2), thoracic, and cervical spine, radiation dose would be limited to 45 Gy, because the spinal cord has a low tolerance of radiation, unless special techniques were employed to keep the dose to the cord at that level. For lesions in the lower lumbar and sacral segments, the dose to the central tumor mass may be increased 50 to 60 Gy; the total dose would depend on tumor size, extent of coverage in the field of sensitive normal tissues (e.g., gastrointestinal, renal), and the age of the patient.

Survival of patients following treatment for spinal lesion was 40 per cent in the Mayo Clinic series.[19] In the Intergroup Ewing's Sarcoma Study series of seven patients with lesions of the sacrum, there were no local failures but four patients developed distant metastasis. Of 37 patients with lesions of the skull and spine, two experienced local recurrences and five patients developed distant metastasis. Our own experience in patients with Ewing's sarcoma of the spine or sacrum is limited to three patients: two cervical spine and one sacrum treated by intensive chemotherapy and radiation. Two patients are alive and well at 33 and 54 months after treatment. In the patient with a sacral tumor, surgical resection was part of the treatment. The one failure, an extensive tumor of the upper cervical spine, recurred at 40 months after treatment.

Ewing's sarcoma of the spine may be quite large. This is shown in the series at St. Bartholomew's Hospital in which two vertebral body lesions were greater than 10 cm and had substantial soft tissue disease. Two of five lesions in the sacrum were greater than 10 cm, and four of the five had very substantial disease outside the bone.[4]

For large Ewing's sarcoma, consideration can be given to resecting the residual lesion or the local site from which the Ewing's sarcoma arose. Ewing's sarcoma of expendable bones is now commonly treated by a trimodality approach (chemotherapy, radiation therapy, and surgery). In most instances, the morbidity associated with an attempted resection of a Ewing's sarcoma of the spine would be excessive for the expected gain.

Primary Lymphoma of Bone

This tumor is less common than Ewing's sarcoma; however, for the spine primary lymphoma of bone appears to be more common than Ewing's sarcoma (Table 9–2). None of our 33 primary lymphomas of bone occurred in the spine.[6] Treatment for these patients would be similar to that for Ewing's sarcoma, in that there would be a combination of multidrug chemotherapy and radiation. The same constraints would apply with reference to avoidance of doses in excess of about 45 Gy to the spinal cord in patients also receiving drug therapy. The local success of treatment of patients with primary lymphoma of bone should be very high (90 per cent) where doses greater or equal to 45 to 50 Gy are realized. Long-term disease-free survival following treatment based upon combination of drugs and radiation should approach 70 to 80 per cent. The exact figure, of course, will depend upon the size and, apparently, the histologic variety of lymphoma of bone.[2, 6]

Solitary Plasmacytoma

In our experience these are not rare tumors. In a recent analysis of the experience at Massachusetts General Hospital (unpublished data, Doran and Suit, 1988) of a total of 22 patients, 12 were in the spine (11) and sacrum (1). In only one patient did the tumor recur locally. Seven of these patients survived free of disease for 50 months or more. Two have no evidence of disease at 59 and 95 months. The disease progressed at 58, 78, 80, 76, and 21 months in the other patients. Radiation dose was generally in the range of 37 to 44 Gy. Our recommendation is 45 Gy in 4.5 weeks. These treatments were well tolerated

and effective. Chemotherapy is not given electively because of the lack of really effective drug regimens.

Osteosarcoma

Results of radiation treatment of osteosarcoma of the spine are poorly documented. Our own experience is minimal. We would expect that radiation combined with grossly complete resection and chemotherapy would provide a worthwhile yield. As shown in Table 9–3, the one patient treated at our institution for osteosarcoma of cervical spine is doing well.

Chordoma of Sacrum

Radiation given preoperatively for massive lesions of the distal sacrum (S3-S5) or for lesions involving parts of S1-S2 is being investigated. The preoperative treatment has two important advantages: it virtually eliminates the risk of transplantation of tumor in the tumor bed if there is a cut-through (not infrequent at this site), and the treatment volume is smaller than if the radiation were given postoperatively. Our experience with several patients has been strongly positive. We are investigating the use of high dose proton radiation (70 to 75 Gy) in the treatment of gross residual disease (incomplete resection) in S1-S2 segments. An analysis of our experience with radiation in the treatment of patients with sacral chordomas is in progress.

Giant Cell Tumors of Bone

Giant cell tumors (GCTs) comprised 24 of the 1317 (approximately 2 per cent) benign tumors of bone in the combined Mayo and NCBT series (Table 9–2). They represented approximately 16 per cent of the benign tumors of the spine and sacrum in those series. GCTs in this anatomic setting are infrequently resectable, and hence radiation is used as treatment. Among 13 GCTs treated at Massachusetts General Hospital (five were in the spine/sacrum) by radiation with or without limited resection, control has been realized in 11. (Control has been achieved in four of the five spinal lesions.) Radiation doses have been in the range of 50 to 60 Gy. These are well tolerated. The experience at Ontario Cancer Institute[3] was reported as control of 14 out of 15 GCTs by radiation alone. We advocate radiation treatment only for the nonresectable lesions.

PROTON BEAM RADIATION THERAPY OF CERVICAL SPINE CHORDOMAS/ CHONDROSARCOMAS AND OF SARCOMA OF THE PARASPINAL TISSUES

Certain histologies require high radiation doses to achieve local tumor control in a high proportion of

TABLE 9–3. SARCOMAS OF THE PARASPINAL TISSUES

Location	Histology	Macroscopic Residual Disease	Chemotherapy	Dose (CGE/days/ fractions)	Sites of Failure	Follow-up Time (mos)
Lumbar	MFH Gr. III	No	No	42/20/32 (+28.7 Gy implant)	—	79
Thoracic	Unclassified Gr. III	No	No	66.5/33/43	—	60
Cervical	Mal. schwannoma Gr. I	No	No	68.4/38/57	DM	17
Cervical	Osteosarcoma Gr. III	Yes	Yes	70.2/39/58	—	12
Cervical/ thoracic	Spindle cell Gr. III	Yes	Yes	64.8/36/55	LF	22
Cervical	Mal. schwannoma Gr. II	No	No	76.2/37/84	MF/DM	6
Thoracic	Fibrosarcoma Gr. III	No	Yes	53.2/29/49	—	106
Lumbar	Liposarcoma Gr. I	No	No	62/31/52	—	35
Cervical/ thoracic	Hemangiopericytoma Gr. II	No	No	67.8/34/55	—	46
Thoracic	MFH Gr. III	No	No	68.7/34/81	—	72
Cervical	Epithelioid sarcoma Gr. II	Yes	No	68.6/38/53	LF/DM	6
Cervical	Ewing's sarcoma	Yes	Yes	59.8/30/48	—	31

CGE = Cobalt gray equivalent; MFH = malignant fibrous histiocytoma; DM = Distant metastases; LF = Local failure; MF = Marginal failure.

subjects. Tumor immediately adjacent to the spinal cord constitutes an important challenge for the radiation oncologist. High energy proton beam treatment is a newer technique that can be quite useful in this situation. Modulated energy proton beams have favorable physical characteristics, namely, a finite range in tissue as a function of energy and a sharply defined lateral beam edge. These properties allow the delivery of a higher tumor than spinal cord dose in many patients.

Since 1974, fractionated proton radiation treatments have been given to patients with malignant disease through a collaborative program between the Department of Radiation Medicine at Massachusetts General Hospital and the Harvard Cyclotron Laboratory (HCL). At HCL, protons are accelerated to 160 MeV and have a maximum penetration in soft tissue of 15.9 cm. The cyclotron produces a fixed horizontal beam. The relative biologic effectiveness of protons compared with cobalt-60 is 1.1. Dose is expressed in the units of cobalt gray equivalent (CGE) and is determined by multiplying the dose in proton gray by 1.1.

Selected patients with paraspinal malignant sarcomas and chordomas have received fractionated proton treatments. Because our proton beam has a penetration of only 15.9 cm, most of these lesions have been in the cervical region. Seventeen patients with spinal chordomas and low grade chondrosarcomas and 12 patients with sarcomas in the paraspinal soft tissues have received proton treatment. All patients had surgical removal of as much tumor as was feasible. In some of the spinal cases, the surgical procedure was a combined neurosurgical/orthopedic effort.

The ability to deliver a higher dose to the tumor than the adjacent spinal cord using proton beam techniques not only depends on the physical characteristics of the proton beam and the exact details of local anatomy, but also on meticulous treatment planning and accurate execution of the treatment plan. Our proton beam treatments are formulated using a computerized multidimensional treatment planning

system. First, the patient is immobilized in the treatment position using alpha cradle mold techniques. Because the cyclotron has a fixed horizontal beam, many of these patients are immobilized in a seated or decubitus position. The immobilized patient then undergoes a treatment planning computed tomography (CT) scan using a scanner that is capable of scanning seated patients. The slice thickness is 3 mm at 3-mm increments through the tumor region.

The tumor volumes and the spinal cord are then outlined on each slice of the treatment planning scan using an interactive computerized system.[9] The operative findings and radiographic studies are essential pieces of information for this task. The position of the spinal cord is determined with the aid of CT with intravenous contrast, magnetic resonance imaging (MRI) studies, or CT with intrathecal contrast, when necessary. These studies are reviewed with a neuroradiologist. Treatment fields for the tumor are designed which minimize the radiation dose to the adjacent spinal cord.[10] Distributions of dose using all treatment fields are computed on each CT slice. The edges of the fields are shaped with brass apertures, and the distal end of the beams are shaped to the distal contour of the tumor with Lucite compensators.[8, 18]

Figure 9–1 shows the dose distribution used for treating a high grade osteosarcoma originating at C2. The smaller volume outlined in the vertebral body represents the residual disease after surgery. The larger volume outlined in the same region is the bed of the original tumor. The dose to the spinal cord was minimized by using complex field arrangements combining matching right lateral fields with a cord block and posterior fields. The 41 CGE isodose line passes through the center of the cord, while the 50 CGE isodose line goes along the left lateral and anterior surfaces of the cord. The stippled area received a dose of 63 CGE or greater. The tumor bed (represented by the larger outlined volume) received a dose of at least 50 CGE except in the regions closest to the cord. The residual tumor (represented by the smaller outlined volume) received a

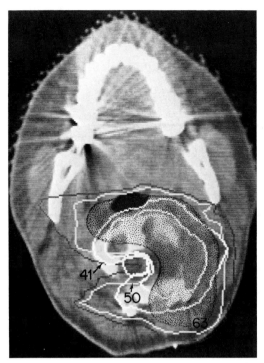

FIGURE 9–1. The dose distribution for treating a high grade osteosarcoma originating at C2.

dose of 70 CGE except in the area adjacent to the spinal cord. The tumor region next to the cord received a gradient of dose; this dose heterogeneity resulted from keeping the cord dose at tolerance levels.

Prior to each treatment the position of the tumor relative to the beam aperture is verified radiographically using an iterative process. The last step in this process is the careful comparison of the portal film and an alignment film generated from the CT data.[10] The field placement accuracy is approximately 2 mm.

Seventeen patients with chordomas[6] or low grade chondrosarcomas[12] of the cervical or thoracic spine have received proton treatment. All of the chordomas occurred in the cervical spine. Two of the low grade chondrosarcomas originated in the cervical vertebrae and two originated in the thoracic spine. Thirteen patients received postoperative radiation and four had preoperative as well as postoperative radiation. All patients had residual tumor; there was no evidence of metastatic disease at the time of proton treatment. None were given chemotherapy.

The final treatment plans employed protons and high energy x-rays. The proton component of the treatment ranged from 100 per cent to 36 per cent, with most patients receiving 70 per cent of the total dose with protons. The median tumor dose delivered with protons and x-rays was 69.8 CGE (range 66.1 to 76.2). The spinal cord dose was considerably less than the tumor dose in all cases. The median follow-up time is 33 months with a range from 6 to 63 months.

Ten of the 17 patients have no evidence of tumor growth. Four patients have had local recurrences at 7 to 39 months after treatment. Three patients have had tumor growth immediately adjacent to the region

of the original tumor (marginal failures). Of these seven patients with either local or marginal failures, three simultaneously developed distant metastases. No radiation-related spinal cord complications have been observed.

Twelve patients with sarcomas of the paraspinal tissues have been treated with protons (Table 9–3). Nine patients received postoperative radiation, while two patients with high grade sarcomas were given pre- and postoperative radiation. One patient received interstitial radiation followed by postoperative radiation. Four patients had macroscopic residual disease after surgery, whereas eight patients had only microscopic residual disease. No patients had evidence of metastatic disease at treatment. Four patients had chemotherapy as a component of the overall treatment.

Both protons and high energy x-rays were used for these treatments. Most patients received 60 per cent of the total proton dose, with a range from 33 per cent to 100 per cent. The median tumor dose was 67.2 CGE, with a range from 42 CGE to 76.2 CGE. The patient receiving 42 Gy also had an implant that gave 28.7 Gy to the tumor bed. The median follow-up time is 33 months, with a range from 6 to 106 months.

Nine of the 12 patients have local and regional control. Two tumors have recurred locally (at 6 and 22 months); the patients had extensive and unresectable tumor. An additional patient had a recurrence immediately inferior to the initial tumor region. This patient as well as one of the patients with local failure also had distant metastases. Further, one patient developed distant metastases only. Overall, eight patients are alive with evidence of any disease. There have been no cases of spinal cord injury in any of these patients. One patient has experienced a late soft tissue necrosis in the treated area.

REFERENCES

1. Alho A, Connor JF, Mankin HJ, et al: Assessment of malignancy of cartilage tumors using flow cytometry. J Bone Joint Surg 65A:779–785, 1983.
2. Bacci G, Jaffe N, Emiliani E, et al: Staging, therapy and prognosis of primary non-Hodgkin's lymphoma of bone and a comparison of results with localized Ewing's sarcoma: Ten years' experience at the Instituto Ortopedica Rizzoli. Tumori 71(4):345–354, 1985.
3. Bell RS, Harwood AR, Goodman SB, et al: Supervoltage radiotherapy in the treatment of difficult giant cell tumors of bone. Clin Orthop 174:208–216, 1983.
4. Brown AP, Fixsen JA, Plowman PN: Local control of Ewing's sarcoma: An analysis of 67 patients. J Radiol 60:261–268, 1987.
5. Dahlin DC: Bone Tumors. 2nd ed. Chicago, Charles C. Thomas, 1970.
6. Dosoretz DE, Raymond AK, Murphy GF, et al: Primary lymphoma of bone: The relationship of morphologic diversity to clinical behavior. Cancer 50:1009–1014, 1982.
7. Gitelis S, Bertoni F, Picci P, Campanacci M: Chondrosarcoma of bone. The experience at the Instituto Ortopedico Rizzoli. J Bone Joint Surg 63A:1248–1257, 1981.
8. Goitein M: Compensation for inhomogeneities in charged particle radiotherapy using computed tomography. Int J Radiat Oncol Biol Phys 4:449–508, 1978.

9. Goitein M, Abrams M: Multidimensional treatment planning. I. Delineation of anatomy. Int J Radiat Oncol Biol Phys 9:777–787, 1983.
10. Goitein M, Abrams M: Multidimensional treatment planning. II. Beam's eye-view, back projection, and projection through CT sections. Int J Radiat Oncol Biol Phys 9:789–797, 1983.
11. Kissane JM, Askin FB, Foulkes M, et al: Ewing's sarcoma of bone: Clinicopathologic aspects of 303 cases from the Intergroup Ewing's Sarcoma Study. Hum Pathol 14:773–779, 1983.
12. Kreicbergs A, Boquist L, Borssen B, Larsson S-E: Prognostic factors in chondrosarcoma. A comparative study of cellular DNA content and clinicopathologic features. Cancer 50:577–583, 1982.
13. Perez CA, Tefft M, Nesbit M, et al: The role of radiation therapy in the management of non-metastatic Ewing's sarcoma of bone. Report of the Intergroup Ewing's Sarcoma Study. Int J Radiat Oncol Biol Phys 7:141–149, 1981.
14. Pritchard DJ, Lunke RJ, Taylor WF, et al: Chondrosarcoma: A clinicopathologic and statistical analysis. Cancer 45:149–157, 1980.
15. Radiological Atlas of Bone Tumors, Vol 1. The Netherlands Committee on Bone Tumors (eds). Baltimore, Williams & Wilkins Co, 1966.
16. Silverberg E, Lubera J: Cancer statistics, 1987. Ca—A Cancer Journal for Clinicians 37:12, 1987.
17. Suit HD, Mankin HJ, Wood WC, et al: Treatment of the patient with stage M_0 sarcoma of soft tissue. J Clin Oncol 6:854–862, 1988.
18. Urie M, Goitein M, Wagner M: Compensating for heterogeneities in proton radiation therapy. Phys Med Biol 29:553–556, 1983.
19. Wilkins RM, Pritchard DJ, Burgert EO, Unni KK: Ewing's sarcoma of bone. Experience with 140 patients. Cancer 58:2551–2555, 1986.

CHEMOTHERAPY

DAVID C. HARMON

Chemotherapy has a growing role in the management of bone tumors. More tumors are showing greater responsiveness to new drugs and schedules. Of the diseases that affect the spine, leukemias respond the most dramatically to chemotherapy. However, because they are systemic illnesses, they are beyond the scope of this chapter. Most of the lesions discussed in this book appear as bulky masses requiring surgery or radiotherapy for local control. Tumors that have a tendency for distant spread may be more completely eradicated by adding systemic chemotherapy. In addition, wide surgical excision or radical radiotherapy of tumors of the spine is often precluded by the tumor's proximity to the spinal cord. A portion of the burden for controlling local tumor may thus rest on chemotherapy, a modality usually reserved for disseminated but microscopic disease.

Chemotherapy alone cannot be relied upon to control most larger masses of tumor because the probability of malignant cells becoming resistant to drugs increases as the tumor grows. Most tumors large enough to be clinically detectable already have subclones resistant to many drugs. Using combinations of selected chemotherapeutic agents may overcome this problem for some tumors, such as lymphomas. However, for most malignancies, we lack agents capable of eradicating all subclones at doses tolerable to patients. Tumor bulk also limits drug penetration. Moreover, in a bulky tumor, a smaller portion of cells will be in the growth fraction where they are susceptible to cytotoxic drugs that target replicating DNA.[51]

Chemotherapy can attack microscopic foci of cancer outside the fields of surgery and radiotherapy and thus can eliminate causes of distant and marginal failure. For most tumors discussed in this book it is this adjuvant role of chemotherapy that is paramount. From a different perspective, chemotherapy can also be used to prevent metastatic tumors of the spine. For example, postoperative adjuvant chemotherapy reduces bone metastases from breast cancer. Moreover, for sensitive tumors like Ewing's sarcoma, preoperative adjuvant chemotherapy can shrink the primary tumor enough to permit less extensive and morbid therapy of local disease.

Since reliable in vitro chemosensitivity assays are currently under development, most patients are treated with drugs shown to have had the highest response rates in earlier series of patients. Whenever possible, combinations are used to overcome resistance to any single agent. Ideally agents having different toxicities are combined so that antitumor effects will add up without additive side effects on normal tissue. The major thrust of most clinical trials is to find new drugs, combinations, or schedules that are maximally tumoricidal but still tolerable.

Because most antineoplastic agents have strong dose-response relationships, regimens aimed at cure generally require doses to be pushed to toxic levels. Limitations of the bone marrow typically demand intermittent courses of therapy to allow recovery of blood counts between treatments. Therefore, bone marrow transplantation and growth factors are being tested to see if they can increase patient tolerance to more intensive therapy. Giving earlier and more aggressive chemotherapy is important to ensure optimal therapeutic activity against rapidly growing tumors for which effective chemotherapy exists.

Because intravenous administration permits more precise blood levels to be achieved, this route is usually preferred for aggressive, cure-oriented regimens. When palliation is the goal, the oral route is often more appropriate. For tumors in the spine, some investigators have preferred the arterial route, hoping to concentrate drug in the area of the tumor while sparing the systemic circulation.[49] Unfortunately, the spine does not lend itself to the kind of isolation-perfusion technique that has experimental and clinical evidence to prove its advantage over the intravenous route.[18] Although some spine tumors have responded to simple arterial infusion, any advantage of intraarterial over intravenous administration is unproven. Unless a tumor avidly takes up a drug on the first pass, most of the drug will enter the systemic circulation just as it would via a vein.[32] Hyperthermia may improve the uptake of a drug but as yet cannot be focused well enough to match the precision of proton beam radiotherapy as described in Chapter 9.

HISTOPATHOLOGIC TYPES OF TUMOR

Osteosarcoma

Since 1970, major advances have been made in the chemotherapy of osteosarcoma. Effective drugs and combinations have been identified and adjuvant chemotherapy has contributed to the dramatic improvement in survival of osteosarcoma of the extremities. Too few reports of osteosarcoma in the spine have been published to judge what impact these advances may have on the curability of this rarer lesion.[72] However, for spine lesions amenable to resection, the same principles of therapy to control systemic spread may apply. For unresectable lesions aggressive chemotherapy can still control disease for a time. Even metastatic disease can sometimes be cured with combined modality therapy.

Alone and in combination, doxorubicin, high dose methotrexate with leucovorin rescue, cisplatinum, and a combination of bleomycin, cyclophosphamide, and actinomycin have produced response rates between 20 and 60 per cent with some complete responses.[15, 37, 54, 56, 68] DTIC and ifosfamide also have activity.[26, 40]

High dose methotrexate with leucovorin rescue appears to work where conventional doses do not.[33] Doses on the order of 12 gm/m^2 may be needed to penetrate tumors and to overcome drug resistance.[67] However, the great expense of this drug contributes to controversy over its optimal dose, as such high doses seem to have value in few other tumors.[1]

Successes with postoperative adjuvant chemotherapy using doxorubicin and high dose methotrexate led the way to a series of increasingly aggressive drug therapies for osteosarcoma.[16, 23, 35] Although there has been controversy, randomized controlled studies now strongly support the role of aggressive adjuvant chemotherapy. In a multiinstitutional randomized study without chemotherapy, the two-year disease-free survival was only 17 per cent compared with 66 per cent for those receiving chemotherapy for high grade osteosarcoma of the extremity.[46] Moreover, studies by Rosen suggest that disease-free survival, up to 90 per cent at two years, can be achieved using preoperative chemotherapy then selecting postoperative therapy based on the degree of response.[64] Although most of the advantage of adjuvant chemotherapy comes from controlling distant metastases, the local failure rate is also reduced, an observation of special interest for marginally resectable lesions like those of the spine.

It may even be possible for preoperative chemotherapy to convert some apparently inoperable tumors into surgically approachable ones.[75, 76] Radiotherapy can provide additional local control.[21] Whether chemotherapy alone can cure completely unresectable tumor remains to be seen. However, useful regression and remissions of disease have been described using combination chemotherapy with or without intraarterial cisplatinum.[6, 34, 36, 65] Intraarterial high dose methotrexate has no advantage over the intravenous adminstration of the drug.[38]

Malignant Fibrous Histiocytoma

Metastatic malignant fibrous histiocytomas have been treated with some success with drugs and regimens that are active in osteosarcoma. Similar adjuvant chemotherapy may be appropriate for the higher grade tumors resembling osteosarcoma.[81] In one series with or without high dose methotrexate, doxorubicin was associated with an improvement in 5-year survival (57 per cent versus 28 per cent) compared with a series treated with surgery alone.[10]

Chondrosarcoma, Fibrosarcoma, Dedifferentiated Mesenchymoma

Higher grade lesions of these histologies have as dismal a prognosis as osteosarcoma treated without chemotherapy. Metastases from these tumors respond to the same drugs used to treat osteosarcoma. Therefore primary lesions may warrant similar adjuvant chemotherapy. However there are few published reports, so the role of chemotherapy in treating these tumors remains unproven.[8]

Vascular Tumors of Bone

Although little is known about the responsiveness of vascular sarcomas of bone, their soft tissue counterparts respond to doxorubicin, DTIC, cyclophosphamide, methotrexate, and ifosfamide.[69]

Chordomas

Although chordomas eventually metastasize in up to one third of patients, chemotherapy has barely been explored, perhaps because recurrent local disease has been the greater problem clinically.[80] Vincristine has shown some activity, and a variety of alkylating agents also have case reports to support their use.[17, 39, 52, 62, 74]

Multiple Myeloma

Although individual painful lytic lesions in the spine are often best treated by radiation, the usually more diffuse spread of myeloma is an indication for chemotherapy. Systemic chemotherapy can slow the spread of disease, counteract complications of hypercalcemia, hyperviscosity, renal failure, and anemia, and thus prolong life.

Probably the most popular drug for treating myeloma is melphalan, but other alkylating agents such as chlorambucil, cyclophosphamide, lomustine, carmustine, and hexamethylmelamine produce responses in 30 to 50 per cent of cases.[3, 12, 14, 41, 73] Higher dose intermittent treatment with melphalan offers convenience but no consistent therapeutic advantage over lower dose continuous schedules.[2] Intravenous therapy provides more precise control of dose, allowing higher dose levels and somewhat higher response rates, but at the cost of more severe myelosuppression.[50] Using bone marrow support, even higher doses can be combined with radiation to achieve yet higher response rates, but also greater toxicity.[58] Even so, cure remains elusive, and such experimental approaches are restricted primarily to the minority of younger patients.

Prednisone is useful for its plasmacytolytic effects and also for its effects on calcium metabolism.[61] Thus prednisone is combined with melphalan in a variety of regimens. It remains uncertain whether adding more drugs initially to this pair adds enough benefit to warrant the increased toxicity and inconvenience. However, some increase in response rate has been claimed for the more complex regimens, especially for patients with more advanced disease.[11, 13, 20, 28, 57, 71]

Alternative therapies include high dose steroids with or without doxorubicin and vincristine.[4] Interferon has definite activity and its role is being investigated.[60] For patients with hyperuricemia, allopurinol is an important adjunct.

Perhaps because current regimens are only moderately efficacious, there is little evidence that patients with solitary plasmacytomas or very early multiple myeloma benefit much from having systemic chemotherapy started early in the course of their disease.[42] Neither is there evidence to support maintenance therapy beyond remission. In fact prolonged alkylating agent therapy is associated with a high risk of secondary leukemia.[7] Nevertheless, when symptomatic disease or complications develop, such as renal impairment, hypercalcemia, hyperviscosity, or advancing cytopenias, the introduction of chemotherapy can make a worthwhile difference.

Neurofibrosarcoma

The literature offers scant information on chemotherapy specific to tumors having neural differentiation but arising in bone. As for vascular tumors of the spine, one might attempt therapy with regimens active in soft tissue counterparts.[69]

Paraspinal Tumors Involving the Spine

Neuroblastoma and peripheral neuroectodermal tumors will be discussed in Chapter 27.

Renal Carcinoma. Renal carcinoma is relatively resistant to chemotherapy. Vinblastine and lomustine have provided a small percentage of worthwhile regressions.[27, 31] Interferon and interleukin-2 with or without lymphokine-activated killer cells or tumor-infiltrating lymphocytes may provide new options for treatment.[24, 55] Hormonal therapies such as megestrol acetate have a very small role.

Lung Carcinoma. Lung cancers of the small cell variety respond frequently and often completely to combinations of cyclophosphamide, doxorubicin, vincristine, etoposide, and cisplatinum as well as to radiotherapy.[22] Cures may be possible. Non–small cell lung cancers respond only partially to these and other drugs.

Retroperitoneal Sarcomas. Retroperitoneal sarco-

mas respond in about half of cases to doxorubicin, DTIC, cyclophosphamide, and ifosfamide. However, adjuvant therapy has not yet proven of value in this setting.[69, 83]

Miscellaneous Tumors

Ewing's Sarcoma

Ewing's sarcoma is especially sensitive to chemotherapy, which is the essential initial component of treatment for all patients. Combinations of cyclophosphamide, doxorubicin, vincristine, and actinomycin are common to a variety of successful programs. Methotrexate, bleomycin, carmustine, 5-fluorouracil, etoposide, DTIC, cisplatinum, and ifosfamide are also useful.[30, 59, 66] While surgery is preferred for easily accessible lesions, moderate dose radiotherapy can control a high percentage of tumors at any site, especially when aided by drug therapy. In one series using aggressive chemotherapy, 65 per cent of patients with axial tumors were disease-free at a median of 41 months.[66] Even patients with metastatic Ewing's sarcoma have a chance of cure with intensive therapy.[30, 59] Adding total body irradiation with or without autologous marrow transplant may improve the cure rate.[53]

Lymphoma

Lymphoma of the spine or epidural space is usually a complication of metastatic disease and occurs occasionally in all types of lymphoma. However, some patients present with apparently solitary lesions in bones, including those of the spine. Local radiotherapy should cure most of these patients, but depending on the histology half or more fail.[19] A possible explanation is that with careful staging more than half of those appearing as isolated lesions will actually have demonstable metastases. Some authors argue for a staging laparotomy to select patients more likely to be cured by radiotherapy alone.[77] Others would prefer at least some adjuvant chemotherapy for all high grade lymphomas of bone.[5, 47] A number of highly effective regimens are available for use as adjuvant with radiotherapy or as salvage for patients relapsing after radiation alone.[9] The more aggressive programs may even eliminate the necessity for radiotherapy in some cases.

Eosinophilic Granuloma

Eosinophilic granuloma that fails to be controlled by surgery or radiation may still respond to chemotherapy with vinblastine and 6-mercaptopurine with or without prednisone.[48] However, since this is seldom an aggressive lesion, intense regimens are rarely justified.

Metastatic Prostate Cancer

Prostate cancer often spreads to bones of the spine. Although radiation provides effective palliation for most patients, in advanced disease hormonal manipulations may also help. Diethylstilbestrol 1 to 3 mg per day, progestational agents, and luteinizing hormone releasing hormone (LHRH) agonists are all effective.[45] Adding an antiandrogen such as flutamide may augment the response rate.[43] Whether and when to add cytotoxic chemotherapy is less clear because of its increased toxicity and modest benefit. Cyclophosphamide is often used and other agents have activity, but no single agent or combination has emerged as clearly superior.[25, 78, 79]

Metastatic Breast Cancer

Those breast cancers possessing estrogen receptors are often managed well with minimal toxicity by hormonal measures. Tamoxifen 10 mg bid, or megestrol acetate 40 mg qid, androgens, and aminoglutethimide are all popular regimens with response rates above 50 per cent.[29, 70, 82] Even in receptor-negative patients, similar response rates are achieved with combination chemotherapy using cyclophosphamide, doxorubicin, 5-fluorouracil, methotrexate, vinblastine, and others. Therapy often relieves symptoms and sometimes prolongs life.[44] More aggressive approaches are under investigation.

CHEMOTHERAPY REGIMENS

Osteosarcoma and Related Tumors

Osteosarcoma, malignant fibrous histiocytoma of bone, high grade chondrosarcoma, fibrosarcoma of bone, and dedifferentiated mesenchymal tumors have been treated with intensive chemotherapy used mostly for osteosarcoma in children. The following regimen is extremely intense and requires very close monitoring by experienced oncologists. Few adults can tolerate full doses. Renal, cardiac, and hepatic function must be good.

D = Doxorubicin 30 mg/M² daily × 3d
d = Doxorubicin 50 mg/M² × 1d
P = Cisplatinum 90 mg/M² × 1d
M = Methotrexate 8–12 gm/M² followed at 24h by leucovorin 15 mg q6h × 10 with adjustments based on methotrexate and creatinine levels
B = Bleomycin 15 U/M² × 2d
C = Cyclophosphamide 600 mg/M² × 2d
A = Actinomycin D 0.6 mg/M² × 2d

(See chart at bottom of page)

Vascular Tumors, Neurofibromas, Paraspinal and Retroperitoneal Soft Tissue Sarcomas

The following regimen has been used in patients with good cardiac and renal function every 3 to 4 weeks for 7 cycles, with modifications for nadir white blood cell counts and for hematuria or elevated bilirubin.

Doxorubicin	15–20 mg/M² daily × 4d
Ifosfamide	2–2.5 gm/M² daily × 3d
Mesna	2–2.5 gm/M² daily × 4d
DTIC	250–300 mg/M² daily × 4d

Chordomas

While no standard chemotherapy is available, vincristine 1.4 mg/M² with a maximum dose of 2 mg might be tried in patients without serious neurologic compromise. Cisplatinum 90 mg/M² may be added or substituted.

Multiple Myeloma

For many patients the simplest and most convenient regimen is probably as good as more intense and complicated ones. Melphalan may be given orally at 0.15 mg/kg daily for 7 days along with prednisone 60 mg per day for 7 days. Cycles are repeated every 6 weeks.

Renal Carcinoma

Vinblastine 10 mg/M² IV every 2 to 3 weeks has a small response rate which may be increased slightly by adding lomustine orally at 100–200 mg/M² every 6 weeks at the expense of increased myelotoxicity.

Lung Carcinoma

Although other histologies may also respond, only small cell lung cancer responds well enough to have a reasonably accepted therapy. A typical regimen includes several cycles at 3-week intervals of cyclophosphamide 1000 mg/M², doxorubicin 40 mg/M², vincristine 1 mg/M², alternating with or followed by cycles of cisplatinum 20 mg/M² and etoposide 100 mg/M² daily for 4 days.

Ewing's Sarcoma

Protocols of various intensity have been tried but most include vincristine 2 mg/M² (max. 2 mg) IV every 1 to 3 weeks, cyclophosphamide 1–1.8 gm/M² IV or orally every 3 weeks, and doxorubicin 45–90 mg/M² IV every 3 weeks up to a cumulative dose of 450 mg/M². Thereafter actinomycin D 1.5 mg/M² is

Week	1	2	3	4	5	6	7	8	9	10	11	12	13	14	15	16	17	18	19	20	21	22	23
	B		M	M	M	M	D			M	M	B		M	M	D			d			d	
	C											C							P			P	
	A											A											
	24	25	26	27	28	29	30	31	32	33	34	35	36	37	38	39	40	41	42	43	44		
		B			M	M			d			d			B			B		M	M		
		C							P			P			C			C					
		A													A			A					

substituted. Newer regimens add cycles of ifosfamide 2 gm/M² and etoposide 100–200 mg/M² daily for 4 to 5 days.

Lymphomas of Bone

High grade, large cell lymphomas respond well to the "CHOP" regimen:

Cyclophosphamide 750 mg/M² IV
Doxorubicin 50 mg/M² IV
Vincristine 1.4 mg/M² (max. 2 mg) IV
Prednisone 100 mg PO daily × 5d

Cycles are repeated every 3 weeks for 6 to 8 cycles.

Eosinophilic Granuloma

Although it seldom requires therapy, this lesion may regress with intravenous vinblastine 6–10 mg/M² every 2 to 3 weeks. Etoposide 100–200 mg/M² IV or PO may also be effective.

Breast Cancer

Several effective protocols can be used. For patients needing radiotherapy near the spinal cord, one might choose one of the "CMF" regimens:

Cyclophosphamide 100 mg/M² daily × 14d
Methotrexate 30–40 mg/M² IV days 1 and 8
5-Fluorouracil 400–600 mg/M² days 1 and 8

When radiosensitization is not an issue, one might substitute doxorubicin 40 mg/M² for methotrexate.

REFERENCES

1. Ackland SP, Schilsky RL: High-dose methotrexate: A critical reappraisal. J Clin Oncol 5:2017–2031, 1987.
2. Ahre A, Bjorkholm M, Mellstedt H, et al: Intermittent high-dose melphalan/prednisone versus continuous low-dose melphalan treatment in multiple myeloma. Eur J Cancer Clin Oncol 19:499–506, 1983.
3. Alexanian R, Haut A, Kahn AU, et al: Treatment for multiple myeloma: Combination chemotherapy with different melphalan dose regimens. JAMA 208:1680–1685, 1969.
4. Alexanian R, Yap BS, Bodey GP, et al: Prednisone pulse therapy for refractory myeloma. Blood 62:572–577, 1983.
5. Bacci G, Jaffe N, Emiliani E, et al: Therapy for primary non-Hodgkin's lymphoma of bone and a comparison of results with Ewing's sarcoma: Ten years' experience at the Instituto Ortopedico Rizzoli. Cancer 57:1468–1472, 1986.
6. Benjamin RS, Murray JA, Wallace S, et al: Intra-arterial preoperative chemotherapy for osteosarcoma: A judicious approach to limb salvage. Cancer Bull 36:32–36, 1984.
7. Bergsagel DE: Plasma cell neoplasms and acute leukemia. Clin Haematol 11:221–234, 1982.
8. Bertoni F, Picci P, Bacchini P, et al: Mesenchymal chondro-sarcoma of bone and soft tissues. Cancer 52:533, 1983.
9. Boyd DB, Coleman M, Papish SW, et al: COPBLAM III: Infusional combination chemotherapy for diffuse large-cell lymphoma. J Clin Oncol 6:425–433, 1988.
10. Capanna R, Bertoni F, Bacchini P, et al: Malignant fibrous histiocytoma of bone: The experience at the Rizzoli Institute: Report of 90 cases. Cancer 54:177–187, 1984.
11. Case DC, Lee BJ, Clarkson BD: Improved survival times in multiple myeloma treated with melphalan, prednisone, cyclophosphamide, vincristine, and BCNU: M-2 protocol. Am J Med 63:897–903, 1977.
12. Cohen HJ, Bertolucci AA: Hexamethylmelamine and prednisone in the treatment of refractory multiple myeloma. Am J Clin Oncol (CCT) 5:21–27, 1982.
13. Cooper MR, McIntyre OR, Propert K: Single, sequential, and multiple alkylating agent therapy for multiple myeloma: A CALGB study. J Clin Oncol 4:1331–1339, 1986.
14. Cornwell GG, Pajak TF, Kochwa S, et al: Comparison of oral melphalan, CCNU and BCNU with and without vincristine and prednisone in the treatment of multiple myeloma. Cancer 50:1669–1675, 1982.
15. Cortes EP, Holland JF, Wang JJ, et al: Doxorubicin in disseminated osteosarcoma. JAMA 221:1132–1138, 1972.
16. Cortes EP, Holland JF, Wang JJ, et al: Amputation and Adriamycin in primary osteosarcoma. N Engl J Med 291:998–1000, 1974.
17. Cummings B, Esses S, Harwood AR: The treatment of chordomas. Cancer Treat Rev 9:299–311, 1982.
18. Didolkar MS, Kanter PM, Baffi RR, et al: Comparison of regional versus systemic chemotherapy with adriamycin. Ann Surg 187:332–336, 1978.
19. Dosoretz D, Raymond AK, Murphy G, et al: Primary lymphoma of bone. The relationship of morphologic diversity to clinical behavior. Cancer 50:1009–1014, 1982.
20. Durie G, Dixon D, Carter S, et al: Improved survival duration with combination chemotherapy induction for multiple myeloma: A Southwest Oncology Group study. J Clin Oncol 4:1227–1237, 1986.
21. Eilber FR, Mirra JJ, Grant TT, et al: Is amputation necessary for sarcomas? A seven-year experience with limb salvage. Ann Surg 192:431–438, 1980.
22. Einhorn LH, Crawford J, Birch R, et al: Cisplatin plus etoposide consolidation following cyclophosphamide, doxorubicin, and vincristine in limited small-cell lung cancer. J Clin Oncol 6:451–456, 1988.
23. Ettinger L, Douglas H, Higby D, et al: Adjuvant Adriamycin and cis-diamminedichloroplatinum (cis-platinum) in primary osteosarcoma. Cancer 47:248–254, 1981.
24. Fisher RI, Coltman CA, Doroshow JH, et al: Metastatic renal cancer treated with interleukin-2 and lymphokine-activated killer cells. Ann Intern Med 108:518–523, 1988.
25. Gibbons RP, Beckley S, Brady M, et al: The addition of chemotherapy to hormonal therapy for treatment of patients with metastatic carcinoma of the prostate. J Surg Oncol 23:133–142, 1983.
26. Gottlieb JA, Baker LH, O'Bryan RM, et al: Adriamycin (NSC-123 127) used alone and in combination for soft tissue and bony sarcomas. Cancer Chemother Rep 6:271–282, 1975.
27. Hahn DM, Schimpff SC, Ruckdeschel JC, et al: Single agent chemotherapy for renal cell carcinoma: CCNU, vinblastine, thiotepa or bleomycin. Cancer Treat Rep 61:1585–1587, 1977.
28. Harley JP, Pajak TF, McIntyre OR, et al: Improved survival of increased-risk myeloma patients on combined triple-alkylating agent therapy: A study of the CALGB. Blood 54:13–21, 1979.
29. Harris A, Powles T, Smith I: Aminoglutethimide for the treatment of advanced postmenopausal breast cancer. Eur J Cancer 19:11–17, 1983.
30. Hayes FA, Thompson E, Hustu H, et al: The response of Ewing's sarcoma to sequential cyclophosphamide and Adriamycin induction therapy. J Clin Oncol 1:45–51, 1983.
31. Hrushesky WJ, Murphy GP: Current status of the therapy of advanced renal carcinoma. J Surg Oncol 9:227–288, 1977.
32. Hsiao-Sheng GC, Gross JF: Intra-arterial infusion of anti-cancer drugs: Theoretic aspects of drug delivery and review of responses. Cancer Treat Rep 64:31–40, 1980.
33. Jaffe N: Recent advances in the chemotherapy of metastatic osteogenic sarcoma. Cancer 30:1627–1631, 1972.
34. Jaffe N, Bowman R, Wang Y-M, et al: Chemotherapy for primary osteosarcoma by intra-arterial infusion. Cancer Bull 36:37–42, 1984.
35. Jaffe N, Frei E, Traggis D, et al: Adjuvant methotrexate and citrovorum-factor treatment of osteogenic sarcoma. N Engl J Med 291:994–997, 1974.

36. Jaffe N, Knapp J, Chung VP, et al: Osteosarcoma: Intra-arterial treatment of the primary tumor with cis-diammine-dichloroplatinum II (CDP). Cancer 51:402–407, 1983.

37. Jaffe N, Link MP, Cohen D: High-dose methotrexate in osteosarcoma. NCI Monogr 56:201–206, 1981.

38. Jaffe N, Prudich J, Knapp J, et al: Treatment of primary osteosarcoma with intra-arterial and intravenous high-dose methotrexate. J Clin Oncol 1:428–431, 1983.

39. Karakousis C, Park J, Fleminger R, Friedman M: Chordomas: Diagnosis and management. Am Surg 47:497–501, 1981.

40. Klein HO, Dias W, Coerper C: Treatment of advanced soft tissue and osteosarcomas with continuous infusion of ifosfamide and mesna. Cancer Chemother Pharmacol 18(Suppl 2):19s, 1986.

41. Korst DR, Clifford GO, Fowler WM, et al: Multiple myeloma. II. Analysis of cyclophosphamide in 165 patients. JAMA 189:758–762, 1964.

42. Kyle RA, Greipp PR: Smoldering multiple myeloma. N Engl J Med 302:1347–1349, 1980.

43. Labrie F, Dupona A, Belanger A, et al: New approach in the treatment of prostate cancer: Complete instead of only partial withdrawal of androgens. Prostate 4:579–594, 1983.

44. Legha S, Buzdar A, Smith T, et al: Complete remissions in metastatic breast cancer treated with combination drug therapy. Ann Intern Med 91:847–852, 1979.

45. Lepor H, Ross A, Walsh P: The influence of hormonal therapy on survival of men with advanced prostatic cancer. J Urol 128:335–340, 1982.

46. Link M, Goorin A, Miser A, et al: The effect of adjuvant chemotherapy on relapse-free survival in patients with osteosarcoma of the extremity. N Engl J Med 314:1600–1606, 1986.

47. Loeffler JS, Tarbell NJ, Kozakewich H, et al: Primary lymphoma of bone in children: Analysis of treatment results with adriamycin, prednisone, oncovin (APO), and local radiation therapy. J Clin Oncol 4:496–501, 1986.

48. Matus-Ridley M, Raney B, Therwani H, Meadows A: Histiocytosis X in children: Patterns of disease and results of treatment. Med Pediatr Oncol 11:99–105, 1983.

49. Mavligit GM, Benjamin R, Patt YZ, et al: Intraarterial cis-platinum for patients with inoperable skeletal tumors. Cancer 48:1–4, 1981.

50. McElwain TJ, Powles RL: High-dose intravenous melphalan for plasma-cell leukaemia and myeloma. Lancet 2:822–824, 1983.

51. Mendelsohn ML: The growth fraction: A new concept applied to tumors. Science 132:1496, 1960.

52. Mensi F, Bombara R, Massari A, et al: The chordoma: Description of 2 clinical cases and results of oncolytic chemotherapy. Minerva Med 70:2759–2766, 1979.

53. Miser J, Kinsella T, Triche T, et al: Preliminary results of treatment of Ewing's sarcoma of bone in children and young adults: Six months of intensive combined modality therapy without maintenance. J Clin Oncol 6:484–490, 1988.

54. Mosende C, Gutierrez M, Caparros B, et al: Combination chemotherapy with bleomycin, cyclophosphamide and dactinomycin for the treatment of osteosarcoma. Cancer 40:2779–2786, 1977.

55. Neidhart JA: Interferon for the treatment of renal cancer. Cancer 57:1696–1699, 1986.

56. Ochs JJ, Freeman AI, Douglas HO, et al: Cis-dichlorodiamineplatinum (II) in advanced osteogenic sarcoma. Cancer Treat Rep 62:239–245, 1978.

57. Oken NM: Multiple myeloma. Med Clin North Am 68:757–787, 1984.

58. Osserman EF, DiRe LB, DiRe J, et al: Identical twin marrow transplantation in multiple myeloma. Acta Haematol 68:215–223, 1982.

59. Pilepich MV, Vietti TJ, Nesbit M, et al: Radiotherapy and combination chemotherapy in advanced Ewing's sarcoma—Intergroup study. Cancer 47:1930–1936, 1981.

60. Quesada JR, Alexanian R, Hawkins M, et al: Treatment of multiple myeloma with recombinant alpha interferon. Blood 67:275–278, 1986.

61. Raisz LG, Luben RA, Mundy GR, et al: Effect of osteoclast activating factor from human leukocytes on bone metabolism. J Clin Invest 56:408–413, 1975.

62. Razis DV, Tsatsaronis A, Kyriazides I, Triantafyllou D: Chordoma of the cervical spine treated with vincristine sulfate. J Med 5:274–277, 1974.

63. Reimer RR, Chabner B, Young RC, et al: Lymphoma presenting in bone: Results of histopathology, staging and therapy. Ann Intern Med 87:50–55, 1977.

64. Rosen G: Preoperative (neoadjuvant) chemotherapy for osteogenic sarcoma: A ten year experience. Orthopedics 8:659–664, 1985.

65. Rosen G, Caparros B, Huvos A, et al: Preoperative chemotherapy for osteogenic sarcoma: Selection of postoperative adjuvant chemotherapy based on response of the primary tumor to preoperative chemotherapy. Cancer 49:1221–1230, 1982.

66. Rosen G, Caparros B, Nirenberg A, et al: Ewing's sarcoma: Ten year experience with adjuvant chemotherapy. Cancer 47:2204–2213, 1981.

67. Rosen G, Nirenberg A: Chemotherapy for osteogenic sarcoma: An investigative method, not a recipe. Cancer Treat Rep 66:1687–1697, 1982.

68. Rosen G, Suvanisirikul S, Kwon C, et al: High-dose methotrexate with citrovorum factor rescue and Adriamycin in childhood osteogenic sarcoma. Cancer 33:1151–1163, 1974.

69. Rosenberg SA, Suit HD, Baker LH: Sarcomas of soft tissues. In DeVita V, Hellman S, Rosenberg SA (eds): Cancer Principles and Practice of Oncology. 2nd ed. Philadelphia, JB Lippincott Company, 1985, pp 1243–1291.

70. Ross M, Buzdar A, Blumenshein G: Treatment of advanced breast cancer with megestrol acetate after therapy with tamoxifen. Cancer 49:4133–4137, 1982.

71. Salmon SE, Haut, Bonnet DJD, et al: Alternating combination chemotherapy and levamisole improves survival in multiple myeloma: A Southwest Oncology Group study. J Clin Oncol 1:453–461, 1983.

72. Shives TC, Dahlin DC, Sim FH, et al: Osteosarcoma of the spine. J Bone Joint Surg 68:660–668, 1986.

73. South Eastern Cancer Study Group: Treatment of myeloma: Comparison of melphalan, chlorambucil and azathioprine. Arch Intern Med 135:157–162, 1975.

74. Sundaresan N, Galicich J, Chu F, Huvos A: Spinal chordomas. J Neurosurg 50:312–319, 1979.

75. Sundaresan N, Galicich J, Rosen G, Huvos A: Primary osteogenic sarcoma of the skull: Five-year disease-free survival following surgery and high dose methotrexate therapy. NY State J Med 85:598–599, 1985.

76. Sundaresan N, Rosen G, Fortner JG, et al: Preoperative chemotherapy and surgical resection in the management of posterior paraspinal tumors. J Neurosurg 58:446–450, 1983.

77. Sweet DL, Moss DP, Simon MA, et al: Histiocytic lymphoma (reticulum-cell sarcoma) of bone: Current strategy for orthopedic surgeons. J Bone Joint Surg 63:79–84, 1981.

78. Torti F, Aston D, Lum B, et al: Weekly doxorubicin in endocrine-refractory carcinoma of the prostate. J Clin Oncol 1:447–482, 1983.

79. Torti F, Carter S: The chemotherapy of prostatic carcinoma. Ann Intern Med 92:681–689, 1980.

80. Volpe R, Mazabraud A: A clinicopathologic review of 25 cases of chordoma (a pleomorphic and metastasizing neoplasm). Am J Surg Pathol 7:161–170, 1984.

81. Weiner M, Sedlis M, Johnston A, et al: Adjuvant chemotherapy of malignant fibrous histiocytoma of bone. Cancer 51:25–29, 1983.

82. Westerberg H: Tamoxifen and fluoxymesterone in advanced breast cancer: A controlled clinical trial. Cancer Treat Rep 64:117–121, 1980.

83. Yap B, Baker L, Sinkovics J, et al: Cyclophosphamide, vincristine, adriamycin, and DTIC (CYVADIC) combination chemotherapy for the treatment of advanced sarcomas. Cancer Treat Rep 64:93–98, 1980.

THE ROLE OF CRYOSURGERY

RALPH C. MARCOVE

Based on personal experience of over 25 years, the author has found cryosurgery to be an effective treatment in eradication of benign symptomatic and/or benign aggressively destructive spine tumors. Fully malignant tumors have also been successfully eradicated to help establish the value of this method of treatment. We have advocated a rebiopsy, two to three months later, of a previously treated malignant lesion. This helps ensure that the tumor has been completely destroyed by cryosurgery. Regional arteriography both before and after treatment may also be helpful to ensure the adequacy of the surgery.

Cryosurgery is a local, in situ necrotizing process that may be equivalent to a more extensive radical removal of tumor. The cup-like shell of the residual bone can easily be reexplored to determine if tumor is still present. Unlike the limitations of radiotherapy, cryosurgery can, if necessary, be repeated. In fact, in the spine there may be no alternative but to periodically repeat cryosurgery to control local disease, for example, in the case of patients with unresectable chordomas or chondrosarcomas. However, a limiting factor may be that in some of these patients, the tumor may be too extensive for thorough, complete cryosurgery or even excision. Here cryosurgery offers only a mode of providing palliation. In such lesions in the distal spine the alternative treatment of hemicorporectomy (Theodore Miller) is now rarely offered. Localized, intraarterial chemotherapy and/or local radiotherapy may remain the only other therapy available. In slow-growing tumors (i.e., low grade chondrosarcoma), even with unresectable multiple pulmonary metastasis, the patient may have a relatively long life expectancy. The latter may convert to a fast-growing more lethal variety (Grade III). In our experience, chemotherapy in this instance can be helpful.

Trials of sulfur (S[35]) therapy have resulted in tumor regression of both chordoma and chondrosarcoma, but this treatment has been occasionally complicated by a leukemoid or frank leukemia. After initial clinical tumor regression (Tables 11–1 and 11–2), serial rebiopsies subsequently done on different tissues after previous S[35] therapy have shown that the residual tumor cells may produce less matrix and appear to be progressively more anaplastic.[26] Perhaps che-

motherapy in this latter hypercellular phase would be helpful, as it has been in our anaplastic chondrosarcoma (Grade III) cases. The S[35] trials at Memorial Sloan-Kettering Cancer Center have now been discontinued because of leukemia complications. The author, nevertheless, believes that a trial of S[35] and subsequent chemotherapy have some merit in late or end-stage disease, especially if one uses modern marrow storage techniques.

A wide array of diseases located in the spine or long bones have been treated by cryosurgery. Such diseases include benign simple bone cysts, symptomatic vertebral hemangioma, aneurysmal bone cysts, eosinophilic granuloma, aggressive fibrous dysplasia, fibromyxoma, giant cell tumor, and benign chondroblastoma. Many of the above diseases can be treated at the initial open biopsy phase once a frozen section confirms the diagnosis. Malignant tumors have also been treated by cryosurgery, including malignant fibrous histiocytoma, osteogenic sarcoma, chondrosarcoma, and Ewing's sarcoma. In these cases the size of the tumor and the ability to deliver the liquid nitrogen to the entire lesion are limiting factors. Preoperative chemotherapy (or radiation therapy) will be helpful for larger lesions. When subsequent rebiopsy proves residual disease, cryosurgery may be the only alternative. Nitrogen may be delivered within a double lumen tube directly to the area (Fig. 11–1A).

An alternative and quicker way to freeze tissue is to pour liquid nitrogen directly into a curetted cavity (Fig. 11–1B). A funnel tip is sealed to the tumor with wet Gelfoam. This technique prevents spilling of the nitrogen into the surrounding tissue. The evaporation of the gas should not be impeded.

Another alternative method of using liquid nitrogen is to use it as a spray to direct it to less accessible cavities and to freeze and temporarily control a bleeding vessel. Bleeding should be controlled because it impedes the nitrogen's ability to necrose the tumor. Bleeding also may be controlled by either a direct spray or first surface freezing and then working deeper to the involved area. Another method is packing the hemorrhage of a curetted tumor with Gelfoam and then freezing the pack and the tumor together. The ice pack that develops can be gradually

TABLE 11–1. CHONDROSARCOMA TREATED BY S³⁵ THERAPY

		Cumulative S³⁵		Number		Clinical Time From:				Hematology at Death/March 1977			
						Death		Alive					
Patient	Sex/Age	mCi	mCi/kg	Dose	Wk*	Dx	Rx†	Dx	Rx	Bone Marrow	Hgb g%	WBC × 10³	Plt × 10³
WM	M/51	4126	48.3	8	75	2 yr	2 yr	—	—	Hypercellular with many primitive cells. Slight differentiation, some clearly of erythroid series. Acute erythroid leukemia. Chromosomal abnormalities.	4.1	0.6	18.0
CK	F/56	2140	45.6	8	88	15 yr	3 yr	—	—	Markedly hypocellular section shows low grade chondrosarcoma, abundant chondroid matrix.	10.1	1.7	33.0
RT	M/26	1550	28.3	5	66	—	—	10 yr	6 yr	Pancytopenia '75	11.6	2.0	47.0
JA	M/13	768	21.6	4	22	1 yr	6 mo	—	—	—	7.8	2.8	171
DO	M/12	388	10.7	2	5	4 mo	3 mo	—	—	—	7.2	18.5	35.0
CF	F/72	718	10.0	2	9	1 yr	4 mo	—	—	—	7.0	5.7	221

*Time from administration of first therapy dose to administration of last dose.
†Time from administration of first therapy dose.

chipped or drilled. The freezing is thereby progressively performed deeper and deeper into the involved tissue. It must be emphasized that the diseases mentioned above have to be located in an area that allows the tumor to be adequately exposed to the liquid nitrogen. As already mentioned, another indication for cryosurgery is in conjunction with local resection, especially if one margin cannot be adequately removed. In these cases the liquid nitrogen can be a useful supplement to the local resection and may be lifesaving.

The size of the freeze may be limited to a 2- to 6-inch diameter (Fig. 11–2A), depending on local vascularity and the amount of different number or

TABLE 11–2. CHORDOMA TREATED BY S³⁵ THERAPY

		Cumulative S³⁵		Number		Clinical Time From:				Hematology at Death/March 1977			
						Death		Alive					
Patient	Sex/Age	mCi	mCi/kg	Dose	Wk*	Dx	Rx†	Dx	Rx	Bone Marrow	Hgb g%	WBC × 10³	Plt × 10³
HS	M/66	2823	37.6	6	64	8 yr	3 yr	—	—	Markedly hypocellular. Aplastic anemia.	5.1	1.4	58.0
RL	M/63	1942	32.3	6	67	11 yr	5.3 yr	—	—	Hypocellular, decrease in myeloid series, increase in erythroid precursors. Terminal acute leukemia.	11.2	3.8	78.0
MD	F/75	1519	21.5	4	40	3.3 yr	3 yr	—	—	Myelomonocytic leukemia, ABO type change.	9.1	16.9	12.0
FMcE	M/51	1106	13.2	3	44	6.5 yr	4.5 yr	—	—	Dysplastic erythroid hyperplasia.	8.0 / 10.0	4.0 / 2.2	6.0 / 22.0
PP	M/56	994	12.3	3	28	6.5 yr	1.3 yr	—	—	Sepsis, persistent thrombocytopenia; increased erythroid hyperplasia.	5.6	9.6	8.0
SE	M/71	824	12.4	2	15	3 yr	2.7 yr	—	—	—	10.6	5.0	13.4
FD	M/50	718	10.1	2	9	1 yr	7 mo	—	—	—	10.2	8.2	308

*Time from administration of first therapy dose to administration of last dose.
†Time from administration of first therapy dose.

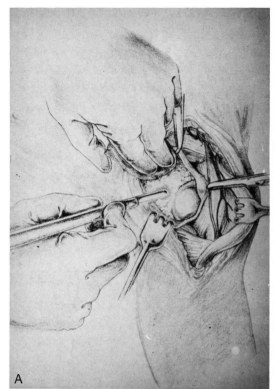

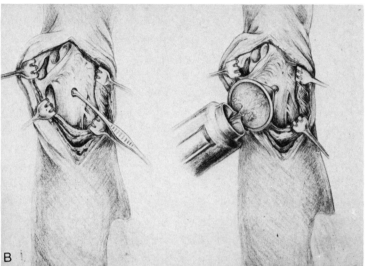

FIGURE 11–1. *A,* The probe method of freezing tumor bone tissue. *B,* The pouring method of freezing tumor bone tissue.

placements of the probe(s). The necrosis (Fig. 11–2B) and regeneration of new bone (Fig. 11–2C and D) have been well documented. Often the tumor (e.g., chordoma) may be enormous and may not therefore be adequately frozen. In addition, where the tumor has contaminated upper sacral margin, this area can be frozen during the resection attempt. Multifocal disease presentation may also limit the benefit of cryosurgery. The dural and spinal nerves may be protected from the cold by placing wet Gelfoam against the structures, and these areas are kept visualized to avoid their freezing. Nerve palsies have been an occasional complication, especially when used in the sacrum or adjacent ilium. For example, one patient with a giant cell tumor at the sacroiliac area of the ilium had both a femoral nerve and a sciatic nerve palsy that resolved completely at two years and three months, respectively. The tumor did not recur and a hemipelvectomy was, therefore, averted.

Giant cell tumors may occur diffuse or localized in the sacrum. Although a giant cell tumor may be local (i.e., of the odontoid) and has been cryosurgically controlled, the author's experience is that giant cell tumors of the spine often may be quite extensive, involving both anterior and posterior spinal elements. It may also be associated with huge areas of aneurysmal bone cyst extending into the adjacent soft tissues. One such case had an additional significant area of unicameral bone cyst as well as a large aneurysmal bone cyst and a third area of giant cell tumor. The surgery had to be supplemented with radiation therapy. (Cryosurgery seemed to be too limited here.) Before cryosurgery or resection attempts, angiography and intravascular plugging with Gelfoam or other agents may be very helpful. When not used,

one patient with a giant cell tumor required transfusion of 60 units of blood to attempt to curette the lesion, and the giant cell tumor could not be frozen because of its size and vascularity. The latter required extensive packing to control hemorrhage. This patient was later advised to undergo a course of radiation therapy, which she declined.

In spine tumors, it may be extremely helpful to perform a fusion connecting unaffected areas of the spine above and below adjacent to the tumor destruction. The fusion may be instrumental in maintaining stability of the patient's spine and may allow recovery without significant morbidity once the tumor is controlled. On comparison, cryosurgery does not interfere with a fusion mass as much as radiation therapy, especially at the higher dose levels (above 3500 cGy). Bone fusions can be supplemented with Steinmann pins and cement at the time of resection.

Ewing's sarcomas often respond dramatically to chemotherapy and/or radiation therapy; however, in 20 to 40 per cent of cases, surgical exploration after "adequate therapy" will give evidence of local persistence of disease. This has been successfully eradicated with cryosurgery as well as local radical resection. Repeat biopsies have subsequently confirmed the successful cryosurgical eradication of a persistent Ewing's sarcoma. The therapeutic approach can be adapted to Ewing's tumor of the spine as well as that occurring in an extremity. Pelvic localization is not uncommon. Surgical eradication of Ewing's sarcoma has repeatedly been shown to result in a doubling of the cure rates when compared with radiation.[33]

Osteogenic sarcoma, which is small and localized, and malignant fibrous histiocytoma have been successfully treated with cryosurgery, even without chemotherapy and without radiation therapy. Four

Text continued on page 108

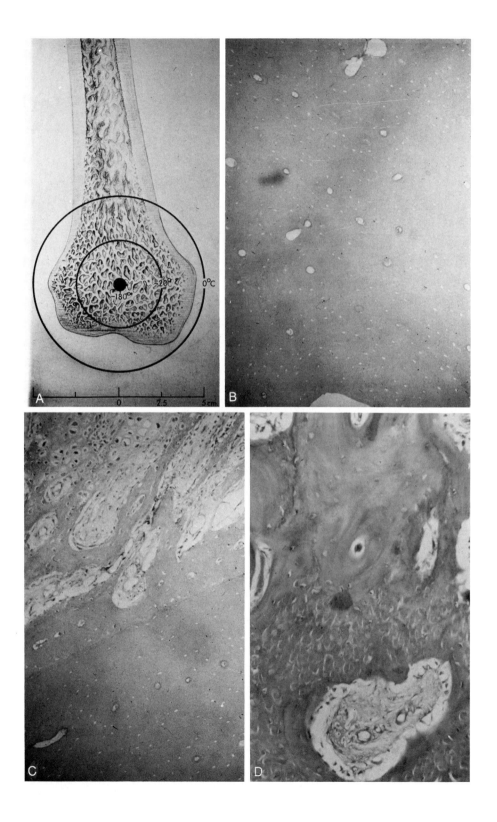

FIGURE 11–2. *A*, The range of visible ice (0° C) and the rapid rise in temperature from the heat sink source (−180° C). Repeated achievement of at least −20° C must be accomplished (three times) to obtain necrosis. *B*, Necrosis of dog cortex is shown by empty lacunae (specimen taken four weeks after cryosurgery). *C*, Periosteal new bone (nonlamellar, hypercellular) is shown developing on the osteonecrotic cortical surface in eight weeks. *D*, Endosteal new bone.

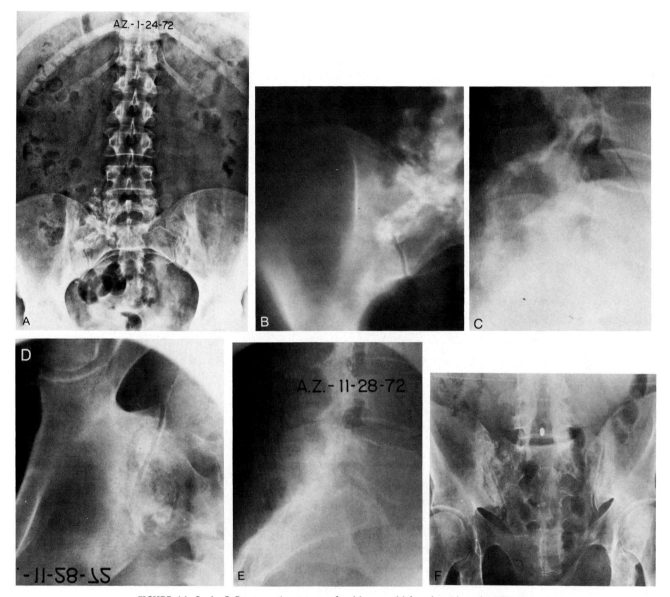

FIGURE 11–3. *A–C,* Preoperative x-rays of a 44-year-old female with a chondrosarcoma of the right iliac crest. *D–F,* Postoperative x-rays of the same patient following en bloc excision of right posterior iliac crest and transverse process of L4 and L5 with cryosurgery. Patient is now 16 years postop with no evidence of disease.

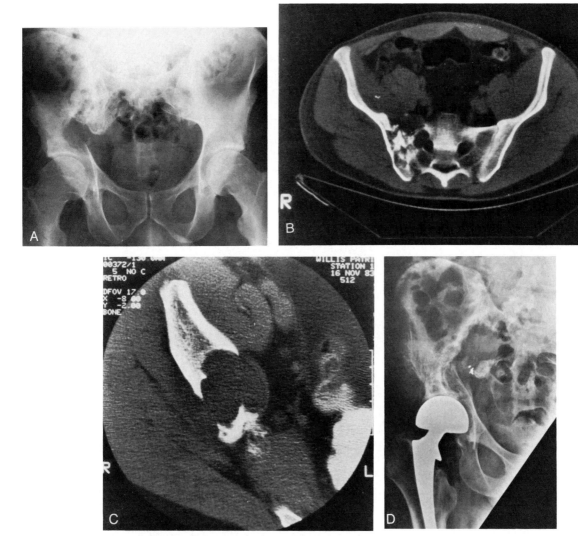

FIGURE 11–4. *A*, Preoperative x-ray of a 24-year-old male with a chondrosarcoma of the left ilium and sacrum. *B* and *C*, Preoperative computed tomography (CT) scan of the same patient. *D*, Postoperative x-ray of the same patient taken 50 months after resection and cryosurgery. Patient has no evidence of disease.

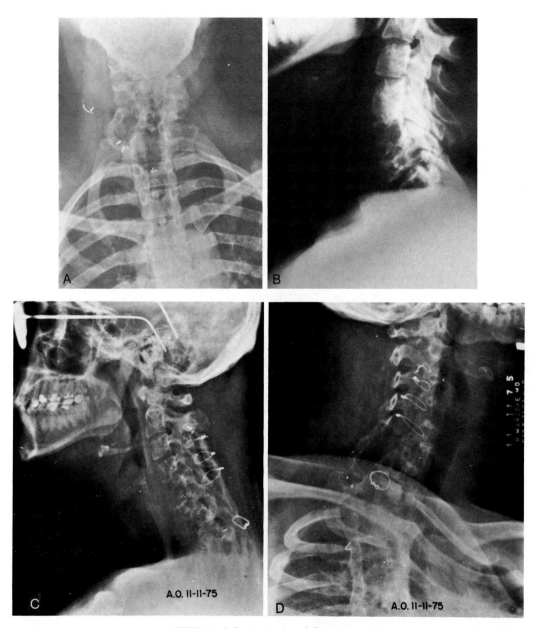

FIGURE 11—5 *See legend on following page*

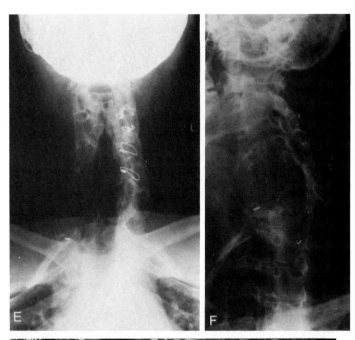

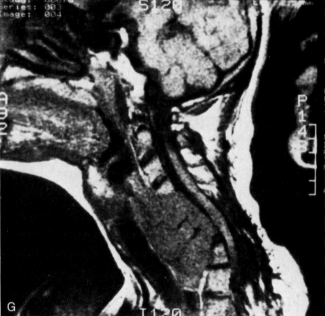

FIGURE 11–5. *A* and *B*, Preoperative x-rays of a 35-year-old male with neurofibromatosis of the cervical spine with spine instability. *C–F*, Postoperative x-rays of the same patient following posterior cervical Robinson fusion using fibula bone grafts. *G*, Postoperative magnetic resonance imaging (MRI) scan of the same patient taken 12 years postfusion. Patient has no evidence of disease and is doing well.

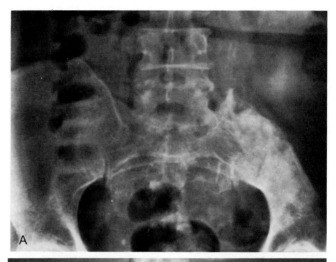

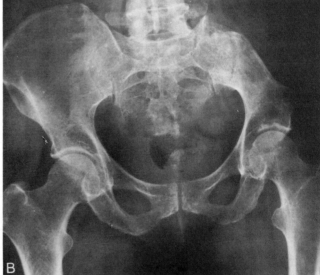

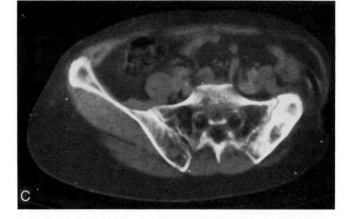

FIGURE 11–6. X-rays (*A* and *B*) and computed tomography (CT) scan *(C)* of a 56-year-old female with a radiation sarcoma of the left sacroiliac joint. Patient underwent resection of wing of ilium and sacrum with cryosurgery.

cases have been reported by the author. Another surgeon's case has had one small suspicious microscopic focus of persistent tumor in the entire specimen postcryosurgery. That instance was particularly favorable for simply repeating cryosurgery following the suspicious rebiopsy.

Low and medium grade chondrosarcoma can be treated by cryosurgery with good results proven by rebiopsies (Fig. 11–3). Among our cases, one patient developed local recurrence three years *after* a negative rebiopsy. Since the alternative treatment to the above failed cryosurgery case was hemicorporectomy, it was decided to repeat the cryosurgery and have the patient resume his normal working and family life (Fig. 11–4). Prior to cryosurgery, this patient had undergone surgical exploration on two occasions in England for a possible hemipelvectomy but was not found resectable because of sacral involvement. Repeat biopsy is again planned. One sacral case has been followed 16 years without evidence of recurrence following cryosurgery. Two negative repeat open biopsies were performed at three months and one year.

In general, the principle of anterior and posterior spinal fusion (Robinson) for pathologic disease is still valid (Fig. 11–5). The author has supplemented such fusions with methyl methacrylate around heavy Steinmann pins. The immediate fixation is valuable following tumor curettage and cryosurgery or resection. This also gives the bone grafts a chance to heal. The fixation should transverse the tumor area from healthy vertebra above to healthy vertebra below. Figure 11–6 illustrates a radiation sarcoma of the spine and ilium with no evidence of disease eight years after local resection and supplemental cryosurgery, where the lumbar spine involvement necessitated cryosurgery in addition to classic tumor resection.

As in any other location, cryosurgery therapy of both benign and malignant tumors as well as resection is possible in the spine. This method is limited by the tumor size. Rebiopsy is recommended in malignant tumors when feasible. Chemotherapy or radiation therapy supplements may be tried. Unlike limitations on radiation dosage, cryosurgery can be repeated multiple times until tumor is controlled.

REFERENCES

1. Ablin RJ, Gonder MJ, Soanes WA: Immunohistologic studies of carcinoma of the prostate. Oncology 29(4):329–334, 1974.
2. Ablin RJ, Soanes WA, Gonder MJ: Prospects for cryo-immunotherapy in cases of metastasizing carcinoma of the prostate. Cryobiology 8(3):271–279, 1971.
3. Albright JA, Gillespie TE, Butaud TR: Treatment of bone metastases. Semin Oncol 7(4):418–434, 1980.
4. Berggren R, Ferraro J, Price B: A comparison of cryophylactic agents for pretreatment of preserved frozen rat skin. Cryobiology 3:272–274, 1966.
5. Biesecker JL, Marcove RC, Huvos AG, Mike V: Aneurysmal bone cysts. A clinicopathologic study of 66 cases. Cancer 26:615, 1970.
6. Cooper IS: Cryogenic surgery: A new method of destruction or extirpation of benign or malignant tissues. N Engl J Med 268:744, 1963.
7. Eckardt JJ, Grogan TJ: Giant cell tumor of bone. Clin Orthop 204:45–58, 1986.
8. Gage AA: Cryosurgery for cancer: An evaluation. Cryobiology 5:241, 1969.
9. Gage AA, Greene JCW, Neiders ME, Emmlings FG: Freezing bone without excision. JAMA 196:770–774, 1966.
10. Goldenberg RR, Campbell CJ, Bonfiglio M: Giant cell tumor of bone. An analysis of two hundred and eighteen cases. J Bone Joint Surg 52A:619, 1970.
11. Goldner JL, Forrest JS: Giant cell tumor of bone. South Med J 54:121, 1961.
12. Gursel E, Roberts M, Veenema RJ: Regression of prostatic cancer following sequential cryotherapy to the prostate. J Urol 108(6):928–932, 1972.
13. Hutter RVP, Worchester JN, Francis KC, et al: Benign and malignant giant cell tumors of bone. Cancer 15:653, 1962.
14. Immenkamp M: Eosinophilic granuloma of the spine. Z Orthop 123(2):227–234, 1985.
15. Jaffe HL, Lichtenstein L, Portis RB: Giant cell tumor of bone: Its pathologic appearance, grading, supposed variants and treatment. Arch Pathol 30:993, 1940.
16. Jennings JW Sr: Production and control of low temperature in cryosurgery. AORN 6:7, 1968.
17. Johnson EW Jr, Dahlin DC: Treatment of giant cell tumor of bone. J Bone. Joint Surg 41A:895, 1959.
18. Johnson EW Jr, Riley LH: Giant cell tumor of bone: An evaluation of 24 cases treated at the John Hopkins Hospital between 1925 and 1955. Clin Orthop 62:187, 1969.
19. Luyet BJ, Grell SM: A study with the ultracentrifuge of the mechanism of death in frozen cells. Biodynamica 1:1–16, 1936.
20. Marcove RC: A 17-year review of cryosurgery in the treatment of bone tumors. Clin Orthop 163:231–234, 1982.
21. Marcove RC, Lyden JP, Huvos AG, Bullough PG: Giant cell tumors treated by cryosurgery. J Bone Joint Surg 55A:1633, 1973.
22. Marcove RC, Miller TR: Treatment of primary and metastatic localized bone tumors by cryosurgery. JAMA 207:1890, 1969.
23. Marcove RC, Miller TR: Treatment of primary and metastatic localized bone tumors by cryosurgery. Surg Clin North Am 49:421, 1969.
24. Marcove RC, Miller TR, Cahan WC: The treatment of primary and metastatic bone tumors by repetitive freezing. Bull NY Acad Med 44:532, 1968.
25. Marcove RC, Stovell PB, Huvos AG, Bullough PG: The use of cryosurgery in the treatment of low and medium grade chondrosarcoma—A preliminary report. Clin Orthop 122:147, 1977.
26. Mayer K, Pentlow KS, Marcove RC, et al: Sulfur-35 therapy for chondrosarcoma and chordoma. *In* Spencer RP (ed): Therapy in Nuclear Medicine. New York, Grune and Stratton, 1978.
27. Mirra JM, Rand F, Rand R, et al: Giant cell tumor of the second cervical vertebra treated by cryosurgery and irradiation. Clin Orthop 154:228–233, 1981.
28. Mnaymneh WA, Dudley H, Mnaymneh LG: Giant cell tumor of bone. An analysis and follow-up study of forty-one cases observed at the Massachusetts General Hospital between 1925 and 1960. J Bone Joint Surg 46A:63, 1964.
29. Pang-fu K, Pu-fan C, Hua-feng T, Tsai-wei S: Cryosurgery in giant cell tumor of bone. Chin Med J 92(2):125–128, 1979.
30. Pegg DE: Cryobiology: Review article. Phys Med Biol 11:209–224, 1966.
31. Rowe AW: Biochemical aspects of cryo-protective agents in freezing and thawing. Cryobiology 3:12–18, 1966.
32. Schwimer SR, Bassett LW, Mancuso AA, et al: Giant cell tumor of the cervicothoracic spine. AJR 136(1):63–67, 1981.
33. Li WK, Lane JM, Rosen G, Marcove RC, et al: Pelvic Ewing's sarcoma—Advances in treatment. J Bone Joint Surg 65A(6):738–747, 1983.

NEW APPROACHES TO MEDICAL MANAGEMENT OF SPINAL TUMORS

RAYMOND P. WARRELL, Jr.

Spinal involvement by malignant tumors, particularly via metastasis, is a frequent occurrence in the course of many patients with cancer. The major problems related to bone metastases are pain, neurologic dysfunction, hypercalcemia, and pathologic fractures. The focus of this chapter is on medical therapies that may reduce the likelihood of developing spinal metastases or palliative treatments that may ameliorate the complications.

PREVENTION

Prevention of spinal metastasis may be primary or secondary. Primary prevention is any maneuver that reduces the likelihood of getting cancer in the first place, or early detection and definitive treatment before metastases have developed. Secondary prevention involves patients who have been diagnosed with cancer but who do not currently have evidence of metastasis. Therapy may involve measures that eradicate potential micrometastasis by tumoricidal treatments. The use of adjuvant cytotoxic chemotherapy after mastectomy for breast cancer is one example of the former method of secondary prevention. These forms of primary or secondary preventive strategies fall beyond the scope of this chapter and will not be reviewed here.

In patients with early-stage cancer, timing of the metastatic event obviously cannot be known. Therefore, secondary prevention may also involve the use of drugs that interfere with the process of metastasis. Such therapy should obviously be directed at populations at highest risk for development of bone metastasis. Highly osteotropic (bone-seeking) tumors include non–small cell lung, breast, and prostate cancer.

Metastasis involves a complex series of events. These steps include separation from the primary tumor, entry into and travel through the lymphatic or vascular system, attachment to and penetration through the basement membrane, and growth and neovascularization of the metastatic tumor. Certain breakdown products of bone (e.g., collagen fragments) are chemotactic for certain tumor cells and may also stimulate tumor growth.[29, 30, 32, 33, 36] Since cancer cells may possess receptors for such molecules on their cell surfaces, these observations may explain the osteotropic behavior of certain types of cancer, particularly breast and prostate cancer. Many tumor cells circulate in blood as clumps together with platelet and fibrin aggregates.[20, 31] There exists an extensive literature on the experimental use of anticoagulants (such as warfarin[10, 24, 51] or other antithrombins[37]), or drugs that affect platelet-tumor cell interactions, such as RA-233[2] and nafazatrom.[48] Theoretically, early initiation of treatment with such agents (i.e., before and during the first operative procedure and for some time thereafter) should increase the circulation time of cancer cells in blood and increase the chance that such cells would be destroyed by the reticuloendothelial system.

Fibronectin and other molecules may be important in the process of attachment to the basement membrane and thus represent potential therapeutic targets for antimetastatic therapy.[9, 26] Invasion of the vascular basement membrane involves tumor-associated enzymes, such as collagenase or plasminogen activator.[11, 35] Thus, invasion might be selectively inhibited by use of protease inhibitors.[12] Neovascularization of the secondary tumor is required, and drugs such as protamine have been shown to inhibit this process. Finally, certain anti-inflammatory drugs (aspirin and flurbiprofen) have also been proposed as inhibitors of bone metastasis.

Despite considerable experimental data, clinical results do not show convincing evidence that adjuvant use of such antimetastatic drugs is useful. These clinical trials are extremely expensive since they necessarily involve large numbers of patients who must be followed for prolonged periods. Persistent efforts should be made to enroll eligible patients in trials designed to evaluate the potential benefit of antimetastatic therapy.

TREATMENT OF ESTABLISHED SPINAL METASTASES

Despite a report that breast cancer cells in culture were able to directly resorb devitalized bone particles,[16] it is generally agreed that tumors cause osteolysis by stimulation of resorption that is mediated by normal bone cells, such as osteoclasts.[34] Therefore, drugs that reduce bone resorption may be useful for reducing specific problems related to accelerated bone loss and also for reducing the incidence of new bone metastases. Ideally, antiresorptive drugs should not adversely affect normal bone nor cause significant toxicity to nontarget tissues. The principal drugs currently available for this purpose are calcitonin, bisphosphonates, and gallium nitrate (Table 12–1).

Calcitonin

Calcitonin is a calcium-regulating hormone derived from chief cells of the thyroid gland. The principal effect of calcitonin is the inhibition of cell-mediated bone resorption by reducing either the number or function of osteoclasts.[14] Calcitonin may also have important effects at the renal level.[25]

Controlled studies in patients with bone metastases are limited. However, preliminary data suggest that therapy with calcitonin can provide important analgesic benefit. In a randomized study, the effects of salmon calcitonin were compared with clodronate and placebo. In this small trial, hydroxyproline excretion was decreased in both treatment groups relative to the placebo group, consistent with inhibition of resorption; onset of pain relief occurred most rapidly in patients who were treated with calcitonin.[21] A randomized, double-blind study versus placebo also showed significantly greater reduction in pain for patients who were treated with calcitonin.[23]

Currently, synthetic salmon calcitonin (Calcimar) is most commonly available. For specialized use in hypersensitive patients, porcine and recombinant human forms are available. Calcitonin is usually injected subcutaneously on a daily basis or three times per week. Experimental studies using calcitonin administered as an intranasal spray have also been reported.

Bisphosphonates

Bisphosphonates (diphosphonates) are analogues of pyrophosphates which are resistant to hydrolysis by pyrophosphatase and thus are stable in vivo for prolonged periods. Bisphosphonates bind to hydroxyapatite and render bone mineral less susceptible to resorption.[19] Many of these drugs also directly inhibit bone cell function and may be directly toxic to osteoclasts.[38] Various bisphosphonates are now in clinical trials, including etidronate, clodronate, and APD.

Etidronate

Etidronate (ethanehydroxy bisphosphonate disodium; Didronel) has been used for several years as treatment for Paget's disease.[28] In patients with cancerous bone metastases, short-term treatment with etidronate administered intravenously has significantly reduced urinary hydroxyproline excretion.[43] Etidronate (Didronel) has also been shown to be significantly more effective than placebo for acute treatment of cancer-related hypercalcemia.[22] This agent is also the only bisphosphonate currently approved for marketing in the United States. Treatment with etidronate administered orally has resulted in reduced bone pain in a small series of patients in an unblinded study.[40] However, even low doses of etidronate are known to cause osteomalacia,[8] which will further compromise bone strength in patients with osteolytic disease. Therefore, etidronate has not been recommended for this use, and research activity has focused on other bisphosphonates.

Clodronate

The most extensive clinical studies with any bisphosphonate have been conducted with clodronate (dichloromethylene bisphosphonate). Metabolic studies in patients with bone metastases show that clodronate increased intestinal calcium resorption with a marginal decrease in bone resorption.[27] In two small series of patients with breast cancer and myeloma, clodronate treatment resulted in decreased urinary hydroxyproline excretion and reduced bone pain.[41, 42] The findings in multiple myeloma were also confirmed in a randomized double-blind study from Europe which involved 13 patients.[15] Symptomatic improvement in bone pain has also been observed with the use of clodronate for bone metastases from prostate cancer.[1]

In a preliminary randomized study, 34 patients with osteolytic metastases from breast cancer received either clodronate or placebo. Patients treated with clodronate experienced significantly greater analgesic relief and required less palliative radiotherapy. A decrease in uptake of radionuclide at the sites of known metastases was observed, along with a significant decrease in the incidence of new pathologic fractures.[17] A surprising finding when this study was updated was the observation of a significant increase in overall survival for patients who received clodronate.[18] These favorable data await confirmation in a larger series.

Clinical investigations with clodronate were suspended after reports of secondary leukemias occurring in patients with multiple myeloma. Although the possibility of an increased incidence of leukemia

TABLE 12–1. DRUGS CURRENTLY AVAILABLE FOR USE AS INHIBITORS OF BONE RESORPTION

Calcitonins
  Salmon calcitonin (Calcimar)
  Recombinant human calcitonin (Cibacalcin)

Bisphosphonates
  Ethanehydroxy bisphosphonate (etidronate disodium; Didronel)
  Dichloromethylene bisphosphonate (clodronate; DCl$_2$MDP)
  Aminohydroxypropylidene bisphosphonate (APD)

Gallium nitrate

was suggested, these findings have not been substantiated in broader clinical trials. Nonetheless, clinical activity with clodronate has largely been superseded by trials with newer bisphosphonates, such as APD.

APD

APD (aminohydroxypropylidene bisphosphonate; Aredia) appears to inhibit bone resorption by inhibiting the function of osteoclasts.[38] Several studies have found that APD administered intravenously is effective treatment for cancer-related hypercalcemia.[6, 7] A preliminary study in patients with osteolytic metastases from myeloma or breast cancer showed that oral treatment with APD reduced urinary excretion of calcium and hydroxyproline, suggesting a direct effect on tumor-induced bone resorption.[44]

In a recent study of 131 women with bone metastases from breast cancer, oral APD significantly reduced bone pain, requirements for palliative skeletal radiation therapy, and the incidence of pathologic fractures relative to placebo.[45] In that study, oral APD was associated with nausea and fever, which reduced compliance with extended use. Nonetheless, this study is important for its confirmation of the beneficial results that can be achieved with the use of bone resorption inhibitors.

Gallium Nitrate

Gallium nitrate was originally developed as an anticancer agent. The drug was unexpectedly found to cause hypocalcemia, and most recent research has been directed toward further elucidation of this effect. Gallium nitrate has been found to be a potent inhibitor of bone resorption in vitro. Gallium nitrate antagonizes the bone resorptive effects of a variety of substances which stimulate bone resorption, including parathyroid hormone,[47] crude lymphokine with "osteoclast activating factor activity,"[47] and recombinant human tumor necrosis factor.[5] Gallium is known to accumulate at very low levels within bone mineral. Such accumulation is associated with the formation of hydroxyapatite crystals that are larger or more "perfect." The physiochemical result is that these crystals are less soluble and more resistant to resorption by osteoclasts.[3] Gallium treatment also increases the uptake of radiolabeled calcium into bone mineral in vivo[39] and increases bone collagen synthesis in vitro.[4] These data suggest not only that gallium decreases bone resorption but also that the drug may enhance bone formation. As such, the agent may be broadly useful for diseases characterized by increased loss of bone mineral.

Preliminary clinical studies have shown that moderate doses of gallium nitrate administered intravenously are acutely effective for control of cancer-related hypercalcemia.[47, 50] These data have since been confirmed in randomized double-blind studies in which gallium was shown to be significantly more potent than salmon calcitonin.[49] These results are depicted graphically in Figure 12–1. Randomized multicenter studies are also in progress to compare the effectiveness of gallium nitrate to etidronate (administered intravenously) for acute therapy of hypercalcemia.

Given the potent effects of gallium nitrate on bone resorption and formation, efforts have been directed toward evaluating whether gallium nitrate could be useful for treatment of bone metastases. In a preliminary study, gallium nitrate was infused intravenously to patients with bone metastases. Gallium was shown to significantly reduce biochemical parameters of accelerated bone loss (i.e., urinary calcium and hydroxyproline).[46] A randomized study has been initiated to evaluate whether chronic (6 months) treatment with low doses of gallium nitrate administered subcutaneously (similar to calcitonin) can restore bone mass in patients with extensive osteolysis due to multiple myeloma. The major outcome determinant will measure total body calcium using neutron activation analysis and total bone mineral with dual

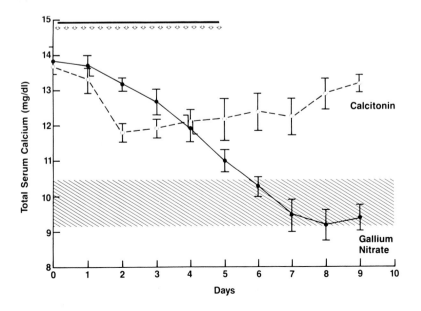

FIGURE 12–1. Comparative effects of gallium nitrate versus maximal doses of salmon calcitonin for acute control of cancer-related hypercalcemia. (From Warrell RP Jr, Israel R, Frisone M, et al: Gallium nitrate for acute treatment of cancer-related hypercalcemia. A randomized, double-blind comparison to calcitonin. Ann Intern Med 108:669–674, 1988.)

photon absorptiometry. These tests—primarily developed as measurements for patients with osteoporosis—are more sensitive, more reliable, and substantially less subjective measures of bone mineralization than conventional radiography or quantitative bone scanning. Preliminary results suggest that gallium nitrate administered subcutaneously may be highly effective in increasing bone calcium content and preventing complications of bone metastasis, including pain, pathologic fractures, and hypercalcemia.[48]

SUMMARY OF CURRENT THERAPY AND RECOMMENDATIONS

The best treatment to avoid complications related to spinal tumors is obviously prevention, either by early diagnosis prior to metastasis or by eradication of micrometastases using cytotoxic chemotherapy. The use of agents that inhibit metastasis formation by circulating tumor cells must be regarded as investigational. Although these agents generally cause few adverse reactions, their use outside of controlled clinical trials cannot be recommended at present.

For patients with established bone disease in the spine, it is becoming increasingly apparent that use of drugs that retard bone resorption may relieve bone pain and reduce the incidence of other complications, such as neurologic dysfunction, pathologic fractures, and hypercalcemia. Clodronate is the best-studied agent for this use, and preliminary results in women with breast cancer appear highly promising. APD administered orally (800 mg twice daily) may be useful for reducing morbidity from skeletal metastases due to breast cancer. Of other bisphosphonates, only etidronate is commercially available in the United States. Use of etidronate in patients with bone metastases is not recommended since even short-term use has been associated with osteomalacia in cancer patients.

Calcitonin (salmon or recombinant human) is widely available. The agent has seen increased use, particularly in the United Kingdom, as a method for relieving bone pain due to skeletal tumors. Although calcitonin has limited potency, further clinical trials to evaluate its efficacy are clearly desirable. In patients with severe bone pain, short-term use of calcitonin (100 to 200 units subcutaneously or intranasally) can be administered daily or three times per week in patients with bone pain to see whether there is any symptomatic response.

Gallium nitrate will be commercially available in 1990 for acute treatment of cancer-related hypercalcemia. While moderate doses are used for this worst-case example of osteolysis, ongoing clinical trials of low doses administered chronically ($20-30$ mg/m²/day, subcutaneously) should definitively establish whether gallium nitrate can retard bone loss or remineralize areas of bone previously eroded by cancer cells.

This area is a focus of intense research interest by many investigators. In the near future, a variety of effective new compounds should become available for palliative medical treatment of patients with spinal involvement by cancer.

REFERENCES

1. Adami S, Salvagno G, Guarrera G, et al: Dichloromethylene diphosphonate in patients with prostatic carcinoma metastatic to skeleton. J Urol 134:1152–1154, 1984.
2. Ambrus JL, Ambrus CM, Gastpar H: Studies on platelet aggregation in vivo. VI. Effect of a pyrimido-pyrimidine derivative (RA-233) on tumor cell metastasis. J Med 9:183–188, 1978.
3. Bockman RS, Boskey A, Blumenthal NC, et al: Gallium increases bone calcium and crystallite perfection of hydroxyapatite. Calcif Tissue Int 39:376–381, 1986.
4. Bockman RS, Israel R, Alcock N, et al: Gallium nitrate stimulates bone collagen synthesis. Clin Res 35:620A, 1987.
5. Bockman RS, Repo MA, Warrell RP, et al: Gallium nitrate inhibits bone resorption induced by recombinant human tumor necrosis factor (TNF). Proc Am Assoc Cancer Res 28:449, 1987.
6. Body JJ, Borkowski A, Cleeren A, Bijvoet OLM: Treatment of malignancy-associated hypercalcemia with intravenous aminohydroxypropylidene diphosphonate. J Clin Oncol 4:1177–1183, 1986.
7. Body JJ, Pot M, Borkowski A, et al: Dose/response study of aminohydroxypropylidene bisphosphonate in tumor-associated hypercalcemia. Am J Med 82:957–963, 1987.
8. Boyce BF, Smith L, Fogelman I, et al: Focal osteomalacia due to low-dose diphosphonate therapy in Paget's disease. Lancet 1:821–824, 1984.
9. Brackenberg R: Molecular mechanisms of cell adhesion in normal and transformed cells. Cancer Metastasis Rev 4:41–58, 1985.
10. Brown JM: A study of the mechanism by which anticoagulation with warfarin inhibits blood-borne metastases. Cancer Res 33:1217–1224, 1973.
11. Carlson SA, Ramshaw IA, Warrington RC: Involvement of plasminogen activator production with tumor metastasis in a rat model. Cancer Res 44:3012–3016, 1984.
12. Cresson DH, Bickman WC, Tidwell RR, et al: In vitro inhibition of human sarcoma cells invasive ability by bis(5-amidino-2-benzimidazolyl) methane—a novel enteroprotease inhibitor. Am J Pathol 123:46–56, 1986.
13. D'Amore PA: Growth factors, angiogenesis and metastases. Prog Clin Biol Res 212:269–286, 1986.
14. Deftos JJ, Furst BP: Calcitonin as a drug. Ann Intern Med 95:192–197, 1981.
15. Delmas PD, Charhon S, Chapuy MC, et al: Long-term effects of dichloromethylene diphosphonate (Cl₂MDP) on skeletal lesions in multiple myeloma. Metab Bone Dis Relat Res 4:163–168, 1982.
16. Eilon G, Mundy GR: Direct resorption of bone by human breast cancer cells in vitro. Nature 276:726–728, 1978.
17. Elomaa I, Blomqvist C, Grohn P, et al: Long-term controlled trial with diphosphonate in patients with osteolytic bone metastases. Lancet 1:146–148, 1983.
18. Elomaa I, Blomqvist C, Porkka L, et al: Diphosphonates for osteolytic metastases. Lancet 1:1155–1156, 1985.
19. Fleisch H, Felix R: Diphosphonates. Calcif Tissue Int 27:91–94, 1979.
20. Gasic GJ, Gasic TB, Galanti N, et al: Platelet-tumor cell interactions in mice: The role of platelets in the spread of malignant disease. Int J Cancer 11:704–718, 1973.
21. Gennari C, Francini G, Gonnelli S, Bigazzi S: Treatment of bone metastasis with antiresorptive drugs. In Garattini S (ed): Bone Resorption, Metastasis, and Diphosphonates. New York, Raven Press, 1985, pp 127–136.
22. Hasling C, Charles P, Mosekilde L: Etidronate disodium for treating hypercalcaemia of malignancy: A double blind, placebo-controlled study. Eur J Clin Invest 16:433–437, 1986.
23. Hindley AC, Hill EB, Leyland MJ, Wiles AE: A double-blind controlled trial of salmon calcitonin in pain due to malignancy. Cancer Chemother Pharmacol 6:71–74, 1982.
24. Hoover HC Jr, Ketcham AS, Millar RC, Gralnick HR: Osteo-

sarcoma: Improved survival with anticoagulation and amputation. Cancer 41:2475–2480, 1978.

25. Hosking DJ, Gilson D: Comparison of the renal and skeletal actions of calcitonin in the treatment of severe hypercalcaemia of malignancy. Q J Med 211:359–368, 1984.

26. Hynes RO: Fibronectins. Sci Am 154:42–51, 1986.

27. Jung A, Chantraine A, Donath A, et al: Use of dichloromethylene diphosphonate in metastatic bone disease. N Engl J Med 308:1499–1502, 1983.

28. Krane SM: Etidronate disodium in the treatment of Paget's disease of bone. Ann Intern Med 96:619–625, 1982.

29. Magro C, Orr FW, Manishen WJ, et al: Adhesion, chemotaxis, and aggregation of Walker carcinosarcoma cells in response to products of resorbing bone. J Natl Cancer Inst 74:829–838, 1985.

30. Manishen WJ, Sivananthan K, Orr FW: Resorbing bone stimulates tumor cell growth: A role for the host microenvironment in bone metastasis. Am J Pathol 123:39–45, 1986.

31. Mehta P: Potential role of platelets in the pathogenesis of tumor metastasis. Blood 63:55–63, 1984.

32. Mundy GR: Chemotactic activity of the gamma-carboxyglutamic acid containing protein in bone. Calcif Tissue Int 35:164–166, 1983.

33. Mundy GR, DeMartino S, Rowe DW: Collagen and collagen-derived fragments are chemotactic for tumor cells. J Clin Invest 68:1102–1105, 1981.

34. Mundy GR, Martin TJ: The hypercalcemia of malignancy: Pathogenesis and management. Metabolism 31:1247–1277, 1982.

35. Nicolson GL: Cancer metastasis: Organ colonization and the cell surface properties of malignant cells. Biochim Biophys Acta 695:113–128, 1982.

36. Orr FW, Mundy GR, Varani J, et al: Chemotactic response of tumor cells to products of resorbing bone. Science 203:176–179, 1979.

37. Pearlstein E, Ambrogio C, Gasic GJ, Karpatkin S: Inhibition of the platelet-aggregating activity of two human adenocarcinomas of the colon and an anaplastic murine tumor with a specific thrombin inhibitor: Dansylarginine N-(3-ethyl-1,5-pentanediyl) amide. *In* Jamieson G (ed): Interaction of Platelets and Tumor Cells. New York, Alan R. Liss, 1982, pp 479–500.

38. Reitsma PH, Teitelbaum SL, Bijvoet OLM, Kahn AJ: Differential action of the bisphosphonates (3-amino-1-hydroxy propylidene)-1,1-bisphosphonate (APD) and disodium dichloromethylidene bisphosphonate (Cl$_2$MDP) on rat macrophage mediated bone resorption in vitro. J Clin Invest 70:927–933, 1982.

39. Repo MA, Bockman RS, Betts F, et al: Effect of gallium on

bone mineral properties. Calcif Tissue Int 43:300–306, 1988.

40. Schnur W: Etidronate for relief of metastatic bone pain. J Urol 131:404–407, 1984.

41. Siris ES, Hyman G, Canfield RE: Effects of dichloromethylene diphosphonate in women with breast carcinoma metastatic to the skeleton. Am J Med 74:401–406, 1983.

42. Siris ES, Sherman WH, Baquiran DC, et al: Effects of dichloromethylene diphosphonate on skeletal mobilization of calcium in multiple myeloma. N Engl J Med 302:310–315, 1980.

43. Urwin GH, Percival RC, Watson ME, et al: Bone turnover in disseminated carcinoma of the prostate and therapy with etidronate (EHDP). Proceedings of the 18th European Symposium on Calcified Tissues 103, 1984.

44. van Breukelen FJM, Bijvoet OLM, van Oosterom AT: Inhibition of osteolytic bone lesions by (3-amino-1-hydroxypropylidene)-1,1-bisphosphonate (A.P.D.). Lancet 1:803–805, 1979.

45. van Holten-Verzantvoort AT, Bijvoet OLM, Cleton FJ, et al: Reduced morbidity from skeletal metastases in breast cancer patients during long-term bisphosphonate (APD) treatment. Lancet 2:983–985, 1987.

46. Warrell RP Jr, Alcock NW, Skelos A, Bockman RS: Gallium nitrate inhibits accelerated bone turnover in patients with bone metastases. J Clin Oncol 5:292–298, 1987.

47. Warrell RP Jr, Bockman RS, Coonley CJ, et al: Gallium nitrate inhibits calcium resorption from bone and is effective treatment for cancer-related hypercalcemia. J Clin Invest 73:1487–1490, 1984.

48. Warrell RP Jr, Bockman RS, Staszewski H, Maiese K: Clinical study of a new antimetastatic compound, Nafazatrom (Bay g 6575): Effects on platelet consumption and monocyte prostaglandin production in patients with advanced cancer. Cancer 57:1455–1460, 1986.

49. Warrell RP Jr, Frisone M, Snyder T, Dilmanian FA, Bockman RS: Gallium nitrate for reversal of osteolysis in multiple myeloma. Blood (Suppl.) 72:259a, 1988.

50. Warrell RP Jr, Israel R, Frisone M, et al: Gallium nitrate for acute treatment of cancer-related hypercalcemia: A randomized double-blind comparison to calcitonin. Ann Intern Med 108:669–674, 1988.

51. Warrell RP Jr, Skelos A, Alcock NW, Bockman RS: Gallium nitrate for acute treatment of cancer-related hypercalcemia: Clinicopharmacologic and dose-response analysis. Cancer Res 46:4208–4212, 1986.

52. Zacharski LR: The biologic basis for anticoagulant treatment of cancer. *In* Jamieson G (ed): Interaction of Platelets and Tumor Cells. New York, Alan R. Liss, 1982, pp 113–127.

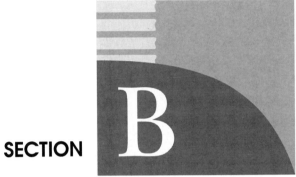

SECTION **B**

SPECIFIC ENTITIES

OSTEOID OSTEOMA AND OSTEOBLASTOMA OF THE SPINE

GEORGE W. SYPERT

INTRODUCTION

Benign primary osteoblastic tumors of the spine may be divided into osteoid osteomas and osteoblastomas.[36, 46–48, 55] In 1953, Jaffe[47] defined osteoid osteoma as a benign bone neoplasm characterized by the formation of a nidus of bone surrounded by fibrovascular tissue and a dense sclerotic bone margin. The term benign osteoblastoma was proposed by Jaffe[48] and Lichtenstein[54] in 1956 to describe a larger bone-forming neoplasm containing abundant normal-appearing osteoblasts. These lesions are therefore histologically identical, and the distinction between these two lesions is based on their respective sizes and differing biologic behavior.[7, 45, 48, 53, 60, 65] An osteoid osteoma is arbitrarily defined as a benign osteoblastic lesion that does not exceed 1.5 cm in size, and a benign osteoblastoma is one that does exceed 1.5 cm in diameter. Osteoid osteomas are thus small, well-confined, and generally self-limited in growth potential. In contrast, osteoblastomas are larger and more extensive, often involving more than one vertebra when arising in the spine, and have the potential for continued local growth; in some cases, the growth may be very aggressive and may mimic a malignant neoplasm.

As with other bone neoplasms, osteoid osteomas and benign osteoblastomas are uncommon. Osteoid osteomas comprise approximately 3 per cent of primary bone tumors and 11 per cent of all primary benign bone tumors.[2, 12] Benign osteoblastomas are less common, representing 1 per cent of all primary bone tumors and 3 per cent of primary benign bone tumors.

OSTEOID OSTEOMA

Approximately 10 per cent of osteoid osteomas are located in the spine, as shown by Jackson's review of 860 cases. Osteoid osteoma tends to present in young patients, with the greatest incidence in the second decade.[49, 58] About 90 per cent of reported cases are less than 30 years of age at the time of diagnosis. There is a clear preponderance in males, with a male:female ratio of 2:1.[36, 49, 58] There does not appear to be any significant racial, ethnic, or familial predilection for these neoplasms.

In 1967, MacLellan and Wilson[57] reviewed 36 cases of spinal osteoid osteomas[9, 10, 21, 23, 24, 33, 39, 43, 46, 66, 68, 89] and added six personal cases. More recently, Janin and colleagues[49] collected 45 subsequently reported cases,[5, 8, 15, 20, 22, 34, 37, 52, 59, 76, 88] and Maiuri and coworkers[58] added 23 cases.[26, 29, 38, 62, 81, 90, 92] In addition, Pettine and Klassen[68a] added 31 patients, such that a total of 141 well-documented cases of symptomatic spinal osteoid osteomas have been described in the literature.

Clinical Presentation

The mean interval between onset of symptoms and diagnosis is about one year, although the range may vary to seven years. In 80 per cent of patients, the diagnosis had been made within two years of onset of symptoms, while 20 per cent of the patients had suffered symptoms for more than two years. Spinal pain was the primary complaint in all reported cases. The pain is generally constant but occasionally may be episodic and is typically localized to the site of the tumor. In the majority, weight-bearing activities aggravate the pain. Nocturnal increase in pain may be noted by one half of the patients. Interestingly, aspirin provided substantial pain relief in approximately one third of the patients. Radicular pain was reported in 50 per cent of cases. Radiculopathic findings, such as paresis, muscle atrophy, reflex changes, and sensory loss, are present in 25 per cent of reported cases.

In some cases, moderate to severe tenderness localized over the tumor present. However, symptoms and signs of myelopathy were noticeably absent in all reported cases of vertebral osteoid osteoma. Lesions involving the fourth and fifth lumbar vertebrae may clinically mimic classic sciatica; some patients have been mistakenly operated upon for disc disease.[12, 23, 79, 80] Scoliosis has been reported to occur in 70 per cent of patients with spinal osteoid osteomas; in fact, osteoid osteoma is the most common cause of painful scoliosis in adolescence.[63, 68a] The curve is almost always convex away from the involved side of the vertebra[57] and is thought to be secondary to muscular spasm. Scoliosis generally occurs with lesions located in the lamina, articular processes, and pedicles, but not when the tumor is located in the spinous processes. Scoliosis varies also with the location of the lesion in the spinal axis and occurs less frequently when located in the cervical spine.

Osteoid osteomas occur at all sites in the axial skeleton. They are most common in the lumbar spine (56 per cent), with the cervical (27 per cent), thoracic (12 per cent), and sacral (2 per cent) spinal regions less frequent sites of involvement. Radiographically, these lesions are confined to a single vertebra, with one half occurring in the lamina or pedicle. In one fifth, it is confined to the articular facet; in another fifth, it is isolated to the transverse process, spinous process, and vertebral bodies.[49, 57, 58, 68a] Involvement of more than one element of the neural arch may occur in 6 per cent of patients. Extension into the soft tissues or epidural space is unusual and is almost never seen.

When positive, conventional radiographs or polytomograms usually demonstrate osteoid osteomas as an isolated radiolucent area, representing the tumor itself, surrounded by a zone of reactive sclerosis. When more mineralized matrix is present within the lesion, it may appear as a radiodense area only, or as a central area of radiosclerosis surrounded by increased radiodensity (Fig. 13–1A).[58] However, conventional radiography[3, 5, 31, 34, 35] and tomography[3, 49, 52, 58] may fail to demonstrate these lesions. Sometimes a subtle lesion with minimal sclerosis may be difficult to recognize because of superimposed surrounding bone. Lesions within less sclerosis may be completely invisible. Thus, conventional radiographic and tomographic imaging may result in false-negative examinations and should be considered inadequate screening studies if osteoid osteoma is suspected.

The radionuclide bone scan is the most reliable screening technique (Fig. 13–1B), with no cases of false-negative bone scans reported in the literature.[26, 31, 35, 56, 68a] The scintigraphic appearance of a spinal osteoid osteoma generally is an oval, well-demarcated focal area of increased activity, occasionally surrounded by a second, less intense zone of radioactive uptake.[3, 31, 35, 58] Given the near 100 per cent positivity with a radioisotopic bone scan, this imaging technique should be considered the screening procedure of choice. Isotopic bone scanning may also be used to facilitate the intraoperative localization of these small lesions.[29, 36] The radionuclide bone scan is useful in detection of small vertebral lesions and can usually localize the lesion to a specific level. It can not distinguish which part of the vertebral segment is affected.

Spinal computed tomography (CT) is the imaging procedure of choice for defining the specific location of the lesion and the exact extent of osseous involvement (Fig. 13–1C). The accuracy of this imaging technique has made it an essential element of surgical planning. Typically, the appearance of an osteoid osteoma CT scan is similar to the plain roentgenographic appearance: well-defined oval area of lucency (nidus) containing a variable amount of mineralized matrix and occasionally surrounded by hyperdense reactive bone. The appearance varies with the windows used to display the CT scan. The nidus can be completely obscured in the sclerosis unless bone windows are used.[26, 41, 58] The nidus may show substantial enhancement if intravenous contrast is used, confirming the high vascularity of this lesion.[58] Contrast enhancement, when present, may be useful in differentiating this lesion from other lesions of the spine.

Conventional myelography is generally normal in cases of spinal osteoid osteoma, as encroachment on the spinal canal is rare. However, CT-myelography may be very helpful in those cases presenting with a radiculopathy. Spinal angiography has been infrequently performed.[25, 34, 51, 91] When carefully performed using subtraction techniques, angiography may confirm the hypervascularity of the lesion as a homogeneous circumscribed blush appearing in the arterial phase and persisting into the venous phase.[25, 51] Grossly at the time of surgery, the nidus of the osteoid osteoma appears as a soft, dark red or firm, yellow-white spherical nodule surrounded by a white margin of dense reactive bone. It may be seen through the center as a red-purple spot. The soft red portion of the nidus contains more blood vessels and bone, whereas the firm and yellow-white portion is principally reactive bone with fewer blood vessels.[10a] The nidus is generally intracortical and may extend into the periosteal or endosteal surface of the bone; it is unusual for the spongiosa to be exclusively affected. The nidus is usually well-circumscribed, less than 1.5 cm in size, and surrounded by sclerotic thickened bone. Generally, the lesion can be readily "shelled out" of the surrounding reactive bone.

Microscopically, the nidus is comprised of irregular, haphazardly arranged woven bone trabeculae embedded in a benign fibrovascular stroma. The nidus is well delineated from the surrounding reactive lamellar bone of the vertebra. Osteoclastic as well as osteoblastic activity is usually prominent. The amount of mineralized woven bone and osteoid (unmineralized bone) varies among lesions. The histologic appearance probably corresponds to the various stages of evolution of the lesion; in the early phases, osteoblastic activity predominates. In the intermediate phases, osteoid is deposited by the osteoblasts; in the later stages, the osteoid becomes well calcified. The histologic features of the lesion do not appear to correlate with the clinical symptoms (Fig. 13–2).

The pathogenesis of osteoid osteoma remains controversial.[10a, 12, 36] Most investigators believe that the lesion is a well-circumscribed neoplasm independent of the surrounding normal bone. Consistent with this hypothesis is the observation that the lesion has its

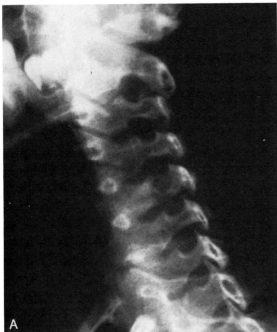

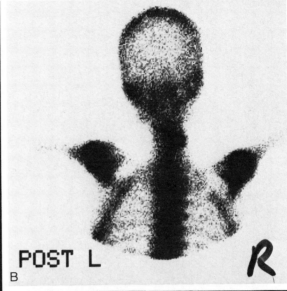

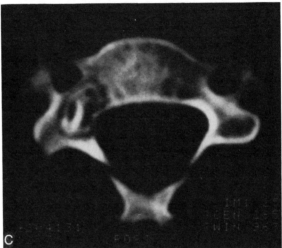

FIGURE 13–1. Osteoid osteoma. A nine-year-old girl presented with a six-week history of progressively intractable and incapacitating right-sided neck and shoulder pain. Her general physical examination and neurologic examination were normal except for neck stiffness, limitation of motion, and right paravertebral cervical tenderness. *A,* Oblique conventional radiograph. The lesion is visible as a well-developed lytic area of the pedicle of C5. *B,* Radioisotopic bone scan. *C,* CT scan of fifth cervical vertebra shows increased uptake at C4. Note the lytic lesion of the right pedicle of CT with a classic central radiodensity on the CT scan.

own blood supply associated with the presence of excessive and atypical growth of bone tissue. Moreover, the classic signs of inflammation are absent microscopically. However, some features are unusual for neoplasia, suggesting a possible infectious or reparative process. These latter features include: (1) small size with limited growth potential, (2) histologic features that appear independent of the duration of the patient's symptoms, (3) immaturity of the central area of the nidus with relative maturity of the osseous tissue in the nidus's periphery, and (4) marginal sclerosis.[10a] Ultrastructural studies, unfortunately, have not been of great help in defining the pathogenesis of osteoid osteoma.[82]

Differential Diagnosis

The differential diagnosis at clinical presentation frequently includes osteomyelitis, other bone tumors, cysts, healing fractures, and occasionally disc disease. Usually, the small size, intracordial location, and homogeneous reactive bone sclerosis help to differentiate osteoid osteomas from these other processes.

However, vertebral lesions can be very difficult diagnostic problems radiographically.

Osteomyelitis typically involves the vertebral body and the disc space; radiographically, it is likely to be characterized by osteolysis and patchy and irregular sclerosis. Patients may show systemic clinical and laboratory evidence of an inflammatory process. Although isotopic scanning with bone-seeking agents is generally positive for both lesions, a gallium scan may be helpful in distinguishing between the two. Gallium is usually taken in strongly by osteomyelitis but shows minimal uptake by osteoid osteoma. Benign bone tumors that require differentiation include osteoblastoma, enostosis (bone island), aneurysmal bone cyst, and eosinophilic granuloma. Benign osteoblastomas and aneurysmal bone cysts are larger, tend to be expansile, and generate less sclerosis. Eosinophilic granuloma is also usually less sclerotic and often results in vertebral collapse. Enostoses are often seen in an older population and are asymptomatic. Malignant bone tumors such as osteosarcoma are larger at presentation than are osteoid osteomas. They have ill-defined, irregular margins with variable sclerosis. Ewing's tumor is usually destructive (osteo-

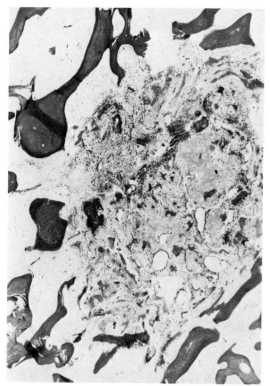

FIGURE 13–2. An osteoid osteoma within the cortex. The cortical bone has been resorbed so that only thin trabecular-like remnants remain. The nidus is a well-circumscribed focus of rich vascular tissue with irregularly arranged woven bone spicules (H & E ×40).

lytic) and predominantly involves the vertebral body, particularly at an early stage. The differential diagnosis can be difficult.

Management

The prognosis of untreated osteoid osteoma remains somewhat uncertain, since the diagnosis is established only after histologic examination of the specimen. Since there have been no reports of malignant transformation or metastases of an osteoid osteoma, the benign nature of this lesion has been inferred.[10a] There have been isolated case reports of spontaneous healing of such lesions in patients diagnosed on clinical and radiographic grounds.[33, 72] The treatment of these lesions is surgical. Radiation therapy is not necessary and may be harmful. Complete excision of the lesion with or without curettage of the surrounding sclerotic bone appears to be curative.[10a, 49, 58, 68a] Optimal surgical treatment produces remission of pain in greater than 95 per cent of cases. Incomplete excision is usually followed by recurrence of the pain. The radionuclide bone scan shows renewed increased local activity. If the lesion recurs, additional attempts at complete excision should be undertaken. Early diagnosis and radical excision of the lesion frequently leads to correction of the antalgic scoliosis. If antalgic scoliosis is to be relieved by excision, the critical duration of symptoms is approximately 15 months.[68a] Patients with symptoms of greater than 15 months' duration tend to

suffer a fixed spinal deformity. The age of the patient appears to be somewhat less important, although the patients who were older at the onset of symptoms and those who were younger at the time of surgical treatment tended to have more spontaneous postoperative correction of the spinal deformity.

OSTEOBLASTOMA

Benign osteoblastomas account for less than 1 per cent of all bone tumors.[55] However, osteoblastoma has a distinct predilection for the spine, especially the posterior elements. More than 40 per cent of reported cases have been located in the spine.[45, 60] Interestingly, more than half of the spinal cases have been associated with scoliosis.[45, 60] Benign osteoblastomas and osteoid osteomas appear to be the most common causes of scoliosis resulting from pain.[64] About 60 per cent of reported cases present in the first two decades of life, predominantly in teenagers.[3] Males are more frequently affected than females. By definition, osteoblastoma is larger than osteoid osteoma at presentation (usually greater than 2 cm) and has a more aggressive growth potential.

In 1981, Janin and colleagues[49] reviewed 39 reported cases of osteoblastoma arising in the spine[6, 13–18, 25, 28, 30, 42, 45, 50, 51, 61, 73, 81, 87] including five cases of their own. The largest personal series are the 10 cases reported by Kirwan and coworkers[53] and the 11 cases reported by Pettine and Klassen.[68a] When these cases are combined with the reports of Akbarnia and Rooholamini,[1] Amacher and Eltomey,[1a] Azouz and colleagues,[3] and Weatherly and coworkers,[89a] a total of 83 well-documented cases of symptomatic spinal osteoblastoma have been described in the literature. An additional 14 patients have been treated at the University of Florida during the past 15 years, yielding a total of 98 cases, which are the basis for this discussion.

Clinical Presentation

The mean interval between onset of symptoms and diagnosis varies from 7 to 14 months. Although the diagnosis was made within two years of symptom onset in 75 per cent of patients, the remainder suffered symptoms for more than two years. Spinal pain is the primary complaint in all patients. The pain is generally constant but may be episodic and is typically localized to the site of the lesion. Weight-bearing activities generally aggravate the pain. Nocturnal pain is common. In contrast to osteoid osteoma, aspirin is less effective in relieving pain associated with this tumor. Scoliosis with the convex side away from the involved side of the vertebrae, generally related to pain-producing lesions in the thoracic spine, has been reported in up to two thirds of such patients. Localized tenderness may be present in many. Radicular pain and signs of radicular compression may occur in 50 per cent of patients, and signs of spinal cord involvement (myelopathy) have been reported in up to 25 per cent of cases. Occasionally, the myelopathy may be severe, and such cases are generally reported in the neurosurgical literature.

The vertebral column is the most frequent site of involvement in osteoblastoma; other frequent locations include the long bones (30 per cent), skull and facial bones (15 per cent), and hands and feet (14 per cent).[41] In the spine, the thoracic and lumbar segments are the most frequent sites, with each region accounting for about 35 per cent of cases. The cervical spine (25 per cent) and sacrum (5 per cent) are less frequent sites of involvement. About one half of spinal osteoblastomas are limited to either the lamina or the pedicle of a single vertebra, with the pedicle being the most frequent site. Isolated lesions of the transverse process, spinous process, and vertebral bodies account for about 20 per cent of cases. Osteoblastomas involve more than one element of the neural arch three times more frequently than do osteoid osteomas, and in 11 per cent a combined lesion of the posterior elements and vertebral body may be present.[49] In about 5 per cent of cases, the tumor involves adjacent vertebrae. Interestingly, the author has treated one case in which the osteoblastoma had extensively involved multiple adjacent vertebrae extending from C4 through T2. A right-to-left side preference ratio of 2:1 has been observed for localized osteoblastomas. Approximately half the reported cases of spinal osteoblastomas have epidural extension of tumor; significant involvement of the paraspinous soft tissues is less frequent.

Neurodiagnostic Imaging

Conventional radiographs may fail to show small localized tumors. When positive, the roentgenographic appearance of osteoblastoma is that of a destructive, expansile lesion in the majority of cases (Figs. 13–3A and 13–4A and C). Sclerosis as the only finding may be present in 15 per cent of cases. Calcification is found within one third of lesions; a calcified shell surrounding the lesion or a paraspinal soft tissue mass is noted in one fifth of osteoblastomas.

The radionuclide bone scan is a reliable screening technique (Fig. 13–3B). As with osteoid osteomas, the author could not find any cases of false-negative bone scans reported in the literature.[31, 49, 91] The scintigraphic appearance of a spinal osteoblastoma is a typical "hot spot."[31, 49, 56, 68a, 70] As with osteoid osteoma, the isotope bone scan is an excellent method for following patients postoperatively and may be used as a guide intraoperatively to localize small lesions.

Spinal CT scan is the best imaging procedure for defining the location of the lesion and the exact extent of the osseous involvement (Figs. 13–3C and 13–4D). This imaging technique is essential to optimally plan the surgical approach, method of excision, and requirement for spinal reconstruction. Typically,

an osteoblastoma appears expansile and destructive on CT scan. There may be evidence of internal bone formation within confluent areas of lucency and surrounding sclerosis. In patients who present with neural compression syndromes, CT-myelography (Fig. 13–3E) should be performed to accurately define the location(s) of neurologic compression so that appropriate surgical decompression can be planned. Conventional myelography may also be useful if there are symptoms or signs of compression of the nerve roots or spinal cord (Fig. 13–3D). If intravenous contrast is also given at the time of CT scan, it typically demonstrates a vascular blush in the area of bone destruction.

The role of magnetic resonance imaging (MRI) (Fig. 13–3D) in the evaluation of patients presenting with primary tumors of the spine is not completely established. Based on personal experience, it is the author's opinion that MRI will be an exceedingly useful imaging procedure and may even replace myelography and CT in the evaluation of patients with neural compression syndromes.

Pathology

Grossly at the time of surgery, osteoblastomas present a variable picture consisting of either a cystic lesion with dense strips of bone separated by large spaces of hypervascular red-gray tissue, which hemorrhage profusely, or an expansile, homogeneous, friable granular mass, varying from red to purple, which is well demarcated from the surrounding normal or reactive bone. Not infrequently, this highly vascular tissue is found to have ruptured through the cortical bone extending into the paraspinous soft tissues or epidural space.

As stated earlier, the histology of osteoid osteoma and osteoblastoma is similar. The tumor is characterized by a rich fibrovascular stroma and abundant prominent osteoblasts rimming interspersed spicules of woven bone arranged in a chaotic fashion. The proportions of osteoid and mineralized woven bone will vary with different tumors and in some instances within an individual tumor. The intervening connective tissue is loosely fibrous and highly vascular (Fig. 13–5). Cartilage formation is not evident. A variable number of multinucleated osteoclast-type giant cells may be seen around areas of hemorrhage or cyst formation and may lead to the erroneous diagnosis of giant cell tumor from a limited sample. More important is the distinction between osteoblastoma and osteosarcoma on small biopsies. In osteosarcomas, cartilage production may be present; the stroma is sparse and sarcomatous spindle cells may be seen with areas of anaplastic giant cells.

There is a variant of osteoblastoma termed aggressive, atypical, malignant, or epithelioid osteoblastoma which is worth mentioning here.[36, 75] Histologically, such tumors are characterized by large atypical osteoblasts (epithelioid osteoblasts) with prominent nucleoli palisading about woven bone trabeculae. Mitoses are frequent. Some pathologists consider this

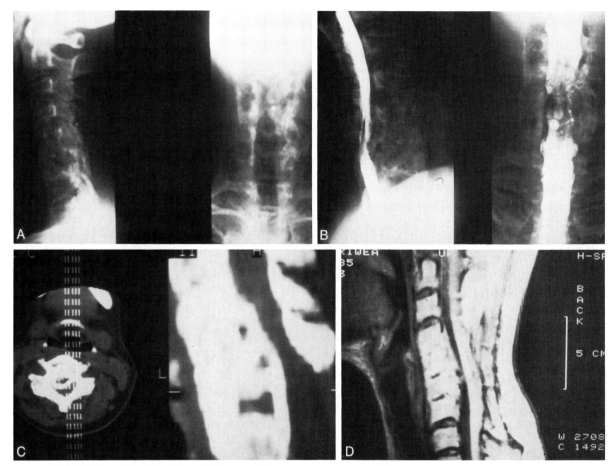

FIGURE 13–3. Osteoblastoma. A 31-year-old woman underwent a diagnostic biopsy of a cervical vertebral lesion 20 years earlier which was consistent with osteoblastoma. This was followed by radiation therapy. She then underwent posterior decompressive laminectomies 16 and 2 years prior to referral to the author to treat progressive cervical myelopathy. On presentation, she had a one-year history of progressive spastic quadriparesis with upper extremity atrophy and a C5 sensory level. There had been a laminectomy of C5–C7. A bone-forming lesion is seen expanding to the C6 contour. *A,* Conventional anteroposterior and lateral radiographs. *B,* Cervical myelogram. There is posterior displacement of the theca by the C6 mass. *C,* CT scan with sagittal reformation shows the extent of spinal cord narrowing. *D,* Midsagittal MRI (proton density image) reveals posterior displacement of the spinal cord.

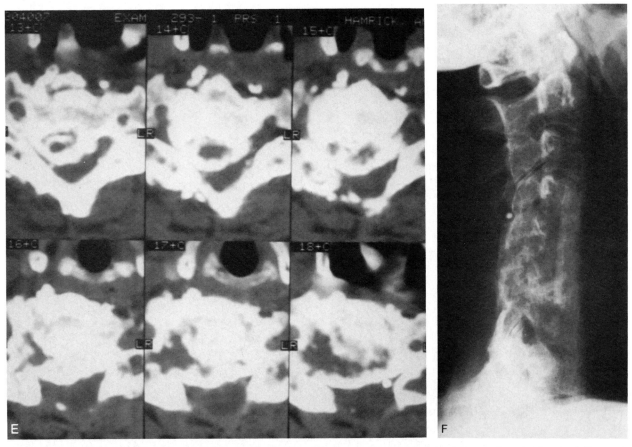

FIGURE 13–3 *Continued E,* CT-myelogram with cuts from C4 to T1 shows almost complete absence of contrast around the cord. *F,* Postoperative lateral radiograph following anterior decompressive corpectomy and fibula allograft reconstruction. The patient made a dramatic recovery of neurologic function. She is now four years postoperative and has resumed all of her normal activities.

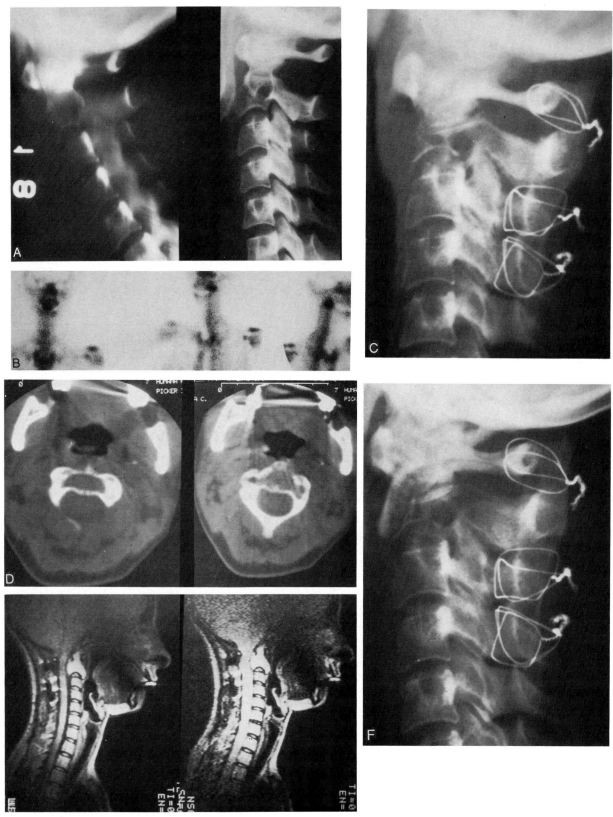

FIGURE 13–4. Osteoblastoma. A 35-year-old woman developed severe suboccipital pain following minor trauma one year earlier. She was initially treated with a halo-vest as she was thought to have a C2 fracture. Due to persistence of symptoms she underwent a posterior C1–C3 fusion. An expansile destructive mass of C2 was recognized after surgery and she was referred to the author for treatment. Her general physical and neurologic examinations were normal except for decreased range of motion of her cervical spine and a well-healed posterior cervical incisional scar. *A,* Conventional lateral radiograph (right) and lateral polytomogram (left) prior to posterior fusion reveal a lytic expansile lesion of the body of C2. *B,* Radioisotope bone scan prior to posterior fusion shows markedly increased uptake of C2. *C,* Conventional lateral radiograph postfusion reveals an anterior soft tissue mass. *D,* CT scan shows the extent of bone destruction. An anterior mass is seen, confined by a partly ossified shell of periosteum. *E,* Midsagittal MRI shows posterior displacement of the spinal cord. *F,* A transoral microsurgical radical corpectomy of C2 was performed with reconstruction of C2 using iliac autograft. She is now two years postoperative and is neurologically normal and working full time with no evidence of recurrence.

variant to be a low grade osteosarcoma, while others believe it is a premalignant lesion. Clearly, in all cases, this lesion is clinically more aggressive and almost always recurs with incomplete surgical procedures or curettage. Therefore, more radial surgical resection is recommended (Fig. 13–6).

Management

The prognosis of benign osteoblastoma is not certain. In most cases, it appears to remain a slowly growing, locally expansile and aggressive, destructive neoplastic process retaining its benign histologic picture when it recurs after surgical therapy. Marginal resection of this lesion appears to be curative.[36, 49] When these lesions arise in vertebrae, intralesional curettage or marginal excision is generally used.

The treatment of spinal osteoblastoma is surgical. Complete surgical excision of the entire lesion with radical curettage of the surrounding normal vertebral bone appears to be curative in the majority of cases.[1, 1a, 16, 36, 44, 49, 68a] In patients with neurologic compression syndromes, radical decompressive surgery is mandatory to preserve neurologic function. When the lesions are large, spinal reconstruction with allograft or autograft bone is necessary after excision of the tumor. With presumed total excision, the recurrence rate appears to be about 10 per cent.[1a] When gross total excision is achieved, greater than 90 per cent of patients will experience relief of their preoperative pain.[1, 16, 36, 44, 68a] Moreover, adequate neurologic decompression results in a high recovery

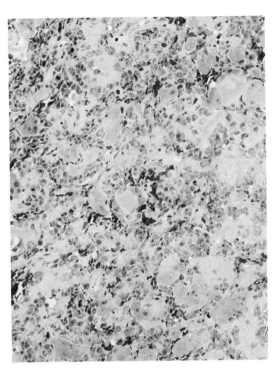

FIGURE 13–6. An atypical osteoblastoma with prominent plump osteoblasts lining irregular woven bone spicules. Compared with Figure 13–5, the larger osteoblasts and prominent nucleoli are striking (H & E × 187).

of neurologic function.[1a, 49, 83a] In patients treated with partial excision of tumor, pain frequently persists, as does neurologic dysfunction when the neural elements are not adequately decompressed.

The role of radiation therapy in the management of osteoblastomas remains controversial. Various investigators have clinical experience that documents the ineffectiveness of radiotherapy.[17, 44, 62a, 74] Radiation therapy should probably be reserved for that rare patient in whom further palliative surgical management is not an option due to either intercurrent illness or recurrence of such magnitude and location that further surgical palliation is of marginal benefit. Radiation therapy is not completely risk free, as tumoricidal doses carry the risk of malignant transformation, spinal cord necrosis, and aggravation of any preexisting spinal cord compression.[12, 13, 72]

REFERENCES

1. Akbarnia BA, Rooholamini SA: Scoliosis caused by benign osteoblastoma of the thoracic and lumbar spine. J Bone Joint Surg 63A:1146–1155, 1981.
1a. Amacher AL, Eltomey A: Spinal osteoblastoma in children and adolescents. Childs Nerv Syst 1:29–32, 1985.
2. Amako T, Maeyama I, Masud M: Atlas on Radiological Diagnosis of Bone and Joint Disease. Vol 3. Bone Tumors. Tokyo, Kimbara, 1968.
3. Azouz EM, Kozlowski K, Marton D, et al: Osteoid osteoma and osteoblastoma of the spine in children. Ped Radiol 16:25–31, 1986.

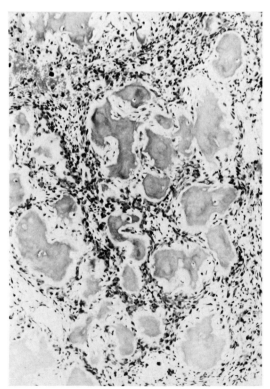

FIGURE 13–5. An osteoblastoma with abundant irregularly arranged woven bone spicules. The background is a benign fibrovascular tissue (H & E × 125).

4. Barwick KW, Huvos AK, Smith J: Primary osteogenic sarcoma of the vertebral column. Cancer 46:595–604, 1980.

5. Blery M, Le Roux B: Osteome osteoide vertebral: À propos de six cas. Ann Radiol (Paris) 21:59–63, 1978.

6. Bloom MH, Bryan RS: Benign osteoblastoma of the spine: Case report. Clin Orthop 65:157–162, 1969.

7. Byers PD: Solitary benign osteoblastic lesions of bone. Osteoid osteoma and benign osteoblastoma. Cancer 22:43–57, 1968.

8. Caldicott WJH: Diagnosis of spinal osteoid osteoma. Radiology 92:1192–1195, 1969.

9. Cameron BM, Friend LF: Osteoid osteoma of the sacrum. J Bone Joint Surg 36A:876–877, 1946.

10. Campos OP: Osteoid osteoma of the cervical spinous process. Report of a case. J Int Coll Surg 9:112–115, 1946.

10a. Cohen MD, Harrington TM, Ginsburg WW: Osteoid osteoma: 95 cases and a review of the literature. Semin Arth Rheum 12:265–281, 1946.

11. Corbettt JM, Wilde AH, McCormack LJ, Evarts CM: Intra-articular osteoid osteoma: A diagnostic problem. Clin Orthop 98:225–230, 1974.

12. Dahlin DC: Bone Tumors: General Aspects and Data on 6,221 Cases. 3rd ed. Springfield, Charles C Thomas, 1967.

13. Dahlin DC, Johnson EW Jr: Giant osteoid osteoma. J Bone Joint Surg 36A:559–572, 1954.

14. Deffebach RR, Phillips TL: Benign osteoblastoma of the vertebra: Report of a case with five year follow up after irradiation. Radiol Clin (Basel) 37:45–52, 1968.

15. De Sousa Dias L, Frost HM: Osteoblastoma of the spine: A review and report of eight new cases. Clin Orthop 91:141–151, 1973.

16. Doron Y, Gruszkiewicz J, Gelli B, Peyser E: Benign osteoblastoma of the vertebral column and skull. Surg Neurol 7:86–90, 1977.

17. Eisenbray AB, Huber PJ, Rachmaninoff N: Benign osteoblastoma of the spine with multiple recurrences: Case report. J Neurosurg 31:468–473, 1980.

18. Epstein N, Benjamin V, Pinto R, Burdzilovich G: Benign osteoblastoma of a thoracic vertebra: Case report. J Neurosurg 53:710–713, 1980.

19. Fagerberg S, Rudstrom P: Osteoid osteoma of a vertebral arch. A case report. Acta Radiol 40:383–386, 1953.

20. Ferrini L: Su due casi di osteoma osteoide della colonna vertebrale. Chir Organi Mov 62:169–174, 1975.

21. Fett HC, Russo VP: Osteoid osteoma of a cervical vertebra. Report of a case. J Bone Joint Surg 41A:948–950, 1959.

22. Fielding JW, Keim HA, Hawkins RJ, Gabrielian J-CZ: Osteoid osteoma of a cervical spine. Clin Orthop 128:163–164, 1977.

23. Fountain EM, Burge CH: Osteoid osteoma of the cervical spine. A review and case report. J Neurosurg 18:380–383, 1961.

24. Frieberger RH: Osteoid osteoma of the spine. A cause of backache and scoliosis in children and young adults. Radiology 75:232–235, 1960.

25. Fukushima T, Kamano S, Sakurai I, Chigasaki H: A case of osteoid osteoma affecting the T8 neural arch; with special reference to selective spinal angiography. No To Shinkei 24:213–219, 1972.

26. Gamba JL, Marinez S, Apple J, et al: Computed tomography of axial skeletal osteoid osteoma. AJR 142:769–772, 1984.

27. Gelberman RH, Olson CO: Benign osteoblastoma of the atlas. J Bone Joint Surg 56A:808–810, 1974.

28. Gertzbein SD, Cruickshank B, Hoffman H, et al: Recurrent benign osteoblastoma of the second thoracic vertebrae: A case report. J Bone Joint Surg 55B:841–847, 1973.

29. Ghelman B, Vigorita VJ: Postoperative radionuclide evaluation of osteoid osteoma. Radiology 146:509–512, 1983.

30. Giachi LM: Osteoblastom dell'arco posteriore cervicale. Chir Organi Mov 58:541–545, 1970.

31. Gilday DL: Diagnosis of obscure childhood osteoid osteomas with the bone scan. J Nucl Med 15:494, 1974.

32. Glasauer FE: Benign osteoblastoma of the cervical spine. NY State J Med 79:1424–1427, 1979.

33. Golding JSR: The natural history of osteoid osteoma. With a report of twenty cases. J Bone Joint Surg 43B:218–229, 1954.

34. Goldstein GS, Dawson EG, Batzdorf U: Cervical osteoid osteoma: A cause of chronic upper back pain. Clin Orthop 129:177–180, 1977.

35. Gore DR, Mueller HA: Osteoid-osteoma of the spine with localization aided by 99 mTc polyphosphate bone scan: Case report. Clin Orthop 113:132–134, 1975.

36. Healey JH, Ghelman B: Osteoid osteoma and osteoblastoma: Current concepts and recent advances. Clin Orthop 204:76–85, 1986.

37. Heiman ML, Cooley CJ, Bradford DS: Osteoid osteoma of a vertebral body: Report of a case with extension across the intervertebral disk. Clin Orthop 118:159–163, 1976.

38. Helms CA, Hartner RS, Volger JB: Osteoid osteoma: Radionuclide diagnosis. Radiology 151:779–784, 1984.

39. Hermann RM, Blount WP: Osteoid osteoma of the lumbar spine. J Bone Joint Surg 43A:567–571, 1961.

40. Herrlin K, Ekelund L, Lovdahl R, Persson B: Computed tomography in suspected osteoid osteomas of tubular bones. Skel Radiol 9:92–97, 1982.

41. Huvos AG: Bone Tumors: Diagnosis, Treatment and Prognosis. Philadelphia, WB Saunders Co., 1979.

42. Irvin GAL: Benign osteoblastoma of spine. NY State J Med 70:687–689, 1970.

43. Jackson IG: Osteoid osteoma of the lamina and its treatment. Am Surg 19:17–23, 1953.

44. Jackson RP: Recurrent osteoblastoma. Clin Orthop 131:229–233, 1978.

45. Jackson RP, Reckling FW, Mantz FA: Osteoid osteoma and osteoblastoma: Similar histologic lesions with different natural histories. Clin Orthop 128:303–313, 1977.

46. Jaffe HL: "Osteoid Osteoma": A benign osteoblastic tumor composed of osteoid and atypical bone. Arch Surg 31:709–728, 1935.

47. Jaffe HL: Osteoid-osteoma. Proc R Soc Med 46:1007–1012, 1953.

48. Jaffe HL: Benign osteoblastoma. Bull Hosp Joint Dis 17:141–151, 1956.

49. Janin Y, Epstein JA, Carras R, Khan A: Osteoid osteomas and osteoblastomas of the spine. Neurosurgery 8:31–38, 1981.

50. Jeanmart L, Brihaye J, Gompel C: Tumeurs rares du rachis. Rhumatol Med Phys 22:317–332, 1967.

51. Kamano S, Fukushima T: Angiographic demonstration of vertebral osteoid osteoma. Surg Neurol 6:167–168, 1976.

52. Keim HA, Reina EG: Osteoid-osteoma as a cause of scoliosis. J Bone Joint Surg 57A:159–163, 1975.

53. Kirwan EOG, Hutton PAN, Pozo JL, Ransford AO: Osteoid osteoma and benign osteoblastoma of the spine. Clinical presentation and treatment. J Bone Joint Surg 66B:21–26, 1984.

54. Lichtenstein L: Benign osteoblastoma: A category of osteoid- and bone-forming tumors other than classical osteoid osteoma, which may be mistaken for giant-cell tumor or osteogenic sarcoma. Cancer 9:1044–1052, 1956.

55. Lichtenstein L, Sawyer WR: Benign osteoblastoma: Further observations and report of twenty additional cases. J Bone Joint Surg 46A:755–765, 1964.

56. Lisbona R, Rosenthall L: Role of radionuclide imaging in osteoid osteoma. Am J Roentgenol 132:77–80, 1979.

57. MacLellan DI, Wilson FC Jr: Osteoid osteoma of the spine. A review of the literature and report of six cases. J Bone Joint Surg 49A:111–121, 1967.

58. Maiuri F, Signorelli C, Lavano A, et al: Osteoid osteomas of the spine. Surg Neurol 25:375–380, 1986.

59. Mallens WMC, Pauwels EKJ, Tetteroo QF: Bone scintigraphy as a guide to the diagnosis of osteoid osteoma. Radiol Clin (Basel) 46:300–306, 1977.

60. Marsh BW, Bonfiglio M, Brady LP, Enneking WF: Benign osteoblastoma: Range of manifestations. J Bone Joint Surg 57A:1–9, 1975.

61. Martin NL, Preston DF, Robinson RG: Osteoblastoma of the axial skeleton shown by skeletal scanning: Case report. J Nucl Med 17:187–189, 1976.

62. Mau H: Das osteoid-osteom der Warbelsaule. Z Orthop 120:761–766, 1982.

62a. McLeod RA, Dahlin DC, Beabout JW: The spectrum of osteoblastoma. Am J Roentgenol 126:321–335, 1976.

63. Mehta MH: Pain provoked scoliosis. Observations on the evolution of the deformity. Clin Orthop 135:58–65, 1978.

64. Mahta MH, Murray RO: Scoliosis provoked by painful vertebral lesions. Skel Radiol 1:223–230, 1977.

65. Merryweather R, Middlemiss JH, Sanerkin NG: Malignant transformation of osteoblastoma. J Bone Joint Surg 62B:381–384, 1980.
66. Mustard WT, DuVal FW: Osteoid osteoma of vertebrae. J Bone Joint Surg 41B:132–136, 1959.
67. Nelson OA, Greer RB III: Localisation of osteoid-osteoma of the spine using computerized tomography. A case report. J Bone Joint Surg 65A:263–265, 1983.
68. Paus BC, Kim TK: Osteoid osteoma of the spine. Acta Orthop Scand 33:24–29, 1963.
68a. Pettine KA, Klassen RA: Osteoid osteoma and osteoblastoma of the spine. J Bone Joint Surg 68A:354–361, 1986.
69. Ransford AO, Pozo JL, Hutton PAN, Kirwan EOG: The behavior pattern of the scoliosis associated with osteoid osteoma or osteoblastoma of the spine. J Bone Joint Surg 66B:16–20, 1984.
70. Rinsky LA, Goris M, Bleck EE, et al: Intraoperative skeletal scintigraphy for localization of osteoid-osteoma of the spine. J Bone Joint Surg 62A:143–144, 1980.
71. Rushton JG, Mulder DW, Lipscomb PR: Neurologic symptoms with osteoid osteoma. Neurology 5:794–797, 1955.
72. Sabanas AO, Bickel WH, Moe JH: Natural history of osteoid osteoma of the spine. Review of the literature and report of three cases. Am J Surg 91:880–889, 1970.
73. Salmon M, Vigouroux C, Argenson C, et al: Osteoblastome du rachis cervical chez un enfant: Problemes diagnostiques et therapeutiques. Chirurgie 96:723–730, 1970.
74. Savitz MH, Rothschild EJ, Chang T, et al: Primary vertebral tumor in an adolescent girl. Mt Sinai J Med (NY) 48:84–88, 1981.
75. Schajowicz F, Lemos C: Malignant osteoblastoma. J Bone Joint Surg 58B:202–211, 1976.
76. Scott M, Lignelli GJ, Shea FJ: Cervical radicular pain secondary to osteoid osteoma of spine. JAMA 217:964–965, 1971.
77. Seltzer RA: Back pain in a young man. JAMA 195:677–678, 1966.
78. Sherman FC, Wilkinson RH, Hall JE: Reactive sclerosis of a pedicle and spondylosis in the lumbar spine. J Bone Joint Surg 59A:49–54, 1977.
79. Sherman MS: Osteoid osteoma. Review of the literature and report of thirty cases. J Bone Joint Surg 29A:918–930, 1947.
80. Sim FH, Dahlin DC, Stauffer RN, Laws ER Jr: Primary bone tumors simulating lumbar disc syndrome. Spine 2:65–74, 1977.
81. Smith TR, Bennett B: Correlation conferences in radiology and pathology: Absent pedicle and back pain. NY State J Med 76:1994–1996, 1976.
82. Steiner GC: Ultrastructure of osteoblastoma. Cancer 39:2127–2136, 1977.
83. Symeonides PP: Osteoid osteoma of the lumbar spine. South Med J 63:975–976, 1970.
83a. Sypert GW: Unpublished data.
84. Tate RC, Kim S-S, Ogden L: Osteoblastoma of the sacrum with intraabdominal manifestation. Am J Surg 123:735–738, 1972.
85. Thompson SK: Benign osteoblastoma of the spine. J R Coll Surg Edinb 25:271–275, 1980.
86. Tonai M, Campbell CJ, Ahn GH, Mankin HJ: Osteoblastoma classification and report of 16 patients. Clin Orthop 167:222–235, 1982.
87. Von Immenkamp M: Ein Benignes osteoblastom des 4. Lendenwirbesl als Urache einer Huftlendenstrecksteife. Orthopade 109:616–625, 1971.
88. Von Steinke H-J, Winkelmann H: Osteoid osteom des Wirbelbogens L IV. Zentralbl Neurochir 30:285–289, 1969.
89. Ward FG: Osteoid osteoma of the transverse process of the fifth cervical vertebra. Proc R Soc Med 50:261, 1957.
89a. Weatherly CR, Jaffray D, O'Brien JP: Radical excision of an osteoblastoma of the cervical spine. J Bone Joint Surg 68B:325–328, 1986.
90. Wedge JH, Chang ST, MacFadyen DV: Computed tomography in localization of spinal osteoid osteoma. Spine 6:423–427, 1981.
91. Winter PF, Johnson PM, Hilal SK, Feldman F: Scintigraphic detection of osteoid osteoma. Radiology 122:177–178, 1977.
92. Zwimpfer TJ, Tucker WS, Faulkner JF: Osteoid osteoma of the cervical spine. Case reports and review of the literature. Can J Surg 25:637–641, 1982.

14

OSTEOSARCOMA OF THE SPINE

NARAYAN SUNDARESAN, ALAN L. SCHILLER,
and DANIEL I. ROSENTHAL

INTRODUCTION

Osteosarcoma is the most common primary malignant tumor of bone (except for myeloma) and accounts for 20 per cent of osseous neoplasms. It is thus twice as common as chondrosarcoma and at least three times as common as Ewing's sarcoma. Its incidence ranges from one to two cases per million in most Western countries, resulting in an estimated 900 to 1500 new cases diagnosed annually in the United States.[17, 47, 57, 109]

Although osteosarcomas may occur at any age, the incidence peaks in the second decade of life.[13, 18, 63] Approximately 40 to 50 per cent of all cases occur between the ages of 10 and 20 years, especially during the adolescent growth spurt. In American blacks, tumors are encountered in a younger age group, corresponding to an earlier growth spurt.[50] Several features suggest a relationship between rapid bone growth and the development of osteosarcoma. (1) There is a predilection of osteosarcoma for the metaphyseal portions of the most rapidly growing bones, that is, the distal femur, proximal tibia, and proximal humerus. (2) Patients with osteosarcoma are generally taller than their age peers. (3) In dogs, osteosarcoma occurs more frequently in larger than in smaller breeds. While the cause of osteosarcoma is unknown, it is interesting that in addition to occurring in rapidly growing bone, it occurs as a secondary neoplasm in a variety of pathologic conditions: Paget's disease, postradiation, fibrous dysplasia, and some benign bone tumors.[14, 22, 23, 41, 42, 45, 48, 49, 67, 86, 87, 96, 102, 104] In general, older patients with osteosarcomas often have secondary tumors—in a series of 117 patients older than 65 years with osteosarcoma, 56 per cent were secondary to other conditions, mainly Paget's disease of bone or radiation therapy.[46] The most common predisposing factor for secondary osteosarcoma is Paget's disease; in a series of 1177 osteosarcomas, Huvos and colleagues noted that 65 (5.5 per cent) were found to be associated with either monostotic or polyostotic Paget's disease.[48] The overall median age at time of diagnosis in patients with Paget's sarcoma was 64 years.

Therapeutic ionizing radiation (RT) is clearly associated with an increased incidence of secondary bone and soft tissue tumors, of which osteosarcoma is the most common histologic type. Both Thorotrast and radioactive radium are also clearly implicated in the production of bone sarcomas.[41] Approximately 40 per cent of radiation-related sarcomas arise within or in the vicinity of the axial skeleton. Less commonly, malignant transformation of benign bone tumors has resulted in secondary osteosarcoma; malignant transformation of exuberant callus formation in osteogenesis imperfecta has also resulted in osteosarcoma. Exceptionally, osteosarcoma may develop in bone that is the site of an infarct.[70]

Apart from these conditions, an increased incidence of osteosarcoma is seen in long-term survivors of bilateral retinoblastoma.[1] Retinoblastoma is a malignant tumor arising in the eyes of newborns and young children. Approximately 10 per cent of patients with retinoblastoma have a family history of the disease, and another 30 per cent have multifocal disease and a negative family history. These two groups (approximately 40 per cent) are capable of transmitting this disease to their offspring, and this tendency is governed by a locus or loci on the long arm of chromosome 13 within band 13q14. In such patients, the observed incidence of osteosarcoma is 2000 times greater than in the rest of the population, an increase that is seen even when no radiation is administered. Recent data also suggest that the retinoblastoma tumor tissue is homozygous for large portions of 13q; this finding implies that homozygosity of 13q may be the fundamental event in the oncogenesis of both retinoblastoma and osteosarcoma.

Osteosarcoma may involve multiple skeletal sites at the same time (synchronous) or may develop consecutively (metachronous).[2, 20, 75] Familial cases have been recorded in siblings, but no documented examples of spinal involvement have been seen in these patients.[27, 69]

Several classifications of osteosarcoma have been proposed based on anatomic site and histologic subtype.[18, 19, 47] Although osteosarcomas classically arise within the marrow cavity (medullary), they may also arise from the surface of long bones (juxtacortical) and occasionally from extraosseous soft tissues or viscera.[90] The histologic subtypes include osteoblastic, fibroblastic, chondroblastic, mixed, and anaplastic variants. Approximately 3 to 11 per cent of osteosarcomas are classified as telangiectatic sarcomas. These tumors radiographically resemble aneurysmal bone cysts and have dilated spaces filled with blood and necrotic tissue, with viable tumor confined to the periphery of the lesion. Telangiectatic sarcomas are often anaplastic, with very little evidence of bone formation. Although previously thought to be associated with an adverse prognosis, it is now recognized that this histologic type has the same biologic behavior as classic osteosarcoma.[47]

Primary osteosarcomas involving the spine present complex therapeutic problems in management, mainly because of the difficulties posed by surgical resection. As a result, the reported median survival of patients with these spinal tumors has ranged from 6 to 10 months.[6, 23, 28, 29, 31, 56, 71, 88] The major advances achieved during the past two decades using combined modality treatment for extremity lesions unfortunately have not translated into similar survival benefits for spinal lesions, because major tumor resection has been believed to be impossible. However, our recent data are more encouraging if complete resection of the involved spine by spondylectomy can be achieved.[98]

CLINICAL FEATURES

Approximately 10 per cent of osteosarcomas arise in the axial skeleton (i.e., skull, ribs, pelvis, and vertebrae); the relative incidence of tumors arising in the spine is reported to be between 0.85 per cent and 3.0 per cent.[13, 18, 77, 102, 105] In a series of 1122 patients treated at the Mayo Clinic between 1909 and 1980, there were 27 patients (2.4 per cent) with primary lesions of the spine.[88] Over a similar time period, 24 patients with osteosarcoma of the spine (approximately 2 per cent of all osteosarcoma cases) were seen at Memorial Sloan-Kettering Cancer Center.[98] Patients with osteosarcoma of the spine were on the average a decade older than patients with extremity lesions, and approximately half the cases were secondary to other conditions.

Most patients with osteosarcoma of the spine present with pain related to the site of the tumor in combination with varying neurologic deficits. Since early symptoms may be nonspecific, such patients are generally diagnosed as having benign disc disease. The median duration of symptoms prior to diagnosis was six months (range: one month to 120 months) in two major series.[88, 98] Two thirds of patients reported in the literature have had neurologic deficits ranging from radiculopathy to complete paraplegia at initial presentation. These clinical findings indicate epidural extension of tumor in all patients at time of diagnosis and have adversely affected the feasibility of curative resection.

RADIOLOGIC FINDINGS

The plain radiographic findings may be variable, owing to the degree of ossification within the tumor.[76] Heavy ossification is characterized by dense areas of sclerosis. In extremity lesions, periosteal response to the tumor may result in transverse or radiating striations in a typical "sunburst" pattern; a triangular periosteal elevation (Codman's triangle) is often seen. These features in association with an ossified soft tissue mass are used to diagnose osteosarcoma, which may be classified on radiographic findings as predominantly osteolytic, sclerotic, or mixed. In the spine, however, the most common finding is that of a mixed osteolytic and sclerotic lesion of the vertebral body. Pathologic fractures may also occur (Fig. 14–1). While suggestive of tumor, these findings provide no indication of histology. In more than 90 per cent of cases, the vertebral body is predominantly involved (Fig. 14–2), but the posterior elements are also affected. The most important differential diagnoses include both osteoblastoma and giant cell tumor of bone in young patients.[10, 64, 66, 67, 79] In the presence of a cystic osteolytic or a coarse trabeculated pattern on x-rays, osteosarcoma may be impossible to distinguish from giant cell tumor unless ossification or calcification is present. In the older age group, the differential diagnosis of lytic lesions includes both metastatic carcinoma and myeloma. In addition, lytic destruction without sclerosis is seen in malignant fibrous histiocytoma, which occurs very rarely in the spine.

Tumor extension into both soft tissues and the spinal canal may be demonstrated by computed tomography (CT) (Fig. 14–3). Besides demonstrating soft tissue extension, CT scans are used to stage the tumor radiologically, ruling out early metastases to the lungs.[4, 15, 21] More recently, magnetic resonance imaging (MRI) is particularly helpful because its multiplanar capability helps to understand the complex anatomy of these lesions. Sagittal and coronal images demonstrate longitudinal extent in a manner more comprehensible than CT.[92] In addition, spinal canal invasion is easier to appreciate, and MRI may be substituted for CT-myelography in many cases. The MR appearance depends heavily on the extent of mineralization: nonmineralized tumor has relatively low signal intensity on T1-weighted images and a bright signal on T2-weighted images. Mineralized tumor appears dark on all sequences.

Radioisotope scans are of help in demonstrating "skip" or "satellite" lesions in tumors of long bones.[4, 33, 62] Following or during therapy, the presence of persistent "hot spots" on bone scans is a reliable indicator of persistent or recurrent tumor. Regular follow-up radionuclide bone scanning is indicated in patients undergoing combination chemotherapy, since many patients now present with relapses in bone.[33, 53, 55] Angiography is currently used to determine tumor neovascularity and to determine the feasibility of limb-sparing resection and intraarterial chemotherapy for extremity tumors.[40, 103, 108] In patients with spinal tumors at the thoracolumbar re-

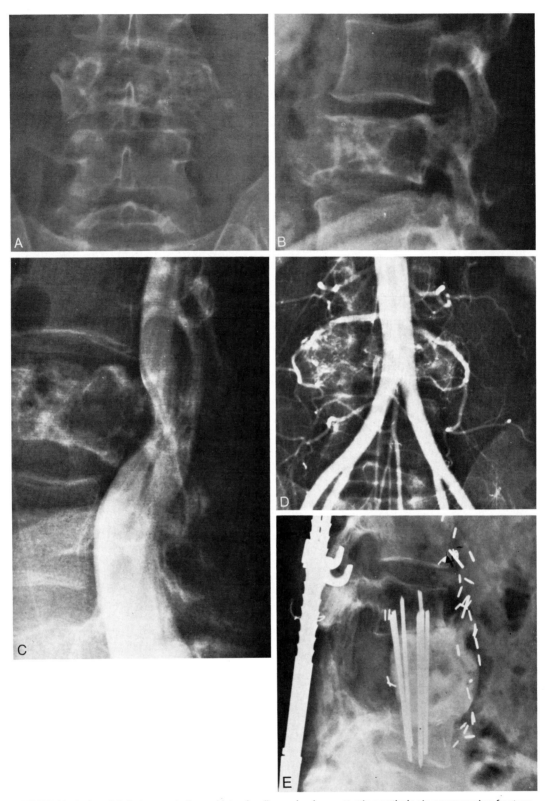

FIGURE 14–1. *A* and *B*, Anteroposterior and lateral radiographs demonstrating pathologic compression fracture. This was originally thought to be a giant cell tumor, in view of the lack of ossification. *C*, Lateral myelogram shows epidural extension and compression of the cauda equina; the patient was initially explored and biopsied through a decompressive laminectomy. *D*, Spinal angiography (nonselective) reveals a hypervascular stain; at present we advocate selective catheterization and embolization prior to definitive surgery. *E*, Complete spondylectomy of the tumor has been achieved using staged procedures. Anteriorly, reconstruction of the resected vertebra was carried out with methyl methacrylate and Steinmann pins. Posteriorly, stabilization was accomplished by the use of Harrington instrumentation and bone grafts. The patient is disease free more than five years.

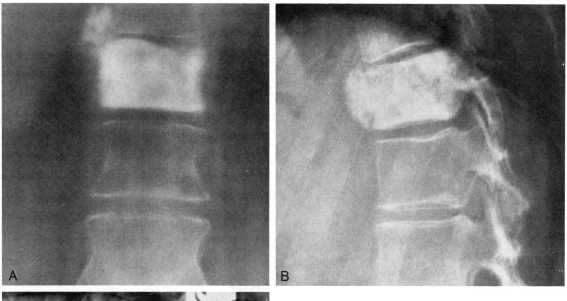

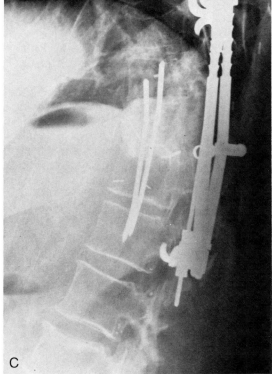

FIGURE 14–2. *A* and *B,* Anteroposterior and lateral radiographs in a patient with "ivory" vertebra involving T11; the initial diagnosis was Paget's disease based on needle biopsy. With the onset of cord compression, laminectomy revealed a high grade spindle cell osteosarcoma compatible with Paget's sarcoma. *C,* Following chemotherapy, complete resection of the vertebra was accomplished in two stages. Patient is disease free more than three years later.

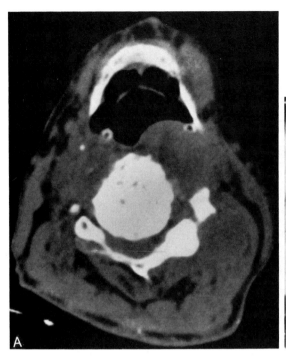

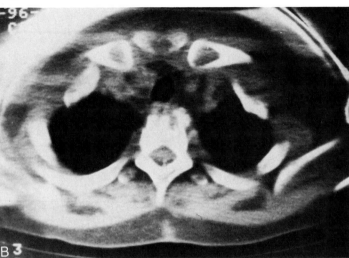

FIGURE 14–3. *A*, CT scan discloses marked sclerosis of the cervical vertebra with anterolateral soft tissue masses. Biopsy revealed osteosarcoma. *B*, CT scan discloses destructive tumor of the T2 vertebra with small soft tissue mass anteriorly; patient was originally thought to have giant cell tumor. Surgery included resection of the vertebra by a transsternal approach.

gion, angiography is indicated to determine the segmental arterial supply to the cord and to identify the artery of Adamkiewicz. In highly vascular neoplasms of the spine, angiography is helpful in obliterating tumor neovascularity and minimizing intraoperative blood loss (see Fig. 14–1*D*). This is accomplished by selective spinal embolization using polyvinyl alcohol (PVA) or absolute alcohol. In addition, arteriography allows selective delivery of chemotherapeutically effective agents such as cisplatin.[52]

BIOPSY

When the diagnosis of osteosarcoma is suspected, tissue confirmation by biopsy is indicated before definitive surgery is undertaken. In extremity lesions, biopsies are performed either by a fine needle aspirate or a Tru-Cut needle. In patients with soft tissue extension of tumor, an accurate diagnosis can be made by needle biopsy in 80 per cent of patients with osteosarcoma. In patients with spinal lesions, needle biopsies (while technically feasible) are not generally used because most patients present with spinal cord compression. Open biopsy is thus frequently used and all too often has been performed by decompressive laminectomy in the past. If the CT scan demonstrates a tumor involving the vertebral body, an *anterior* approach should be used for biopsy rather than a laminectomy.

The surgical approach should be carefully planned and meticulous hemostasis achieved so that postoperative hemorrhage does not result in tracking of tumor along the tissue planes. Prior to biopsy of a suspected malignant spine tumor, the chosen area should be carefully packed off and a small cortical window made with osteotomes. By limiting the initial bony opening in the vertebra, it is often possible to

remove all soft tumor by using intralesional curettage. All soft tissue tumor should be removed. If the pathologist can reliably make the diagnosis of a malignant tumor, a subtotal spondylectomy may be performed. The operation should be complete enough to remove all bone and tumor down to the dura, and it is not enough to merely curette down to normal-appearing bone. It should also be extensive enough so that complete removal of the vertebra can be performed at a subsequent stage. If a reliable diagnosis cannot be made, and if the patient is not in need of neural decompression, the procedure may be terminated at this stage. The bone window from the biopsy site should be closed with a methyl methacrylate plug. The biopsy area itself should be carefully packed off with Gelfoam from surrounding tissues. If the surgeon choses a posterior approach for biopsy, intraoperative radiographic control is essential so that removal of normal bone can be minimized. A small portion of the lamina and facet should be removed, and biopsy should be performed through the pedicle. The biopsy tract should be plugged by hemostatic agents such as Gelfoam and Avitene (microfibrillar collagen) to avoid tissue contamination by tumor cells.

PATHOLOGY

All osteosarcomas, despite their classification as to type, have as their common histologic feature the production of bone by neoplastic osteoblasts. This bone may constitute only a small portion of the tumor but nevertheless is the diagnostic criterion used by the pathologist. Consequently, the gross appearance of such tumors usually is of a gritty granular quality when rubbed because of the bone production.

There are a number of classifications used to

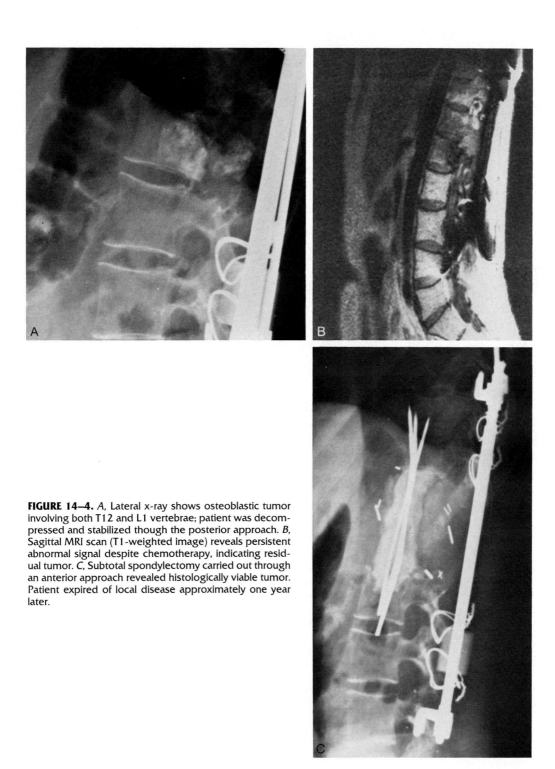

FIGURE 14–4. *A,* Lateral x-ray shows osteoblastic tumor involving both T12 and L1 vertebrae; patient was decompressed and stabilized though the posterior approach. *B,* Sagittal MRI scan (T1-weighted image) reveals persistent abnormal signal despite chemotherapy, indicating residual tumor. *C,* Subtotal spondylectomy carried out through an anterior approach revealed histologically viable tumor. Patient expired of local disease approximately one year later.

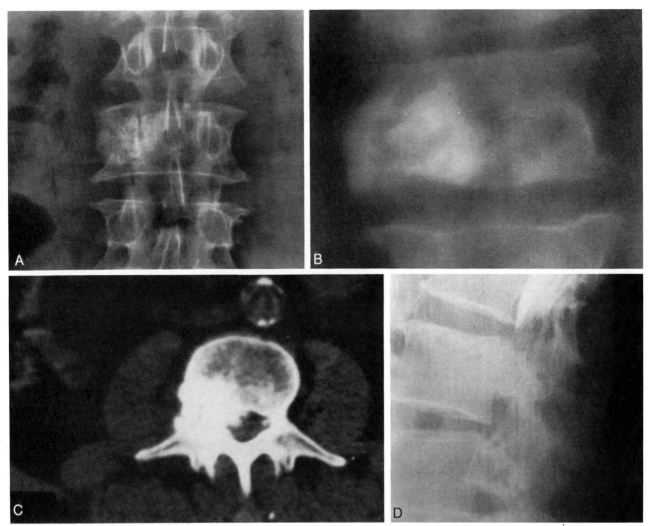

FIGURE 14–5. *A*, An anteroposterior plain film of the lumbar spine demonstrates destruction of the right pedicle at L3. There is an ill-defined pattern of increased density overlying the pedicle and the lateral aspect of the vertebral body. *B*, An anteroposterior tomogram illustrates the poorly organized pattern of neoplastic bone formation as well as distortion of the margins of the vertebral bodies, suggesting a soft tissue mass. *C*, A CT scan reveals a dense bone-forming lesion involving the posterior aspect of the vertebral body, the pedicle, and a small portion of the lamina of L3. There is extension into the spinal canal and the neural foramen. *D*, A myelogram reveals complete block at the L3 level.

subdivide osteosarcoma. For simplicity and particularly related to the spine, four divisions may be found, all of which have bone production by the tumor cells as their common denominator. They are:

1. Osteogenic osteosarcoma
2. Chondrogenic osteosarcoma
3. Fibrogenic osteosarcoma
4. Osteosarcoma secondary to Paget's disease or radiation

Gross Findings

Osteosarcomas are extremely vascular tumors; therefore, foci of hemorrhage and/or large vascular spaces are often found producing a bloody tumor. Sometimes most of the tumor is a bloody mass. There are always areas of grittiness corresponding to the bone production. If the bone is mineralized, calcified or rock-hard areas are apparent. Gray-white tissue

of fibrogenic areas or glistening blue slimy tissue of chondrogenic foci may also be seen.

The tumor in the spine usually extends through the vertebral body cortex into the soft tissues or spinal canal by the time it is diagnosed. The pedicle or transverse processes may also be invaded at surgery with extensive osseous destruction. The classic persistent reactive bone (Codman's triangle) seen in the long bones is not present in the spine.

Microscopic Findings

The production of woven bone, mineralized or unmineralized (osteoid), by malignant osteoblasts is the single diagnostic feature of any kind of osteosarcoma. All osteosarcomas have disorganized, haphazardly arranged spicules or masses of woven bone enmeshed in a richly vascular bed. The cells surrounding the bone spicules are anaplastic spindle or

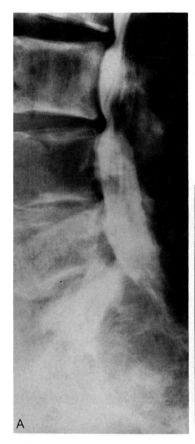

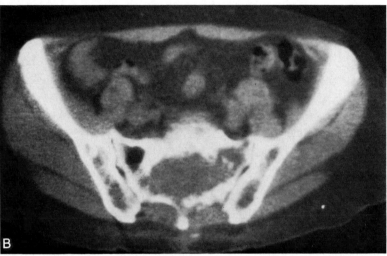

FIGURE 14–6. *A,* Osteogenic sarcoma arising in Paget's disease. A lateral plain film from a myelogram demonstrates an area of destruction involving the 1st, 2nd, and 3rd sacral segments. Notice the coarsening of the trabecular architecture of the sacrum, a finding that is also prominent at L3. Although Paget's disease is common in the spine, degeneration into sarcoma is less frequent than at other sites. *B,* A CT scan demonstrates the destructive lesion of the sacrum. A small amount of tumorous new bone formation is seen in the left sacral ala.

polygonal cells with frequent atypical mitoses. The malignant osteoblasts spring from the background sarcoma; there is no prominent osteoblastic palisading about the bone spicules because there are no significant morphologic differences between the cells. The osteocytes embedded in the bone resemble the background sarcoma cells as well. If cartilage foci are present, the chondrocytes have the malignant features of a standard chondrosarcoma.

Foci of hemorrhage or necrosis are common features of osteosarcoma. In such areas, the woven bone produced by the tumor ("tumor bone") may be more easily seen because the background sarcoma cells have lost their staining affinity. Fibrogenic foci are identical to any spindle cell malignancy, and therefore a diligent search for bone production should be made anytime such foci are seen in a bone tumor (Figs. 14–9 to 14–13).

There are no specific special stains that are diagnostic of osteosarcoma. Immunoperoxidase stains may be used to establish the sarcomatous nature of these tumors and therefore to rule out an epithelial origin, since metastatic carcinomas or even melanoma may rarely be confused with osteosarcoma. Similarly, electron microscopy may be useful in such conditions. However, the simple technique of using polarized light microscopy is extremely useful because it identifies the woven bone production by the tumor. Often such an examination is not necessary since the tumor bone is prominent; however, there are instances in which bone production is scant and a careful search must be done. Under polarized light, the bone collagen is easily seen.

There are a number of cases in which the presence of bone production is not confirmed, and the pathologist is left with a malignant spindle cell tumor producing collagen. If these cells are arranged in whorls as in a pinwheel or storiform pattern, then the diagnosis of malignant fibrous histiocytoma may be made. Particularly common in such tumors are scattered large polygonal cells with prominent bean-shaped nuclei that represent the histiocytic component. Sometimes multinucleate giant cells are also present. In classic fibrosarcoma, the storiform pattern and histiocytic differentiation are not present (Figs. 14–14 and 14–15).

The distinction between an atypical or aggressive osteoblastoma and osteosarcoma may be very difficult. However, features that include foci of necrosis, lack of osteoblastic palisading, and frequent mitotic activity speak more for osteosarcoma than for a benign neoplasm.

TREATMENT

Since there is no standardized protocol for malignant lesions of the spine, it is appropriate to use principles gained in the experience of extremity tumors. Once the diagnosis is established, metastatic disease should be ruled out by chest CT scans and radionuclide bone scans. The standard treatment for osteosarcoma of the extremities is complete surgical resection, which is accomplished either by amputation or by a limb-sparing radical local resection.

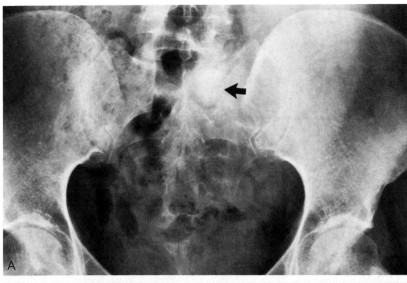

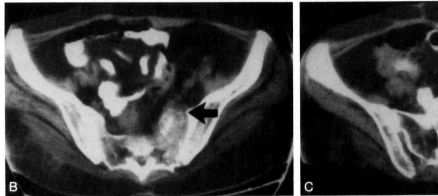

FIGURE 14–7. *A,* An anteroposterior plain film of the pelvis demonstrates an area of amorphous new bone formation involving the left ala of the S1 segment (*arrow*). There is destruction of the left S1 neural foramen. From the plain film, it is impossible to determine whether a soft tissue mass is present. *B* and *C,* CT scans through S1 and S2 show extensive destruction of the left side of the sacrum and a large amount of tumorous new bone. A soft tissue mass is seen extending into the pelvic soft tissues in the area of the destroyed S1 neural foramen (*arrow*).

With the advent of effective chemotherapy, limb-sparing segmental resections along with the use of endoprostheses have become increasingly used for extremity tumors. In many centers, definitive surgery is often delayed so that early systemic chemotherapy can be instituted (neoadjuvant chemotherapy). Rosen proposed that surgery be delayed for up to 16 weeks prior to resection of the primary tumor while the patient receives chemotherapy.[80–84] The rationale for neoadjuvant chemotherapy is based on three premises: first, that systemic micrometastases are already present at the time of initial diagnosis, and thus chemotherapy is instituted when the metastatic tumor burden is relatively small and responsive prior to the emergence of drug-resistant clones. This is particularly important in osteosarcoma in which the doubling time is estimated to be between 30 and 40 days. Second, regression of the primary tumor allows more effective and less radical or mutilating surgical resection because it allows the surgical plane to be carried close to the tumor. This argument is particularly valid in spinal tumors, since only intralesional procedures are feasible. The third advantage is that the effects on the tumor by the chemotherapy regimen can be histologically quantified (Table 14–1), and these observations allow appropriate planning of future therapy.[82]

Surgery for Vertebral Tumors

In patients who have had the diagnosis unexpectedly established by decompressive laminectomy, we favor the use of several cycles of chemotherapy to control metastatic disease if the patient is neurologically stable. We base this on the assumption that the procedure has violated tissue planes and that additional extensive surgery in the immediate postoperative period may produce morbidity that could delay the institution of chemotherapy. Exceptions to this approach are the presence of either severe neurologic deficit, for example, paraparesis, or pain indicating an unstable spine. In such cases, tumor resection and decompression of the spinal cord as well as stabilization may need to be completed prior to chemotherapy.

If the diagnosis is suspected clinically, the initial procedure should be a subtotal spondylectomy

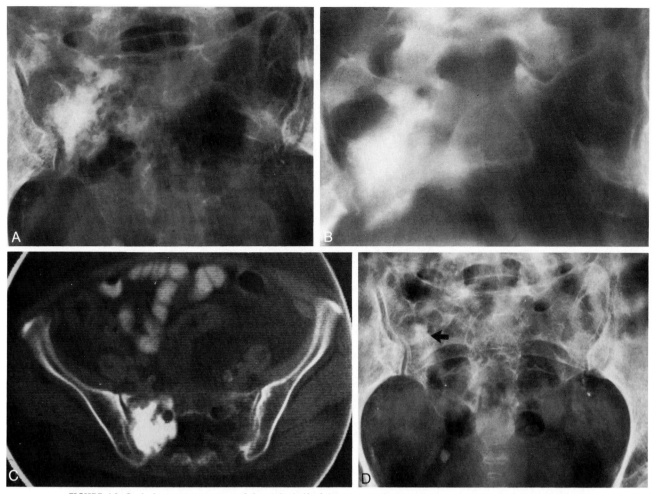

FIGURE 14–8. *A*, An osteosarcoma of the right half of the sacrum demonstrates areas of bone lysis and dense new bone formation. *B*, An anteroposterior tomogram illustrates these findings with great clarity, revealing that the tumor abuts the right sacroiliac joint but does not appear to cross it. *C*, A CT scan illustrates the extensive area of bone destruction and shows no evidence of a soft tissue mass. *D*, In retrospect, the lesion was present on a plain film obtained almost two years earlier (*arrow*).

through an anterolateral approach. This requires resection of the involved vertebral body and reconstruction of the resected segments with methyl methacrylate and instrumentation using approaches that we have previously described.[93–95] At the time of resection, a sufficient amount of the vertebral body should be removed so that the procedure of spondylectomy (removal of the entire vertebra) can be completed at a subsequent procedure. Patients are continued on combination chemotherapy with serial evaluation of the local tumor by radionuclide bone scans and CT scans. In addition, serial evaluation of serum alkaline phosphatase levels is useful in monitoring response to therapy.[58, 101] At the time of second operation, the decision to control local tumor either by chemotherapy or by RT should be based on the presence or absence of viable tumor in the resected specimen. Local RT should be used in all cases where neoadjuvant chemotherapy has failed to eradicate all microscopic disease.

Whenever possible, RT treatments should be coordinated by discussion with the radiation oncologist and administered in such a manner as to spare the midline. In our experience, strictly posterior RT ports are associated with a high potential for wound breakdown, especially when instrumentation and bone grafts are subsequently used through midline incisions. If the patient experiences side effects from chemotherapy which delay its use, local RT may be used prior to operation as well, with the caveat that this may increase morbidity from later surgery.

Results of Treatment

Most studies of osteosarcoma of the spine are limited to single case reports, and only three large institutional series have been reported to date.[6, 88, 98] In 1980, Barwick and colleagues reported a series of 10 patients with osteosarcoma of the spine (excluding the sacrum) seen over a 67-year period.[6] The overall median survival was 6 months, and there was only one long-term survivor. A three-year-old boy with a thoracic tumor was treated by external RT and chemotherapy (nitrogen mustard) and survived 6 years and 2 months. Several other reports suggest the feasibility of long-term survival in the occasional patient. Mnaymneh reported a patient treated by

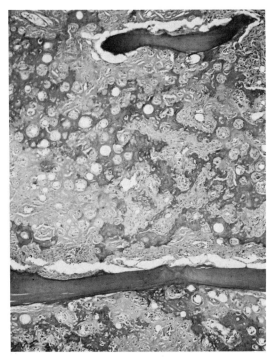

FIGURE 14–9. A low power view of an osteosarcoma invading between preexisting trabecular bone. The tumor produces numerous small irregular spicules of woven bone (tumor bone). The background marrow tissue is of malignant spindle cells (H & E ×55).

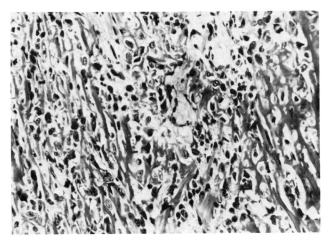

FIGURE 14–11. Osteosarcoma with prominent woven bone production. Note the atypical pleomorphic sarcoma cells which produce the woven bone (tumor bone). H & E ×200.

partial resection, external RT, and chemotherapy; this patient subsequently died of doxorubicin toxicity approximately 2 years later.[71] Ogihara and coworkers reported the case of a 15-year-old boy with osteosarcoma of the fourth thoracic vertebra.[74] This patient was paraplegic at the time of diagnosis. Following laminectomy, he was treated with 30 mg of intraar-terial doxorubicin (Adriamycin) daily for 3 days through the feeding intercostal artery. He received three further courses at 6-week intervals through the intraarterial route and then received systemic chemotherapy—the Compadri-III regimen (vincristine, methotrexate, phenylalanine mustard, Adriamycin). Four months following treatment, he became ambulatory and was free of disease at last follow-up (6 years). Poppe and colleagues reported a patient who was treated only with external radiation and survived for more than 10 years, but no further details of therapy were given.[77] Shives and coworkers reported a median survival of 10 months in a series of 27 patients with osteosarcoma of the spine, but none of their patients had been treated intensively with the modern combination chemotherapy regimens cur-

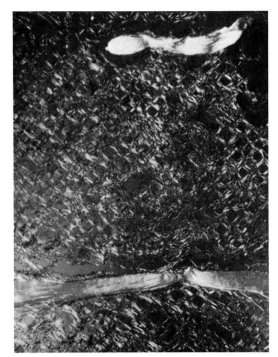

FIGURE 14–10. The same field seen under polarized light. The tumor bone is seen as irregular arranged woven bone spicules, whereas the preexisting trabecular bone is lamellar (H & E ×55).

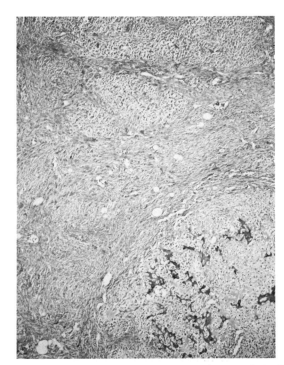

FIGURE 14–12. A fibrogenic osteosarcoma with a prominent fibroblastic spindle cell background. Tumor bone production is present in the lower left portion of the field (H & E ×50).

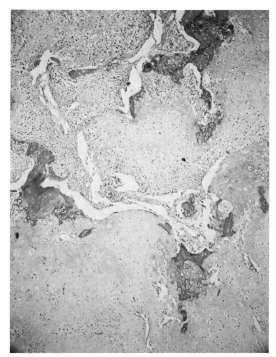

FIGURE 14–13. Chondrogenic osteosarcoma with lobules of neoplastic cartilage admixed with foci of sarcoma producing tumor bone (H & E ×50).

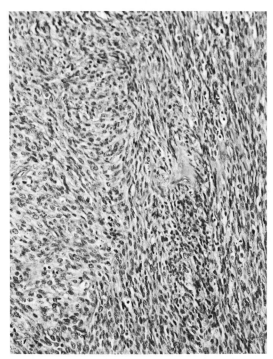

FIGURE 14–15. Fibrosarcoma with interdigitating bundles of malignant spindle cells (H & E ×175).

rently available.[88] More recently, we have updated our experience at Memorial Sloan-Kettering Cancer Center to include sacral tumors as well.[98] The 24 patients treated over a 35-year period (1949 to 1984) were divided into two groups. The earlier 13 patients were treated primarily with laminectomy and radiation; in this group, the median survival was 6 months and there was only one long-term survivor. The more

recent 11 patients were treated by more aggressive surgery (including spondylectomy) and received combination chemotherapy. The chemotherapy regimens were based on the T-7 and T-10 protocols described by Rosen. Multiple operations to remove residual or recurrent tumor were carried out in four patients. In this group, there were five long-term survivors (> 5 years), of whom three are completely disease-free. Only one patient developed metastatic disease while receiving chemotherapy. We believe that these results, achieved by using principles of chemotherapy and surgery for extremity lesions, represent a useful model for the treatment of osteosarcoma of the spine. These results are summarized in Table 14–2.

Role of Chemotherapy

Although the principles of chemotherapy for osteosarcoma are dealt with elsewhere, several points deserve emphasis. Prior to 1972 the outlook for patients with extremity lesions was bleak, despite the fact that primary tumors had been adequately treated by amputation. The 5-year survival in several large

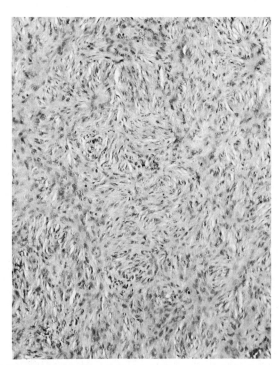

FIGURE 14–14. Malignant fibrous histiocytoma with spindle cells arranged in a pinwheel or storiform pattern. Such foci are characteristic in such tumors (H & E ×125).

TABLE 14–1. HISTOLOGIC GRADING OF TUMOR RESPONSE TO CHEMOTHERAPY

GRADE	RESPONSE
I	Little or none
II	Areas of acellular tumor bone, necrosis, or fibrosis, with other areas of histologically viable tumor
III	Predominant areas of acellular tumor, bone, necrosis, or fibrosis, with scattered foci of histologically viable cells
IV	No evidence of viable tumor in specimen

TABLE 14–2. CLINICAL FEATURES AND RESULTS OF TREATMENT (AUTHOR'S SERIES)

CASE NO.	AGE/SEX	LOCATION	PREEXISTING CONDITION	SURGERY	RT	CT	STATUS (Months)
1	15 M	S	—	Wide Excision	+	T-7	60 ANED
2	17 M	S	—	Biopsy	+	ADR, CTX, VCR	12 DOD
3	44 M	L	—	Lam	+	T-7	60 DOD
4	31 F	T	—	VBR	+	T-7	48 AWD
5	67 M	S	Paget's	Biopsy	+	HDMTX, ADR, c'p DDD	21 DOD
6	30 M	L	—	VBR	+	T-10	66 ANED
7	59 F	T	RT	VBR	−	T-7	6 DOD
8	71 F	T	Paget's and RT	VBR	−	ADR, c'p DDD	14 DOD
9	66 M	C	—	VBR	+	ADR, c'p DDD	12 DOD
10	59 F	T	Paget's	VBR	+	ADR, c'p DDD	36 ANED
11	59 F	L	Paget's	Biopsy	+	T-7	18 DOD

S = sacral; L = lumbar; T = thoracic; C = cervical; Lam = laminectomy; VBR = vertebral body resection; RT = radiation therapy; CT = chemotherapy; ADR = Adriamycin; CTX = cytoxan; VCR = vincristine; c'p DDD = cisplatin; HDMTX = high dose methotrexate; ANED = alive, no evidence of disease; AWD = alive with disease; DOD = died of disease.

series was approximately 20 per cent, with most patients relapsing with pulmonary metastases within the first 2 years of treatment.[37, 47, 63] The presumptive evidence therefore suggested that 80 per cent of patients with osteosarcoma had micrometastases at the time of diagnosis.

During the early 1970s, the use of high dose methotrexate was seen to produce remissions in 30 to 40 per cent of patients with osteosarcoma.[51] With the concomitant use of leucovorin rescue, toxicity from mucositis and myelosuppression was minimized. Similarly, doxorubicin was found to produce tumor regression in 30 per cent of patients with metastatic osteosarcoma.[16] Both these drugs have a steep dose-response curve, and despite the fact that they were initially established as the two most active single agents, there are few studies combining the drugs in patients with evaluable disease. These drugs produced a disease-free survival that reached a plateau at 40 per cent at 5 years.

At the same time, Rosen introduced a variety of combination chemotherapy regimens, named the T-4, T-7, and T-10 protocols, to treat osteosarcoma in both the adjuvant and neoadjuvant setting. Since 1973, 185 patients with primary osteosarcoma of the extremities were treated with adjuvant chemotherapy; 48 per cent of the originally treated 52 patients remained free of disease for a median of 7 years. The T-4 chemotherapy consisted of the sequential administration of high dose methotrexate with leucovorin rescue, doxorubicin, and cyclophosphamide. The T-7 protocol consisted of high dose methotrexate with leucovorin rescue given initially in four weekly doses and then given sequentially following the combination of BCD (bleomycin, cyclophosphamide, and dactinomycin) and doxorubicin given at a dose of 90 mg/m^2 per course. Preoperative chemotherapy was used in all patients who were referred prior to amputation. High dose methotrexate was used at doses of 12 gm/m^2 for patients who had not completed their growth spurt and at doses of 8 gm/m^2 in fully grown individuals. Using the T-7 protocol, 43 of 54 patients (80 per cent) remained free of disease for a median of 4 years. In 1978, cisplatin at a dose of 100 to 120 mg/m^2 on a 1-day or 5-day treatment schedule was noted to have a 55 per cent response rate; it was therefore added to the treatment regimens of patients at risk of developing metastases as determined by partial or poor effect or preoperative chemotherapy.[82–84] Patients having a good response to preoperative chemotherapy were not subjected to the potential additional morbidity or permanent renal toxicity of cisplatin, since such patients remained free of disease if they continued on the preoperative regimen. This protocol, in which the postoperative chemotherapy was based on the response of the primary tumor to chemotherapy, was termed the T-10 protocol. The T-10 protocol uses high dose methotrexate with leucovorin rescue, BCD, and ADR (Adriamycin) as preoperative treatment. In those who respond (see Table 14–1), the histologic effects observed are quantified into four grades. Patients showing Grade 3 or 4 responses continue on the same drugs used preoperatively. In those patients showing Grade 1 or 2 responses, cisplatin is added and high dose methotrexate is omitted. With this approach, 80 per cent of patients have remained continuously free of disease at 3 years.[83]

A number of other studies have confirmed the effectiveness of chemotherapy regimens using methotrexate.[12, 30, 32, 36, 39, 43, 102] At the present time, the role of high dose methotrexate therapy is complicated by many variables that may affect outcome, including dose, schedules, length of infusion, and leucovorin rescue schemata.[39] As such, high dose methotrexate is considered an investigational agent and is available through the National Cancer Institute only for clinical research trials. Green and colleagues have carefully reviewed the published data on the contribution of methotrexate to these chemotherapy regimens and have concluded that the only way of answering this question would be deletion of methotrexate in future studies. They believe that there is little justification for this since high dose methotrexate is one of the most tolerable agents used. With careful monitoring of drug levels, the incidence of renal toxicity is low, and the only serious toxicity of high dose methotrexate is chronic or acute encephalopathy. High dose methotrexate therapy is extremely expensive; the cost of a dozen treatments may range from $40,000 to $50,000 excluding indirect expenses.

Of the other experimental approaches, the use of intraarterial therapy represents an attractive option because it offers the possibility of increasing local concentration of the antineoplastic agent while minimizing systemic toxicity. Although intraarterial doxorubicin appeared to be effective through this route, it has not been abandoned in favor of the systemic route. Intraarterial cisplatin was first administered for osteosarcoma by Benjamin and associates and is currently used at the MD Anderson Cancer Institute. Jaffe reported the use of intraarterial cisplatin at a dosage of 150 mg/m[2] every two weeks. He analyzed the effect of repeated courses of therapy on the development of Grade 3 to 4 necrosis; overall 16 of 42 patients (38 per cent) had at least 90 per cent tumor necrosis. In addition, he compared intraarterial cisplatin and high dose methotrexate as primary single agent chemotherapy for osteosarcoma. The overall response rate of patients treated with intraarterial cisplatin (60 per cent) was superior to that of patients treated with methotrexate (27 per cent); the complete response rate for intraarterial cisplatin was 47 per cent and for methotrexate 20 per cent. In a more recent study, Jaffe has noted that eradication of tumor depends on both the concentration of cisplatin reaching the target organ, and the cumulative deposition associated with the increased number of courses. His current recommendation is to administer seven courses of preoperative intraarterial cisplatin at two-week intervals to augment the number of patients who will achieve greater than 90 per cent necrosis.[54a]

The protocol used by Jaffe is as follows: criteria for entry include normal values of hemogram, liver function, electrolytes, and creatinine clearance. Patients are hospitalized and hydrated with a maintenance infusion of 5 per cent dextrose in 0.5 per cent saline administered as 300 ml/m[2] for 12 to 24 hours. Immediately prior to the infusion, 50 ml of 20 per cent mannitol is administered intravenously over 15 minutes. The infusion procedure requires intraarterial insertion of a catheter percutaneously using the Seldinger technique. The tip of the catheter is then positioned into the vessel supplying the tumor. A volumetric infusion pump primed with 120 ml of saline and 2000 units of sodium heparin is attached to the catheter, and the infusion is initiated at 20 ml per hour. The initial dose of cisplatin should be 100 mg/m[2]. This is escalated to 150 mg/m[2]. The cisplatin is mixed in 300 ml of normal saline and 3000 units of aqueous sodium heparin and is infused over two hours. Concurrently, the intravenous maintenance infusion is altered to 1000 ml of 5 per cent dextrose in 0.5 per cent saline plus 200 ml of mannitol administered over 8 hours. When this is completed, 5 per cent dextrose in 0.5 per cent saline at 300 ml/m[2] for 24 hours is reinstituted. Treatment is repeated at two-week intervals for seven courses. This protocol, based on Jaffe's experience, should produce good to excellent responses in all primary tumors.

Although the rationale for chemotherapy now appears established, some studies have questioned the value of adjuvant treatment. In several reports, it was suggested that the disease-free survival without adjuvant chemotherapy increased from 20 per cent in the 1960s to 30 to 40 per cent in the 1970s.[89, 99] One possible explanation was the more accurate staging studies done to identify patients with metastatic disease by either chest CT scan or lung tomography as well as the intrinsic biologic heterogeneity of the tumor. The Mayo Clinic conducted a prospective study in which patients were assigned to high dose methotrexate or no chemotherapy following amputation. At five years, the disease-free survival was approximately 40 per cent in both groups.[24]

To determine the role of adjuvant chemotherapy, several controlled multiinstitutional studies were conducted. Eilber reported a randomized study at the University of California in patients with extremity osteosarcoma who were randomized to either aggressive adjuvant chemotherapy or no treatment after preoperative intraarterial doxorubicin therapy and radiation therapy to the primary tumor.[25] The adjuvant chemotherapy arm employed methotrexate at a dose of 100 mg/kg during the first exposure and 200 mg/kg thereafter. At 24 months' median follow-up, the disease-free and overall survival rates were significantly in favor of immediate postadjuvant chemotherapy. Forty-five per cent of patients relapsed and 20 per cent died on the chemotherapy arm compared with relapse in 80 per cent and death in 52 per cent on the observation arm.[25]

Link and coworkers reported the results of MIOS (multiinstitutional osteosarcoma study) of 156 patients with high grade osteosarcoma of the extremities; of these, 113 were found eligible for randomization and 36 patients accepted randomization.[60] There were six patients with axial tumors who were considered ineligible for the study. The postoperative adjuvant chemotherapy was based on Rosen's protocols. Of the 18 patients assigned to chemotherapy, 12 remain disease-free and 5 had recurrences; one patient died from chemotherapy toxicity. Of the 18 patients assigned to observation without adjuvant chemotherapy, only 3 have remained free of disease and 15 have had relapses. The two-year relapse-free interval was 17 per cent for the control group and 6 per cent in the adjuvant chemotherapy group. A similar difference was seen in those patients who declined randomization. Of the 59 who elected treatment, 43 remain relapse-free and 16 have had relapses. Of the 18 who elected observation, 3 remain relapse-free and 15 have relapsed. There were two deaths—one during remission attributed to chemotherapy, and one after relapse due to a combination of toxicity and progressive tumor. With the intensive chemotherapy treatment, hematologic toxicity was severe in 33 per cent of patients and was life-threatening in an additional 16 per cent. Elevation of serum enzymes was common and resulted in fatal hepatic failure in one patient. Toxic effects of the central nervous system including seizures and raised intracranial pressure were also observed. The authors concluded that adjuvant chemotherapy has definite benefit in producing relapse-free survival but cautioned that more than one third of patients without metastases would relapse despite the best possible treatment. Morbidity from combination chemotherapy is considerable, and treatment is expensive.

The only new drug that has emerged in the treatment of osteosarcoma is ifosfamide. Ifosfamide is an analogue of cyclophosphamide and, in animal experiments, was shown to be more effective and less toxic than cyclophosphamide. In the absence of uroprotection, the dose-limiting factor is hemorrhagic cystitis. It is therefore given with Mesna (2-mercaptoethanesulfonate sodium). Previous studies in Europe by Marti and others have suggested response rates ranging from 38 to 83 per cent for ifosfamide alone in pretreated sarcomas.[3, 65] In a phase II study, Antman and colleagues noted a 40 per cent response rate for ifosfamide in previously treated bony sarcomas.[3]

Ifosfamide is generally used at an initial rate of 2.0 gm/m^2 on days 1 to 4. The dose can be escalated to 2.5 gm/m^2 if toxicity is acceptable. It is generally given intravenously over 4 hours daily. Mesna is given at a dose of 20 per cent of the ifosfamide dose 15 minutes prior to ifosfamide therapy and every 4 hours thereafter for 5 doses. If urine output drops, 20 mg of furosemide is given intravenously. Major side effects of ifosfamide include somnolence or confusion, metabolic acidosis, gross or microscopic hematuria, elevated creatinine levels, and myelosuppression. Of these, myelosuppression is potentially dose limiting. Investigators are currently evaluating the use of ifosfamide in combination with methotrexate and doxorubicin in the preoperative treatment of primary and metastatic osteosarcoma.

How does one extrapolate these data into the management of spinal tumor? We believe that combination chemotherapy currently offers the best potential for control of metastatic disease and allows intralesional resection of tumor to be performed without fear of dissemination. For spinal lesions, the major problem remains one of achieving local control; for complete resection, the entire vertebra has to be removed (spondylectomy) and this requires a two-stage operation. However, sacral tumors can be resected by wide local excision in a single procedure.

Treatment of Metastatic Disease

Clinically evident metastatic disease in lungs or bones is present at diagnosis in 10 to 20 per cent of patients with osteosarcoma. The presence of metastatic disease at onset does not necessarily preclude long-term survival, although the survival rate is significantly lower than for patients with localized disease. In the early years, 80 per cent of relapses occurred in the lung and approximately 20 per cent occurred in bone, heart, brain, and other sites. The majority of relapses generally occur within two years. However, alterations in the patterns and incidence of metastatic disease following adjuvant chemotherapy have been noted.[33, 53, 55] In the series reported by

Guiliano,[33] 59 of 111 patients (53 per cent) with osteosarcoma of the extremities developed clinically evident distant metastases. Of these, 36 developed pulmonary metastases as the initial site of recurrence. Eighteen of 19 patients (95 per cent) treated between 1971 and 1974 by amputation alone developed pulmonary relapse; only 18 of 40 (45 per cent) treated after 1974 with surgery and adjuvant chemotherapy developed pulmonary metastases alone as the initial site of recurrence. In the latter group, 11 of 50 patients (22 per cent) developed extrapulmonary metastases as the initial site of recurrent disease, and 11 patients developed simultaneous pulmonary and extrapulmonary metastases. Of the extrapulmonary sites, bone lesions were found in 14, spine and epidural lesions in three, brain alone in two, and other sites in four. Similarly, Jaffe has noted that patients with adjuvant chemotherapy developed pulmonary metastases later and that these nodules were fewer in number.[53]

Current recommendations for treatment of metastatic disease include aggressive resection of pulmonary metastases, which includes multiple thoracotomies when necessary.[35, 68, 80, 100] Pooled data analyzed by Goorin show that 41 per cent of patients with pulmonary metastases can be rendered disease-free and can survive for long periods following surgery.[35] Complete resection of metastatic lesions can now be accomplished even when the spine is involved, although the prognosis is considerably poorer. Our experience suggests that the strategy for resecting metastatic foci should be used for osteosarcoma involving the spine and that the operation should be performed once radionuclide bone scans or CT scans demonstrate early spinal involvement. Recent data also suggest that flow cytometry of the tumors may be of considerable help in predicting metastatic potential and the need for more intensive therapy.[6, 44, 61] Patients with near diploid stem lines have considerably better prognosis and a lowered potential for metastatic disease compared with those with marked aneuploidy. These exciting developments in therapy should encourage all spinal surgeons to adopt a more aggressive and optimistic attitude in caring for patients with lesions involving the spine. A cure rate of 80 per cent is now envisioned for patients with extremity tumors using combined modality treatment.

REFERENCES

1. Abramson DH, Ellsworth RM, Zimmerman LE: Non-ocular cancer in retinoblastoma survivors. Trans Acad Ophthalmol Otolaryngol 81:454–457, 1976.
2. Amsutz HC: Multiple osteogenic sarcoma—metastatic or multicentric? Report of 2 cases and review of the literature. Cancer 24:923–931, 1969.
3. Antman KH, Ryan L, Elias A, et al: Response to ifosfamide and mesna: 124 previously treated patients with metastatic or unresectable sarcoma. J Clin Oncol 7:126–131, 1989.
4. Bacci G, Picci P, Calderoni P, et al: Full-lung tomograms and bone scanning in the initial workup of patients with osteogenic sarcoma: A review of 126 cases. Eur J Cancer 18:967–971, 1982.

5. Ballance WA, Mendelsohn G, Carter JR, et al: Osteogenic sarcoma: Malignant fibrous histiocytoma subtype. Cancer 62:763–771, 1988.
6. Barwick KW, Huvos AG, Smith J: Primary osteogenic sarcoma of the vertebral column: A clinico-pathologic correlation of ten patients. Cancer 46:595–604, 1980.
7. Bauer HCF, Kreicsberg A, Silversward C, Tribukait B: DNA analysis in the differential diagnosis of osteosarcoma. Cancer 61:2532–2540, 1988.
8. Beck JC, Wara WM, Boyhill EG Jr, et al: The role of radiation therapy in the treatment of osteosarcoma. Radiology 120:163–165, 1976.
9. Bentzen SM, Poulsen HS, Kaae S, et al: Prognostic factors in osteosarcomas: A regression analysis. Cancer 62:194–202, 1988.
10. Bertoni F, Unni KK, McLeod KA, Dahlin DC: Osteosarcoma resembling osteoblastoma. Cancer 55:416–426, 1985.
11. Braddock GTF, Hadlow VD: Osteosarcoma in enchondromatosis (Ollier's disease). Report of a case. J Bone Joint Surg 40(B):145–149, 1966.
12. Burgers JMV, Van Glabbeke M, Busson A, et al: Osteosarcoma of the limbs: Report of the EORTC-SIOP 03 trial 20781. Cancer 61:1024–1031, 1988.
13. Campanacci M, Cervellati G: Osteosarcoma. A review of 345 cases. Ital J Orthop Traumatol 1:5–22, 1975.
14. Campbell E, Whitfield RD: Osteogenic sarcoma of the vertebra secondary to Paget's disease. Report of 3 cases with compression of the spinal cord and cauda equina. NY State J Med 43:931, 1943.
15. Cohen M, Grosfeld J, Baehner R, Weetman R: Lung CT for detection of metastases: Solid tissue neoplasms in children. Am J Roentgenol Rad Ther Nucl Med 139:895–898, 1982.
16. Cortes EP, Holland JF, Wang JJ, et al: Amputation and adriamycin in primary osteosarcoma. N Engl J Med 291:998–1000, 1974.
17. Dahlin DC: Bone Tumors: General Aspects and Data on 6221 Cases. Springfield, IL, Charles C Thomas, 1978.
18. Dahlin DC, Coventry MB: Osteogenic sarcoma: A study of 600 cases. J Bone Joint Surg 49(A):101–110, 1967.
19. Dahlin DC, Unni KK: Osteosarcoma of bone and its important recognisable variables. Am J Surg Pathol 1:61–77, 1977.
20. Davidson JW, Chacha PB, James W: Multiple osteosarcomata: Report of a case. J Bone Joint Surg 47(B):537–541, 1965.
21. De Santos LA, Bernadino ME, Murray JA: Computed tomography in the evaluation of osteosarcoma: Experience with 25 cases. AJR 132:535–540, 1979.
22. Dorfman HD: Malignant transformation of benign bone lesions. Proc Natl Cancer Conf 7:901–913, 1977.
23. Dowdle JA Jr, Winter RB, Dehner LP: Post-radiation osteosarcoma of the cervical spine in childhood. J Bone Joint Surg 59A:969–971, 1977.
24. Edmonson JH, Green SJ, Ivins JC, et al: A controlled pilot study of high dose methotrexate as postsurgical adjuvant treatment for primary osteosarcoma. J Clin Oncol 2:152–156, 1986.
25. Eilber FR, Giuliano A, Eckardt J, et al: Adjuvant therapy for osteosarcoma. J Clin Oncol 5:21–26, 1987.
26. Enneking WF, Spanier SS, Goodman MA: A system for the surgical staging of musculo-skeletal sarcomas. Clin Orthop Rel Res 153:106–120, 1980.
27. Epstein LI, Bixler D, Bennett JE: An incidence of familial cancer, including 3 cases of osteogenic sarcoma. Cancer 25:889–891, 1970.
28. Kathie K, Grant KB, Hess JF: Osteogenic sarcoma of the neck (atlas). J Iowa Med Soc 61:728–730, 1971.
29. Fielding JW, Fietti VG Jr, Hughes JEO, Gabrielian JC: Primary osteogenic sarcoma of the cervical spine. A case report. J Bone Joint Surg 58(A):892–894, 1976.
30. French Bone Tumor Study Group: Age and dose of chemotherapy as major prognostic factors in a trial of adjuvant chemotherapy of osteosarcoma combining two alternating drug combinations and early prophylactic lung irradiation. Cancer 61:1304–1311, 1988.
31. Gandolfi A, Bordi C: Primary osteosarcoma of the cervical spine causing neurological symptoms. Surg Neurol 21:441–444, 1984.
32. Gehan EA, Sutow WW, Uribe-Botero G, et al: Osteosarcoma: The M.D. Anderson experience 1950–1974. *In* Terry WD, Wirdhorst D (eds): Immunotherapy of Cancer: Present Status of Trials in Man. New York, Raven Press, 1978, pp 271–282.
33. Guiliano AE, Feig S, Eilber FR: Changing metastatic patterns of osteosarcoma. Cancer 54:2160–2164, 1984.
34. Goldman AB, Becker MH, Braunstein P, et al: Bone scanning osteogenic sarcoma. Correlation with surgical pathology. Am J Roentgenol Rad Ther Nucl Med 124:83–90, 1975.
35. Goorin AM, Delorey MJ, Lack EE, et al: Prognostic significance of complete surgical resection of pulmonary metastases from osteogenic sarcoma: Analysis of 32 patients. J Clin Oncol 2:425–431, 1984.
36. Goorin AM, Delorey M, Gelber R, et al: The Dana Farber Cancer Institute/The Children's Hospital Adjuvant Chemotherapy trials for osteosarcoma; three sequential studies. Cancer Treat Symp 3:155–159, 1985.
37. Goorin AM, Abelson HT, Frei E III: Osteosarcoma: Fifteen years later. N Engl J Med 313:1637–1643, 1986.
38. Goorin AM, Perez-Atayde A, Gebhardt M, et al: Weekly high dose methotrexate and doxorubicin for osteosarcoma: The Dana Farber Cancer Institute Study III. J Clin Oncol 5:1178–1187, 1987.
39. Green JL, King SA, Wittes RE, Leyland Jones B: The role of methotrexate in osteosarcoma. J Natl Cancer Inst 80:626–656, 1988.
40. Halpern M, Freiberger RH: Arteriography as a diagnostic procedure in bone disease. Radiol Clin North Am 8:277–288, 1970.
41. Harrist TJ, Schiller AL, Trelstad RL, et al: Thorotrast associated sarcoma of bone: A case report and review of the literature. Cancer 44:2049–2058, 1979.
42. Hastrup J, Jensen TS: Osteogenic sarcoma arising in non-osteogenic fibroma of bone. Acta Pathol Microbiol Scand 63:493–499, 1965.
43. Henson J, Sutow WW, Elder K, et al: Adjuvant chemotherapy in non-metastatic sarcoma: A Southwest Oncology Group Study. Med Pediatr Oncol 8:343–352, 1981.
44. Hiddeman W, Roesner A, Worman B, et al: Tumor heterogeneity in osteosarcoma as identified by flow cytometry. Cancer 59:324–328, 1987.
45. Huang TL, Cohen NJ, Sahgal S, Tseng CH: Osteosarcoma complicating Paget's disease of the spine with neurologic complications. Clin Orthop Jun (141):260–265, 1979.
46. Huvos AG: Osteogenic sarcoma of bones and soft tissues in older patients: A clinico-pathologic analysis of 117 patients older than 60 years. Cancer 57:1442–1449, 1986.
47. Huvos AG: Bone Tumors: Diagnosis, Treatment and Prognosis. Philadelphia, WB Saunders Co., 1979, pp 47–93.
48. Huvos AG, Butler A, Bretsky SS: Osteogenic sarcoma associated with Paget's disease of bone: A clinico-pathologic study of 65 patients. Cancer 52:1489–1495, 1983.
49. Huvos AG, Woodard HQ, Cahan WG, et al: Post-radiation osteogenic sarcoma of the bone and soft tissue: A clinico-pathologic study of 66 patients. Cancer 55:1244–1255, 1985.
50. Huvos A, Butler A, Bretsky SS: Osteosarcoma in the American black. Cancer 52:1959–1965, 1983.
51. Jaffe N, Frei E III, Traggis D, Bishop Y: Adjuvant methotrexate and citrovorum-factor treatment of osteogenic sarcoma. N Engl J Med 291:994–997, 1974.
52. Jaffe N, Robertson R, Ayala A, et al: Comparison of intra-arterial cis-diamine-dicholoroplatinum II (CDP) with high dose methotrexate and citrovorum factor rescue in the treatment of primary osteosarcoma. J Clin Oncol 3:1101–1104, 1985.
53. Jaffe N, Smith HT, Abelson HT, Frei E III: Osteogenic sarcoma: Alterations in the pattern of pulmonary metastases with adjuvant chemotherapy. J Clin Oncol 1:251–254, 1983.
54. Jaffe N, Spears R, Eftekhari F, Robertson R, et al: Pathologic fractures in osteosarcoma: Impact of chemotherapy on primary tumor and survival. Cancer 59:701–709, 1987.
54a. Jaffe N: Effects of cumulative courses of intra-arterial cis-diammine dichloroplatin-II on the primary tumor in osteosarcoma. Cancer 63:63–67, 1989.

55. Jeffree GM, Price CHG, Sissions HA: The metastatic patterns of osteosarcoma. Br J Cancer 32:87–107, 1975.

56. Lang G, Kehr P, Paternotte H, Aeb J: Radiation induced sarcoma of the sixth cervical vertebra. Rev Chir Orthop 67:691–693, 1981.

57. Larsson SE, Lorentzon R: The incidence of malignant primary bone tumors in relation to age, sex and site. A site of osteogenic sarcoma, chondrosarcoma and Ewing's sarcoma diagnosed in Sweden from 1958–1968. J Bone Joint Surg 56:534–540, 1974.

58. Levine AM, Rosenberg SA: Alkaline phosphatase levels in osteosarcoma tissue are related to prognosis. Cancer 44:2291–2293, 1979.

59. Lievre JA, Darcy M, Pradat P, et al: Tumeur à cellules giantes du rachis rachis lumbaire, spondylectomie totale en deux temps. Rev Rhum Mal Osteoartic 35:125–130, 1968.

60. Link MP, Goorin AM, Miser AW, et al: The effect of adjuvant chemotherapy on relapse free survival in patients with osteosarcoma of the extremity. N Engl J Med 314:1600–1606, 1986.

61. Look AT, Douglass EC, Meyer WH: Clinical importance of near diploid tumor stem lines in patients with osteosarcoma of an extremity. N Engl J Med 318:1567–1572, 1988.

62. Malawer MM, Dunham WK: Skip metastases in osteosarcoma: Recent experiences. J Surg Oncol 22:236–245, 1983.

63. Marcove RC, Mike V, Hajek JV, et al: Osteogenic sarcoma under the age of 21 years. A review of 145 operative cases. J Bone Joint Surg 52(A):411–423, 1970.

64. Marsh HO, Choi CB: Primary osteogenic sarcoma of the cervical spine originally mistaken for benign osteoblastoma: A case report. J Bone Joint Surg 52A:1461–1471, 1970.

65. Marti C, Kroner T, Kemagen W, et al: High dose ifosfamide in advanced osteosarcoma. Cancer Treat Rep 69:115–117, 1985.

66. McLeod RA, Dahlin DC, Beaubout JW: The spectrum of osteoblastoma. Am J Roentgenol 126:321–325, 1976.

67. Merryweather R, Middlemiss JH, Sanerkin NG: Malignant transformation of osteoblastoma. J Bone Joint Surg 62(A):381–384, 1980.

68. Meyer WH, Schell MJ, Kumar PM, et al: Thoracotomy for pulmonary metastatic osteosarcoma: An analysis of prognostic indicators of survival. Cancer 59:374–379, 1987.

69. Miller CW, McLaughlin RE: Osteosarcoma in siblings. Report of two cases. J Bone Joint Surg 59(A):261–262, 1977.

70. Mirra JM, Bullough PG, Marcove RC: Malignant fibrous histiocytoma and osteosarcoma in association with bone infarcts. Report of four cases, two in caisson workers. J Bone Joint Surg 50(A):932–940, 1974.

71. Mnaymneh W, Brown M, Tejada F, Morrison G: Primary osteogenic sarcoma of the second cervical vertebra. Case report. J Bone Joint Surg 61(A):460–462, 1979.

72. Morse D Jr, Reed JO, Bernstein J: Sclerosing osteogenic sarcoma. Am J Roentgenol Rad Ther Nucl Med 88:491–495, 1962.

73. Nachman J, Simm SA, Dean L, et al: Disparate histologic responses in simultaneously resected primary and metastatic sarcoma following intravenous neoadjuvant chemotherapy. J Clin Oncol 5:1185–1190, 1987.

74. Ogihara Y, Sekiguchi K, Tsuruta T: Osteogenic sarcoma of the fourth thoracic vertebra. Long term survival by chemotherapy only. Cancer 53:2615–2618, 1984.

75. Parham DM, Pratt CB, Parvey LS, et al: Childhood multifocal osteosarcoma: Clinico-pathologic and radiologic correlates. Cancer 55:2653–2658, 1985.

76. Patel DV, Hammer RA, Levin B, Fisher MA: Primary osteogenic sarcoma of the spine. Skeletal Radiol 12:276–279, 1984.

77. Poppe E, Liverud K, Efskind J: Osteosarcoma. Acta Chir Scand 134:549–556, 1968.

78. Putnam JG Jr, Roth JA, Wesley MN, et al: Survival following aggressive resection of pulmonary metastases from osteogenic sarcoma: Analysis of prognostic factors. Ann Thorac Surg 36:516–523, 1983.

79. Roessner A, Metze K, Heymer B: Aggressive osteoblastoma. Pathol Res Pract 179:433–438, 1985.

80. Rosen G, Huvos AG, Mosende C, et al: Chemotherapy and thoracotomy for metastatic osteogenic sarcoma: A model for adjuvant chemotherapy and the rationale for the timing of thoracic surgery. Cancer 41:841–846, 1978.

81. Rosen G, Marcove RC, Caparros B, et al: Primary osteogenic sarcoma. The rationale for preoperative chemotherapy and delayed surgery. Cancer 43:2163–2177, 1979.

82. Rosen G, Caparros B, Huvos AG, et al: Preoperative chemotherapy for osteogenic sarcoma: Selection of postoperative adjuvant therapy based on the response of the primary tumor to preoperative chemotherapy. Cancer 49:1221–1230, 1982.

83. Rosen G, Marcove RC, Huvos AG, et al: Primary osteogenic sarcoma: Eight year experience with adjuvant chemotherapy. J Cancer Res Clin Oncol 106:55–67, 1983.

84. Rosen G, Nirenberg A, Caparros B, et al: Osteogenic sarcoma: Eighty percent, three year disease-free survival with combination chemotherapy (T7). Natl Cancer Inst Monogr 56:213–220, 1981.

85. Schajowicz F, Lamos C: Malignant osteoblastoma. J Bone Joint Surg 58B:202–211, 1976.

86. Scheiden R, Oberthaler W: Radiation induced osteosarcoma of the sacrum following radiation of an undiagnosed bone lesion. Acta Orthop Trauma Surg 102:128–130, 1983.

87. Shannon FT, Hopkins JS: Paget's sarcoma of the vertebral column. Acta Orthop Scand 48:385–390, 1977.

88. Shives TC, Dahlin DC, Sim FH, et al: Osteosarcoma of the spine. J Bone Joint Surg 68(A):660–668, 1986.

89. Simon MA: Causes of increased survival of patients with osteosarcoma: Current controversies. J Bone Joint Surg 66(A):306–309, 1984.

90. Sordillo PP, Hajdu SI, Magill GB, Golbey RB: Extraosseous osteogenic sarcoma: A review of 48 patients. Cancer 51:727–734, 1983.

91. Strander J, Adamson U, Aparisi T, et al: Adjuvant interferon treatment of human osteosarcoma. Recent Results Cancer Res 68:40–44, 1979.

92. Sundaram M, McGuire MH, Herbold DR: Magnetic resonance imaging of osteosarcoma. Skeletal Radiol 16:23–29, 1987.

93. Sundaresan N, DiGiacinto GV, Hughes JEO: Surgical approaches to primary and metastatic tumors of the spine. In Schmidek HH, Sweet WH (eds): Operative Neurosurgical Techniques: Indications, Methods, Results. Vol 2. Orlando, Grune & Stratton, 1988, pp 1525–1537.

94. Sundaresan N, Galicich JH, Lane JM, Scher H: Stabilisation of the spine involved by cancer. In Dunsker SB, Schmidek HH, Frymoyer J, Kahn A III (eds): The Unstable Spine. Orlando, Grune & Stratton, 1986, pp 249–274.

95. Sundaresan N, Galicich JH, Lane JM, et al: Treatment of neoplastic cord compression by vertebral body resection and stabilisation. J Neurosurg 63:676–684, 1985.

96. Sundaresan N, Huvos AG, Rosen G, Lane JM: Post radiation sarcoma of the spine following treatment of Hodgkin's disease. Spine 11:90–92, 1986.

97. Sundaresan N, Krol G, Hughes JEO: Malignant tumors of the spine. In Youmans JR (ed): Neurological Surgery. 3rd ed. Philadelphia, WB Saunders Co., 1990 (in press).

98. Sundaresan N, Rosen G, Huvos AG, Krol G: Combined modality treatment of osteosarcoma of the spine. Neurosurgery 23:714–719, 1988.

99. Taylor WF, Ivins JC, Dahlin DC, et al: Trends and variability in survival among patients with osteosarcoma: A seven year update. Mayo Clin Proc 60:91–104, 1985.

100. Telander RL, Pairolero PC, Pritchard DJ, et al: Resection of pulmonary metastatic osteogenic sarcoma in children. Surgery 84:335–341, 1978.

101. Thorpe WP, Reilly JJ, Rosenberg SA: Prognostic significance of alkaline phosphatase measurements in patients with osteogenic sarcoma receiving chemotherapy. Cancer 43:2178–2181, 1979.

102. Uribe-Botero G, Russell WD, Sutow WW: Primary osteosarcoma of bone. A clinico-pathologic investigation of 243 cases, with necropsy studies in 54. Am J Clin Pathol 67:427–435, 1977.

103. Voegeli E, Fuchs WA: Arteriography in bone tumors. Br J Radiol 49:407–415, 1976.

104. Weatherby RP, Dahlin DC, Ivins JC: Post-radiation sarcoma of bone: Review of 78 Mayo Clinic cases. Mayo Clinic Proc 56:294–306, 1981.
105. Weinfeld MS, Dudley HR Jr: Osteogenic sarcoma. A follow up study of the 94 cases observed at Massachusetts General Hospital from 1920 to 1980. J Bone Joint Surg 44(A):269–276, 1962.
106. Williams AH, Schwinn CP, Parker JW: The ultrastructure of osteosarcoma. A review of 20 cases. Cancer 37:1293–1301, 1976.
107. Winkler K, Beron G, Kotz R, et al: Neoadjuvant chemotherapy for osteosarcoma: Results of a cooperative German/Austrian study. J Clin Oncol 2:617–624, 1984.
108. Yaghmai I: Angiographic features of osteosarcoma. Am J Roentgenol Rad Ther Nucl Med 129:1073–1081, 1977.
109. Young JL, Percy CL, Asire AJ: National Cancer Institute Monograph No 57—Surveillance, Epidemiology, End Results 1973–1977 Cancer Mortality & Statistics. Bethesda, 1981.

15 BENIGN CARTILAGE TUMORS OF THE SPINE

DALE B. GLASSER, FRANK P. CAMMISA, JR.,
and JOSEPH M. LANE

Benign cartilage tumors rarely occur in the spine. Both osteochondroma and enchondroma are thought to be derived from cartilaginous rests left behind by the advancing epiphyseal or apophyseal growth plate. This may account for the rarity of osteochondromas and enchondromas of the spine (< 1 per cent of the approximately 800 combined cases at the Hospital for Special Surgery and Memorial Sloan-Kettering Cancer Center).

OSTEOCHONDROMA

A solitary osteochondroma is a noninherited malformation, not a true neoplasm. It consists of a hyalin cartilage–capped bony growth on either a broad base or a stalk first appearing in relationship to the epiphyseal growth plate.[2, 3] Most cases are painless and become noted during the first two decades of life. Benign lesions are often elongated and point toward the metaphysis of the involved bone. They usually cease growth within one to three years of closure of the adjacent growth plate, and their cartilaginous caps become very thin over the years. Surgical intervention is indicated for suspected malignant transformation (see below), pain from pressure on adjacent tissues (e.g., nerves), or dysfunction from tumor entrapment of nerves or vessels. Surgical resection should include the perichondral soft tissue covering (perichondrium) and all cartilage extending to normal cortical bone.

The diagnostic histologic findings include a hyalin cartilage cap covered by a fibrous membrane (perichondrium) and an underlying bony stalk directly connected to the cortex of the parent bone. There is *no cortex between the lesion and the parent bone,* resulting in direct continuity of the marrow space of the lesion and the parent bone. The degree of active endochondral ossification beneath the cartilage cap is related to age; older lesions have less activity. Therefore, endochondral ossification may be very active in teenagers, and the lesions should not be confused

Supported by the Greenwall Foundation

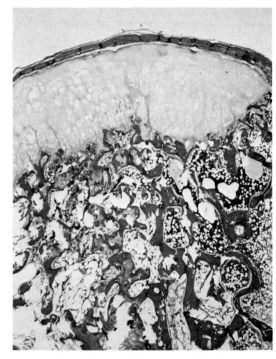

FIGURE 15–1. Osteochondroma with a prominent hyalin cartilage cap covered by a fibrous perichondrium. Endochondral ossification is occurring deep to the cartilage cap (H & E ×16).

with more aggressive forms of cartilage or bone-forming lesions[4] (Fig. 15–1).

Hereditary multiple osteochondromatosis is an autosomal dominant disorder involving the development of multiple osteochondromas at the ends of enchondrally formed bones.[1–3] This entity is associated with bony modeling abnormalities, shortening of limbs, and misalignment. Rarely a patient may develop malignant degeneration of an osteochondroma. Vertebral involvement is rare even in widespread multiple osteochondromatosis. Wide surgical excision is the treatment for troublesome lesions as indicated above.

ENCHONDROMA

A solitary enchondroma is a benign intramedullary tumor composed of hyalin cartilage arising from

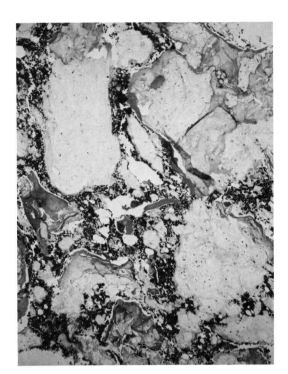

FIGURE 15–2. An enchondroma with well-formed hyaline cartilage nodules rimmed by bone (H & E ×60).

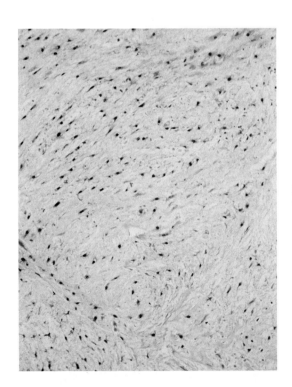

FIGURE 15–3. An enchondroma with a focus of myxoid cartilage in enchondromatosis (H & E ×150).

cartilaginous growth rests, usually discovered from the first to the sixth decades.[1-3] It most commonly occurs in the short tubular bones of the hands and feet and only rarely in the vertebral column (less than 1 per cent of the 289 combined cases at the Hospital for Special Surgery and Memorial Sloan-Kettering Cancer Center). Benign tumors usually do not require treatment. Those lesions suspected of malignant degeneration need biopsy and appropriate treatment (see below). Multiple enchondromatosis and Maffucci's syndrome (multiple enchondromatosis with soft tissue hemangiomas) rarely affect the spine but can result in progressive and debilitating deformity. Up to 50 per cent of patients with these conditions may develop chondrosarcoma. Various surgical methods have been employed in the treatment of multiple enchondromatoses. These have included simple curettage, curettage with autologous/homologous bone grafting, and en bloc excision with reconstruction. Treatment of sarcomatous degeneration is discussed in Chapter 16.

Histologically, an enchondroma is composed of hyalin cartilage nodules rimmed by bone (lamellar or woven) with little or no chondrocyte atypia. There may be some foci of endochondral ossification, but this should not be confused with a malignant bone-forming tumor. Occasionally, myxoid cartilage may be seen in those cases of enchondromatosis of Maffucci's syndrome[4] (Figs. 15–2 and 15–3).

REFERENCES

1. Aprin H: Chondrosarcoma in children and adolescents. Clin Orthop 166:226, 1982.
2. Huvos AG: Bone Tumors: Diagnosis, Treatment and Prognosis. Philadelphia, WB Saunders Co., 1979, pp 206–237.
3. Lane JM, Boland PJ: Tumors of bone and cartilage. *In* Goldsmith HS (ed): Practice of Surgery. Philadelphia, Harper and Row, 1983, pp 1–26.
4. Schiller AL: Diagnosis of borderline cartilage lesions of bone. Semin Diagn Pathol 2:42–62, 1985.

CHONDROSARCOMA OF THE SPINE:

Memorial Sloan-Kettering Cancer Center Experience

FRANK P. CAMMISA, JR., DALE B. GLASSER,
and JOSEPH M. LANE

INTRODUCTION

Chondrosarcoma is a malignant tumor in which the malignant chondrocytes form cartilage without bone.[30] They may arise de novo as a primary malignancy or, rarer still, may occur secondary to a preexisting benign cartilaginous tumor (e.g., enchondroma, osteochondroma)[7, 10, 11, 21] or subsequent to radiation therapy.[19, 30] Although they are not common tumors, they are second only to osteosarcoma in frequency of primary sarcomas of bone.

As with other primary tumors of bone, males are at somewhat higher risk than females. The mean age at presentation is approximately 40 years, with patients ranging from the first to the ninth decades of life.[2, 30] The most common sites are the pelvis, femur, humerus, and scapula. Chondrosarcoma is very rare in the spine, as are most other primary tumors. Fewer than 4 per cent of lesions arise in the spine or sacrum.[30]

An aberration in carbohydrate metabolism has been noted in up to 75 per cent of patients, which may take the form of normal blood glucose levels in the face of an abnormal glucose tolerance curve and high insulin levels.[41] Increased glycolysis may be noted in tumor cells. Insulin and insulin growth factor (IGF) are documented stimulators of cartilage metabolism. High binding rates of IGF have been demonstrated by Tripell.[64] The contribution of insulin and IGF to the etiology of chondrosarcoma is unknown.

Histologically, chondrosarcomas may be divided into three grades of increasing virulence. Low grade, or Grade I, lesions have mild cellular atypia, some double nuclei, and abundant hyalin matrix. These may be difficult to differentiate solely on histologic grounds from an actively growing enchondroma. Radiographic and clinical criteria (see below) may help in this regard. Grade 2 lesions have significant atypia and are more densely cellular, with multiple nuclei in some cells, multiple cells per lacuna, and foci of necrosis. Grade 3 lesions display marked atypia, mitotic figures, multinucleate cells, very little matrix, and areas of necrosis. The presence of myxoid cartilage matrix is an ominous finding since these lesions tend to be more aggressive. *All* chondrosarcomas invade between existing bony structures, whereas enchondromas do not. This last point is often useful in distinguishing between a Grade 1 (low grade) chondrosarcoma and an enchondroma. Even in low grade chondrosarcoma, the cartilage lobules may become peripherally calcified and undergo endochondral ossification. This is less apt to happen in higher grade lesions[57] (Figs. 16–1, 16–2, and 16–3).

DNA analysis using flow cytometry is a recent technique that may help to provide additional prognostic information. Kreicbergs[33, 34] has determined that lesions with a normal DNA content are associated with a significantly higher survival rate than tumors displaying aneuploidy (abnormally increased nuclear DNA content). Polyploidy (increased chromosome number) is associated with a poor prognosis. Patients with diploid tumors had a 10-year survival probability of 81 per cent compared with 29 per cent for those with hyperploid lesions. Unfortunately, these techniques have thus far been unable to shed much additional light on the most difficult problem of differentiating benign lesions from borderline or low grade malignancies. Mankin and coworkers have attempted to define malignancy by specific matrix alterations.[37, 38] Although high water content tends to be identified in malignant tumors, the overlap with benign tumor matrix analysis precludes unequivocal

Supported by the Greenwall Foundation.

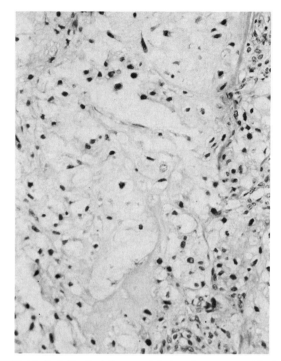

FIGURE 16–1. A Grade 1 (low grade) chondrosarcoma with abundant hyalin matrix, cellular atypia, and mild pleomorphism. The nuclei have nucleoli, and some lacunae are empty, indicating necrotic foci (H & E ×215).

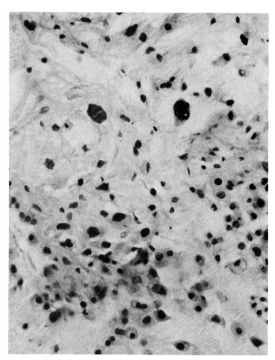

FIGURE 16–3. A Grade III chondrosarcoma with little cartilage matrix, marked pleomorphism, binucleate cells, and necrotic foci. Giant tumor cells are easily seen (H & E ×280).

designation of malignancy solely in terms of matrix composition, particularly in borderline lesions.

RADIOGRAPHIC CHARACTERISTICS

Chondrosarcomas arising centrally within the bone produce large areas of radiolucency. The lobular growth of cartilage results in the appearance of trabeculation and multilocular medullary bone destruction. Scalloping of the endosteal surface may be seen for the same reason. Cortical destruction occurs only later. There are often foci of spotty calcification. Peripheral chondrosarcomas produce large soft tissue masses and variable amounts of destruction of

the underlying bone. There are often calcified shadows with radiating spicules arranged at right angles to the cortex. In both types of chondrosarcoma heavy calcification is not usual. Rapid enlargement, decreasing intralesional calcifications, and aggressive bone/tumor borders favor chondrosarcoma over benign chondromas.

Rosenthal has attempted to determine features on radiographs and computed tomography (CT) scans which are useful in predicting high versus low grade chondrosarcomas. The most useful features include the characteristics of the tumor/bone margin on radiograph, the morphology of the calcification on both modalities, the pattern of the soft tissue extent on CT scan, and the presence of necrosis on CT scan.[53] Briefly, the more calcification and the more sharply defined bone bodies with no necrotic foci, the more low grade the tumor.

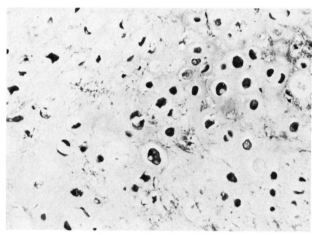

FIGURE 16–2. A Grade II chondrosarcoma with marked pleomorphism but with abundant cartilage matrix. There is chondrocyte necrosis as well (H & E ×200).

CLINICAL PRESENTATION

The most common presenting symptom is pain, often worse at night and when reclining. Frequently there has been a long history of pain, with a recent exacerbation. Patients in our series and in others have been mistakenly thought to have a herniated disc and have been subjected to laminectomy.[6, 58] Almost 4 per cent of 1000 patients at the Mayo Clinic with vertebral bone tumors were originally diagnosed as having protruded disc.[58] They emphasize that intractable, progressive pain that is exacerbated in the supine position favors the diagnosis of a neoplasm. A mass may be present in posteriorly based lesions or in the cervical spine. Neurologic involve-

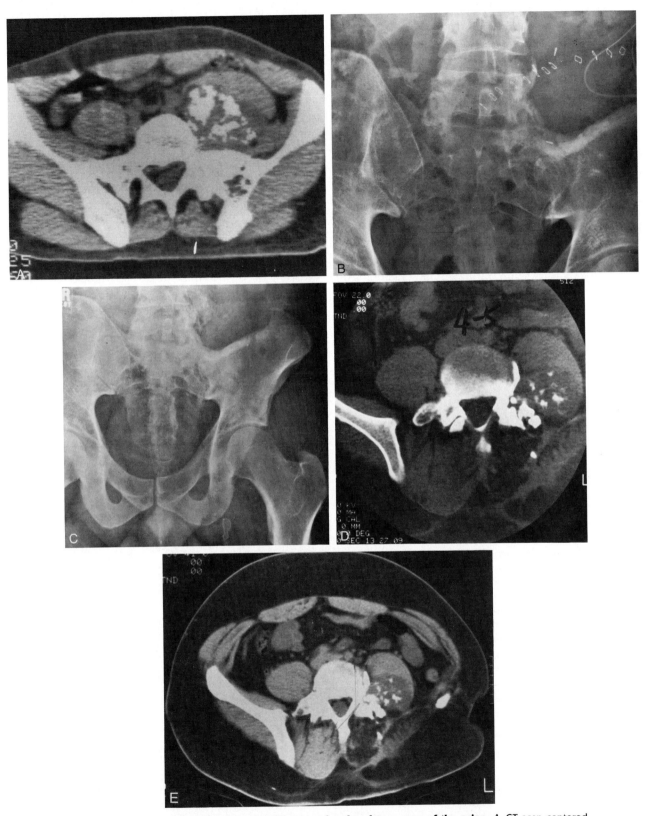

FIGURE 16–4. Multiple radiographs and CT scans of a chondrosarcoma of the spine. *A,* CT scan centered on S1 demonstrates an intermediate grade chondrosarcoma. There are calcifications extending anterior to the sacral ala. *B,* Patient was treated with a local excision of the sacral ala and part of the ilium (anteroposterior lumbosacral spine). *C,* Several years later a recurrence at the L4-5 area is identified by laterally placed calcifications. *D* and *E,* Two CT cuts through L4-5 demonstrate the recurrent calcification. Following a second resection, the patient has remained without evidence of disease for three years.

ment including sciatica and radiculopathy may bring the patient to medical attention.

Patients with known preexisting benign conditions such as osteochondromatosis or Ollier's disease (multiple enchondromatosis) should be carefully evaluated if they complain of back pain. In a recent review of our own series of chondrosarcomas, 14 consecutive patients with lesions of the spine or sacrum were studied.[6] Four lesions arose in preexisting benign cartilaginous tumors. Four lesions were located in the cervical spine, three in the lumbar spine, six in the sacrum, and one in the coccyx. The overall survival (disease-free at 60 months) was 67 per cent.

STAGING AND PREOPERATIVE EVALUATION

Preoperative studies for the extent of local disease should begin with radiographs of the axial spine in the anteroposterior, lateral, and oblique projections.[35, 36] Conventional tomography may be used to delineate extent of tumor; however, we prefer computerized tomography with reformatted sagittal views.[44] Myelography, both conventional and in conjunction with CT scan, is useful to determine the presence of extradural compression by tumor. Bone scan may help to define the extent of local disease as well as to determine the presence of multifocal or metastatic disease.[27, 28, 58] Magnetic resonance imaging (MRI) may prove to be the single best modality,[61] although we have had limited experience with this modality in these rare lesions. It can clearly identify in axial, sagittal, and coronal planes the soft tissue extent of the lesion, marrow involvement, and spinal canal impingement. Bony architecture is less easily studied.

The lung is the most common site of metastasis of chondrosarcoma. Either CT scan or conventional tomography may be used to look for evidence of metastatic disease. At Memorial Hospital, we prefer tomography for sarcomas of bone, which yields fewer false-positive results. All tumors are staged according to the method of the Musculoskeletal Tumor Society, based on histologic grade, anatomic (compartmental) extent, and distant spread.[15] At Memorial Hospital, the majority (79 per cent) of chondrosarcomas of the spine and sacrum were Stage IB (low grade, extracompartmental), with the remainder (21 per cent) Stage IIB (high grade, extracompartmental).[6]

SURGICAL TREATMENT

Biopsy techniques should follow the same principles as for other tumor surgery. The incision must be placed so that it may be entirely excised en bloc with the specimen at definitive surgery. For suspected malignant lesions, incisional biopsy is preferable to excisional biopsy. The soft tissue extent of the lesion may be sampled, and a frozen section should be performed to determine the adequacy of tissue to avoid having to biopsy bone. Needle biopsies provide

extremely limited tissue for analysis. Since it is difficult to differentiate malignant from benign cartilage tumors with small samples of material, percutaneous biopsy has been less successful with cartilage tumors than with other lesions.

Benign tumors of the spine require surgical treatment if they are increasing in size, causing intractable pain, neurologic deficit, or instability. Activity of the lesion (latent, active, or aggressive) as well as its location will determine the necessary procedure. Latent lesions (no growth) usually do not require treatment. However, intrapelvic osteochondromas of large size (> 4 cm) that grow after age 20 or contain a cartilaginous cap of greater than 0.5 cm after age 25 should be excised outside the perichondral soft tissue lining cap. For an active intraosseous benign cartilaginous lesion that is not in an area likely to cause neurologic or mechanical deficit, thorough curettage to normal bone may suffice. Aggressive cartilaginous lesions require wide excision. Intralesional resections may be augmented by adjuvant cryosurgery, but recurrence rates may be higher than with wide excision.

Malignant cartilaginous tumors of the spine require an aggressive approach to surgical treatment.[8, 16, 22, 25, 29, 39, 43, 59, 60] Histologic grade of lesion is the most significant determinant of local recurrence. Many surgeons perform less aggressive surgical procedure for low grade tumors; however, recurrence of chondrosarcoma may have a more aggressive histologic appearance, and the best hope for cure is at the initial procedure. The anatomy of the spine and sacrum does not lend itself to the classic principles of musculoskeletal tumor surgery. Radical resection (entire compartment) is not possible and not desired. Optimal treatment is wide excision, although the result is often a marginal or intralesional procedure owing to tumor location. Even when wide excision is possible, intraoperative contamination often occurs. Local adjuvant techniques such as cryosurgery may be useful to extend the margin and prevent or delay recurrence in cases in which wide excision is not possible.

For tumors arising in the posterior arch, the excision is dictated by the location and size of the tumor. If the facet joints are sacrificed, stabilization is required. This may consist of lateral fusion between the transverse processes utilizing autogenous and/or allogeneic bone in combination with internal fixation. Method of fixation should be individualized and is dependent upon the resection as well as the surgeon's facility with the techniques. Currently, various centers have used pedicle screw/plates, rods with sublaminar wiring, and CD instrumentation.

Anteriorly based tumors can be treated with resection of the entire involved vertebral segment(s). Stabilization is always required and consists of interbody fusion utilizing autogenous fibula, tricortical iliac, or rib strut grafts. Allograft diaphyseal sections may be utilized.

Some lesions require combined anteroposterior approaches. This may be performed in a one- or two-stage procedure, and again one must utilize appropriate stabilization techniques.

Postoperative management including immobilization and rehabilitation should be individualized according to the surgical procedure and fixation techniques used.

Cryosurgery has been reported to be useful in preventing local recurrence in chondrosarcomas.[42] A recent review of chondrosarcoma of the spine and sacrum reported no local recurrences when cryosurgery was added to intralesional or marginal procedures, as compared with 43 per cent recurrence rate when cryosurgery was not used (p < 0.05).[6] The technique must be precise owing to the proximity of vital neurologic structures. Protection of the dural sac and nerve roots may be provided by a barrier of Gelfoam. Liquid nitrogen is applied in a controlled manner using either a probe or funnel. Three complete freeze-thaw cycles are recommended for adequate tumor kill. The use of cryosurgery did not seem to have a detrimental effect on wound healing in our experience.

Several investigators have looked at the efficacy of other adjuvant treatments in experimental models.[13, 17, 20, 45, 64] Systemic chemotherapy and radiation therapy have not proven to be of great benefit in human chondrosarcoma,[8, 16, 22, 24, 32, 47] and therefore the patient's best hope lies in complete surgical extirpation.

MALIGNANT SUBGROUPS

Several subgroups of chondrosarcoma have been described recently, including clear cell, mesenchymal, and dedifferentiated chondrosarcoma. Although at Memorial Hospital we have not encountered these rare tumors in the vertebral column, they are discussed for completeness.

Clear cell chondrosarcomas superficially resemble chondroblastoma and are particularly noted for a high local recurrence rate and frequent metastases.[66] Since they have a high predilection for secondary ossification centers and demonstrate many similar histologic characteristics of chondroblastoma, they may be a malignant form of chondroblastoma. *Mesenchymal chondrosarcoma* is a small cell sarcoma with cartilaginous elements.[3, 31] Thirty per cent are extraosseous and only rarely present in the spine. The limited number of cases precludes firm therapeutic recommendations, but these tumors have responded to a Ewing's sarcoma chemotherapeutic program. Dedifferentiated chondrosarcomas arise by transformation of low grade chondrosarcoma to high grade spindle cell tumors.[12, 49] The long-term prognosis is poor. Wide excision and adjuvant chemotherapy may prove to be effective in some.

REFERENCES

1. Alho A, Connor JF, Mankin HJ, et al: Assessment of malignancy of cartilage tumors using flow cytometry. J Bone Joint Surg 65A:779, 1982.
2. Aprin H: Chondrosarcoma in children and adolescents. Clin Orthop 166:226, 1982.
3. Bertoni F: Mesenchymal chondrosarcoma of bone and soft tissues. Cancer 52:533, 1983.
4. Buckwalter JA: The structure of human chondrosarcoma proteoglycans. J Bone Joint Surg 65A:958, 1983.
5. Camins MB, Duncan AW, Smith J, Marcove RC: Chondrosarcoma of the spine. Spine 3:202–209, 1978.
6. Cammisa F, Glasser D, Lane J, et al: Chondrosarcoma of the spine and sacrum. Orthop Trans 11:578, 1987.
7. Campanacci M: Malignant degeneration in fibrous dysplasia. Ital J Orthop Traumatol 5:373, 1979.
8. Campanacci M, Guernelli N, Loenessa D: Chondrosarcoma: A study of 133 cases, 80 with long-term follow-up. Ital J Orthop Traumatol 1:387, 1975.
9. Chan HSL, Turner-Gomes SO, Chuang SH, et al: A rare cause of spinal cord compression in childhood from intraspinal mesenchymal chondrosarcoma. A report of two cases and review of the literature. Neuroradiology 26:323, 1984.
10. Coley BL, Higinbotham NL: Secondary chondrosarcoma. Ann Surg 139:547, 1954.
11. Cowan WK: Malignant change and multiple metastases in Ollier's disease. J Clin Pathol 18:650, 1965.
12. Dahlin DC, Beabout JW: Dedifferentiation of low-grade chondrosarcomas. Cancer 28:461, 1971.
13. Eisenbarth GC, Wellman DK, Lebowitz HE: Prostaglandin A, inhibition of chondrosarcoma growth. Biochem Biophys Res Commun 60:1302, 1974.
14. Enneking WF, Dunham WK: Resection and reconstruction for primary neoplasm involving the innominate bone. J Bone Joint Surg 60A:731, 1978.
15. Enneking WF, Spanier SS, Soodman M: Current concepts review: Surgical staging of musculoskeletal sarcoma. J Bone Joint Surg 62A:1027, 1980.
16. Eriksson, AI, Schiller A, Mankin JH: The management of chondrosarcoma of bone. Clin Orthop 153:44, 1980.
17. Ettlin R: HIstologic changes during regression induced by retinoic acid in a transplantable rat chondrosarcoma. Virchows Arch [Pathol Anat] 396:1, 1982.
18. Evans HL, Ayala AG, Romsdahl MM: Prognostic factors in chondrosarcoma of bone. A clinicopathologic analysis with emphasis on histologic grading. Cancer 40:818, 1977.
19. Fitzwater JE, Cabaud HE, Farr GH: Irradiation-induced chondrosarcoma. J Bone Joint Surg 58A:1037, 1976.
20. Foley TP Jr: Demonstration of receptors for insulin and insulin-like growth factors on swarm rat chondrosarcoma chondrocytes. Evidence that insulin stimulates proteoglycan synthesis through the insulin receptor. J Biol Chem 257:663, 1982.
21. Garrison RC, Unni KK, McLeod RA, et al: Chondrosarcoma arising in osteochondroma. Cancer 49:1890, 1982.
22. Gitelis S, Bertoni F, Picci P, Campanacci M: Chondrosarcoma of bone. The experience at the Istituto Ortopedico Rizzoli. J Bone Joint Surg 63A:1248, 1981.
23. Harsh GR, Wilson CB: Central nervous system mesenchymal chondrosarcoma. J Neurosurg 61:375, 1984.
24. Harwood AR: Radiotherapy of chondrosarcoma of bone. Cancer 45:2769, 1980.
25. Henderson ED, Dahlin DC: Chondrosarcoma of bone: A study of 288 cases. J Bone Joint Surg 45A:1450, 1963.
26. Hirsh LF, Thanki A, Spector HB: Primary spinal chondrosarcoma with eighteen-year follow-up: Case report and literature review. Neurosurgery14:6, 1984.
27. Hudson TM: Radionuclide bone scanning of medullary chondrosarcoma. AJR 139:1071, 1982.
28. Hudson TM: Scintigraphy of benign exostoses and exostotic chondrosarcoma. AJR 140:581, 1983.
29. Huth JF, Dawson EG, Eilber FR: Abdominosacral resection for malignant tumors of the sacrum. Am J Surg 148:157, 1984.
30. Huvos AG: Bone Tumors: Diagnosis, Treatment and Prognosis. Philadelphia, WB Saunders Co., 1979, pp 206–237.
31. Huvos AG: Mesenchymal chondrosarcoma: A clinicopathologic analysis of 35 patients with emphasis on treatment. Cancer 51:1230, 1983.
32. Kim RY: High energy irradiation in the management of chondrosarcoma. South Med J 76:729, 1983.
33. Kreicbergs A, Boquist L, Borssen B, Larsson S: Prognostic factors in chondrosarcoma. A comparative study of cellular

DNA content and clinicopathologic features. Cancer 50:577, 1982.

34. Kreicbergs A, Soderberg G, Zetterberg A: The prognostic significance of nuclear DNA content in chondrosarcoma. Anal Quant Cytol 4:271, 1980.

35. Lane JM: Malignant bone tumors. *In* Alfonson AE, Gardner B (eds): The Practice of Cancer Surgery. New York, Appleton-Century-Crofts, 1982, pp 307–324.

36. Lane JM, Boland PJ: Tumors of bone and cartilage. *In* Goldsmith HS (ed): Practice of Surgery. Philadelphia, Harper and Row, 1983, pp 1–26.

37. Mankin HJ, Cantley KP, Lippiello L, et al: The biology of human chondrosarcoma. I. Description of the cases, grading, and biochemical analyses. J Bone Joint Surg 62A:160, 1980.

38. Mankin HJ, Cantley KP, Schiller AL, Lipiello L: The biology of human chondrosarcoma. II. Variation in chemical composition among types and subtypes of benign and malignant cartilage tumors. J Bone Joint Surg 62A:176, 1980.

39. Marcove RC: Chondrosarcoma: Diagnosis and treatment. Orthop Clin North Am 8:811, 1977.

40. Marcove RC, Mike V, Hutter RVP: Chondrosarcoma of the pelvis and upper end of the femur. An analysis of factors influencing survival time in 113 cass. J Bone Joint Surg 54A:561, 1972.

41. Marcove RC, Shaji H, Arlen M: Altered carbohydrate metabolism in cartilaginous tumors. Contemp Surg 5:53, 1974.

42. Marcove RC, Stovell PB, Huvos AG, Bullough PG: The use of cryosurgery in the treatment of low and medium grade chondrosarcoma. Clin Orthop 122:147, 1977.

43. Martin NS, Williamson J: The role of surgery in the treatment of malignant tumours of the spine. J Bone Joint Surg 52B:227, 1970.

44. Mayes GB: Computed tomography of chondrosarcoma. Comput Tomogr 5:345, 1981.

45. McCumbee WD: Hormonal and metabolic regulation of human chondrosarcoma in vitro. Cancer Res 43:513, 1983.

46. McFarland GB Jr, McKinley LM, Reed RJ: Dedifferentiation of low grade chondrosarcoma. Clin Orthop 122:157, 1977.

47. McNaney D: Fifteen year radiotherapy experience with chondrosarcoma of bone. Int J Radiol Oncol Biol Phys 8:187, 1982.

48. Meachim G: Editorials and annotations: Histological grading of chondrosarcomata. J Bone Joint Surg 61B:393, 1979.

49. Miller DR: A comparison of collagen synthesis by different categories of human chondrosarcoma in organ culture. Clin Orthop 168:252, 1982.

50. Nilsonne U: Function after pelvic tumor resection involving the acetabular ring. Int Orthop 6:27, 1982.

51. Pritchard DJ, Lunke RJ, Taylor WF, et al: Chondrosarcoma: A clinicopathologic and statistical analysis. Cancer 45:149, 1980.

52. Rengachary SS, Kepes JJ: Spinal epidural metastatic "mesenchymal" chondrosarcoma. J Neurosurg 30:71, 1969.

53. Rosenthal D, Schiller AL, Mankin HJ: Chondrosarcoma: Correlation of radiological and histological grade. Radiology 150:21, 1984.

54. Sanerkin NG: The diagnosis and grading of chondrosarcoma of bone. A combined cytologic and histological approach. Cancer 45:582, 1980.

55. Sanerkin NG, Gallagher P: A review of the behavior of chondrosarcoma of bone. J Bone Joint Surg 61B:395, 1979.

56. Schajowicz F: Juxtacortical chondrosarcoma. J Bone Joint Surg 59B:473, 1977.

57. Sim FH, Dahlin DC, Stauffer RN, Laws ER: Primary bone tumors simulating lumbar disc syndrome. Spine 2:65, 1977.

58. Smith FW, Nandi SC, Mills K: Spinal chondrosarcoma demonstrated by Tc-99m-MDP bone scan. Clin Nucl Med 7:111, 1982.

59. Smith WS, Simon MA: Segmental resection for chondrosarcoma. J Bone Joint Surg 57A:1097, 1975.

60. Stener B: Total spondylectomy in chondrosarcoma arising from the seventh thoracic vertebra. J Bone Joint Surg 53B:288, 1971.

61. Sundaram M, McGuire MH, Herbold DR, et al: Magnetic resonance imaging in planning limb-salvage surgery for primary malignant tumors of bone. J Bone Joint Surg 68A:809, 1986.

62. Swelt MB, Thonar EJ, Immelman AR: Glycosaminoglycans and proteoglycans of human chondrosarcoma. Biochem Biophys Acta 437:71, 1976.

63. Theim R: Sensitivity of cultured human osteosarcoma and chondrosarcoma cells to retinoic acid. Cancer Res 42:4771, 1982.

64. Trippel S: Personal communication, 1989.

65. Unni KK, Dahlin DC, Beabout JW: Chondrosarcoma: Clearcell variant. A report of 16 cases. J Bone Joint Surg 58A:676, 1976.

66. Wilkes LL, Cannon CL, Ham OE: Malignant tumors of the pelvic girdle mimicking the herniated disk syndrome. Clin Orthop 138:217, 1979.

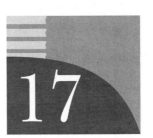

CHONDROSARCOMA OF THE SPINE:

Mayo Clinic Experience

FRANKLIN H. SIM, FRANK J. FRASSICA,
LESTER E. WOLD, and RICHARD A. McLEOD

INTRODUCTION

Chondrosarcoma is a malignant tumor that produces hyaline cartilage. Of all primary malignant tumors of bone, it is third in frequency, after multiple myeloma and osteosarcoma, and accounts for approximately 10 per cent of all bone sarcomas. In the United States, approximately 380 new cases of chondrosarcoma are reported each year.

In a Mayo Clinic series,[5] 85 per cent of 634 chondrosarcomas were primary and 15 per cent were secondary to malignant degeneration of a preexisting benign cartilage lesion. In the latter group, referred to as secondary chondrosarcoma, the original lesion is usually an osteochondroma (Fig. 17–1), particularly in patients with multiple familial osteochondromatosis. Less often, the original lesion is an enchondroma. Because of their distinctive histologic appearances and different biologic behaviors, chondrosarcomas have several different variants.

The ages of patients with chondrosarcoma range from 3 to 80 years, with a mean of 45 years in most studies. The peak incidence is in the fifth and sixth decades. In fact, excluding myeloma, chondrosarcoma is the most frequent primary malignant tumor of bone affecting middle-age patients. Patients with chondrosarcoma of the spinal column are reportedly younger than patients with chondrosarcoma of other sites. Males are more frequently affected, with ratios ranging from 1.5:1 to 2:1.

INCIDENCE OF VERTEBRAL CHONDROSARCOMA

Although more than three fourths of the chondrosarcomas in the Mayo Clinic series occurred in the trunk and proximal limb girdles, the lesions occasionally involved the spinal column—occurring at this site in 55 of the 634 cases. Most authors have reported a uniform distribution in the vertebral column, but others have noted a higher incidence in the thoracic spine. Among the 55 spinal chondrosarcomas in the Mayo Clinic series, 9 involved the cervical spine, 18 the thoracic spine, and 12 the lumbar spine. In addition, there were 16 sacral lesions.

Of the 265 chondrosarcomas reported from Memorial Hospital,[16] 27 involved the vertebrae and 3 the sacrum. In Camins and associates'[3] report of 19 spinal chondrosarcomas, there were six in the cervical spine, five in the thoracic spine, three in the lumbar spine, and five in the sacrum. Törmä[32] noted 11 spinal lesions among 250 chondrosarcomas: four cervical, four thoracic, one lumbar, and two sacral. In the series of 81 chondrosarcomas reported by Evans and colleagues,[9] there were five vertebral lesions, one of which was located in the sacrum. Eriksson and coworkers[8] and Stener[28] each reported four vertebral chondrosarcomas. In a series of 133 cases of chondrosarcoma at the Rizzoli Institute, Campanacci and associates[4] noted three of spinal involvement: one in the thoracic spine, one in the lumbar spine, and one in the sacrum.

CLINICAL FEATURES

The signs and symptoms depend on the location of the chondrosarcoma. They tend to be insidious in onset. In lesions of the extremity, the most frequent symptom is pain, although there may be a palpable mass, swelling, tenderness, or pathologic fracture. In the spinal column, the pain is usually localized at the initial presentation. Movement of the spinal column may increase the pain, but it becomes relentless, even at rest. Radicular pain usually follows and is more prominent when the tumor is in the cervical or lumbosacral region. When present in these regions, the radicular pain is frequently unilateral. Thoracic radicular pain is often bilateral and bandlike. Frequently, the pain is worse at night.

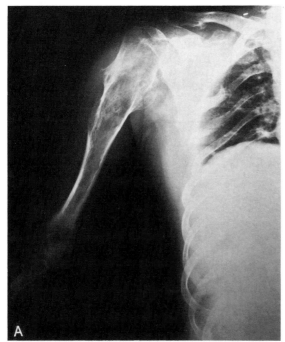

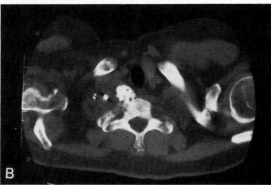

FIGURE 17–1. Chondrosarcoma in cervical spine of patient with multiple familial osteochondromatosis. *A,* Anteroposterior radiograph of humerus demonstrating extensive involvement with exostoses. *B,* CT scan of lower cervical spine showing degeneration of an exostosis into a chondrosarcoma with a soft tissue mass.

With further progression of the tumor, weakness gradually ensues; the pattern of weakness depends on the location of the tumor. Compression of the spinal cord produces upper motor neuron weakness with spasticity, increased reflexes, and Babinski responses. Because the spinal cord ends at L1–L2, cord compression can occur only with epidural lesions above L1. Lesions below that level do not compress the spinal cord but do compress the nerve roots of the cauda equina. Nerve root compression produces lower motor neuron weakness with flaccid tone and decreased or absent muscle stretch reflexes but does not produce Babinski responses.

Sensory disturbances also may be the result of spinal cord or nerve root involvement. Radicular involvement produces numbness, paresthesia, or dysesthesia in a dermatomal pattern, indicating the level of the lesion. Arm symptoms occur with cervical lesions, trunk symptoms with thoracic lesions, leg symptoms with lumbar lesions, and saddle-area symptoms with sacral lesions.

Autonomic impairment is the initial complaint of only a small percentage of patients, although it often can be detected at the time of diagnosis. Bowel dysfunction usually presents as obstipation or constipation. Stool incontinence is usually seen only in patients with advanced disease. Orthostatic hypotension, impotence, and decreased sweating are other signs of autonomic impairment.

A thorough general examination of a patient with back pain or neurologic dysfunction who is suspected of having a chondrosarcoma is important. Examination of the spinal column generally reveals percussion tenderness over the involved vertebrae. The range of motion of the spinal column may be decreased owing to pain and spasm of the paravertebral muscles. Straight leg raising or the femoral stretch test may exacerbate the pain. Extension of the cervical or lumbar spinal column may reproduce radicular pain. The neurologic findings in patients with spinal chondrosarcoma depend on the site as well as the extent of the lesion. As noted, cord compression occurs when the lesion is located above L1. Cord compression produces not only weakness with increased muscle stretch reflexes and tone below the level of the lesion but also a positive Babinski sign. Spinal cord lesions produce impaired vibratory, joint position, temperature, and pain sensations below the level of the lesion. Light touch is the last sensory modality to be lost.

A lesion at or below L1 produces compression of the nerve roots of the cauda equina, resulting in decreased muscle tone and muscle stretch reflexes and weakness in the legs. The sensory loss involves all modalities, including light touch. With a cauda equina lesion that persists for more than a few weeks, atrophy and denervation, which may be confused with peripheral neuropathy, are detected on an electromyelogram of the lower extremity muscles.

DIAGNOSTIC AND STAGING STUDIES

General Considerations

When an osseous spinal lesion is discovered, an organized and systematic approach to its evaluation, integrating all the clinical and radiographic information, is mandatory. Once a reasonable differential diagnosis has been established from the clinical-radiologic correlation, additional studies may be indicated to assess the extent of tumor involvement and spinal stability. An isotope bone scan is helpful in detecting other unsuspected lesions.[1, 19, 20, 27] Computed tomography (CT) and magnetic resonance imaging (MRI) are invaluable in imaging the local extent of involvement of the tumor in the vertebrae or sacrum, as well as in determining the soft tissue extension. Excretory urography or cystography will show deviation of the ureter and bladder, while a barium enema study will indicate the relationship of a sacral tumor to the large bowel. Routine myelography or CT-myelography is useful in assessing the relationship of a spinal tumor to the neural contents.

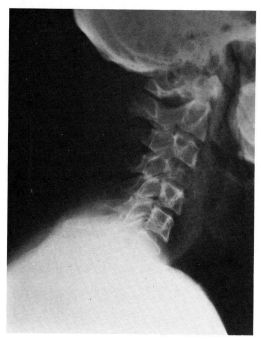

FIGURE 17–2. Chondrosarcoma of C4. Poorly marginated lytic destruction of vertebral body combined with anterior soft tissue mass indicates malignancy.

Roentgenographic Evaluation

Spinal chondrosarcomas may present as an area of lytic destruction involving the body or the dorsal elements or both (Fig. 17–2). Margination of these tumors varies widely, although most often the margin is poorly defined, supporting a diagnosis of malignancy. Matrix calcification is the most important diagnostic finding and is noted in about two thirds of the lesions (Fig. 17–3). Typically, the calcification consists of multiple densities that are discrete and punctate. When the lesion is purely lytic,[14, 23] which is more common in high grade lesions, the radiographic presentation is usually nonspecific. Once a chondrosarcoma reaches the cortical bone, it may cause cortical erosion or expansion. Eventually, most chondrosarcomas break through the cortex and extend into the soft tissues. Like the extraosseous portion of these tumors, the soft tissue component may either be unmineralized or show various degrees of calcification.

About one fourth of chondrosarcomas are located peripheral to the vertebrae, usually arising from a previously existing osteochondroma that may be either a solitary lesion or one of many lesions in multiple hereditary exostoses (Fig. 17–4). Secondary chondrosarcoma is readily diagnosed when there is evidence of an underlying osteochondroma. Distinguishing between a secondary and a periosteal chondrosarcoma may not be possible when the tumor has destroyed all evidence of the previous lesion.

Chondrosarcomas may be missed on routine radiographs. When this occurs, tomography, isotope bone scan, CT scan, or MRI may be required (Fig. 17–5). In selected cases, plain film tomography is useful to show more detail of the vertebral changes, especially when overlap obscuration has occurred. The isotope bone scan is sometimes useful for detection and localization and may be useful in excluding other sites of abnormality. Routine myelography or CT-myelography is useful in demonstrating the intraspinal component of a tumor and its effect on the dura, cord, and nerve roots.

Computed tomography and MRI are the techniques of choice for the demonstration of tumor extent locally, regionally, and systemically. CT is well suited to the imaging of spinal chondrosarcomas because it simultaneously demonstrates the pathologic anatomy of both bone and soft tissue structures. The excellent density resolution, in combination with the cross-sectional display, allows an accurate deter-

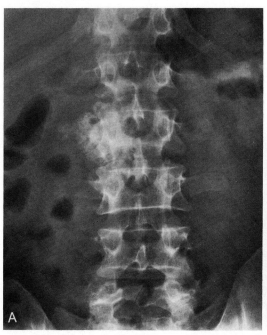

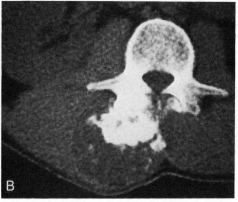

FIGURE 17–3. Chondrosarcoma of L2. *A*, Heavily mineralized tumor of dorsal elements. *B*, CT scan shows larger soft tissue component with subtle calcification beyond densely mineralized region that was seen on radiographs.

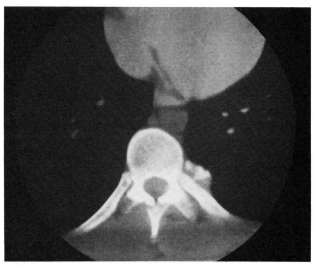

FIGURE 17–4. CT scan shows chondrosarcoma of thoracic vertebrae. Chondrosarcoma arose in osteochondroma in patient with multiple hereditary exostoses. Note intraspinal component.

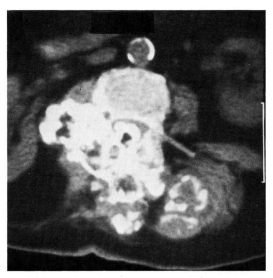

FIGURE 17–6. Chondrosarcoma of lumbar spine. CT scan demonstrates extent of this large, heavily mineralized tumor.

mination of the tumor extent and its effect on adjacent neurovascular structures and organs (Fig. 17–6). MRI has the further advantage of having unsurpassed tissue contrast and the ability to image directly in the axial, coronal, sagittal, and oblique planes. CT is superior to radiography for the detection of matrix calcification, whereas MRI usually fails to detect lesional mineralization.

Low grade chondrosarcomas are relatively avascular, but the higher the grade the more vascular the tumor in general. Angiography can be useful in defining the major feeding vessels and in determining the relationship of the tumor to the adjacent blood vessels. Angiography is most helpful in the cervical spinal column, but this invasive technique is rarely necessary.

Biopsy

Biopsy is a critical aspect of staging. The biologic potential of the chondrosarcoma varies with the his-

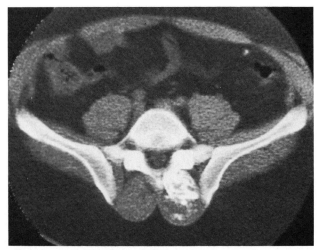

FIGURE 17–5. Chondrosarcoma of S1. CT scan shows partially mineralized peripheral chondrosarcoma arising posteriorly. Radiographs failed to detect this tumor.

tologic grade and influences the planned surgical procedure. While the biopsy is generally incisional, with a carefully planned skin incision that can be completely removed at definitive treatment, we utilize a needle biopsy for cervical and thoracic lesions and an open biopsy for other, more readily accessible lesions.

Surgical Staging

Recent advances in preoperative investigative measures have improved the ability to determine the precise location and extent of the tumor. Important factors used to predict the outcome of treatment and to design the treatment itself include the tumor grade (G), site (T) (including location, size, recurrence), and presence or absence of metastasis (M). In the surgical staging system[7] adopted by the Musculoskeletal Tumor Society (Table 17–1), the tumor grade is based on histologic findings, radiographic evaluation, and clinical presentation. This system describes two grades of lesions: low grade (G_1) and high grade (G_2). The tumor site has been divided into intracompartmental (T_1) and extracompartmental (T_2) for staging purposes and is determined by the natural barriers to tumor extension. For surgical purposes, the lesion includes the tumor, pseudocapsule, and reactive zone. Patients with extracompartmental lesions (extraosseous extension) are at a higher risk for local recurrence and metastasis.

Pathologic Features

Hyaline cartilage tumors usually have an opalescent quality on gross examination. Cystic and myxoid changes are most frequently identified in malignant hyaline cartilage tumors, whereas benign enchondromas are more uniform in their gross appearance. In the Mayo Clinic files, only 7 endochondromas (6 vertebral, 1 sacral) and 20 osteochondromas (17

TABLE 17–1. SURGICAL STAGING SYSTEM OF THE MUSCULOSKELETAL TUMOR SOCIETY

STAGE	GRADE	SITE		METASTASIS
I				
A	Low (G$_1$)	Intracompartmental	(T$_1$)	None (M$_0$)
B	Low (G$_1$)	Extracompartmental	(T$_2$)	None (M$_0$)
II				
A	High (G$_2$)	Intracompartmental	(T$_1$)	None (M$_0$)
B	High (G$_2$)	Extracompartmental	(T$_2$)	None (M$_0$)
III				
A	Low (G$_1$)	Intra or extra	(T$_{1-2}$)	Regional or distant (M$_1$)
B	High (G$_2$)	Intra or extra	(T$_{1-2}$)	Regional or distant (M$_1$)

From Enneking WF: Musculoskeletal Tumor Surgery. Vol 1. New York, Churchill Livingstone, 1983, p 81; by permission.

vertebral and 3 sacral) have been noted. Of the 39 chondrosarcomas of vertebral and sacral locations, approximately one half are secondary chondrosarcomas. All of these lesions represent malignant degeneration or transformation of an osteochondroma. The diagnosis of secondary chondrosarcoma is entertained if residual features of osteochondroma are identifiable. This problem frequently is more easily solved by review of the radiographs.

Since osteochondroma is the most common benign cartilage tumor of the vertebrae and sacrum, special attention should be paid to identifying secondary chondrosarcoma arising in an osteochondroma. Generally, the cartilage cap of an osteochondroma is less than 1 cm thick, whereas a secondary chondrosarcoma has a cap of 3 or 4 cm, at least focally.

Dedifferentiated chondrosarcoma[6, 10] also may be identified by its gross pathologic features. This high grade lesion has regions of typical hyaline cartilage tumor abutting on areas of more fleshy tumor that may have the histologic appearance of fibrosarcoma, malignant fibrous histiocytoma, or osteosarcoma.

Although the gross examination is important, the final diagnosis requires careful histologic evaluation. The most important histologic features used to differentiate a benign from a malignant hyaline cartilage tumor are its local pattern of growth (invasive versus circumscribed), cellularity, nuclear pleomorphism, presence of binucleated chondrocytes, necrosis, and the presence or absence of myxoid changes. As previously mentioned, malignant hyaline cartilage tumors outnumber chordomas.

Two benign cartilage tumors that histologically may be confused with chondrosarcoma occur in the vertebrae and sacrum. Both chondroblastoma (two) and chondromyxoid fibroma (two) have been identified in these locations in the Mayo Clinic files. The hypercellularity of these lesions and the presence of myxoid foci may result in misdiagnosis. This risk is amplified if the clinical and radiographic features are not taken into consideration before a final diagnosis is rendered.

Another malignant tumor in the histologic differential diagnosis of chondrosarcoma is chordoma.[24] Chordomas are about as common as chondrosarcomas in the vertebrae but outnumber chondrosarcomas approximately 10 to 1 in the sacrum. Both chordomas and chondrosarcomas grow in a lobulated low-power pattern and may have myxoid regions. However, a chordoma usually has a greater cytologic and nuclear pleomorphism than does chondrosarcoma and also tends to be more cellular. In addition, the abundant foamy cytoplasm of the diagnostic physaliferous cells is absent in the chondrosarcoma.

From a pathologic perspective, when a hyaline cartilage tumor is encountered in a vertebral or sacral location, chondrosarcoma is the most likely diagnosis. A chondrosarcoma in these regions shows the same features, such as hypercellularity, local invasion, necrosis, cellular pleomorphism, and nuclear atypia, as in its more common long-bone and pelvic locations.

TREATMENT

The treatment of chondrosarcoma is surgical removal.[2, 15, 26] Control of the primary lesion is very important because local recurrence will adversely affect survival. A long follow-up is necessary because recurrence can develop many years after the initial treatment. The aggressiveness of the surgical procedure depends on the histopathologic grade and size of the lesion, as well as on its location. Four basic types of surgical oncologic margins have been adopted by the Musculoskeletal Tumor Society (Table 17–2). These are based on the relationship of the margin to the natural barriers to extension and not on an absolute physical distance between the lesion and the wound margin. The margins may be achieved by either local (excision) or ablative (am-

TABLE 17–2. CLASSIFICATION OF WOUND MARGINS ACCORDING TO THE MUSCULOSKELETAL TUMOR SOCIETY*

TYPE	PLANE OF DISSECTION	RESULT
Intracapsular	Piecemeal debulking or curettage	Leaves macroscopic disease
Marginal	Shell out en bloc through pseudocapsule or reactive zone	May leave either satellite or skips
Wide	Intracompartmental en bloc with cuff of normal tissue	May leave skips
Radical	Extracompartmental en bloc entire compartment	No residual

*The table shows the types of wound margins, how they are obtained, and the result in terms of residual disease. This classification is based upon the relationship of the margin to the natural barriers to extension rather than on the physical distance between the edge of the lesion and the margin of the wound.

From Enneking WF: Musculoskeletal Tumor Surgery. Vol 1. New York, Churchill Livingstone, 1983, p 90; by permission.

putation) surgical procedures. Eriksson and colleagues[8] have outlined the ideal procedures for chondrosarcoma based on various stages.

When small, the lesion can be resected and a fusion performed as necessary. Resectability is based on the sparing of vital neural structures and on the ability to completely remove the lesion with a margin of normal tissue (Fig. 17–7). Large lesions that abut vital structures are unresectable (Fig. 17–8).

Whereas the treatment of choice for chondrosarcoma is early surgical excision with a wide margin of uninvolved tissue, this treatment is rarely feasible for vertebral chondrosarcomas because of such vital structures as the spinal cord, nerves, aorta, vena cava, bowel, and bladder. Thus, spinal chondrosarcoma

has usually been removed piecemeal, and foci of tumor are often left behind. This type of incomplete excision has led to a higher incidence of recurrence and a decreased survival of patients with vertebral chondrosarcoma. However, new methods of reconstructive surgery and improved instrumentation have increased the number of tumors that are resectable with clear margins. In addition, advances that may help control the foci of tumor left behind are being made in adjuvant therapy.

Since its description by Lièvre and coworkers in 1968,[18] total spondylectomy for giant cell tumor has been popularized by Stener,[28, 29] and this has led to the application of more aggressive surgical techniques for chondrosarcomas of the spinal column.

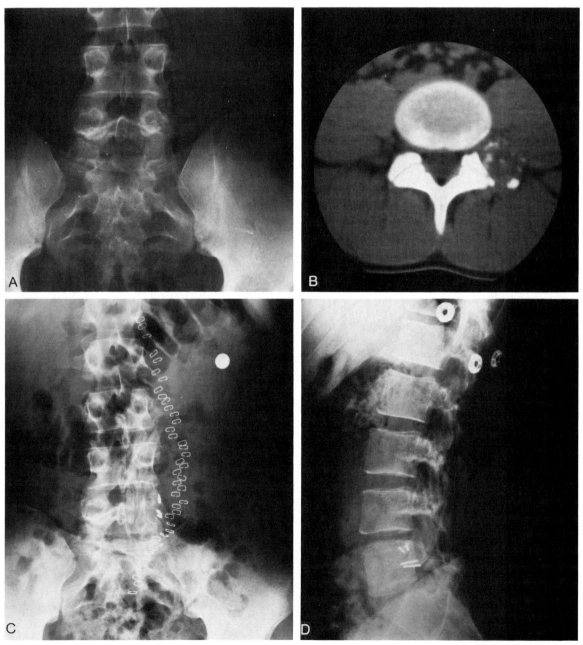

FIGURE 17–7. *A,* Anteroposterior radiograph of lower lumbar spine and sacrum demonstrating a mineralized soft tissue mass arising from transverse process of L5. *B,* CT scan demonstrating small size of lesion with no involvement of spinal cord. *C* and *D,* Lesion was resected, and L4 to sacrum was fused.

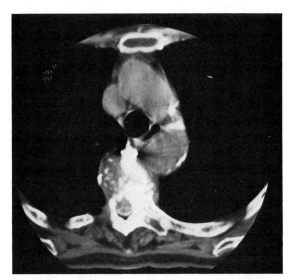

FIGURE 17–8. CT scan of chest demonstrating large chondrosarcoma in intimate juxtaposition to arch of aorta, trachea, and esophagus.

Many lesions require both anterior and posterior approaches to remove the tumor, followed by spinal stabilization using autogenous bone grafts (ilium, fibula, tibia, and ribs), frozen bone, and various instrumentation. Each has advantages and disadvantages, such as morbidity of additional surgery, cost, and interference with further evaluation of tumor recurrence.

Indications for spinal stabilization include removal of articular facets, pedicles, or vertebral bodies that produce instability. Spinous processes, transverse processes, and lamina can be excised without requiring stabilization. Anterior as well as posterior stabilization is necessary when several adjuvant vertebral (complete or specific) parts are removed.

Radiotherapy

Chondrosarcoma is generally regarded as a radioresistant tumor because of the slow rate of DNA synthesis. Several studies indicate that radiotherapy is indicated for nonsurgical candidates, for patients with inadequate surgical margins,[30] and as a primary method of treatment in selected patients. Studies show that patients with high grade lesions generally do not benefit from radiotherapy in terms of survival, but they do benefit from the palliative standpoint. McNaney and colleagues[21] indicated that patients with incomplete margins benefited from radiotherapy. However, the series was small and follow-up was short. Saunders and associates[25] reported the use of high dose helium ions in the treatment of five patients with spinal chondrosarcomas. The beam can be precisely directed, with excellent localization of radiation, and hence a dose in excess of spinal cord tolerance can be delivered to the vertebral column. The early results of their study are promising; however, follow-up was short (average, 22 months), and histologic grade was not mentioned in the report. Harwood and coworkers[11] evaluated radiotherapy in

a series of 31 patients with incompletely resected tumors. Six patients with Grade 1 lesions (three pelvis, one rib, one skull, one sinus) received 5000 cGy postoperatively, and three patients are free of disease 5 to 15 years later. Five patients with Grade 2 lesions were evaluated, and two of the five are disease-free—one at 4 years and the other at 15 years. The results of treatment of high grade lesions are extremely poor. Kim and colleagues[17] reported similar findings.

Chemotherapy

No patient studies to date have demonstrated a benefit using chemotherapy. Retinoic acid stimulates the release of chondrocyte lysosomal enzyme and has been proposed as a possible therapeutic agent.[12, 31] It inhibits the growth of cultured chondrosarcoma lines (also osteosarcoma), but there are no reports of human trials to date.

Radioactive sulfur (^{35}S) is another agent that has been found to inhibit chondrocyte and chondrosarcoma growth by its incorporation into cells and by the inhibition of glycosaminoglycan synthesis.

DISCUSSION

Overall, the five-year survival rate in chondrosarcoma of bone is approximately 50 per cent.[4, 13, 22] Although the histologic interpretation of these tumors is often difficult, a definite correlation exists between histologic grade of the tumor and overall survival. Patients with low grade lesions have distinctly improved disease-free and overall survival rates compared to patients with high grade lesions. Patients with central lesions (spine and pelvis) have a poorer prognosis than do patients with lesions located in the limbs. In addition to the histologic grade, the size of the lesion seems to be the other significant prognostic factor.

When chondrosarcoma occurs in its usual location, as in the proximal limb girdles, it is difficult to treat. However, the therapeutic problems are much greater when it involves the spine or sacrum. While the prognosis of patients with chondrosarcoma involving the vertebral column has been poor in the past, a more favorable outcome has resulted because of improvements in imaging techniques, which show the precise localization of the tumor, and the application of more aggressive surgical techniques to the spinal lesions, along with combined anterior and posterior excision, supplemented as needed by anterior and posterior fusion.

REFERENCES

1. Abello R, Lomena F, Garcia A, et al: Unusual metastatic chondrosarcoma detected with bone scintigraphy. Eur J Nucl Med 12:306–308, 1986.
2. Blaylock RL, Kempe LG: Chondrosarcoma of the cervical spine. Case report. J Neurosurg 44:500–503, 1976.

3. Camins MB, Duncan AW, Smith J, Marcove RC: Chondrosarcoma of the spine. Spine 3:202–209, 1978.

4. Campanacci M, Guernelli N, Leonessa C, Boni A: Chondrosarcoma: A study of 133 cases, 80 with long term follow-up. Ital J Orthop Traumatol 1:387–414, 1975.

5. Dahlin DC, Unni KK: Bone Tumors: General Aspects and Data on 8,542 Cases. 4th ed. Springfield, IL, Charles C Thomas, 1986.

6. de Lange EE, Pope TL Jr, Fechner RE: Dedifferentiated chondrosarcoma: Radiographic features. Radiology 161:489–492, 1986.

7. Enneking WF: Limb salvage. *In* Enneking WF (ed): Musculoskeletal Oncology. New York, Churchill Livingstone, 1987, p 81.

8. Eriksson AI, Schiller A, Mankin HJ: The management of chondrosarcoma of bone. Clin Orthop 153:44–66, 1980.

9. Evans HL, Ayala AG, Romsdahl MM: Prognostic factors in chondrosarcoma of bone: A clinicopathologic analysis with emphasis on histologic grading. Cancer 40:818–831, 1977.

10. Frassica FJ, Unni KK, Beabout JW, Sim FH: Dedifferentiated chondrosarcoma. A report of the clinicopathologic features and treatment of seventy-eight cases. J Bone Joint Surg [Am] 68:1197–1205, 1986.

11. Harwood AR, Krajbich JI, Fornasier VL: Radiotherapy of chondrosarcoma of bone. Cancer 45:2769–2777, 1980.

12. Healey JH, Lane JM: Chondrosarcoma. Clin Orthop 204:119–129, 1986.

13. Henderson ED, Dahlin DC: Chondrosarcoma of bone—a study of two hundred and eighty-eight cases. J Bone Joint Surg [Am] 45:1450–1458, 1963.

14. Hermann G, Sacher M, Lanzieri CF, et al: Chondrosarcoma of the spine: An unusual radiographic presentation. Skeletal Radiol 14:178–183, 1985.

15. Hirsch LF, Thanki A, Spector HB: Primary spinal chondrosarcoma with eighteen-year follow-up: Case report and literature review. Neurosurgery 14:747–749, 1984.

16. Huvos AG: Bone Tumors: Diagnosis, Treatment and Prognosis. Philadelphia, WB Saunders Co., 1979, p 209.

17. Kim RY, Salter MM, Brascho DJ: High-energy irradiation in the management of chondrosarcoma. South Med J 76:729–731, 735, 1983.

18. Lièvre JA, Darcy M, Pradat P, et al: Tumeur à cellules géantes du rachis lombaire, spondylectomie totale en deux temps. Rev Rhum Mal Osteoartic 35:125–130, 1968.

19. McLean RG, Choy D, Hoschl R, et al: Role of radionuclide imaging in the diagnosis of chondrosarcoma. Med Pediatr Oncol 13:32–36, 1985.

20. McLean RG, Murray IP: Scintigraphic patterns in certain primary malignant bone tumours. Clin Radiol 35:379–383, 1984.

21. McNaney D, Lindberg RD, Ayala AG, et al: Fifteen year radiotherapy experience with chondrosarcoma of bone. Int J Radiat Oncol Biol Phys 8:187–190, 1982.

22. Pritchard DJ, Lunke RJ, Taylor WF, et al: Chondrosarcoma: A clinicopathologic and statistical analysis. Cancer 45:149–157, 1980.

23. Rosenthal DI, Schiller AL, Mankin HJ: Chondrosarcoma: Correlation of radiological and histological grade. Radiology 150:21–26, 1984.

24. Salisbury JR, Isaacson PG: Distinguishing chordoma from chondrosarcoma by immunohistochemical techniques (letter to the editor). J Pathol 148:251–252, 1986.

25. Saunders WM, Chen GT, Austin-Seymour M, et al: Precision, high dose radiotherapy. II. Helium ion treatment of tumors adjacent to critical central nervous system structures. Int J Radiat Oncol Biol Phys 11:1339–1347, 1985.

26. Sim FH: Chondrosarcoma. *In* Uhthoff HK (ed): Current Concepts of Diagnosis and Treatment of Bone and Soft Tissue Tumors. Berlin, Springer-Verlag, 1984, pp 405–410.

27. Smith FW, Nandi SC, Mills K: Spinal chondrosarcoma demonstrated by Tc-99m-MDP bone scan. Clin Nucl Med 7:111–112, 1982.

28. Stener B: Surgical treatment of giant cell tumors, chondrosarcomas, and chordomas of the spine. *In* Uhthoff HK (ed): Current Concepts of Diagnosis and Treatment of Bone and Soft Tissue Tumors. Berlin, Springer-Verlag, 1984, pp 233–242.

29. Stener B: Musculoskeletal tumor surgery in Goteborg. Clin Orthop 191:8–20, 1984.

30. Suit HD, Goitein M, Munzenrider J, et al: Definitive radiation therapy for chordoma and chondrosarcoma of base of skull and cervical spine. J Neurosurg 56:377–385, 1982.

31. Thein R, Lotan R: Sensitivity of cultured human osteosarcoma and chondrosarcoma cells to retinoic acid. Cancer Res 42:4771–4775, 1982.

32. Törmä T: Malignant tumours of the spine and the spinal extradural space: A study based on 250 histologically verified cases. Acta Chir Scand Suppl 225:1–176, 1957.

GIANT CELL TUMORS OF THE SPINE

M. CAMPANACCI, S. BORIANI, and A. GIUNTI

INTRODUCTION

Giant cell tumor of bone is a histologically benign tumor whose clinical behavior is sometimes unpredictable and capricious. Its malignant counterpart—the so-called giant cell sarcoma—is best defined as a high grade sarcoma with scattered giant cells, which rarely presents at the same time as initial diagnosis but often appears at the site of a previous histologically benign giant cell tumor, usually after radiation therapy.[16, 18] Giant cell tumor must be distinguished from other lesions containing giant cells, such as aneurysmal bone cysts and osteoblastoma, which frequently originate in the spine.

The difficulties in diagnosis and treatment of giant cell tumor of the spine are compounded not only by the problems of this condition but also by specific pitfalls related to the anatomic sites within the vertebral column.

A major problem in the management of giant cell tumor at all locations is the correlation of the stage at presentation with the prognosis. A histologic grading[9] has proved unreliable; the surgical staging proposed by Enneking[6] is still to be appraised but probably offers a reasonable basis for deciding treatment.

The unpredictable clinical behavior of giant cell tumor is shown by three features: (1) a 30 to 50 per cent local recurrence rate is seen after intralesional procedures regardless of stage[3, 4]; (2) malignant transformation especially after radiotherapy varies from 5 per cent to 15 per cent[7, 10, 12, 18] and may approach 29 per cent in cases that are treated by doses exceeding 45 Gy[2]; and (3) a benign giant cell tumor may produce pulmonary metastases without clear biologic relationship to its radiologic aggressiveness.[1, 15, 21] Such metastases may on occasion spontaneously regress or be controlled by marginal surgical excision, but can be lethal in 25 per cent of cases.

In giant cell tumor of the limbs, an intralesional procedure may be performed even in Stage 2 and 3 lesions in association with local adjunctive therapy, when en bloc excision is thought to be contraindicated. The high risk of local recurrence (about 30 per cent) may be acceptable, since en bloc resection can be offered as definitive treatment of local recurrence (provided that vascular and nerve bundles are not involved).

In giant cell tumor of the spine and sacrum, intralesional procedures are almost always unavoidable—regardless of the stage—owing to the relative surgical inaccessibility of such regions. Local recurrence, however, represents a potential threat to neurologic function and life. Moreover, the diagnosis of giant cell tumor in the spine and sacrum is frequently delayed due to the difficulties in radiographic appraisal of a spinal tumor producing local or referenced pain. Often a small tumor lesion, not visible, may cause severe pain, whereas the sacral tumors grow to extremely large sizes before manifesting symptoms.

CLINICAL PRESENTATION

In our experience (398 cases observed at Istituto Rizzoli until 1985), about 60 per cent of giant cell tumors arise around the knee (distal femur, proximal tibia, proximal fibula). Proximal humerus and distal radius are frequent sites (about 8 to 10 per cent), whereas the incidence of proximal femur and distal tibia lesions is about 5 per cent. The spine is a rare location: 12 cases (3 per cent) arose in the spine cranial to the sacrum; a similar incidence is reported in the literature,[5, 8, 12, 14, 19] ranging from 2 per cent to 5 per cent. The sacrum itself is even less frequently involved (9 cases, 2 per cent); it is noteworthy to mention from the literature[5, 8, 12, 14, 19] that there is a wider range of incidence in this site (from 1.2 per cent to 8.7 per cent).

The sex and age distributions are the same as for tumors at other locations: there is a slight predominance of females, with a peak incidence in the third decade. No specific segment is preferentially involved in the spine. Among our 12 cases, only one arose in the posterior arch; the remaining 11 originated from the vertebral body. In four cases the whole vertebra was involved; in seven cases the tumor destroyed half the vertebra extending to the ipsilateral arch, with a well-defined margin. An analogy may be seen with the epiphyseal asymmetric sites of giant cell tumor of the limbs.[4, 5, 19] In two aggressive cases, the tumor invaded two adjacent vertebrae.

For sacral tumors, the following radiologic extensions are evaluated for surgery: the superior limit of the tumor, expansion across the midline, and involvement of the sacroiliac joint. Three of our cases were limited to the half-sacrum, two tumors crossed the midline and the sacroiliac joint, four involved the whole sacrum with anterior expansion. The superior limit was the disc space L4–L5 in three aggressive lesions, L5 and S1 in five active lesions, and S3 in one latent tumor.

Three different modes of clinical presentation are recorded in our series:

1. A painless, slowly enlarging mass was the only complaint in one sacral case.

2. A moderate intermittent pain, long-lasting in five sacral sites (median 14 months), shorter in six vertebral sites (median 6 months) with peripheral irradiation in three associated with moderate stiffness. In two cases, the patients were hospitalized for acute sharp pain resulting from compression fractures and reported a history of slight pain lasting several months.

3. A short course of pain and stiffness and neurologic symptoms with tender masses were observed in seven cases (four vertebral cases, two beginning with paraplegia, median 9 months; three sacral cases with incomplete neurologic compression, median 4 months).

The most frequent clinical finding in vertebral sites is paraspinal muscular spasm; a mass may be noticed frequently in cervical tumors. An enormous mass in a lumbar giant cell tumor (13 × 11 × 12 cm) was observed in a single case (Fig. 18–1), radiographically and histologically characterized by wide aneurysmal bone cyst–like areas. Sacral tumors were frequently misdiagnosed as disc disease, with patients (three) undergoing surgery for disc prolapse.

A special note should be made on the case of a man aged 54 who had a radiographically typical Paget's disease. He began to complain of radicular pain, and some weeks later an x-ray showed an osteolytic aggressive lesion of the body of L5. The histologic findings confirmed the diagnosis of typical Paget's disease. The patient refused treatment and died after four years because of enormous local extension of tumor.

RADIOGRAPHIC FINDINGS

Vertebral Sites. All lesions were radiographically lytic and were well circumscribed (active) (see Fig. 18–6) or widely expanded (aggressive). Often these lesions were limited to a hemivertebra (Fig. 18–2) by a rim that appeared faint on plain radiography but was well defined on conventional film and computed tomography (CT). No sclerotic margin or periosteal reaction was seen. Balloon-like enlargement of the vertebra (aneurysmal bone cyst–like) was sometimes found in parts of the tumor.

Even in cases of total vertebral involvement, the tumors were well defined from the residual bone, and the expansile, noninvasive growth was limited by a thin pseudocapsule, which was seldom ossified. This demarcation was always shown by CT scan (Fig. 18–3). This slow tumoral growth rarely provoked neurologic compression, whereas true aggressive lesions were more commonly seen with aneurysmal bone cyst–like areas developing within the tumor (see Fig. 18–1).

A pathologic fracture sometimes occurred in lesions involving the whole vertebral body. However, the height and symmetry of the vertebral body were preserved owing to the peripheral expansion of the tumor. In one patient, the tumor eroded two of the three columns (body and one articular column), resulting in subluxation (Fig. 18–4).

Sacral Sites. The radiographic picture was similar to giant cell tumor of the limbs. Homogeneous oval or round lytic lesions, sometimes trabeculated, with no ossification or calcification were observed (Fig. 18–5). The margins were indistinct, like those of a water puddle in the sand, without a sclerotic rim or periosteal reaction (Fig. 18–7). On plain x-rays, it may be quite difficult to see a lytic lesion in the thickness of the sacrum. Consequently, giant cell tumors of the sacrum—like chordoma and epithelial lytic metastases—are diagnosed late, when the edges of sacral foramina are eroded or the sacroiliac joint is involved (Fig. 18–8). CT scans are more accurate, thus playing an important role in staging studies.

Pathologic Features

Grossly the tissue of giant cell tumor may vary considerably in the same specimen: varying in color from light to dark brown to bloody; the consistency is usually soft and homogeneous, associated with focal cystic, necrotic, or rubbery areas. No bone reaction is found at margins of the lesions. A reactive, hypervascular zone may be a feature of active or aggressively growing tumors. Some lesions appear grossly as an aneurysmal bone cyst if the cyst formation predominates. The main histologic features are the mononuclear cells, interposed with numerous multinucleated osteoclast-like giant cells. The shape of mononuclear cells is variable, whereas the nuclei are oval or plump with a prominent nucleolus. The multinucleated giant cells contain nuclei with the same features. Bone may be present but is reactive. It is never a product of the tumor cells. Cystic areas filled with blood and lined by mononuclear cells or fibrous tissue, similar to those of aneurysmal bone cyst, are common.

The three main diagnostic features of giant cell tumor are: (1) sheets of mononuclear round cells, (2) randomly scattered osteoclast-type giant cells (multinuclear cells), and (3) identical nuclei found in the mononuclear cells and multinuclear cells. At present there are no immunoperoxidase staining methods or

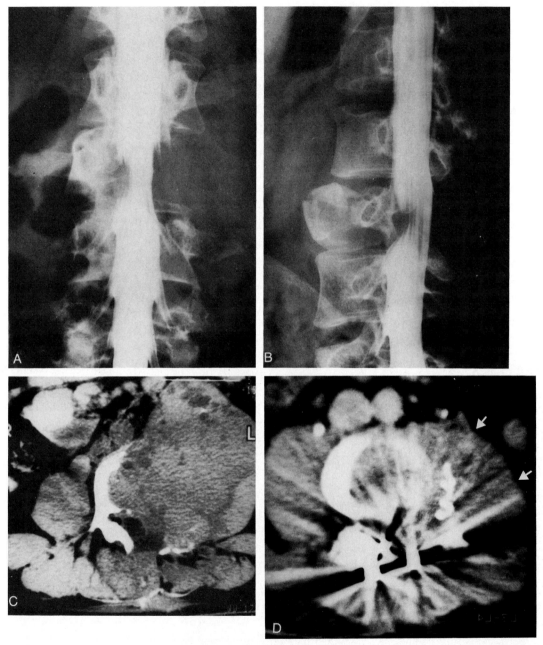

FIGURE 18–1. C.T., a 25-year-old male. Enormous giant cell tumor of L2 with compression of the cauda (*A* and *B*) expanding to the abdominal wall (*C*). CT scan shows many aneurysmal bone cyst–like areas. A posterior segmental instrumentation was performed; after radiotherapy and twice-repeated embolization, the mass was found dramatically reduced (*D*) and the case was elected for anterior stabilization. At 18-month follow-up, no recurrence developed.

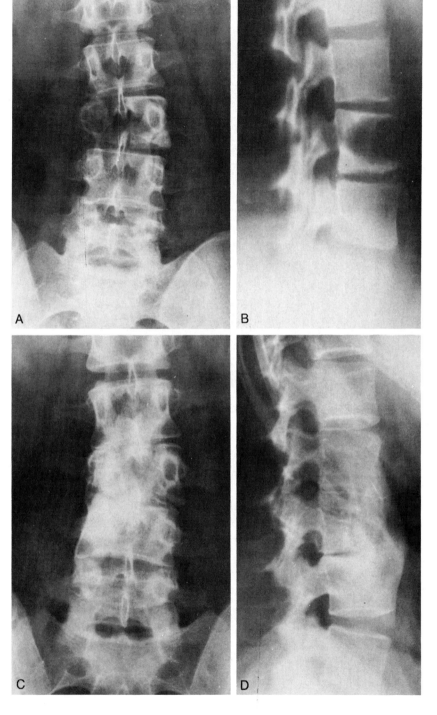

FIGURE 18–2. L.G., a 23-year-old female. Giant cell tumor of L3 involving half of the body and the corresponding pedicle. A lytic lesion with a sharp margin in the vertebral spongiosa and a faint limit anteriorly is evident on plain film (*A*) and computed tomogram (*B*). Intralesional wide excision via anterolateral approach was performed, followed by iliac graft. Eight years after treatment (*C* and *D*) no sign of recurrence was found; a sound fusion was obtained.

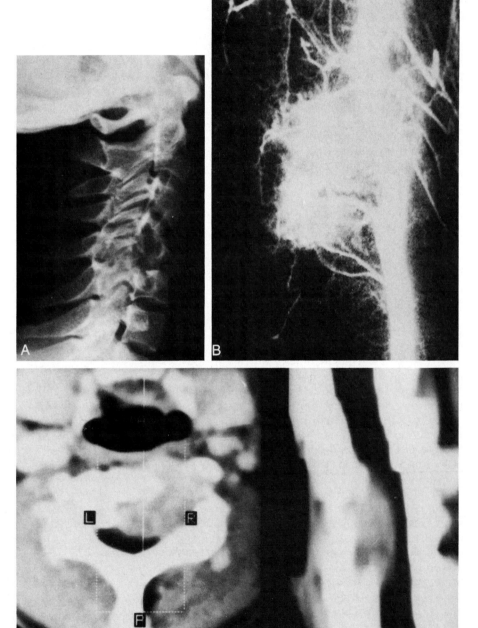

FIGURE 18–3. G.M., a 23-year-old female. Giant cell tumor of C3 and C4 without neurologic involvement. The patient complained of a short course of pain and growing mass. The radiograph (A) shows a pathologic compression fracture; on angiogram (B) a highly vascularized mass is evident. The extracompartmental expansion is confirmed by CT scan (C). All these data indicated—with histologic confirmation—a Stage 3 giant cell tumor.

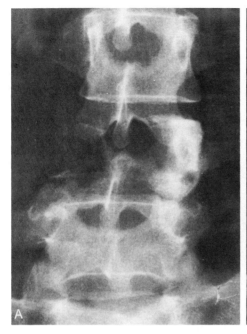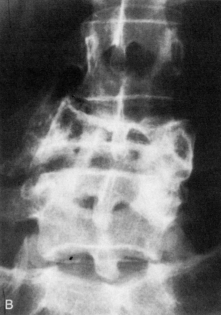

FIGURE 18–4. D.C., a 36-year-old female. Giant cell tumor of L4, involving the right half of the body and the arch, provokes a lateral subluxation (A). Five years after radiotherapy (B), there was increased ossification with persistence of morphologic alteration and dislocation.

electron microscopic techniques to distinguish between aneurysmal bone cyst and giant cell tumor.

Histologically, a grading system using three grades of malignancy—low, intermediate, and high[9]—has been described, but has not proven useful for prognosis.

Differential Diagnosis

In the true vertebrae, giant cell tumor must be distinguished from aneurysmal bone cysts, which exhibit a peculiar balloon-like appearance. This feature may also be observed in limited parts of a giant cell tumor. Densitometry on CT scan may be helpful in detecting blood-filled, cystic areas (see Fig. 18–1). Since it is possible to find such areas in some giant cell tumors, CT scan can be used to obtain needle biopsies of solid areas. Histology, however, is not always definitive. The diagnosis of giant cell tumor is suggested when the tumor has large areas that are solid and very cellular, alternating with blood-filled cyst-like spaces.

Chordoma is another radiographic consideration; this tumor is more destructive, has no internal septations, and is sometimes calcified. Older patients are usually affected. Osteoblastoma of the spine may also be confused with giant cell tumor; tumoral osteogenesis is often visible on plain radiographs.

Metastatic carcinoma generally develops in an older age group. Metastases are usually located in the vertebral body. The margins are indistinct, and frequently there is vertebral collapse. Isotope scans may reveal multiple sites of involvement.

Primary hyperparathyroidism may produce osteolytic lesions in the sacrum radiographically similar to giant cell tumor, while in the true vertebrae the presence of such "brown tumors" is exceptional. The brown tumor may also be histologically similar or

identical to giant cell tumor. The diagnosis relies on the clinical complaints, radiographic features of involvement of other bones, and laboratory findings. Solitary or multiple myeloma is typical of late adulthood, characterized by rounded osteolytic central lesions with faint margins, often presenting with compression fractures of the vertebral bodies. A skeletal survey including the calvarium may reveal the typical "punched-out" lesions.

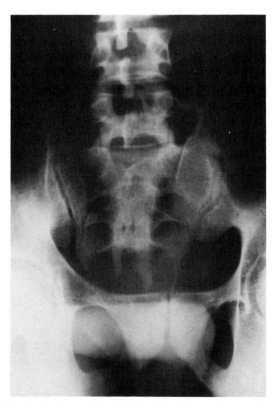

FIGURE 18–5. T.I., a 22-year-old male. Giant cell tumor distal to S3, well confined (Stage I), thus eligible for en bloc resection.

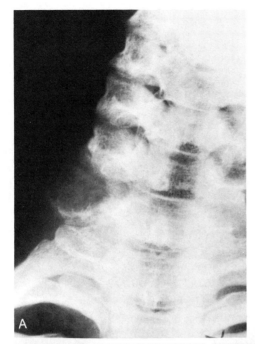

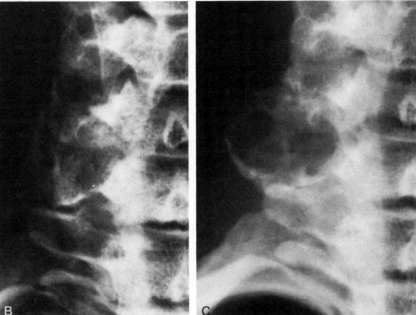

FIGURE 18–6. T.G., a 21-year-old female. Giant cell tumor of the lateral articular process of C7. At the beginning, a radiolucent well-marginated mass is evident on plain radiogram (*A*). Six months after radiotherapy, the sclerotic rim is better defined (*B*). Seven years later (*C*), there was more ossification.

Finally, it should be remembered that many malignant tumors, such as osteosarcoma, fibrosarcoma, and malignant fibrous histiocytoma, may be characterized by the presence of reactive giant cells and may thus resemble giant cell tumor histologically. Their rarity in the spine, different radiographic appearances, and biologic behavior usually make distinction possible.

Staging Studies and Surgical Indications

For staging purposes CT and isotope scans and sometimes magnetic resonance imaging (MRI) and angiography are required. CT scan shows the exact extent of the tumor (see Fig. 18–3) and its expansion beyond anatomic borders. Isotope scans are used to detect subtle lesions and to exclude multiple lesions. The uptake of isotope generally extends beyond the limits seen on plain radiographs in the more rapidly growing tumors.

Magnetic resonance imaging can show intraosseous and extraosseous tumor extent in multiple planes. Spinal angiograms (see Fig. 18–3) generally show modest vascularity in the central portion, surrounded by a reactive neovasculature at the edges of the lesion. This effect is particularly prominent in aggressive lesions. Angiography can also be used for purposes of embolization as an adjuvant to surgery or as the definitive form of treatment. Myelography—especially when followed by CT scans with contrast me-

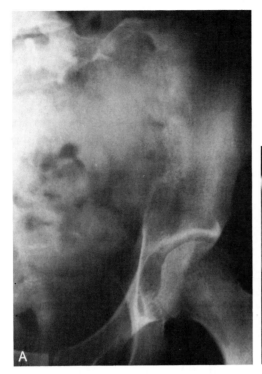

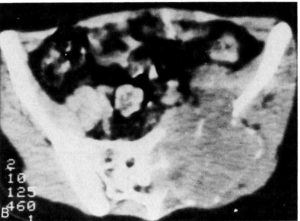

FIGURE 18–7. M.R., a 23-year-old female. Stage 3 giant cell tumor involving the whole left half of the sacrum, expanding across the sacroiliac joint and occupying the ischial incisure. *A*, plain film; *B*, CT scan.

dium—is particularly important in detecting the limit of the tumor toward the dura (see Fig. 18–1). This is quite important, since wide resection may not be possible in cases of involvement of the epidural space.

The staging studies must be completed by a biopsy confirming the diagnosis, but excisional biopsy may contaminate the surgical planes. Needle biopsy may be a better alternative, provided that it is possible to obtain pathologic tissue without undue morbidity. We perform needle biopsy under CT scan control, thus obtaining representative specimens and preserving the possibilities of an uncontaminated treatment.

A significant correlation exists between clinical presentation and radiographic studies. In fact, an indolent or intermittently painful clinical course corresponds to a tumor confined within the bone (intraosseous), not surrounded by hypervascularized areas, and characterized by moderate isotope uptake. A tumor characterized by pain has the radiographic appearance of a lytic expanding lesion, extruding through the cortex but contained by a thin layer of reactive bone. The isotope scan is intensely positive. Finally, a rapid-growing lesion appears radiographically as a mass widely expanding in the soft tissues, while the angiogram shows a marked hypervascularity around the tumor with possible satellite nodules in neighboring tissues. Isotope scan is hot beyond the limits of the tumor. These features make it possible to define the lesions, respectively, as latent, active, and aggressive and are applicable to spinal giant cell tumor.[6]

The major purpose of staging is to decide whether the lesion is best managed by intralesional excision, marginal resection, or wide resection. The surgical anatomy of vertebrae and sacrum, however, is such that en bloc resection is feasible only in the sacrum distally to S2 or in Grade 1 and 2 lesions located in the posterior arch. In selected cases of sacral tumors

that do not cross the median line, resection may be performed even at a higher level, possibly including the sacroiliac joint, without loss of urogenital function (compensated by the contralateral sacral nerves). In considering therapy, it should be noted that untreated or recurrent giant cell tumor of the sacrum will eventually involve neural structures, thus compromising bladder and bowel function and threatening life. In our experience, it is better to decide upon a curative surgical procedure at original diagnosis, rather than to expose the patient to progressive pain and paralysis due to the unremitting progression of the disease. Vertebral body resections are mentioned in the literature,[11, 17, 20] but these procedures cannot be defined as marginal or wide en bloc procedures; intralesional one- or two-stage excisions of the vertebrae are possible but result in local tissue contamination.

Curettage is an adequate treatment of Grade 1 giant cell tumor, provided that it is performed using accepted oncologic techniques (excision of pseudocapsule and removal of all the pathologic and reactive tissues). In Grade 2 lesions, local adjunctive measures are advised, such as phenol, cement, or cryosurgery, in order to achieve deeper control of the tumor margins. Embolization and radiotherapy should be considered for Grades 2 and 3 lesions of the spine. The former is valuable in reducing intraoperative bleeding and is particularly useful in lesions with wide aneurysmal bone cyst–like areas, provided that selective angiography does not reveal any substantial connection with the medullary arteries.

Radiotherapy may be considered only in unresectable or nonembolizable lesions. In any case, the minimum effective dose (no more than 30 Gy ideally) should be used to minimize the risk of radiation-induced sarcoma. In one sacral patient, who underwent orthovoltage therapy in 1952 at the age of 21,

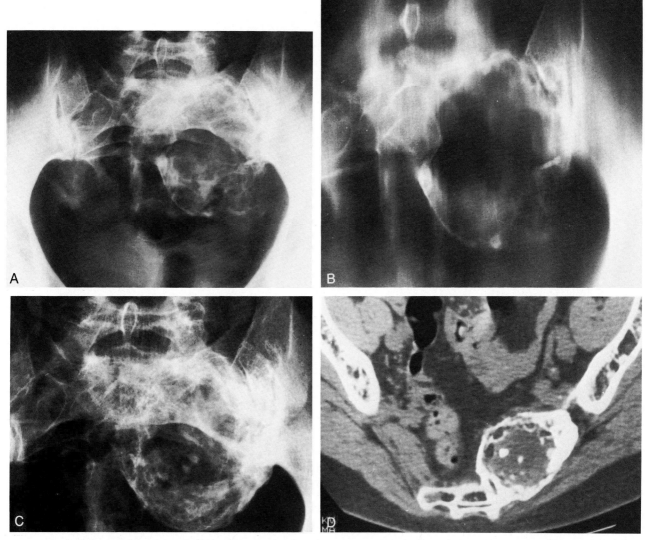

FIGURE 18–8. D.P.F., a 41-year-old female. *A*, Plain film Stage 2 giant cell tumor. *B*, Sclerotic rim surrounds the tumor, well defined by plain tomogram. Four years after radiotherapy, the mass is widely ossified. *C*, Plain film; *D*, CT scan.

a highly malignant sarcoma developed 9 years later. Four other patients were submitted to megavoltage therapy: one subsequently died intraoperatively, two died one year after treatment for local progression, and one has no evidence of disease 7 years after treatment. Grade 3 giant cell tumor should not be managed by intralesional procedures, as the risk of recurrence rises to 80 per cent. As previously stated, one should not hesitate in considering definitive treatment for fear of unavoidable neurologic deficit. If en bloc resection is not feasible, all adjunctive measures should be used.

REFERENCES

1. Bertoni F, Present D, Enneking WF: Giant cell tumor of bone with pulmonary metastases. J Bone Joint Surg 67A:890–900, 1985.

2. Boriani S, Sudanese A, Baldini N, Picci P: Evoluzione sarcomatosa del tumore a cellule giganti. Ital J Orthop Traumatol 12:203–211, 1986.

3. Campanacci M: Tumori delle ossa e delle parti molli. Bologna, A. Gaggi, 1981.

4. Campanacci M, Baldini N, Boriani S, Sudanese A: Giant cell tumor of bone. J Bone Joint Surg 69A:106–113, 1987.

5. Dahlin DC: Bone tumors. General aspects and data on 6221 cases. Springfield, IL, Charles C Thomas, 1978.

6. Enneking WF: Musculoskeletal Tumor Surgery. New York, Churchill Livingstone, 1983.

7. Hutter RVP, Worcester JN, Francis KC, et al: Benign and malignant giant cell tumors of bone; a clinico-pathological analysis of the natural history of the disease. Cancer 15:653–690, 1962.

8. Huvos AG: Bone Tumors: Diagnosis, Treatment and Prognosis. Philadelphia, WB Saunders Co., 1979.

9. Jaffe HL, Lichtenstein L, Portis RB: Giant cell tumor of bone. Its pathologic appearance, grading, supposed variant and treatment. Arch Pathol 30:993–1031, 1940.

10. Jaffe HL: Tumors and Tumorous Conditions of the Bones and Joints. Philadelphia, Lea and Febiger, 1958.

11. Lièvre JA, Camus JP, Darcy M, Pradat P: Spondylectomie

totale (exerese extra-ligamentaire d'une vertebre). Deux observations. Ann Med Interne 123:887–894, 1972.

12. Mirra JM, Gold RH, Marcove RC: Bone Tumors. Diagnosis and Treatment. Philadelphia, JB Lippincott Co., 1980.

13. Nascimento AG, Huvos AG, Marcove RC: Primary malignant giant cell tumor of bone. Cancer 44:1393–1402, 1979.

14. The Netherlands Committee on Bone Tumors: Radiological Atlas on Bone Tumors. Paris, Mouton, 1973.

15. Rock MG, Pritchard DJ, Unni KK: Metastases from histologically benign giant cell tumor of bone. J Bone Joint Surg 66A:269–274, 1984.

16. Rock MG, Sim FM, Unni KK, Witrak GA, et al: Malignant giant cell tumor of bone: Clinicopathological assessment of nineteen patients. J Bone Joint Surg 68A:1073–1079, 1986.

17. Roy-Camille R, Sailant G, Bisseric M, et al: Resection vertebrale totale dans la chirurgie tumorale au niveau du rachis dorsal par voie posterieure pure. Rev Chir Orthop 67:421–430, 1981.

18. Sanerkin NG: Malignancy, aggressiveness and recurrence in giant cell tumor of bone. Cancer 46:1641–1649, 1980.

19. Schajowicz F: Tumors and Tumor-Like Lesions of Bone and Joints. New York, Springer Verlag, 1981.

20. Stener B: Surgical treatment of giant cell tumor, chondrosarcomas and chordomas of the spine. *In* Uhthoff HK (ed): Current Concepts of Diagnosis and Treatment of Bone and Soft Tissue Tumors. Berlin, Springer Verlag, 1984.

21. Vanel D, Contesso G, Rebibo G, et al: Benign giant cell tumors of bone with pulmonary metastases and favourable prognosis. Skeletal Radiol 10:221–226, 1983.

GIANT CELL TUMORS OF THE SPINE AND SACRUM:

Mayo Clinic Experience

FRANKLIN H. SIM, DOUGLAS J. McDONALD, RICHARD A. McLEOD, and K. KRISHNAN UNNI

INTRODUCTION

Giant cell tumor of bone is a distinctive and challenging neoplasm with an aggressive clinical course. It is a relatively common tumor, accounting for 18.2 per cent of the benign tumors in the Dahlin and Unni series.[9] In its usual location—at the end of a long bone, and particularly in the region of the knee—giant cell tumor poses a difficult treatment problem. However, this problem is greatly magnified when the tumor involves the spinal column or sacrum. Localization in vertebrae is not common, ranging from 2 to 10 per cent in the reported series.[11, 12, 14, 16, 25, 27, 28, 32] Most series[10] indicate that the sacrum is most commonly involved, but Larsson and colleagues[18] and others[17, 24] found more giant cell tumors involving the vertebrae above the sacrum. Neurologic involvement is frequent, depending on the location and aggressiveness of the lesion.[19] Moreover, there is no consensus as to the best method of treatment of spinal giant cell tumor.

CLINICAL FEATURES

The bone tumor registry at our institution includes 407 patients with a diagnosis of giant cell tumor based on histologic sections. The 411 tumors in this series illustrate the rarity of multifocal involvement. The age and sex distributions are shown in Figure 19–1. In this overall series there was a slight predilection for females (56 per cent), which was more marked in patients under age 20. Eighty-five per cent of the patients in our series were over age 20 at the time of diagnosis. The peak incidence was in the third decade. When the giant cell tumor involved the spine or sacrum, the female predilection was more marked (70 per cent), and the patients tended to be younger (30 per cent under age 20).

In this series, the distal femur was the most common site of occurrence, followed by the proximal tibia (Fig. 19–2); these two sites accounted for more than 50 per cent of the tumors. The distal radius was the third most common location, followed by the sacrum, which accounted for 33 tumors. In the Dahlin and Unni series of bone tumors,[9] giant cell tumor was by far the most common benign tumor of the sacrum. However, giant cell tumor was less common in the spine above the sacrum, being the fourth most common benign tumor of the vertebral column in the Dahlin and Unni series.[9] In our current series of giant cell tumors, 16 lesions were in the spine above the sacrum: 6 in the cervical region, 6 in the lumbar region, and 4 in the thoracic region.

Pain is the most common presenting complaint and is usually associated with spinal tenderness. Initially the pain can be localized to the spine or sacrum, but soon a pattern of nerve root referred pain develops. Neurologic involvement is also common and varies from areas of numbness to paraparesis and loss of bowel and bladder function. Depending on the exact location, neurologic involvement can be the result of cord compression or varying degrees of root compression. Lumbosacral radiculopathy secondary to root compression is present in a high percentage of

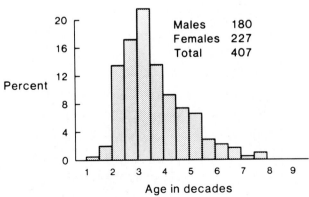

FIGURE 19–1. Age distribution of 407 patients with giant cell tumors.

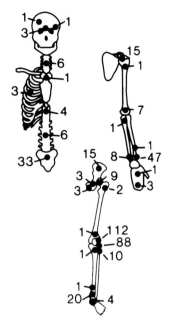

FIGURE 19–2. Distribution of giant cell tumors by site.

sacral lesions. A presacral mass occasionally is noted in patients with sacral lesions.

Radiographic Features

Spinal giant cell tumors are characterized by their purely lytic destruction, having neither surrounding reactive sclerosis nor matrix mineralization (Fig. 19–3). Some tumors have sharp margination and cortical expansion, whereas others are poorly marginated and may exhibit cortical destruction and a soft tissue mass. This latter presentation may be radiologically indistinguishable from that of malignancy. About one fourth of the patients have an associated pathologic compression fracture. Unlike most other tumors of the spine, these neoplasms have a predilection for the vertebral body.

Sacral tumors are more commonly located in the upper segments and often extend to the sacroiliac joint. This eccentric location may be useful in distinguishing giant cell tumor from sacral chordoma. Superiorly located sacral tumors may extend across the joint to involve the adjacent ilium (Fig. 19–4).

Computed tomography (CT) is used routinely to characterize and to stage these tumors preoperatively and is especially useful with sacral lesions. The cross-sectional display provided by CT scan is well suited for demonstration of tumor extent and status of adjacent organs and neurovascular structures. Magnetic resonance imaging (MRI) can help define the relationship to intraspinal structures. Giant cell tumors may recur within the bone or may implant within the soft tissues. Serial radiographs and tomograms aid in the detection of intraosseous recurrence. CT scan or MRI is best for soft tissue recurrence. These latter lesions may have peripheral "egg-shell" ossification (easier to recognize on CT scan than on MRI), which helps in their identification.

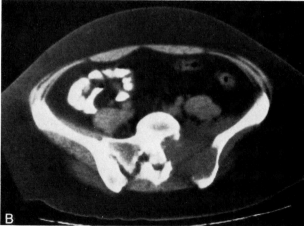

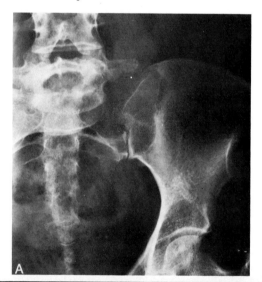

FIGURE 19–4. Pelvis with giant cell tumor in body of sacrum and extending across to involve nearby ilium. *A,* Anteroposterior radiograph. *B,* Computed tomography scan of same lesion.

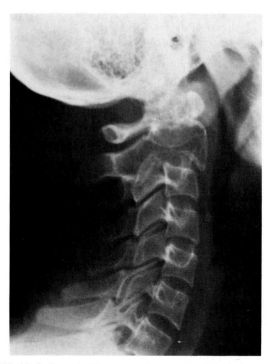

FIGURE 19–3. Lateral radiograph of the spine showing extensive destruction of C2.

TABLE 19–1. SUMMARY OF CLINICAL DATA: 27 PATIENTS WITH GIANT CELL TUMOR OF SPINE OR SACRUM

CASE	SEX; AGE (YR)	SITE	SYMPTOMS*	TREATMENT	RESULT
			Tumor in Spine		
1	F;24	T10	Pain (6 mo)	Excision, arthrodesis with rib graft	No evidence of disease at 21 yr
2	F;66	L3	Pain (3 mo), root compression	Excision, arthrodesis with rib graft	No evidence of disease at 7 yr
3	F;17	C4	Pain (2 mo)	Excision	No evidence of disease at 14 yr
4	F;17	C2	Pain (4 mo)	Excision, radiation for recurrence (4500 cGy)	No further recurrence at 9½ yr
5	F;25	C5	Pain (1 mo)	Excision	No evidence of disease at 7 yr
6	M;26	L4	Pain (3 mo), root compression	Excision, anterior and posterior arthrodesis, Harrington rod, fibula graft	No evidence of disease at 4 yr
7	F;22	C2	Pain (1 yr)	Excision, arthrodesis	No evidence of disease at 2 yr
8	F;22	L1	Pain (1 yr)	Excision, anterior and posterior arthrodesis, fibula and rib grafts	No evidence of disease at 2 yr
9	M;34	T4 and T5	Pain (1 mo), cord compression	Radiation (4400 cGy), excision, anterior and posterior arthrodesis, fibula and rib grafts	Death at 1 yr†
10‡	F;28	T10	Pain (4 mo), root compression	Excision, radiation (3500 cGy, elsewhere), excision	No evidence of disease at 9 yr
11‡	F;15	C2, distal radius	Pain (2 mo), cord compression	Excision (elsewhere, twice), excision (here), fusion (three times), excision (elsewhere, three times)	Status unclear, possible persistent tumor
12‡	F;19	L4	Pain (onset), root compression	Excision, L3 to L5 fusion, radiation (5075 cGy, elsewhere), excision, anterior and posterior arthrodesis	No evidence of disease at 3 yr
13‡	M;33	L5	Pain (6 mo), root compression	Excision (elsewhere, twice), radiation (4660 cGy, elsewhere), debulking	Alive at 4 yr
			Tumor in Sacrum		
14	F;21	S	Pain (1 mo), root compression	Debulking, excision for recurrence (three times)	No further recurrence at 16 yr
15	F;25	S	Pain (2 yr), mass, root compression	Excision	No evidence of disease at 17 yr
16	M;20	S	Pain (5 mo), root compression	Excision	No evidence of disease at 17 yr
17	F;27	S	Pain (1 mo), root compression	Radiation (3900 cGy)	No evidence of disease at 8 yr
18	M;18	S	Pain (onset), root compression	Excision	No evidence of disease at 13 yr
19	M;25	S	Pain (onset), root compression	Debulking, radiation (4000 cGy), radial lumbosacral resection (elsewhere), thoracotomy, chemotherapy	Benign metastasis, no further disease at 5 yr
20	F;28	S	Pain (6 mo), mass, root compression	Excision, radiation (5000 cGy)	No evidence of disease at 6 yr
21	F;17	S	Pain (onset), root compression	Excision, radiation (5000 cGy), excision for recurrence, thoracotomy, chemotherapy	Benign metastasis, death at 1 yr due to progressive sacral and pulmonary involvement

Table continued on following page

TABLE 19–1. SUMMARY OF CLINICAL DATA: 27 PATIENTS WITH GIANT CELL TUMOR OF SPINE OR SACRUM *Continued*

CASE	SEX; AGE (YR)	SITE	SYMPTOMS*	TREATMENT	RESULT
22	F;23	S	Pain (1 mo), root compression	Excision, radiation recommended	Lost at 1 mo
23	M;18	S	Pain (3 mo), root compression	Excision, radiation	No evidence of disease at 2 yr
24	M;45	S	Pain (2 mo), root compression	Biopsy, radiation (5000 cGy, elsewhere), excision	No evidence of disease at 2 yr
25‡	F;29	S	Pain (onset), mass, root compression	Excision, radiation (elsewhere), excision	No evidence of disease at 7 yr
26‡	F;33	S	Pain (3 yr), root compression	Radiation (2550 cGy, elsewhere), T2 and T3 chordotomy	Alive at 8 yr
27‡	F;45	S	Pain (onset), mass, root compression, rectal hemorrhage	Debulking (elsewhere), biopsy, radiation (3000 cGy)	Malignant, alive with metastasis at 1 yr

*Duration is shown in parentheses.
†Radiation-induced fibrosarcoma.
‡Patient referred for recurrent tumor.

Pathologic Features

Grossly, there are no distinctive features that distinguish giant cell tumor from other vertebral tumors. Typically, however, giant cell tumors are characteristically soft, friable, and gray to brown-red, and they often penetrate into adjacent tissues. Histologically, these lesions are similar to giant cell tumors in other locations (Fig. 19–5). Typical zones show sheets of mononuclear cells with many benign multinucleate giant cells, commonly containing 20 to 30 nuclei, scattered more or less uniformly about the field. The nuclei of giant cells have the same appearance as nuclei of the mononuclear cells in the background. These are round or oval and are not spindly. Mitotic activity is common in the stromal cells of benign giant cell tumors. Necrosis is found relatively frequently in giant cell tumors (Fig. 19–5). The benign giant cell tumors in our series are not graded because we have

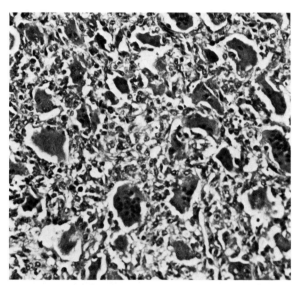

FIGURE 19–5. Microscopic view of giant cell tumor with sheets of mononuclear cells and scattered multinucleate giant cells. (H & E, ×158).

not found any reliable grading system, nor has grading been helpful in predicting tumor behavior.

TREATMENT

The treatment alternatives for giant cell tumor are numerous and remain controversial. When the lesion is in a long bone, there is universal agreement that surgical excision is the best treatment, but controversy continues as to the type of operation: the extent of surgery and subsequent functional deficit are weighed against the risk of recurrence. Excision by curettage preserves the adjacent joint and maintains joint function, but it is associated with an increased incidence of local recurrence, ranging from 25 to 58 per cent in the literature.[5, 8, 13, 22, 30, 31] In the series from our institution,[21] lesional curettage was associated with a 34 per cent recurrence. On the other hand, en bloc resection provides the least chance of recurrence for a long bone lesion (7 per cent in our series), but it generally requires an extensive reconstruction with subsequent loss of function.

The planning of optimal treatment for a giant cell tumor in the spine or sacrum involves a difficult decision. It is agreed that complete removal gives the best result.[6, 8, 13, 15, 22] However, when the lesion is in the spine or sacrum, it is often difficult to achieve an adequate margin with surgical excision, and, in the past, palliative treatment has been carried out, often with inadequate radiation therapy. Since total spondylectomy for giant cell tumor was described by Lièvre and colleagues[20] in 1968 and was popularized by Stener and Johnsen,[29] more aggressive surgical techniques have been used to treat these spinal lesions—for example, combined anterior and posterior excision supplemented, as needed, by anterior and posterior fusion[26, 33] (Fig. 19–6). When a lesion involves the lower portion of the sacrum and complete en bloc resection can be carried out with preservation of the S2 and S3 nerve roots, this is preferred. However, when resection would cause significant

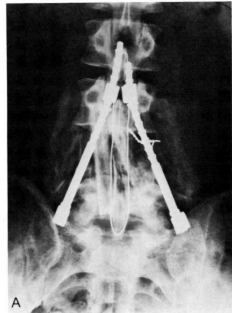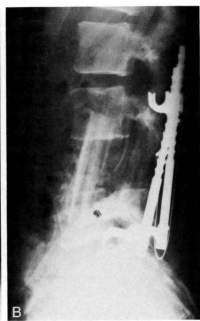

FIGURE 19–6. Anteroposterior (*A*) and lateral (*B*) radiographs showing extensive anterior and posterior reconstruction after resection of a large giant cell tumor in the body of L4.

neurologic deficit or when en bloc resection of a spine lesion is not possible, a pessimistic outlook may not be warranted. In both Dahlin's series[7] and the experience from the Rizzoli Institute reported by Savini and associates,[26] patients with spine lesions appeared to do better than patients with tumors of other sites, even with incomplete excision with or without radiation.

Therefore, in patients whose tumors do not appear to be amenable to complete resection (such as an extensive sacral lesion), a more limited operation with gross removal of the tumor and careful curettage of remaining tumor, decompression of the neural elements, and radiation therapy to eliminate the residual tumor cells may be appropriate. We think that radiation therapy generally should be considered whenever incomplete excision is carried out. If extensive bone grafting is used to stabilize the spine, it is advisable to delay the postoperative radiation therapy for approximately six weeks to facilitate early incorporation of the grafts.[3, 26]

Although earlier reports suggested that radiation therapy was ineffective in preventing local progression,[13, 22, 23] series utilizing adequate doses of modern supervoltage radiation have shown the effectiveness of this technique.[2, 3] The potential for malignant transformation[4, 8, 13, 22, 23] dictates that radiation therapy not be used as routine treatment for all giant cell tumors, but this caution must be balanced against the consequences of tumor progression when the lesion is in the spine or sacrum. Our results with incomplete surgical excision and decompression for large sacral lesions were similar to those of Larsson and coworkers,[19] who reported favorable results with supervoltage radiation therapy.

Our 49 patients with giant cell tumor involving the spine or sacrum were seen over the course of many decades and were treated with various techniques and by a number of surgeons. In order to gain more meaningful insight into the behavior of giant cell tumor in the spine and sacrum, we analyzed the results of treatment in the more recent cases that had been evaluated and treated according to modern concepts. In this series of 27, 14 involved the sacrum and 13 the spine (5 in the lumbar region, 5 in the cervical region, and 3 in the thoracic region). The clinical data from all 27 of these patients are shown in Table 19–1. The mean age was 26 years (range, 15 to 66 years), and the mean duration of symptoms was 3.5 months (range, 0 to 36 months).

Treatment included subtotal excision followed by radiation therapy in one patient with a vertebral lesion and in one patient with a sacral lesion. Complete resection was carried out for 11 vertebral and 10 sacral lesions. Adjuvant radiation therapy was utilized for nine patients in this group. Radiation alone after histologic confirmation by biopsy was given to three patients with giant cell tumor of the sacrum. When radiation was utilized, usually 4,000 to 5,000 cGy were administered over a four-week period. In most instances, this was followed by radiographic evidence of gradual sclerosis, particularly at the margins.

Overall, control was noted in 11 of the 13 vertebral giant cell tumors (85 per cent). This included 10 of the 11 patients treated with complete en bloc excision and one of two patients treated with subtotal excision with or without radiation therapy. One patient died of his disease; this patient had a malignant giant cell lesion in the thoracic area which may have been induced by radiation therapy (Case 9). Twelve patients were alive and well at the time of follow-up (mean, 7.0 years). Six patients were free of disease more than 5 years after diagnosis, and two have remained free of disease more than 10 years after diagnosis.

Tumor control was achieved in 12 (86 per cent) of the 14 patients with sacral lesions. This included 9

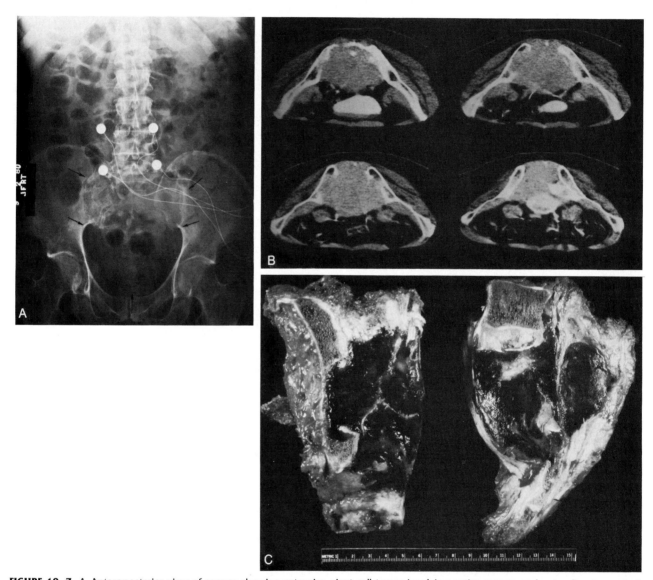

FIGURE 19–7. *A,* Anteroposterior view of sacrum showing extensive giant cell tumor involving entire sacrum and extending to posterior ilium. *B,* Computed tomography scans showing extent of involvement; a large soft tissue mass is present. *C,* Surgical specimen showing red-brown lesion extending into L5 vertebra and spinal cord.

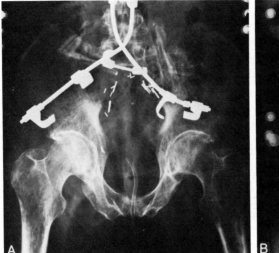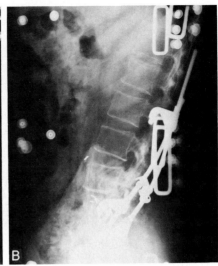

FIGURE 19–8. Same patient as in Figure 19–7, 6 months after fusion. Anteroposterior (*A*) and lateral (*B*) radiographs of lumbar spine.

of the 10 patients treated by complete en bloc excision and one patient treated with subtotal excision with radiation therapy. Radiation alone achieved control in two of three patients (67 per cent). In the sacral tumor group there were two patients with benign metastasis; one (Case 21) died with progressive pulmonary involvement. One patient (Case 27) had a malignant course and was alive with metastatic disease at one year after treatment; however, this patient was lost to follow-up. Nine patients with sacral lesions were free of their disease at 5 years, and four of them were free of disease at 10 years after diagnosis.

Recurrences were noted in 5 of 27 patients (18 per cent) after treatment at our institution. Two of these recurrences were from spinal lesions (Cases 4 and 11), and three were from sacral lesions (Cases 14, 19, and 21). One of the recurrences in the spine was successfully treated with radiation alone; all of the sacral recurrences were treated with a second excision.

For recurrent sacral lesions that have not responded to local excision and radiation therapy, radical removal of the entire sacrum and lower lumbar spine may be necessary for cure (Figs. 19–7 and 19–8). By the time this is necessary, bowel and bladder functions are already compromised. However, this operation does necessitate sacrifice of sciatic nerve function and requires an extensive reconstructive procedure. In these instances, resection is facilitated by an anterior and posterior approach with ligation of the internal iliac arteries to reduce vascularity. Moreover, embolization before surgery has been effective in reducing vascularity.

CONCLUSION

Giant cell tumor of the spine is not common—the incidence ranges from 1.2 to 3.8 per cent of all vertebral tumors.[1, 6, 27] The sacrum, however, is the fourth most common location for this tumor. Lesions located in these areas pose challenging treatment problems in orthopedic oncology and require a team approach to management. Complete surgical resection is preferred. However, the location and extent of the tumor often mandate incomplete excision with supervoltage radiation therapy postoperatively.

REFERENCES

1. Arseni C, Horvath L, Maretsis M, Carp N: Giant cell tumors of the calvaria. J Neurosurg 42:535–540, 1975.
2. Bell RS, Harwood AR, Goodman SB, Fornasier VL: Supervoltage radiotherapy in the treatment of difficult giant cell tumors of bone. Clin Orthop 174:208–216, 1983.
3. Berman HL: The treatment of benign giant-cell tumors of the vertebrae by irradiation. Radiology 83:202–207, 1964.
4. Cahan WG, Woodard HQ, Higinbotham NL, et al: Sarcoma arising in irradiated bone: Report of eleven cases. Cancer 1:3–29, 1948.
5. Campanacci M, Giunti A, Olmi R: Giant-cell tumours of bone: A study of 209 cases with long-term follow-up in 130. Ital J Orthop Traumatol 1:249–277, 1975.
6. Cohen DM, Dahlin DC, MacCarty CS: Vertebral giant-cell tumor and variants. Cancer 17:461–472, 1964.
7. Dahlin DC: Giant-cell tumor of vertebrae above the sacrum: A review of 31 cases. Cancer 39:1350–1356, 1977.
8. Dahlin DC, Cupps RE, Johnson EW Jr: Giant-cell tumor: A study of 195 cases. Cancer 25:1061–1070, 1970.
9. Dahlin DC, Unni KK: Bone Tumors: General Aspects and Data on 8,542 Cases. 4th ed. Springfield, IL, Charles C Thomas, 1986.
10. Di Lorenzo N, Spallone A, Nolletti A, Nardi P: Giant cell tumors of the spine: A clinical study of six cases, with emphasis on the radiological features, treatment and follow-up. Neurosurgery 6:29–34, 1980.
11. Ellis F: Treatment of osteoclastoma by radiation. J Bone Joint Surg [Br] 31:268–280, 1949.
12. Geschickter CF, Copeland MM: Tumors of Bone. 3rd ed. Philadelphia, JB Lippincott Co., 1949, pp 303–304.
13. Goldenberg RR, Campbell CJ, Bonfiglio M: Giant-cell tumor of bone: An analysis of two hundred and eighteen cases. J Bone Joint Surg [Am] 52:619, 1970.
14. Hutter RVP, Worcester JN Jr, Francis KC, et al: Benign and malignant giant cell tumors of bone: A clinicopathological analysis of the natural history of the disease. Cancer 15:653–690, 1962.
15. Jaffe HL: Tumors and Tumorous Conditions of the Bones and Joints. Philadelphia, Lea & Febiger, 1958.
16. Johnson EW Jr, Dahlin DC: Treatment of giant-cell tumor of bone. J Bone Joint Surg [Am] 41:895–904, 1959.
17. Keplenger JE, Bucy PC: Giant-cell tumors of the spine. Ann Surg 154:648–660, 1961.

18. Larsson JE, Lorentzon R, Boquist L: Giant-cell tumor of bone. A demographic, clinical and histopathological study of all cases recorded in the Swedish Cancer Registry for the years 1958 through 1968. J Bone Joint Surg [Am] 57:167–173, 1975.

19. Larsson JE, Lorentzon R, Boquist L: Giant-cell tumors of the spine and sacrum causing neurological symptoms. Clin Orthop 111:201–211, 1975.

20. Lièvre J-A, Darcy M, Pradat P, et al: Tumeur a cellules géantes du rachis lombaire, spondylectomie totale en deux temps. Rev Rhum Mal Osteoartic 35:125–130, 1968.

21. McDonald DJ, Sim FH, McLeod RA, Dahlin DC: Giant-cell tumor of bone. J Bone Joint Surg [Am] 68:235–242, 1986.

22. McGrath PJ: Giant-cell tumour of bone: An analysis of fifty-two cases. J Bone Joint Surg [Br] 54:216–229, 1972.

23. Mnaymneh WA, Dudley HR, Mnaymneh LG: Giant-cell tumor of bone: An analysis and follow-up study of the forty-one cases observed at the Massachusetts General Hospital between 1925 and 1960. J Bone Joint Surg [Am] 46:63–74, 1964.

24. Netherlands Committee on Bone Tumours: Localization in the Skeleton of Fourteen Hundred and Two Primary Tumours and Tumour-Like Lesions. Paris, Mouton & Company, 1966.

25. Prossor TM: Treatment of giant-cell tumours of bone: With a review of twenty-five cases. J Bone Joint Surg [Br] 31:241–251, 1949.

26. Savini R, Gherlinzoni F, Morandi M, et al: Surgical treatment of giant-cell tumor of the spine. J Bone Joint Surg [Am] 65:1283, 1983.

27. Schajowicz F: Giant-cell tumors of bone (osteoclastoma): A pathological and histochemical study. J Bone Joint Surg [Am] 43:1–29, 1961.

28. Spjut HJ, Dorfman HD, Fechner RE, Ackerman LV: Tumors of bone and cartilage. In Atlas of Tumor Pathology. Section 2, Fascicle 5. Washington, DC, Armed Forces Institute of Pathology, 1971, pp 201–232.

29. Stener B, Johnsen OE: Complete removal of three vertebrae for giant-cell tumour. J Bone Joint Surg [Br] 53:278, 1971.

30. Sung H, Kuo DP, Shu WP, et al: Giant-cell tumor of bone: Analysis of two hundred and eight cases in Chinese patients. J Bone Joint Surg [Am] 64:755, 1982.

31. Takechi H, Eto S, Taguchi R: Follow-up study of giant cell tumor of bone. Acta Med Okayama 365:349, 1982.

32. Windeyer BW, Woodyatt PB: Osteoclastoma: A study of thirty-eight cases. J Bone Joint Surg [Br] 1:252–267, 1949.

33. Yuan-zhang M, Hua-feng T, Ben-fu C, Yan-qing Y: Radical resection of dorsolumbar vertebra and prosthetic replacement in giant cell tumor. Chin Med J [Engl] 95:537, 1982.

20

VASCULAR TUMORS OF THE SPINE

T. FORCHT DAGI and HENRY H. SCHMIDEK

INTRODUCTION

Primary tumors of the vertebral bodies are rare, and vascular tumors—with the exception of hemangiomas—are even rarer. Nonetheless, recent advances in neuroimaging, interventional radiology, and techniques of spinal resection and stabilization mandate a reconsideration of this group of lesions and their current management.

During embryologic development, the mesenchymal layer of the embryo differentiates into fibroblasts, chondroblasts, and osteoblasts. This same tissue also gives rise to the vertebral bodies. In the course of maturation, the sclerotome becomes intimately involved with vascular, neuronal, lipomatous, and hematopoietic elements.[39] Any of these can become the origin of benign or malignant tumors in which vascular elements will be represented to a greater or lesser extent.

CLASSIFICATION OF VASCULAR TUMORS THAT INVOLVE THE SPINE

The classification of vascular tumors that involve the spine is shown in Table 20–1. There are two basic categories of primary bone tumors: benign and malignant. This chapter will focus on hemangiomas, angiolipomas, angiosarcomas, and hemangiopericytomas. The latter are often simply referred to as a subcategory of angiosarcomas. Disappearing bone disease, also called massive or essential osteolysis, Gorham's disease, and Jackson-Gorham's disease, may represent multiple hemangiomas confined to a single bone or appearing in several adjacent bones

TABLE 20–1. CLASSIFICATION OF VASCULAR TUMORS OF THE SPINE

Benign
Hemangioma
Disappearing bone disease
Angiolipoma

Malignant
Hemangioendothelioma (angiosarcoma)
Hemangiopericytoma

and is included for this reason.[33, 34] Huvos suggests that Kümmell's disease—wedging of the vertebral body without obvious cause—may be a related phenomenon.

Hemangioma of the Osseous Spine

A hemangioma (benign hemangioendothelioma) is a benign lesion of bone, occasionally hamartomatous, but at other times a true neoplasm, consisting of newly formed capillary, cavernous, or venous blood vessels.[33]

Most hemangiomas of bone are asymptomatic. Huvos[33] cites an overall incidence of 11 per cent in five large autopsy series; Dahlin reported 47 symptomatic hemangiomas in a series of 3987 (1.2 per cent). Jacobson cites a similar figure: 0.9 per cent of 1650. In long bones, hemangiomas can cause pulsating pain. In the vertebral column, localized pain and muscle spasm with variable neurologic symptomatology are characteristic.[45, 50] The pedicles and spinous processes may be preferentially involved,[72] and neurologic deficits can occur specifically from expansion of the neural arch (ref. 45, Case 4), from enlargement of the vertebral body,[42] and from neural compression by epidural tissue or epidural hemorrhage[7, 37] (also, ref. 56, Case 1). Alternatively, the spine may be deformed because it becomes biomechanically unstable. This results in kyphosis or scoliosis. An important characteristic of hemangiomas is that they rarely cause compression fractures, perhaps because the coarse trabeculations within the body buttress the weaker parts.[45] Curvature of the spine occurs because of mechanical forces on a single involved body at a critical point, rather than from compression fracture.[5, 7, 21] Although the *absence* of cortical fractures has been emphasized as an important differential radiographic sign, high resolution computed tomography (CT) has indicated that cortical disruptions can occur in affected vertebrae[42] and that, in contradistinction to other pathologic fractures, compression fractures that accompany spinal hemangioma often heal with time.[3] This observation suggests that treatment by immobilization may suffice in particular cases.

In the spine, the thoracic region is most commonly involved by these lesions.[55] Women are affected slightly more frequently. The incidence seems to increase after middle age, but in the clinically significant group, young adults predominate.[33] In an autopsy series of 409 spinal hemangiomas, the incidence of single lesions was 66.5 per cent; of two to five tumors, 32.8 per cent; and of more than five tumors, 0.7 per cent.[35] Rarely do osseous hemangiomas arise outside of the spine or in the craniofacial bones.

Symptomatic hemangiomas have been misdiagnosed as herniated discs. Multiple lesions can mimic spinal metastases.[72] Hemorrhage can arise from large dilated vessels in the bone, from the soft tissue component in the epidural canal, or from anomalous vessels draining or feeding the lesion.[33, 36] Spinal cord compression may occur from expansion of the vertebral bodies or the neural arch, from extension along a nerve root or into the epidural space, from compression fractures, or from hematoma.[3] The lesion can also present primarily as a vascular epidural mass.[3, 7, 29, 37, 45, 56]

Vertebral hemangiomas have been reported in association with various systemic conditions and congenital anomalies. For example, a 13-year-old boy presented with scoliosis and multiple vertebral cavernous hemangiomas.[43] He was shown to have systemic hemangiomatosis with both skeletal and extraskeletal hemangiomas. This condition can be complicated by consumptive coagulopathy. In another report, a 16-month-old male presented with subarachnoid hemorrhage in the late stages of *Haemophilus influenzae* meningitis (ref. 9, Case 2). There was an 8 × 3 cm congenital port-wine nevus over the right lumbar region. A soft tissue mass was palpable under the nevus, and a thrill was present in the mass. Weakness of the right lower extremity had been recognized since one month of age. Angiography demonstrated an intraspinal arteriovenous malformation (AVM) extending from T6 and L3 as well as a large capillary hemangioma eroding the 12th thoracic and first three lumbar vertebrae. Following partial embolization, the hemangioma was removed without difficulty. The AVM was left for a second stage. The child proved to have Klippel-Trenaunay-Weber syndrome, a form of angiomatosis related to other neurocutaneous syndromes and associated with cutaneous nevi, cutaneous and subcutaneous hemangiomata, phlebectasia, and hypertrophy of the affected parts of the body.

Radiographic Features

Plain spinal radiographs are often diagnostic (Figs. 20–1 and 20–2), although sometimes a differential diagnosis will have to be considered. These studies demonstrate vertically striated vertebral bodies owing to reactive ossification around areas of hemangioma and producing a "honeycomb" or "corduroy cloth" appearance. At least one third of the body must be involved for the classic findings to be recognizable on plain film.[29] The tumor generally involves the body primarily, but it can extend to the posterior elements and even to the ribs. Erosion of these

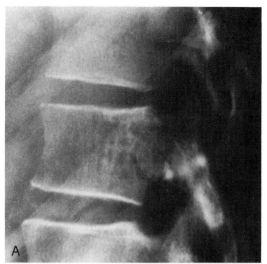

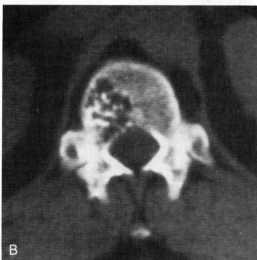

FIGURE 20–1. *A,* A lateral plain film of T12 demonstrates vertically oriented lucencies separated by thickened trabecular bone occupying the posterior half of the vertebral body. There is no evidence of vertebral expansion or cortical destruction. A small amount of contrast material is present within the spinal canal from a previous myelogram. *B,* A CT scan demonstrates that the lucent lesion is confined to the right half of the vertebral body and extends into the base of the pedicle. The low attenuation values seen within this lesion represent intralesional fat, a common finding in hemangioma. When cut in cross-section by the CT scan, the vertically oriented trabeculations appear as punctate regions of increased density.

structures is not specific, but the honeycombed expansion of the vertebral body and the neural arch is highly characteristic. The cortices and disc spaces are usually intact, although in one unusual case reported by Leehey and coworkers[42] the degree of cortical disruption was quite striking. Collapse of the vertebral body is equally unusual and is more characteristic of metastatic disease than of hemangioma. Vertebral body collapse obscures the characteristic radiographic findings of spinal hemangioma and invalidates these diagnosis criteria. Healy and colleagues claim that approximately one third of involved spines have multiple vertebrae—up to five—affected.[29]

Paravertebral soft tissue masses can be seen in conjunction with vertebral hemangiomas. These masses may represent paravertebral hematomas[3] or extravertebral tumor extension (Fig. 20–2).

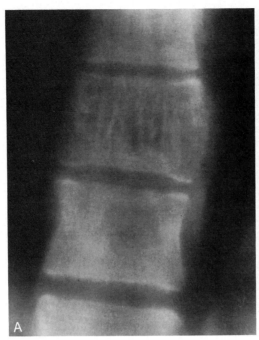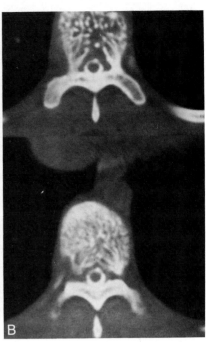

FIGURE 20-2. *A,* An anteroposterior tomogram of T10 demonstrates the typical findings of hemangioma occupying the entire vertebral body. There is a very small paravertebral soft tissue mass. *B,* CT scan sections from this patient demonstrate the coarsened trabeculations to good advantage. There is contrast within the spinal canal from a myelogram. There is no evidence of epidural mass effect.

Tuberculosis may also cause paravertebral masses; unlike hemangiomatous vertebrae, tuberculous vertebrae usually collapse. But even before they collapse, tuberculous vertebral bodies can usually be identified by destruction of the intervertebral disc and anterior vertebral erosions. Vertical striations are not seen with tuberculosis. Metastatic changes can be distinguished from bony spinal hemangiomas by the presence of cortical erosion, by the degree of osteolysis, and by the tendency to collapse. Bony expansion is rare in metastatic disease (except for renal cell carcinoma and myeloma), and destruction or erosion of the pedicle at noncontiguous levels other than the one under scrutiny is quite common when multiple sites are affected by a metastatic process. Paget's disease, especially the monostotic variant, creates trabeculations in bone that are superficially similar to those induced by hemangiomas. On detailed examination, however, they are far more coarse and are accompanied by cortical thickening, giving a "picture frame" appearance to the vertebral body. In addition, Paget's disease usually involves other bony structures and is accompanied by an elevated serum alkaline phosphatase level. Other causes of trabeculated bone include multiple myeloma, lymphoma, and blood dyscrasias.[42]

Examination by CT scan demonstrates the bony changes of hemangioma to best advantage.[9, 11, 44, 56] The expansion of the body and the involvement of the arch can be clearly seen. Hemangiomas may or may not be enhanced by the injection of intravenous contrast material. Soft tissue expansion into the paravertebral space and soft tissue incursion into the epidural space can be identified. The soft tissue mass is usually enhanced. Brooks and colleagues demonstrate the usefulness of modified bolus injection technique for contrast enhancement (ref. 9, Case 1). Schnyder and associates recommend additional CT examination after intrathecal contrast injection to delineate the epidural component of the tumor (ref. 56, Case 1).

The diagnosis can be refined angiographically.[45] Typically, a hemangioma is fed by the intercostal arteries through branches proximal to the radicular vessels. There is usually a very prominent and very extensive tumor blush.[71] Multiple pools of contrast medium in the lesion coalesce and opacify the tumor (ref. 45, Cases 7, 8, and 9). Eisenstein and colleagues reported one case in which the angiographically delineated extent of the tumor was not appreciated on CT soon.[16] Schnyder and coworkers, in contrast, reported two cases in which angiography was normal or nonconclusive while CT scan was diagnostic. In both cases, acute myelopathy was caused by hemorrhage, and the hematoma impeded angiographic visualization of the lesion.[56] Feuerman and colleagues treated a radiographically similar case of subacute myelopathy in which angiography did not disclose a major brush.[19] Angiography is not ipso facto diagnostic of hemangioma and cannot reliably distinguish between hemangioma and other equally vascular tumors. Nonetheless, selective spinal angiography is necessary if surgical resection is contemplated. The artery of Adamkiewicz should be identified in lesions of the lower thoracic spine.

Myelography, historically the most useful technique for localizing compressive lesions in the spine, has been eclipsed by CT scan. Myelographic findings are not specific in hemangiomatous compression of neural elements.[45] Radioisotope bone scans may be negative in hemangiomas and are of little use except to distinguish metastatic disease from hemangiomas.[4, 45, 72]

Pathology

Grossly, the lesion may arise either in the marrow spaces or in the periosteum, with secondary resorption of underlying bone producing a honeycomb

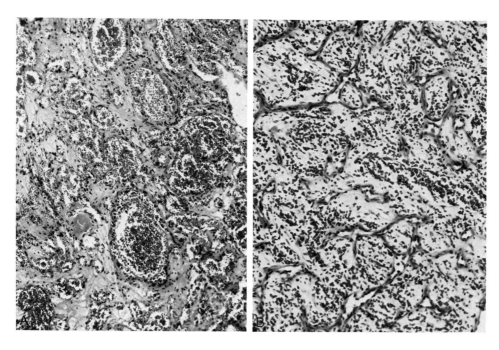

FIGURE 20–3. *A,* Hemangioma composed of large dilated vascular spaces filled with blood. The intervening stroma is coarse fibrous tissue (H & E ×125). *B,* A higher power view of a hemangioma with interconnecting vascular spaces lined by prominent, but flat, endothelial cells (H & E ×157).

bloody mass. Microscopically, the capillary hemangiomas have numerous capillary channels with occasional larger feeding vessels. The endothelial lining is composed of small, flat, uniform, endothelial cells. The cavernous type comprises multiple, large, thin-walled, vascular spaces lined by flat endothelial cells. The venous type has small, thick-walled, venous vessels intermixed with arterioles, capillaries, or large feeding vessels[33] (Figs. 20–3 and 20–4). Aneurysmal bone cysts, sometimes grossly similar to hemangiomas, are distinguished by the lack of endothelial cells lining the large hemorrhagic spaces. The presence of fibrous tissue and reactive bone with multinucleated giant cells also speaks for aneurysmal bone cyst.

Treatment

Hemangiomas are radiosensitive lesions showing changes following the administration of 3000 to 4000 cGy.[18, 22] Historically, treatment often consisted of radiation, sometimes combined with decompressive laminectomy.[7] This form of treatment was used particularly to treat pain. Of eight patients with radiographically demonstrated hemangiomas and back pain (but without a tissue diagnosis) treated by Faria and associates, 77 per cent reported significant pain relief over 6 to 44 months following x-ray therapy.[18] Glanzmann and associates reported a similar experience with a series of 62 patients accumulated over a 36-year period.[22] Another large series, that of Yang and colleagues, reports pain relief in 87.5 per cent of 16 patients in whom pain was the primary complaint. Five of seven patients with paraplegia of several weeks' duration recovered function: three allegedly became normal, although detailed neurologic information is not provided.[70] Although radiotherapy is effective for treatment of pain without neurologic deficit, this approach is controversial.[16] The complications of radiation for this indication have not been tabulated. Faria and coworkers observed that the appearance of the affected bone may not change despite the achievement of symptomatic relief.[18]

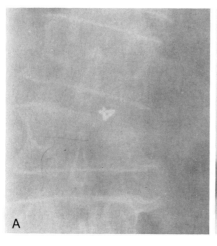
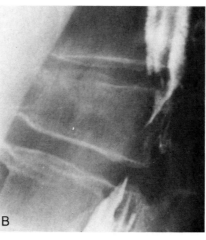

FIGURE 20–4. Anteroposterior and lateral views of L2 demonstrate a destructive lytic process involving the left pedicle and the left side of the vertebral body. There is complete destruction of the superior end plate and the left natural vertebral margin. The borders of the lesion are poorly seen and are highly irregular. No definite soft tissue mass can be appreciated on these plain films. There is residual contrast material within the spinal canal from a previous myelogram. The appearances are entirely nonspecific and could represent any malignant neoplasm.

Because the operative morbidity and mortality in the past were unacceptably high, decompression was recommended only for symptomatic cord compression.[33, 43, 45] Currently, fine needle biopsy techniques are capable of confirming the diagnosis while minimizing the risk of hemorrhage, even from highly vascular lesions such as spinal hemangioblastomas.[57] With or without biopsy as a preliminary step, surgical treatment of symptomatic cases can be achieved through a combination of staged intravascular techniques and vertebral body resection.

Therapeutic approaches that combine endovascular techniques with surgical resection or radiation have evolved over the past 15 years. Hekster and coworkers first demonstrated that spinal cord compression by vertebral hemangioma could be reversed by percutaneous embolization of feeding vessels.[30] Radiotherapy was administered afterward for a definitive treatment. Benati and colleagues combined embolization with laminectomy for decompression.[6] Gross and associates reported one patient with a T9 level and progressive spastic paraparesis following two operative decompressions in whom embolization was used to treat recurrent disease. Percutaneous embolization with Gelfoam slivers (2 × 6 mm) suspended in saline relieved a myelographic block and was followed by clinical improvement.[26] Actual resection of a hemangiomatous vertebral body following embolization was first reported in 1977.[31] Embolization alone can relieve subarachnoid block, provide symptomatic relief of pain, and render a highly vascular lesion amenable to surgery at lower risk. Nonetheless, there is, to date, insufficient long-term follow-up to determine whether embolization alone can cure hemangiomas definitively or whether, like cerebral AVMs, endovascular techniques should be considered essentially a preoperative (or preradiative) modality. Gelfoam particles, for example, produce only temporary occlusion of tumor vessels and are usually followed by recanalization.[8]

Recent reports have emphasized the success of aggressive surgical approaches including preoperative embolization, radical tumor resection, and spinal reconstruction and stabilization for individual cases of hemangioma occupying the vertebral body.[25, 31] Combined anterior and posterior approaches have been utilized. No large series has been reported to date, however. Graham's case was unusual in that the patient, an elderly woman, presented with a back pain, a compression fracture at the site of a previously biopsied but unresected T12 hemangioma, and generalized osteoporosis.[25]

In the presence of only modest tumor vascularity, or in the absence of discernible feeders, vertebral body resection may proceed without embolization. Feuerman and coworkers successfully treated a 62-year-old woman with radiating back pain and symptoms of neurogenic claudication whose T10 vertebral body had been replaced by hemangioma. Despite the presence of a myelographic block, spinal angiography showed that the tumor, fed by the T10 intercostal vessels, was only minimally vascular. The affected body was resected transthoracically and replaced with

an iliac crest strut graft with a blood loss of approximately 1000 cc.[19] Fusion proceeded without difficulty. Laminectomy, the traditional surgical approach to compressive spine lesions, should be restricted to lesions lying posteriorly and sparing the vertebral body. In the case of hemangiomas, only those that uniquely affect the neural arch should be approached in this manner.[12] The authors have had no personal experience with transpedicular or costotransversectomy approaches to the vertebral body for hemangiomatous invasion, and the literature is silent on this point. By analogy with other anteriorly situated lesions, however, it seems preferable to choose a transthoracic approach if at all possible.

Angiolipoma of the Osseous Spine

An angiolipoma is a benign neoplasm of adipose tissue with a prominent vascular component.[67] These tumors constitute a biologically distinct, exceedingly rare, subgroup of spinal lipomas that have also been called, at times, angiolipoma, angiomyolipoma, hemangiolipoma, and fibrolipoma. Six epidural angiolipomas have been reported to involve the vertebral body or neural arch. Two manifested trabeculated changes in the vertebral body suggestive of hemangioma; four did not.[24, 51, 54, 67] Most of the angiolipomas described presented with a dorsal or dorsolaterally situated epidural mass and neural compression, although those cases that invaded the vertebral body were associated with a more anterior or anterolaterally situated epidural component.

The lesions are unencapsulated and are permeated with small and medium caliber vessels. Some of these vessels may be arteries showing abnormal variation in the thickness of the media and a marked degree of smooth muscle proliferation extending into the adjacent fat. Large venous spaces and numerous thin-walled blood vessels are evident.[54, 67] The bony trabeculations of the vertebra are invaded. The prominence of other mesenchymal elements in some reported cases reflects a continuum between the angiolipomas and the angiomyolipomas. In the absence of an obvious lipoma, it might be very difficult or even impossible to differentiate this tumor from hemangioma extending into the (otherwise normal) epidural space.[67] This entity appears to be distinct from neoplastic angioendotheliosis.[4] The CT scan in the case reported by von Hanwehr and associates was not enhanced after contrast injection.[67]

Gross total removal appears to result in cure.[51, 54] Whereas neurologic improvement has followed decompression in reported cases, it is not clear whether complete resection is always possible, or even necessary.

Angiosarcoma of the Osseous Spine

Angiosarcoma (hemangioendothelioma, malignant angioma, angioendothelioma, angiofibrosarcoma, hemangiosarcoma, hemangioblastoma, angioblastic

TABLE 20–2. DIFFERENTIATING CHARACTERISTICS: HEMANGIOMA AND ANGIOSARCOMA

	HEMANGIOMA	ANGIOSARCOMA
Gross appearance	Brown-red, soft	Rubbery, fleshy, sponge-like organizing clot
Origin	Vertebral body, marrow, periosteum	Cortex or medulla
Microscopic appearance	Sparsely cellular, thickly trabeculated	Bone invaded by cellular tumor
Vessels	Capillary spaces	Small capillaries dominant structure
Endothelium	Small flat uniform, inconspicuous with rare mitoses	Plump, pleomorphic, hyperchromatic endothelial cells, "buds," mitoses, stroma infiltrated by sarcoma cells

sarcoma, hemangioendothelioblastoma, malignant angioblastoma, intravascular endothelioma, and multiple endothelioma) is a malignant tumor composed primarily of neoplastic blood vessels. This categorization does not include spinal hemangioblastomas associated with von Hippel-Lindau disease or other varieties of multiple hemangiomatosis (e.g., Wyburn-Mason disease). Hemangioblastomas are classically intramedullary and do not involve the vertebral bodies. There is one case, however, reported by Stevens[60] of a histologically proven solitary hemangioblastoma involving the pedicles and body of T9 with a soft, extremely vascular mass. It produced a bony texture much like that accompanying cavernous hemangioma.

Angiosarcoma refers to a solitary or multifocal neoplasm characterized by irregular anastomosing vascular channels lined by one or more layers of anaplastic, endothelial cells.[33] This is an exceedingly rare lesion, constituting less than 1 per cent of all primary malignant bone tumors and having a calculated annual incidence of one case per 14,000,000.[33] Of 39 cases with solitary bone involvement at Memorial Hospital in New York (representing approximately one third of all documented angiosarcomas), two (5.1 per cent) involved the vertebral column. Several individual cases have been reported recently, bringing the number of histologically confirmed examples to 14.[10, 14, 23, 38, 41, 47]

Multifocal angiosarcomas tend to cluster in one anatomic region, even to the extent of remaining monostotic. Unifocal lesions are less likely to appear in the vertebrae than elsewhere. There is no discernible sex or age preference except in multifocal disease, for which the age of presentation is 10 years younger and males predominate. Unifocal lesions, in general, are more poorly differentiated. Differentiation of angiosarcomas from hemangiomas is generally straightforward. The differentiating characteristics are summarized in Tables 20–2 and 20–3.

Presentation in the vertebral body is not character-

TABLE 20–3. DEMOGRAPHICS: HEMANGIOMA VS. ANGIOSARCOMA

	INCIDENCE	DEMOGRAPHICS
Hemangioma	11% spine tumors, 1% all bone tumors (Mayo)	F > M, symptomatic in younger adults
Angiosarcoma	5% all bone tumors (Mayo), no valid estimate of incidence in spine	Monofocal: F = M; polyostotic: F > M, younger onset

ized by any pathognomonic symptom complex. The duration of symptoms is variable.

Radiographic Features

These tumors are osteolytic and erode the cortex. An occasional zone of sclerosis surrounds the tumor. The borders vary from well demarcated to indistinct. Their general appearance in the vertebral column is not specific and cannot be well differentiated from solitary plasmacytoma or metastasis. Metastatic renal cell and thyroid carcinoma rank high in the differential diagnosis (Fig. 20–4).

Angiography clearly demonstrates the vascularity of these lesions, although they occasionally stain poorly in the periphery. It is uncommon to find evidence of arteriovenous shunting. Extension into neighboring soft tissues is well delineated, especially by magnetic resonance imaging (MRI).

Bone scan was negative in a case of angiosarcoma of the sacrum reported by Lee, who notes that false-negative studies are occasionally encountered in aggressive, lytic tumors.[41]

Pathology

These are soft, fleshy tumors that give the gross appearance of an organizing rubbery blood clot. Tumor nodules are often well delineated and appear in the cortex or in the medulla. Microscopically, there is great capillary proliferation. Although the inherent neoplastic quality of the hyperchromic, plump endothelial lining is debated, this cell type clearly predominates. In large lesions, the central portions may be of spindle or polygonal sarcoma cells, whereas the periphery demonstrates continuing vascular proliferation. Pleomorphic endothelial cells line the vascular channels. Cystlike changes can occur (Fig. 20–5).

The biologic activity of these tumors is variable. Many authors, beginning with Thomas in 1942 and Stout one year later, have emphasized the existence of a spectrum of malignancy.[14, 38, 47, 61, 66, 69] Benign angiosarcomas are encapsulated and "pseudoinvasive," according to Neumärker, and are synonymous with capillary hemangioma. The histologic appearance of malignant hemangioendotheliomas (angiosarcoma), however, is more protean, and their behavior is sarcomatous.[47] In a histologic study of 29 tumors, including four of spinal origin, Campanacci and colleagues identified three categories based on histologic differentiation and natural history.[10] Grade I behaves as hemangioma.[38] Grade III is sarcomatous. Grade II is transitional and unpredictable. Two cases

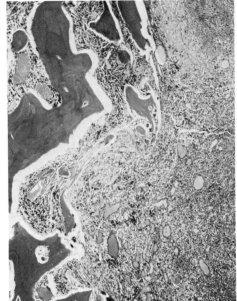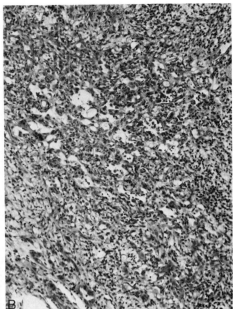

FIGURE 20–5. *A,* A low power view of an angiosarcoma showing invasion into the cortex and infiltration into the haversian channels. Such a pattern is often seen with malignant tumors (H & E ×50). *B,* Angiosarcoma composed of small irregular vascular spaces lined by plump atypical endothelial cells (H & E ×125).

of spinal origin in Campanacci's series were Grade II, and two were Grade III. Lange's case was Grade I, although it was particularly unusual in that a benign hemangioendothelioma arose adjacent to an osteoblastoma.[38]

Unifocal lesions contain anaplastic lining and stromal endothelial cells with atypical mitoses suggestive of a high grade sarcoma. In Huvos' series, the multifocal lesions are less anaplastic with a more restrained cellular pleomorphism.

The differential diagnosis of this lesion includes aneurysmal bone cysts as well as other vascular bone tumors, both primary and metastatic (Table 20–2).[33]

Treatment

Prolonged survival has been reported following forequarter or hindquarter amputation or total en bloc resection of peripheral lesions. Vertebral body lesions have traditionally been treated with radiation therapy after subtotal excision. Radical removal utilizing combined endovascular and microsurgical approaches should be considered.[46] Torrential bleeding may be anticipated if the blood supply is unmodified: one of Lange and colleagues' patients lost an estimated 5200 cc during the subtotal curettage of a one-level lesion; Edinger was forced to terminate the procedure because of hemorrhage (cited as Example 4 in ref. 47). The survival in unifocal extravertebral disease is 18 per cent over five years using current treatment modalities.[33] With vertebral involvement survival has exceeded three years in two patients: Lange's case[38] of a hemangioma at T10 (Campanacci Grade I) remains well 45 months after diagnosis, and Edinger's case at T4-T6 which was classified as frankly malignant remains unchanged after four years. The first case was not irradiated; the second received 1600 cGy. There is one reported case of metastasis to lung and kidney in a 67-year-old woman with an inoperable malignant lesion at C6-C7. Survival in this case was 22 weeks.[65]

Hemangiopericytoma

There are approximately 30 cases of vertebral hemangiopericytoma reported in the literature.[1, 13, 28, 44, 46, 58] This entity, first described by Stout and Murray in 1942, is believed to originate from the Zimmermann pericyte, a contractile cell related to smooth muscle.[64] Tumor cells are outside the connective tissue sheaths of blood vessels and capillaries; this feature is one of two that distinguish hemangiopericytomas from a typical angiosarcoma.[44] The other is the lack of Factor VIII–related antigen immunoperoxidase staining[13] (Table 20–4). There is no sex or age preponderance. One reported case had the

TABLE 20–4. HEMANGIOPERICYTOMAS AND ANGIOSARCOMAS: MICROSCOPIC DIFFERENTIAL DIAGNOSIS

	HEMANGIOPERICYTOMA	ANGIOSARCOMA
Infiltration	Diffuse	Diffuse
Gross appearance	Vascular	Soft, friable, and vascular
Encapsulation	Poor	Very poor
Dominant cell type	Pericyte	Malignant endothelial cells and pericytes
Necrosis	Not prominent	Prominent
Hemosiderin deposits	Not prominent	Prominent
Intracellular HGE	Not prominent	Prominent
Anastomotic channels	None	May be present
Mitoses	Variable	Common
Distinguishing features seen with reticulum stain	Tumor cells *outside* connective tissue sheaths of blood vessels	Hyperchromatic nuclei, bizarre mitotic figures, and vessels plugged by tumor; tumor cells *inside* connective tissue sheath of blood vessels

same histologic appearance in the vertebra of C4 as a previously excised angioblastic meningioma.[1]

These tumors are exceedingly rare in bone. Most of the available information is derived from reports of systemic hemangiopericytomas. Between 15 and 57 per cent of tumors metastasize, usually within five years but as late as 26 years after presentation.[1, 17, 28, 32, 44, 46, 49]

Pathology

Hemangiopericytomas contain two separate histologic components. The vascular component consists of capillaries with normal endothelial cells and intact basement membranes, whereas the neoplastic element is composed of ovoid to spindle-shaped cells forming cords or sheets between the vascular elements[28, 62, 63] (Fig. 20–6). The pericyte is frequently referred to as a cell capable of differentiating into endothelial, smooth muscle, or glial elements.[1, 17] Pitlyk and associates suggest that 1 per cent of meningiomas occurring in the spinal canal may be hemangiopericytomas.[52] Transitional forms between hemangiopericytomas, hemangioepitheliomas, and other mesenchymal neoplasms may occur.[13, 46] Fine structure analysis suggests that these tumors are histologically similar to hemangioblastomas and ontogenically distinct from meningiomas,[53] although tissue culture may be needed to differentiate these entities definitively. It may be possible to distinguish hemangiopericytomas from meningiomas by means of differences in the basement membrane and by the presence or absence of cytoplasmic glycogen filaments, cytoplasmic condensations, and desmosomes. Hemangiopericytomas typically have a basement membrane, cytoplasmic filaments of 60 to 80 nm in width, and cytoplasmic condensations, but no desmosomes; whereas meningiomas have prominent desmosomes and lack a basement membrane, intracellular filaments, and cytoplasmic condensations.[12]

Natural History and Treatment

The 10-year survival rate is generally estimated to be on the order of 70 per cent. Specific information for spinal lesions has not been collected.[28] Surgery alone inevitably leaves residual tumor; as with other varieties of angiosarcoma, bleeding can be severe. A case recently encountered at the University of Vermont involved a 20-year-old female with myelopathy, anisocoria, destruction of the C7 and T1 vertebral bodies and partial destruction of the first rib, a myelographic block at the level of T1-T2 from below, and a right-sided paraspinous soft tissue mass extending into the thoracic apex and being enhanced on CT. The tumor was first approached posteriorly via C7-T2 laminectomy and decompressed with a blood loss of 7500 cc. At a second stage with the combination of thoracotomy and a posterior approach, definitive tumor resection was attempted. Despite a 24-hour procedure that required 83 units of packed red cells, 107 units of fresh frozen plasma, 80 units of cryoprecipitate, 64 liters of crystalloid, 40 units of platelets, 2 units of hetastarch, and 2100 cc of autotransfusion, the tumor could not be extirpated. The patient made an excellent neurologic and surgical recovery and was fused posteriorly for stability during a third procedure. There has been no evidence of recurrence over three years.

Although radiation therapy has been recommended on empiric grounds after subtotal decompression, no change in outcome has been demonstrated. Embolization preceding surgery may reduce operative bleeding but risks an increase in neurologic deficit from acute swelling of the mass.[46]

CONCLUSION

The most common presenting symptom of vertebral neoplasms is persistent pain that is unrelieved by rest or positional adjustment. The pain accompanies invasion or displacement of the vertebral body or the adjacent and surrounding tissues, including periosteum, pleura, peritoneum, nerve roots, neural plexus, and spinal cord. The origin of the pain is often difficult to establish, although suggestions have included irritation of these tissues, gross or microscopic pathologic fractures, and vertebral instability.[20] Vascular tumors are often expansile and erode bone.[9]

The presence and the degree of neurologic involvement in association with primary vascular spinal tumors are unpredictable and depend on the location of the tumor, its size, its biologic activity, and the individual anatomy of the spinal canal. Epidural hemorrhage arising from vascular tumors has resulted in acute neurologic deterioration.[7, 37] On the other hand, most hemangiomas are completely asymptomatic.

The process of differential diagnosis should in-

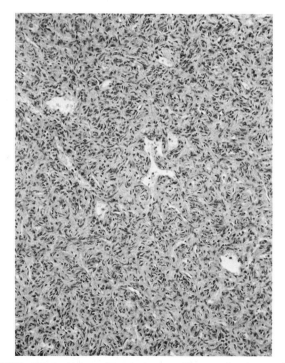

FIGURE 20–6. Hemangiopericytoma with prominent vascular spaces lined by flat endothelial cells. The intervening cells are neoplastic pericytes external to the endothelial lining cells (H & E × 125).

clude complete blood count, sedimentation rate, calcium, phosphorus, total protein, alkaline phosphatase, and skin test for tuberculosis, as well as routine urinalysis and chest x-ray. A serum electrophoresis, assay for prostatic fraction of serum acid phosphatase, and HTLV-III titers are needed in certain settings.

Whenever a primary vertebral neoplasm is suspected, the entire skeleton should be surveyed radiographically. This can be done most simply with a technetium bone scan. Certain lesions produce a false-negative bone scan; thus, 50 per cent of multiple myeloma and certain endocrine disorders will be silent. Vascular lesions are generally well demonstrated, but hemangiomas may fail to take up isotope.[44, 72] A gallium scan may be more sensitive in inflammatory and lymphomatous lesions but provides no advantage in vascular tumors.[20] With nonvascular lesions, the discussion on whether to biopsy the lesion prior to or following a metastatic work-up turns on the age of the patient, the location and accessibility of the tumor, and the clinical setting. Because of the dangers inherent in biopsying vascular tumors, every effort should be made to arrive at a reasonable diagnosis by employing noninvasive measures. This can often be achieved because the radiographic characteristics of these lesions are relatively distinct (Table 20–5). Several imaging modalities will delineate the three-dimensional structural characteristics of a spinal (osseous) tumor. It is also necessary to determine whether the lesion is solitary or multifocal, how it has distorted the normal anatomy, and whether it is associated with any other changes in bony or soft tissue. Standard radiographs with anteroposterior, lateral, and oblique projections; linear or hypocycloidal polytomography; technetium and gallium bone scanning; computed tomography; magnetic resonance imaging; and regional angiography of the conventional or digital variety may all be needed to fully assess the nature of these lesions and attempt to establish their characteristics, often as an antecedent to operation.[20, 68]

Magnetic resonance imaging is now widely used as a general screening technique for the spine. Images are obtained in T1, T2, and balanced (proton-weighted) modes. Vascular tumors on MRI will show a signal dropout in proportion to flow through the lesion. MRI has been known to miss small intraspinal lesions, however, and its sensitivity and specificity for vertebral lesions have not yet been established. For planning a surgical approach, the three-dimensional perspective obtained with MRI is unsurpassed.

Computed tomography has distinct and obvious advantages for assessing bone, particularly in the axial plane. Reformatted sagittal and coronal images, however, are less satisfactory than the images that can be obtained directly on MRI. CT scan demonstrates the extent of bony disruption, the relationship of thecal contents to any masses, and the relationship of the posterior and lateral vertebral elements to the anterior ones. In addition, characteristic and pathognomonic features, such as the thickened bony trabeculations of hemangiomatous vertebrae, are well appreciated on CT scan.[42]

Magnetic resonance imaging may be used as a noninvasive screening procedure to assess the bony and soft tissue compartments prior to (and possibly instead of) myelography. At present, however, a positive MRI should still be supplemented by contrast myelography, in which one combines the fluoroscopic examination with CT scanning of areas of interest. In addition, contrast-enhanced CT scan using intravenous iodine may provide information concerning the nature of the total involvement.

Angiography is always directed at specific sites of interest. Certain digital units have begun to approach cut film angiography in resolution. High speed capabilities (up to 30 frames per second) make digital units invaluable for defining the vascular anatomy when combined with selective arterial injections. The contrast requirements are also reduced.

Finally, physical examination should encompass a search for systemic and local evidence of the nature of the disease. A search for retinal angiomas, hemangiomas, or papilloedema via indirect ophthalmoscopy should be carried out. The skin should be examined to detect cutaneous vascular lesions such as cutaneous hemangiomas, port-wine stains, and soft tissue masses overlying areas of tenderness or of radiographic pathology. As a rule, clinical findings are rarely specific and are often characterized by tenderness, scoliosis, limitation of movement due to spasm or pain, and, much more rarely, neurologic compromise appropriate to the level of the lesion. The general physical examination may be more productive, particularly if other skeletal abnormalities or tumors are discovered.

TABLE 20–5. RADIOGRAPHIC FINDINGS OF PRIMARY VASCULAR SPINE TUMORS

Hemangioma	Angiosarcoma	Hemangiopericytoma
Axial sclerotic strands	Osteolytic	Cortical erosion
Coarse trabeculations	Minimal periosteal reaction	Reactive ossification
Vertical linear reactive ossifications	Borders vary: well demarcated to indistinct	Bone expands
"Corduroy cloth" pattern	Solitary lesions are nonspecific	
Primary site: vertebral body		
Secondary sites: laminae, spinous and transverse processes, disc space, and ribs		
Bone expands		
Vertebra rarely disintegrates		
Collapsed vertebra not pathognomonic		
Frequently accompanied by paravertebral mass		

REFERENCES

1. Anderson C, Rorabeck CH: Skeletal metastases of an intracranial malignant hemangiopericytoma. J Bone Joint Surg (Am) 62:145–148, 1980.
2. Ash P, Loutit JF: The ultrastructure of skeletal haemangiosarcomas induced in mice by strontium-90. J Pathol 122:209–218, 1977.
3. Baker ND, Greenspan A, Neuwirth M: Symptomatic vertebral hemangiomas: A report of four cases. Skeletal Radiol 15:458–463, 1986.
4. Beal MF, Fisher CM: Neoplastic angioendotheliosis. J Neurol Sci 53:359–375, 1982.
5. Bell RL: Hemangioma of a dorsal vertebra with collapse and compression myelopathy. J Neurosurg 12:575–576, 1955.
6. Benati A, Da Pian R, Mazza C, et al: Preoperative embolization of a vertebral hemangioma compressing the spinal cord. Neuroradiology 7:181–183, 1974.
7. Bergstrand A, Hook O, Lidvall H: Vertebral haemangiomas compressing the spinal cord. Acta Neurol Scand 39:59–66, 1963.
8. Berenstein A, Russel E: Gelatin sponge in therapeutic neuroradiology: A subject review. Radiology 141:105–112, 1981.
9. Brooks BS, El Gammal T, Beveridge WD: Erosion of vertebral pedicles by unusual vascular causes. Report of three cases. Neuroradiology 23:107–112, 1982.
10. Campanacci M, Boriani S, Giunti A: Hemangioendothelioma of bone: A study of 29 cases. Cancer 46:804–814, 1980.
11. Cerullo LJ: Commentary on Healy M, Herz DA, Pearl L: Spinal hemangioma. Neurosurgery 13:691, 1983.
12. Ciappetta P, Celli P, Palma L, Mariotini A: Intraspinal hemangiopericytomas. Report of two cases and review of the literature. Spine 10:27–31, 1985.
13. Cuccurulo L, Mignini R, Moraci A, et al: Hemangiopericytoma of the cervical spine. Acta Neurol (Napoli) 6:472–478, 1984.
14. De Santis E, Sessa V: Emangioendotelioma primitivo dell'osso. Chir Organi Mov 66:331–337, 1980.
15. DiLorenzo N, Nardi P, Ciappetta P, Fortuna A: Benign tumors and tumorlike conditions of the spine. Radiological features, treatment and results. Surg Neurol 25:449–456, 1986.
16. Eisenstein S, Spiro F, Browde S, et al: The treatment of a symptomatic vertebral hemangioma by radiotherapy. Spine 11(6):640–642, 1986.
17. Enzinger FM, Smith BH: Hemangiopericytoma: An analysis of 106 cases. Hum Pathol 7:61–82, 1976.
18. Faria SL, Schlupp WR, Chiminazzo H Jr: Radiotherapy in the treatment of vertebral hemangiomas. Int J Radiat Oncol Biol Phys 11:387–390, 1985.
19. Feuerman T, Dwan PS, Young RF: Vertebrectomy for treatment of vertebral hemangioma without pre-operative embolization. J Neurosurg 65:404–406, 1986.
20. Friedlaender GE, Southwick WO: Tumors of the spine. In Rothman, RH, Simeone FA (eds): The Spine. Philadelphia, WB Saunders Co., 1974, pp 1022–1040.
21. Ghormley RK, Adson AW: Hemangioma of vertebrae. J Bone Joint Surg 23:887–895, 1941.
22. Glanzmann G, Rust M, Horst W: Irradiation therapy of vertebral angiomas: Results in 62 patients during the years 1939 to 1975. Strahlentherapie 153:522–525, 1977.
23. Glenn JN, Reckling FW, Mantz FA: Malignant hemangioendothelioma in a lumbar vertebra. A rare tumor in an unusual location. J Bone Joint Surg 56:1279–1282, 1974.
24. Gonzales-Crussi F, Enneking WF, Areau VM: Infiltrating angiolipoma. J Bone Joint Surg (Am) 48A:1111–1124, 1966.
25. Graham JJ, Yang WC: Vertebral hemangioma with compression fracture and paraparesis treated with preoperative embolization and vertebral resection. Spine 9:97–101, 1984.
26. Gross CE, Hodge CJ, Binet EF, Kricheff II: Relief of spinal block during embolization of a vertebral body hemangioma. Case report. J Neurosurg 45:327–330, 1976.
27. Gunterberg B, Kindblom LG, Laurin S: Giant-cell tumor of bone and aneurysmal bone cyst. A correlated histologic and angiographic study. Skeletal Radiol 2:65–74, 1977.
28. Harris DJ, Fornasier VL, Livingston KE: Hemangiopericytoma of the spinal canal. Report of three cases. J Neurosurg 49:914–920, 1978.
29. Healy M, Herz DA, Pearl L: Spinal hemangioma. Neurosurgery 13:689–691, 1983.
30. Hekster REM, Luyendijk W, Tan TI: Spinal cord compression caused by vertebral haemangioma relieved by percutaneous catheter embolization. Neuroradiology 3:160–164, 1972.
31. Hemmy DC, McGeem DM, Armbrust FH, Larson SJ: Resection of a vertebral hemangioma after preoperative embolization. Case report. J Neurosurg 47:282–285, 1977.
32. Herrmann HD, Hess H, Kridde OE: Hämangiopericytoma des Armes mit Wirbelmetastasierung und Querschnittssyndrom. Arch Orthop Unfall-Chir 63:267–272, 1968.
33. Huvos AG: Bone Tumors. Diagnosis, Treatment, and Prognosis. Philadelphia, WB Saunders Co., 1979.
34. Johnson PM, McClure JG: Observations on massive osteolysis. A review of the literature and report of a case. Radiology 71:28–42, 1958.
35. Junghanns H: Ueber die Haufigkeit gutartiger Geschwulste in den Wirbelkörpern (Angiome, Lipome, Osteome). Arch Klin Chir 169:204–212, 1932.
36. Kosary IZ, Braham J, Shacked I, Shacked R: Spinal epidural hematoma due to hemangioma of vertebra. Surg Neurol 7:61–62, 1977.
37. Lang EF, Peserico IL: Neurologic and surgical aspects of vertebral hemangiomas. Surg Clin North Am 40:817–823, 1960.
38. Lange TA, Zoltan D, Hafez GR: Simultaneous occurrence in the spine of osteoblastoma and hemangioendothelioma. Spine 11:92–95, 1986.
39. Langman J: Medical Embryology. Baltimore, Williams & Wilkins Co., 1975, pp 66–68, 145–146.
40. Larsson SE, Lorentzon R, Boquist L: Malignant hemangioendothelioma of bone. J Bone Joint Surg (Am) 57:84–89, 1975.
41. Lee S: Hemangioendothelial sarcoma of the sacrum. CT findings. Comput Radiol 10:51–53, 1986.
42. Leehey P, Naseem M, Every P, et al: Vertebral hemangioma with compression myelopathy: Metrizamide CT demonstration. J Comput Assist Tomogr 9(5):985–985, 1985.
43. Lozman J, Holmblad J: Cavernous hemangiomas associated with scoliosis and a localized consumptive coagulopathy. A case report. J Bone Joint Surg 58:1021–1024, 1976.
44. Mao P, Angrist A: Hemangiopericytoma of heart with metastasis to vertebra. Arch Pathol 83:466–470, 1967.
45. McAllister VL, Kendall BE, Bull JW: Symptomatic vertebral hemangiomas. Brain 98:71–80, 1975.
46. Muraszko KM, Antunes JL, Hilal SK, Michelsen WJ: Hemangiopericytomas of the spine. Neurosurgery 10:473–479, 1982.
47. Neumärker Von K-J, Tennstedt A, Lehmann R: Ein Beitrag zum zervikalen Hämangioendotheliom im Kindesalter. Zentralb Neurochir 46:290–303, 1985.
48. Netherlands Committee on Bone Tumours: Radiological Atlas of Bone Tumours. Vol I. Baltimore, Williams & Wilkins Co., 1966, pp 191–193.
49. O'Brien P, Brassfield RD: Hemangiopericytoma. Cancer 18:249–252, 1965.
50. Paige ML, Hemmati M: Spinal cord compression by vertebral hemangioma. Pediatr Radiol 6:43–45, 1977.
51. Pearson J, Stellar S, Feigin I: Angiolipoma. Long term cure following radical approach to malignant appearing benign intraspinal tumor. Report of 3 cases. J Neurosurg 33:466–470, 1970.
52. Pitlyk PJ, Dockery MB, Miller RH: Hemangiopericytoma of the spinal cord. Neurology 15:649–653, 1965.
53. Popoff PJ, Malinin TI, Rosomoff HL: Fine structure of intracranial hemangiopericytoma and angiomatous meningioma. Cancer 34:1187–1197, 1974.
54. Rivkind A, Margulies JY, Lebensart P, et al: Anterior approach for removal of a spinal angiolipoma. Spine 11:623–625, 1986.
55. Robbins LR, Fountain EN: Hemangioma of cervical vertebras with spinal cord compression. N Engl J Med 258:685–687, 1958.
56. Schnyder P, Fankhauser H, Mansouri B: Computed tomography in spinal hemangioma with cord compression. Report of two cases. Skeletal Radiol 15:372–375, 1986.
57. Silverman JF, Dabbs DJ, Leonard JR, Harris LS: Fine needle

aspiration cytology of hemangioblastoma of the spinal canal. Report of a case with immunocytochemical and ultrastructural studies. Acta Cytol 30:303–308, 1986.

58. Stern MB, Grode ML, Goodman MD: Hemangiopericytoma of the cervical spine: Report of an unusual case. Clin Orthop Rel Res 151:201–204, 1980.

59. Stjernvall L: Vertebral angiosarcoma: A case report. Acta Orthop Scand 41:165–168, 1970.

60. Stevens AU, Love J, Davis C, Kendall BE: Capillary hemangioblastoma of bone resembling a vertebral hemangioma. Br J Radiol 56:571–575, 1983.

61. Stout AP: Hemangio-endothelioma: A tumor of blood vessels featuring vascular endothelial cells. Ann Surg 118:445–464, 1943.

62. Stout AP: Hemangiopericytoma: A study of twenty-five new cases. Cancer 2:1027–1035, 1949.

63. Stout AP, Lattes R: Tumors of soft tissues. In Atlas of Tumor Pathology, Series 2, Fascicle 1. Washington, DC, Armed Forces Institute of Pathology, 1967.

64. Stout AP, Murray MR: Hemangiopericytoma: A vascular tumor featuring Zimmerman's pericytes. Ann Surg 116:20–33, 1942.

65. Sweterlitsch PR, Torg JS, Watts H: Malignant hemangioen-

dothelioma of the cervical spine: A case report. J Bone Joint Surg (Am). 52:805–808, 1970.

66. Thomas A: Vascular tumors of bone. A pathological and clinical study of twenty-seven cases. Surg Gynecol Obstet 74:777–795, 1942.

67. von Hanwehr R, Apuzzo ML, Ahmadi J, Chandrasoma P: Thoracic spinal angiomyolipoma: Case report and literature review. Neurosurgery 16:406–411, 1985.

68. White AA III, Johnson RM, Punjabi MM, Southwick WO: Biomechanical analysis of clinical stability in the cervical spine. Clin Orthop 109:85–96, 1975.

69. Wu KK, Guise ER: Malignant hemangioendothelioma of bone: A clinical analysis of 11 cases treated at Henry Ford Hospital. Orthopaedics 4:58–62, 1981.

70. Yang Z-Y, Zhang L-J, Chen Z-X, Hu H-Y: Hemangioma of the vertebral column. A report on twenty-three patients with special reference to functional recovery after radiation therapy. Acta Radiol Oncol 25(Fasc. 2):129–132, 1985.

71. Zander E, Foroglou G: Processus vasculaires vertebromedullaires. Schweiz Arch Neurol Neurochir Psychiatr 98:56–70, 1966.

72. Zito G, Kadis GN: Multiple vertebral hemangiomas resembling metastases with spinal cord compression. Arch Neurol 37:247–248, 1980.

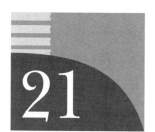

CHORDOMAS

NARAYAN SUNDARESAN, DANIEL I. ROSENTHAL, ALAN L. SCHILLER, and GEORGE KROL

INTRODUCTION

Chordomas are rare primary malignant tumors arising predominantly from the axial skeleton. They are traditionally considered slow-growing, locally invasive neoplasms and constitute between 1 and 4 per cent of malignant bone tumors in several large series.[32, 79, 80, 81, 90, 91] Although more than 1000 cases have been reported to date, the only true epidemiologic data are two studies published in the Scandinavian literature. In the Swedish Registry, Eriksson noted an annual incidence of 0.5 per cent per million population, with chordomas accounting for 17.5 per cent of all primary malignant tumors of bone.[14] Over a 12-year period (1958 to 1970), 979 tumors were registered, of which 290 were malignant tumors arising from the axial skeleton. Of these, chordomas accounted for close to 20 per cent of such neoplasms. A similar incidence in Finland was noted by Paavolainen.[55] Approximately 50 per cent of all chordomas arise in the sacrococcygeal region, 35 per cent in the sphenooccipital region in the region of the clivus, and 15 per cent in the true vertebrae above the sacrum.[12, 13, 36, 50, 90] This distribution of lesions is due to the persistence of notochord in the fused bones of the sacrum and basiocciput, whereas in the spine osseous notochordal tissue tends to disappear. In addition, there are reports of "ectopic" chordomas arising outside the skeletal axis within the maxilla, sinuses, larynx, and other soft tissues.[4, 6, 25, 32, 58, 59, 66, 78, 95, 97]

The site of origin of chordomas is presumed to be the embryonic notochord.[17, 23, 26, 27] Among animals of the phylum Chordata, the notochord is the first skeletal structure to be formed. It gives way to the axial skeleton in the subphylum Vertebrata. Portions of notochord persist in fishes in the trunk and tail, but only vestiges remain in modern reptiles, birds, and mammals. Embryologically, the notochord itself is seen in the somite period of the embryo, that is, from the 20th to the 30th day of human development. It originates as a group of cells that pass laterally from the primitive streak to form the intraembryonic mesoderm. During the formation of the intraembryonic mesoderm, thickening of the ectoderm at one end forms the Hensen's node or primitive knot. A chord of cells migrates forward from the Hensen's node between the entoderm and ectoderm, which is termed the head process. As development proceeds, the notochordal process fuses with and intercalates in the embryonic endoderm. Ultimately, a flattened plate of columnar cells is formed, which is termed the notochordal plate. The notochord itself develops from the notochordal plate by a longitudinal folding of the latter and by separation from endoderm. This separation proceeds in a cranial-caudal direction, leaving rests of notochordal cells closely associated with the developing pharynx.

During the development of the axial skeleton, the vertebral bodies themselves are formed from loose mesenchymal cells that are laid segmentally from the paraaxial mesoderm (sclerotomes). The sclerotome gives rise to all skeletal elements, connective tissue, cartilage, as well as bone. The organization of the sclerotome into segmental levels results in the development of a cranial portion that is less condensed and a caudal portion that is condensed. Fusion of adjacent segments traps the notochord within the disc, and thus the nucleus pulposus is the only adult derivative of notochord. However, Willis and others have noted that remnants of notochord are found within the clivus and the parapharyngeal structures in up to 2 per cent of autopsies.[91] Virchow erroneously believed that these remnants were of cartilaginous origin.[87] He is, however, credited for the term "physaliphorous," which describes the large, vacuolated cells that are typical of the tumor. In 1858, Muller was the first to suggest that these remnants were persisting notochordal relics and named them "ecchordosis physalifora."[51] Further support for the theory of notochordal origin also rests on Ribbert's and Congdon's experiments in which they punctured intervertebral disc tissue in young rabbits and showed that the proliferating disc tissue resembled chordoma.[8, 63, 64] Electron microscopy and tissue culture studies also suggest a histologic similarity between chordoma and disc tissue.[18, 19, 26, 28, 48, 74, 96] It is curious, however, that chordomas arise from the vertebral body and the sacrum and have not been associated with the one structure traditionally associated with the notochord, that is, the nucleus pulposus. More recently, Ulich and Mirra have reported finding a microscopic ectopic remnant of notochord and hyaline cartilage within the vertebral body and postulate that these remnants may be the origin of chordomas developing in the spine.[84]

PATHOLOGY

Grossly, chordomas are lobulated, gray, partially translucent, glistening, cystic or solid masses that resemble cartilage tumors or occasionally a mucin-producing carcinoma.[13] The consistency varies from firm and focally ossified or calcified tissue, to extremely soft, myxoid, gelatinous, or even semifluid material. These tumors appear to be well circumscribed owing to pseudocapsule formation within soft tissue, but this is not evident within bone.[32] In all sacral tumors, intact and elevated periosteum anteriorly forms the pseudocapsule of the tumor. In the bone itself, the tumor appears to be multifocal invading between trabeculae without a clear margin of reactive bone (Fig. 21–1).

Microscopically, the tumors are characterized by a distinct, lobular architecture that is formed by the physaliphorous ("soap bubble") cells with ample vacuolated cytoplasm as well as by the "signet ring" type of cells. A thick layer of fibrous tissue is usually seen secondary to soft tissue compression, which is focally incomplete, and is invaded by infiltrating tumor cells. The intracytoplasmic mucus droplets vary greatly in size, and they stain positively for both glycogen and mucin. The smaller, better preserved tumor nodules often have polygonal cells in close proximity to each other similar to carcinoma cells with mucin production. In addition, larger tumor lobules have ample

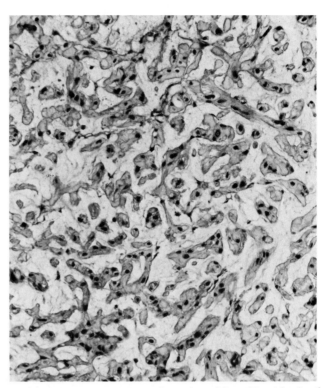

FIGURE 21–2. A chordoma with cords and branching islands of large vacuolated polygonal cells (physaliphorous cells) separated by abundant mucopolysaccharide matrix (H & E, × 157).

extracellular mucin with only a few stellate cells scattered about especially in the peripheral areas. Marked variation in nuclear size and chromatin may be seen. Binucleate forms and multinucleated giant cells are also seen in some areas. Mitotic figures are rare, and cellular anaplasia and increased mitotic activity do not seem to correlate with a more virulent clinical course (Fig. 21–2). In fact, the only histologic feature that corresponds to a more indolent course is the finding of cartilaginous differentiation especially in skull tumors.[24, 86] Frequently, the histologic distinction between chondrosarcoma and chordoma may be difficult especially in the clival region. The tendency for both intra- and extracellular mucin production helps to distinguish them from cartilaginous tumors. Cartilage lesions have a positive staining reaction with phosphotungstic acid hematoxylin (PTAH), while chordomas are mostly negative for PTAH.[10] Chordomas are readily impregnated by silver-staining reticulin fibers which support the tumor cells.[65] In limited biopsy specimens, histologic diagnosis may be confused with mucin-producing adenocarcinoma, myxosarcoma, or chondrosarcoma. Histologic variations of chordoma include chondroid chordoma, which occurs particularly at the skull base. In a review of 155 tumors, 22 patients were shown to have this cartilaginous differentiation, and 19 of the 22 lesions were located in the sphenooccipital region.[24] Of interest is the fact that the average survival for patients with chondroid chordoma was 15.8 years, compared with the average 4.1-year survival for patients with typical chordoma.

Ultrastructural studies of the tumor have been carried out by several authors.[18, 52, 56, 74, 86] These show

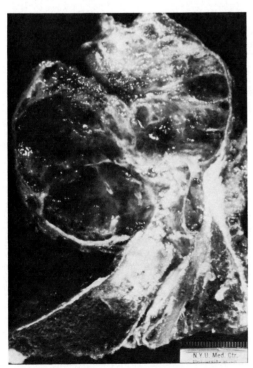

FIGURE 21–1. A sacral chordoma composed of lobulated, gelatinous, well-circumscribed tissue arising from the bone.

the presence of two cell types: the stellate and the physaliphorous cells with many transitional forms. The small, compactly arranged stellate cells appear to be the primary cell type, with elongated indented nuclei and sparse cytoplasmic organelles including agranular endoplasmic reticulum, occasional profiles of rough endoplasmic reticulum, and mitochondria. The physaliphorous cells are identified by the abundant cytoplasm containing vesicles or vacuoles for different types. It has been suggested that the stellate cell is the primary neoplastic cell, which subsequently evolves into the physaliphorous cell and accounts for the autonomous growth of the tumor.[52] The evolution of the stellate cell into the physaliphorous cell supposedly occurs through a process of cisternal dilatation and internal secretion, a process that has been observed in the developing notochord.

Although the typical chordoma is easy to recognize, it is important to remember that this tumor may show a wide range in its histologic appearance and pattern; in addition to the areas showing physaliphorous cells, an occasional tumor may show a typical spindle cell sarcomatous arrangement and a round cell pattern, and yet others may show an epithelial arrangement.[88] Following treatment with radiation therapy, areas of spindle cell sarcoma formation may be seen; on occasion, the chordoma may be transformed into a malignant fibrous histiocytoma.[5, 21, 38, 43, 47, 81] In difficult cases, immunoperoxidase studies may be helpful in distinguishing chordoma from adenocarcinoma and cartilage tumors.[1, 37, 46, 54, 68] Chordomas are usually positive for keratin and S-100 protein, whereas cartilage tumors are keratin negative and adenocarcinomas are S-100 negative.

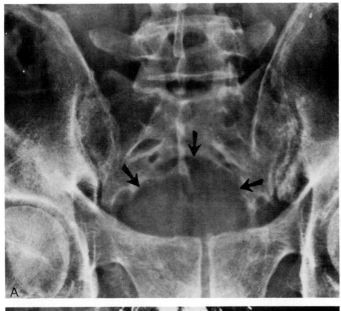

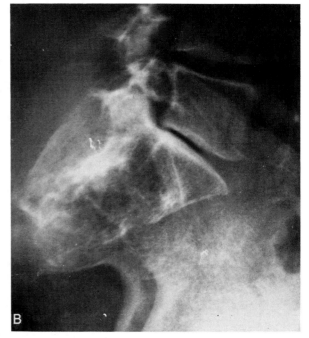

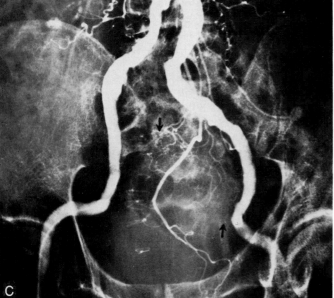

FIGURE 21–3. *A,* Anteroposterior view showing destruction of sacrum (*arrows*). *B,* Lateral view of sacrum showing lytic destruction, often difficult to appreciate because of overlying gas shadows. *C,* Nonselective arteriography reveals areas of tumor blush as indicated by arrows.

CLINICAL FEATURES

Over a 36-year period (1949 to 1985), a total of 88 patients with histologically verified spinal chordomas were treated at Memorial Sloan-Kettering Cancer Center. Of these, 54 patients were treated in the earlier 27 years, and the more recent 34 patients were treated within the latter 7 years.[78, 81] In the entire series, there were 60 males and 28 females, with a male:female ratio of 2:1 reported in most series. Fifty-six lesions were located in the sacrococcygeal region, and 30 involved the vertebral column at a higher level (true vertebrae). There were two tumors involving the clivus and skull base. The youngest patient was 2½ years old, and the oldest was 74 years old. The mean age of the sacrococcygeal group was approximately 56 years, whereas tumors originating in the true vertebre (vertebral chordomas) occurred in a younger age group (mean 47 years). In the literature, chordomas have been reported from infancy through advanced ages.[93] Approximately half the cases are encountered in the fifth through the seventh decades of life.

The clinical symptoms and signs varied with the location and extent of the tumor. In general, symptoms associated with sacrococcygeal tumors were present 6 months to a year before diagnosis. The most frequent symptom was pain, located either in the low back or in the sacrum or coccyx, which was reported in 75 per cent of our patients. Occasionally, patients complained of pain in the buttocks or perineum. There were no specific characteristics of the pain, which was described variously as dull, sharp, continuous, or intermittent. Since these early symptoms were insidious and nonspecific, they were frequently ignored by the patient or the physician. Fifteen per cent of the patients related the pain to a prior history of trauma to the lower back. Rectal dysfunction (change in bowel habits, tenesmus, or rectal bleeding) was noted as an additional symptom in approximately 20 per cent of the patients. Occasionally, patients reported urinary incontinence, but this symptom is less common than in the past, since diagnosis is established by computed tomography (CT) scan at an earlier stage of the disease.

Twelve patients in the early series noted a mass over the coccyx, and on several occasions this mass was presumed to be a pilonidal cyst. In addition, radicular pain in the sciatic distribution, sensory loss, and other neurologic deficits were present in 10 patients. Frequently, pain was referred along the corresponding dermatome; thus, patients with L1-L2 lesions generally complained of pain in the hip, knee, groin, or sacroiliac region. Many of these patients were treated for degenerative arthritis, disc disease, coccydynia, or hemorrhoids for several months before the true diagnosis was established. In every sacral tumor when examined, there was a palpable presacral mass that did not involve the rectal mucosa. The longest time to clinical detection in our more recent series of 34 patients was an asymptomatic lytic lesion of the sacrum that had been followed for more than 10 years prior to clinical growth and onset of symptoms. There appeared to be no tendency toward earlier clinical detection in the recent group of 34 patients when compared with the previous group of 54 patients.

Patients with vertebral chordomas generally presented with a shorter duration of symptoms; while radicular pain and neurologic deficits are common, the prevertebral mass may frequently become symptomatic, especially in the cervical and nasopharyngeal regions. Thus, dysphagia or nasal obstruction may lead to the erroneous diagnosis of a nonosseous retropharyngeal tumor.[4, 53, 58, 60, 95] Two of the lumbar chordomas in our previous series presented as intraabdominal masses for which exploratory laparotomies were performed without the spinal origin of the tumor being recognized. Fortunately, it is now rare that a patient is completely paralyzed secondary to spinal cord compression, since most spinal tumors are now diagnosed earlier with magnetic resonance imaging (MRI).

RADIOLOGIC FEATURES

The most consistent radiologic finding in sacral chordomas is destruction of several segments of the sacrum associated with a soft tissue tumor mass anterior to it.[13, 25, 29, 72, 94] The degree of calcification in the tumor may vary from 40 to 80 per cent, depending on whether this is sought on plain radiographs or CT scans.[39, 73, 94] The soft tissue mass is disproportionately larger than the area of bone destruction, and frequently the superior limit of the mass may be above the level of bone involvement. Generally, the calcification is amorphous and peripheral in location. Tumors involving the true vertebrae generally originate in a single vertebral body and are lytic with surrounding reactive sclerosis[78] (Figs. 21–3 through 21–5). Involvement of adjacent vertebral bodies is a common feature of chordomas with sparing of the intervertebral discs. An anterolateral paraspinal mass is seen in all these patients, and in a few the intraosseous extension is barely perceptible. Myelography was carried out in all our patients and disclosed epidural extension of tumor in more than 90 per cent of patients with tumors involving the true vertebrae.

Radionuclide bone scans, when performed in this group of patients, rarely show positive uptake in the tumor. Spinal angiography was performed in some patients, often to determine whether the tumor was vascular.[16, 78] In the majority, the tumor was relatively avascular, but selective angiography frequently revealed a focal tumor blush.

Although traditional radiographic methods of tumor staging include intraosseous pyelography, barium studies, and even angiography and venography, it is clear that CT scans are capable of disclosing the total extent of tumor mass without the need for additional studies (Figs. 21–6 and 21–7). No enhancement is seen with the administration of intravenous contrast, which is therefore not recommended for patients with spinal lesions.[39] With the

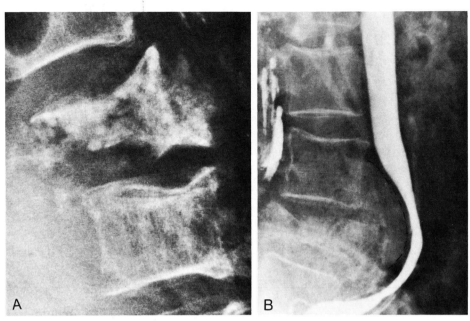

FIGURE 21–4. *A*, Note collapse of the lumbar vertebra and sclerosis secondary to chordoma. *B*, Inferior vena cavogram illustrating anterior soft tissue involvement (pre-CT era).

introduction of MRI, another useful radiodiagnostic tool is available.[67] MRI allows tumor evaluation in the axial, sagittal, and coronal planes. Recently, Rosenthal and colleagues have shown that MRI provides superior contrast to CT scan because of the prolonged T1 and T2 times of the tumors.[67] The soft tissue tumor masses are especially well shown by MRI scan, with long TR and TE (T2-weighted) images (Figs. 21–8 through 21–11). Rectal invasion is easily visualized—a site that is rarely involved by these tumors. MRI cannot detect the effects of radiation or the small polyp-like extension of tumor into the surrounding pseudocapsule described by Hudson and Galcerran.[30] The radiologic findings are so characteristic—that is, the presence of a soft tissue extension with bone involvement—that there should rarely be difficulty in making the radiologic diagnosis. Although these tumors grow strictly in the midline, diagnostic confusion may occasionally result if the

tumor grows eccentrically and presents as a pelvic mass with minimal or no apparent intraosseous involvement (Figs. 21–12 through 21–14).

METASTASES

Whereas the tendency of chordomas to recur locally is well known, the propensity for these tumors to metastasize may not be. Earlier reports suggested that approximately 10 per cent of patients with chordomas developed distant metastases.[7, 13, 50] In Utne and Pugh's review of cases, only 3 out of 71 patients were discovered to have developed metastatic lesions.[85] In our earlier series, 11 of 18 vertebral chordomas and 10 of 36 sacral chordomas were found to have disseminated metastases.[78] The difference in incidence between the two groups was statistically significant. Metastases appeared uniformly

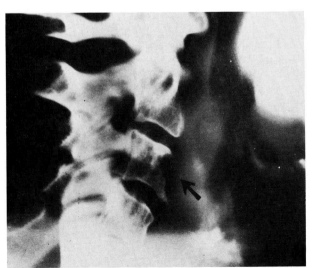

FIGURE 21–5. Early lytic destruction of the C3 vertebra (*arrow*), which on biopsy proved to be chordoma.

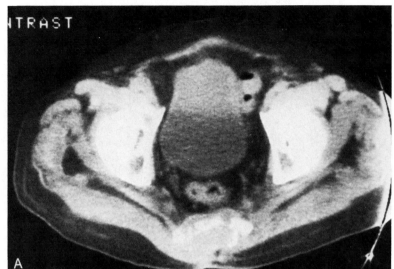

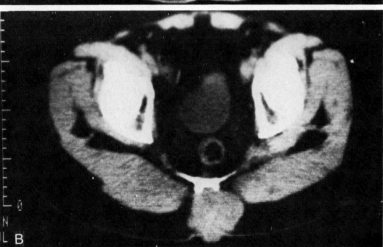

FIGURE 21–6. *A* and *B,* With the advent of CT scan, smaller tumors are being diagnosed. CT scan through lower end of sacrum shows destructive lesion with extension into posterior gluteal region.

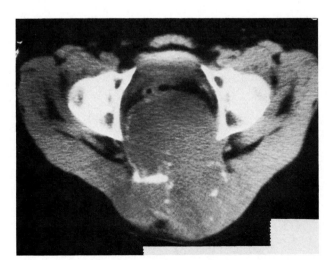

FIGURE 21–7. CT scan reveals large presacral tumor with calcification at periphery. Approximately 80 per cent of sacral tumors are shown to exhibit peripheral calcification.

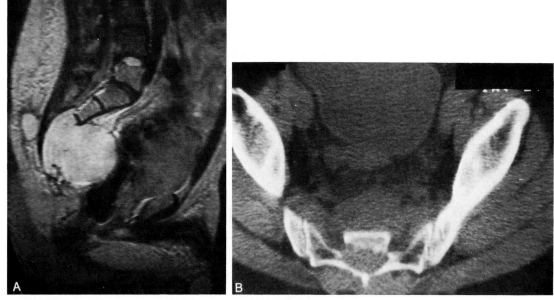

FIGURE 21–8. *A,* Sagittal SE 1500/60 image on MRI. Tumor contrasts strongly with adjacent tissues. Note extension of tumor into posterior biopsy specimen. This was also seen on CT scan but was difficult to distinguish from scar formation. Soft tissue mass clearly extends anterior to S2. *B,* Axial CT scan. Loss of fat plane between tumor and rectum. Despite this appearance, rectal wall was not involved at surgery.

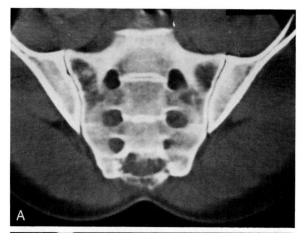

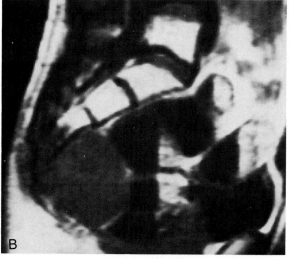

FIGURE 21–9. *A,* Direct coronal CT scan. Tumor within body of S4 segment. First three sacral roots are spared bilaterally. *B,* Sagittal SE 500/30 image after rectal air insufflation. No fat plane between tumor and rectum. Despite this, rectum was free of tumor at surgery. Tumor can be seen within central parts of body of S3, but its relationship to sacral nerves cannot be appreciated at this projection.

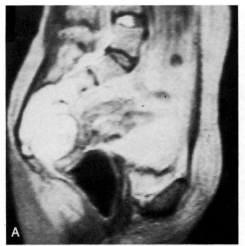

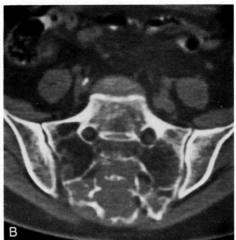

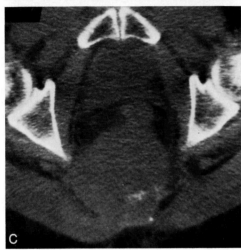

FIGURE 21–10. *A,* Sagittal SE 1500/60 image. Large mass arises from sacrum and extends into second sacral segment. *B,* Direct coronal CT scan. Tumor invades S2 neural foramina bilaterally. At surgery, nerves could be dissected free of tumor. *C,* CT scan in corrected axial projection. Invasion of right coccygeus muscle. Tumor cannot be distinguished from rectal wall, raising possibility of invasion. At surgery, lesion was adherent to rectum but was not invasive. (From Rosenthal DI, Scott JA, Mankin HJ, et al: Sacrococcygeal chordoma: Magnetic resonance imaging and computed tomography. AJR 145:143–147, 1985; © by the American Roentgen Ray Society.)

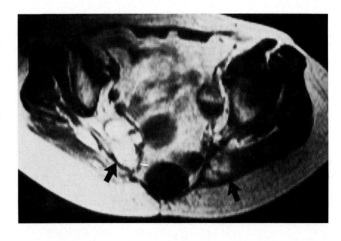

FIGURE 21–11. Axial SE 1500/60 image. Tumor recurrence within gluteus muscles bilaterally (*arrows*). Tumor is easily recognized by brightness on the image.

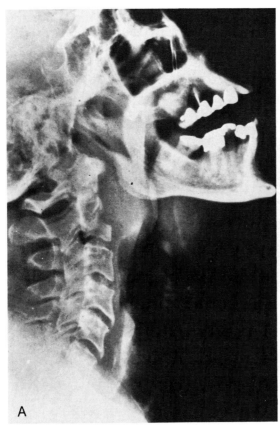

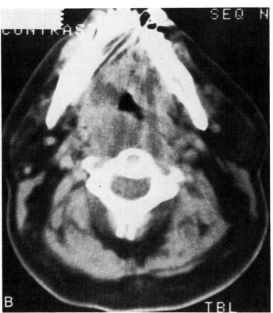

FIGURE 21–12. *A,* Lateral cervical spine. Note retropharyngeal soft tissue mass with minimal involvement of the C2 vertebra. *B,* Axial CT scan. Note parapharyngeal soft tissue extension of tumor.

throughout the course of therapy and were discovered as early as one year and as late as 10 years after tissue diagnosis, and therefore did not merely reflect a long follow-up period. There was no obvious correlation between the incidence of metastases and the mode of treatment of the primary tumor. Sites of metastases included soft tissues, lymph nodes, lung, bone, liver, and other intraabdominal viscera. Occasionally, widely disseminated metastases to organs including the heart, pleura, and brain were found. In our more recent experience, 30 per cent of the patients developed metastases, similar to what has been reported in several different series.[33, 65, 81] Chambers and Schwinn found an incidence of 30 per cent in 27 cases, but curiously the metastases in their study were predominantly to skin and bone.[7] In two of three patients with dermal metastases, the lesions in the skin were diagnosed even prior to the primary tumor. In their study, the histologic appearance of the tumor—anaplasia and the degree of mitosis—did appear to correlate with the presence of metastases. Metastatic lesions in chordoma have little impact on overall survival because death frequently results from complications of local treatment failure.

The presence of metastatic disease has offered the opportunity to study the biologic doubling time of chordoma. In patients with primary tumors, Cummings and coworkers estimated a doubling time of the primary lesion of approximately 6 months.[12] Metastatic tumor nodules on the other hand may have much shorter doubling times, ranging from 9 to 36 days; in another report metastatic nodules in the lung had average doubling times of 3.3 months.

TREATMENT

There is general agreement that complete surgical resection is the treatment of choice in chordomas,[3, 20, 25, 34, 35, 41, 50] but this type of surgery may not always be technically feasible in advanced cases or in patients with medical contraindications. In early years, the majority of patients with sacrococcygeal tumors presented with involvement of the second sacral segment, which was then considered a contraindication for curative resection. This was based on the assumption that an intact first sacral segment was necessary for maintenance of pelvic strength and stability. Further, disruption of the second through fourth sacral nerves leads to complete and irreversible loss of bladder and bowel function, often considered unacceptable in a seemingly benign tumor.

Although Mabry[41] had suggested in 1935 that the anatomy of the sacrum did not permit very radical surgery, Mixter and Mixter described extensive radical treatment by a preliminary defunctioning colostomy and subsequent en bloc resection through a posterior approach, with removal of the lower three segments of the sacrum and preservation of the first few sacral nerves. This surgical approach was expanded by McCarty and colleagues in 1952,[42] and we recommend this approach for sacral tumors involving the third sacral segment and below.

The posterior approach is done with the patient in a Kraske position. A midline incision is made over the sacrum and coccyx, with skin flaps fashioned. Both the midline skin and a portion of the subcutaneous tissue may have to be resected with the sacrum

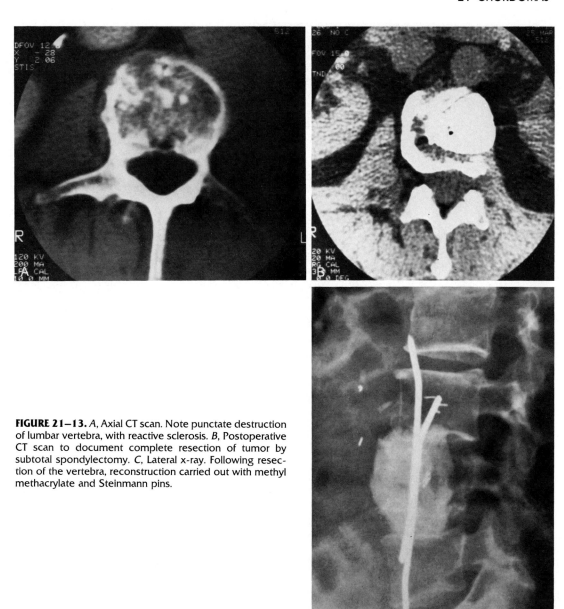

FIGURE 21–13. *A,* Axial CT scan. Note punctate destruction of lumbar vertebra, with reactive sclerosis. *B,* Postoperative CT scan to document complete resection of tumor by subtotal spondylectomy. *C,* Lateral x-ray. Following resection of the vertebra, reconstruction carried out with methyl methacrylate and Steinmann pins.

if the tumor extends posteriorly. The gluteal muscles and piriformis muscles are divided to reach the sacroiliac joint. With a perianal skin incision and perineal dissection (Fig. 21–15*A*), the rectum and pelvic organs are mobilized to protect them during later sacral resection. The sacrum and ilium are then osteotomized, usually at the S2-S3 level, unless the tumor extends more proximally (Fig. 21–15*B*). The sacral resection should be carried above the tumor in order to avoid contaminating the wound with tumor cells. The proximal nerve roots including the pudendal nerve and sacral nerves are carefully identified and preserved. The sacrum is removed, leaving a large space into which suction drains are placed. The coccyx is removed with the specimen. If the caudal sac of the spinal cord is cut, this is carefully repaired. The gluteal muscles may be rotated to fill in the defect.

Of the 50 patients in the Mayo Clinic series who

had excision of the tumor using this approach, 25 patients had wide local excision without the tumor being entered, while the remainder had inadvertent incision of tumor during resection.[33] For those patients with violation of tumor, the recurrence rate was 64 per cent; for those patients in whom the tumor was removed en bloc, the recurrence rate was 28 per cent. Complications related to surgically treated patients consisted of bladder dysfunction in 40 per cent most of which cleared spontaneously. Fecal incontinence was noted in 20 per cent, but all had gradual clinical improvement. Wound-related complications occurred in another 8 per cent. In the overall series of 63 patients, 25 per cent were continuously free of disease.

The only modification of this surgical approach that we advocate is that the mobilization of the rectum and the anal canal should be performed by positioning the patient in the lithotomy position. Following

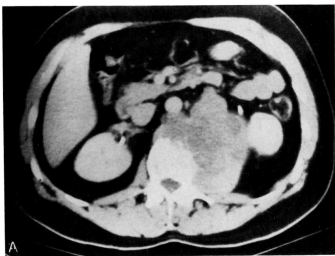

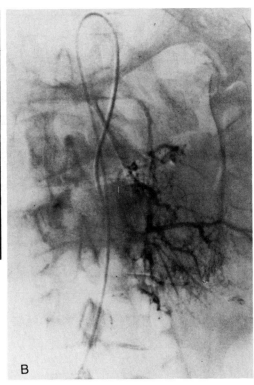

FIGURE 21–14. *A*, Axial CT scan. Note large soft tissue paraspinal component with apparently minimal bone involvement. *B*, Selective arteriogram showing moderately hypervascular tumor. Tumor was embolized prior to operation to minimize blood loss.

careful bowel preparation in the operating room, a purse-string suture is placed around the anus. A posterior perineal incision is made (Fig. 21–15A), and the anal canal and rectum are mobilized away from the presacral space. Positioning a lap pad behind the rectum after dissection allows the osteotomy of the sacrum to be performed without injury to the rectum. We also recommend removal of the biopsy tract through which the diagnosis was established. We generally complete the posterior sacrectomy by positioning the patient in the prone position.

Variations on the surgical approach include the one-stage abdominosacral approaches used by Localio[40] and more recently by Huth.[31] Localio and Eng have suggested this combined approach with the patient positioned in the lateral position (Fig. 21–16). An oblique incision is made from the left iliac crest and costal margin; the left colon is mobilized along with the rectum and is displaced anteriorly and to the patient's right. The left ureter is identified. The iliac vessels are also mobilized and are held by tapes for temporary occlusion. The middle sacral vessels and lateral sacral veins are suture ligated. Posteriorly, a transverse incision is made over the sacrum and skin flaps are developed. The gluteal muscles are dissected free from their iliac attachments. The anococcygeal ligaments are incised and the presacral space is entered to join the abdominal dissection. Surgery proceeds with sectioning of the sacroiliac, sacrotuberous, and sacrospinous ligaments. The piriformis muscles are cut. To mobilize the sacrum, osteotomies have to be performed through the sacroiliac articulations and the sacrum. Nerve roots below the level of the sacral osteotomy are included in the resection. The tumor specimen is then completely mobilized. The wounds are then closed with suction drains.

Profuse blood loss may accompany such procedures, and therefore the use of hypotensive anesthesia or a cell saver is recommended. In Localio's series of five patients, there were four long-term survivors. In view of the propensity for blood loss, a preliminary laparotomy during which time both internal iliac vessels are secured and ligated has been recommended.[25] During the initial abdominal exploration, the tumor itself is completely mobilized and freed from the rectum, and the middle sacral vessels are ligated. The abdominal incision is then closed, and the patient undergoes posterior sacral resection after being placed in a prone position. In our view, ligation of the internal iliac vessels does not reduce bleeding from the sacral osteotomies, which is the major cause of blood loss during operation. The critical decision of whether the tumor should be approached by an abdominal or perineal approach should be based on whether the examining finger can reach the superior limit of the tumor from the perineal approach. The majority of sacral chordomas that have been diagnosed within the past decade are generally small and are located below the level of the second segment. In such cases, it is not necessary to perform an initial abdominal exploration.

In Huth's technique,[31] patients are placed in the lateral decubitus position, and the abdomen, thigh, buttocks, and perineum are prepared and draped. With a midline incision, the abdomen is explored and the rectum is mobilized laterally (Fig. 21–17). The middle sacral vessels are ligated, and the internal iliac vessels are isolated with vessel loops. Posteriorly, the incision begins at the sacrococcygeal junction and extends to the first sacral segment, after which it is extended over the iliac crest. The skin incision is deepened down to the periosteum, and the erector spinalis muscles are dissected subperiosteally from

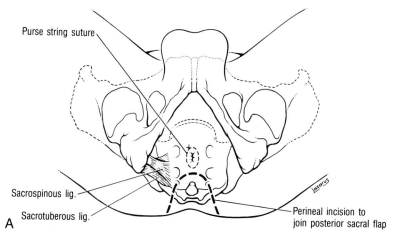

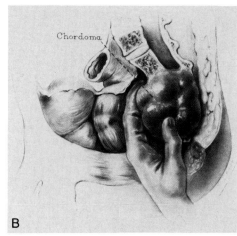

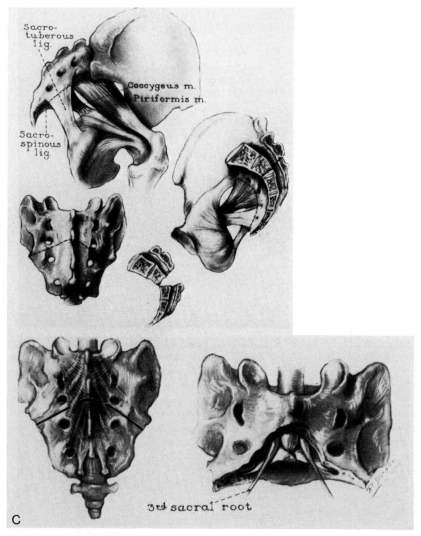

FIGURE 21–15. *A*, For small tumors below the S3 segment, the patient is placed in the lithotomy position as shown. After rectal preparation, a purse-string suture is placed around the anus. The perineal incision is then opened along dotted lines, and the presacral space is developed to mobilize rectum from tumor. *B*, and *C*, The upper limit of the chordoma should be identified by the palpating finger, and sacral osteotomy should then be completed by division of the sacrum and its associated ligaments. (Reproduced with permission from McCarty CS, Waugh JM, Mayo CW, Coventry MB: The surgical treatment of presacral tumors: A combined problem. *Proceedings of the Staff Meetings of the Mayo Clinic* 27(4):73–84, 1952.)

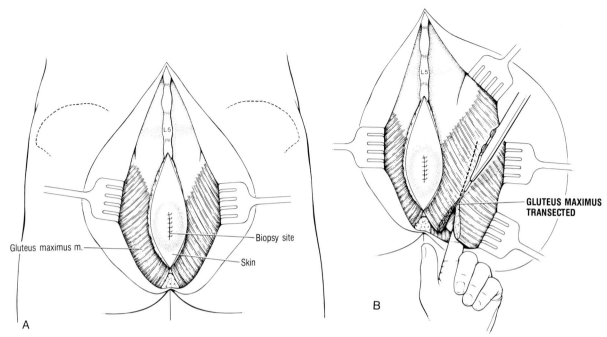

FIGURE 21–16. Posterior incisions and flaps are designed vertically for small tumors *(A)*, and should leave the biopsy tract with the tumor mass. For larger tumors, a transverse incision is recommended. The gluteus maximus is transected by protecting the undersurface with the surgeon's finger *(B)*.

the bone and are retracted laterally. The dura is identified at the L5-S1 interspace, and a sacral laminectomy is performed with Kerrison rongeurs. The cephalic extent of the tumor is identified, and nerve roots that are to be included in the dissection are carefully clipped and ligated at their exit from the dura. The inferior portion of the gluteus maximus is then detached from the sacrum, and the sacroiliac ligaments are divided. Similarly, the sacrospinous, piriformis, and coccygeus muscles are divided. The sciatic notches are then visualized, and care is taken to protect the superior gluteal vessels. With a wide osteotome, a transverse osteotomy is performed, the abdominal surgeon protecting the iliac vessels. The osteotomy is then continued obliquely into the sciatic notch, and the anterior longitudinal ligament is divided. This then permits mobilization of the entire specimen. The erector spinalis and gluteus maximus muscles are then closed with interrupted sutures, and the skin and subcutaneous tissues are closed with a drain.

For much larger tumors, the approach described by Stener and Gunterberg should be used.[75] At least one vertebra proximal to the radiologic limit of the tumor should be removed to ensure tumor-free margins (Fig. 21–18). In younger patients, the argument that preservation of bladder and bowel function is important does not take into account the fact that the majority of recurrent tumors will cause an irreversible loss of bladder and bowel function, with death resulting from local tumor. Stener has shown that if all sacral nerves are sacrificed on one side, there may be little clinical impairment of urogenital and anorectal function. Furthermore, transection of the sacrum above the level of the first sacral foramina does not lead to loss of pelvic stability and strength and is compatible with ambulation in the upright

posture. In Stener's series of eight patients with chordoma, five have remained free of tumor for more than 5 years.

The surgical approach that we use for large tumors in which the soft tissue component is above S2 is essentially the same. After careful bowel preparation, the abdomen is initially opened through a large semicircular incision that runs parallel to the iliac crests bilaterally (Fig. 21–19). The tendon of the rectus abdominis is cut above the incision of the pubic bone, and the abdominal muscle wall is cut on either side at the lateral border of the rectus sheath. An anterior extraperitoneal approach is thus used, and the parietal peritoneum can be retracted on either side to expose the bifurcation of the common iliac artery and vein. The dissection is then carried medially behind the peritoneum, and the ureter is displaced anteriorly. The two dissections from both sides should meet behind the rectum and thus expose the promontory and the upper part of the sacrum (Fig. 21–20).

If the rectum has to be included, then a midline abdominal incision and a lower rectal transection through the rectosigmoid junction are carried out. The internal iliac vessels on either side including the vein should be suture ligated and divided. Both lateral and median sacral arteries and veins are divided and ligated. The periosteum is then stripped off the sacrum, and this subperiosteal dissection should continue down to the level chosen for the sacral osteotomy. During this dissection, the sympathetic trunk should be cut. The lumbosacral trunks that pass anterior to the sacral area should be freed so that they can be protected when the sacral osteotomy is performed. The beginning of the sacral osteotomy can be marked out by cutting the bone

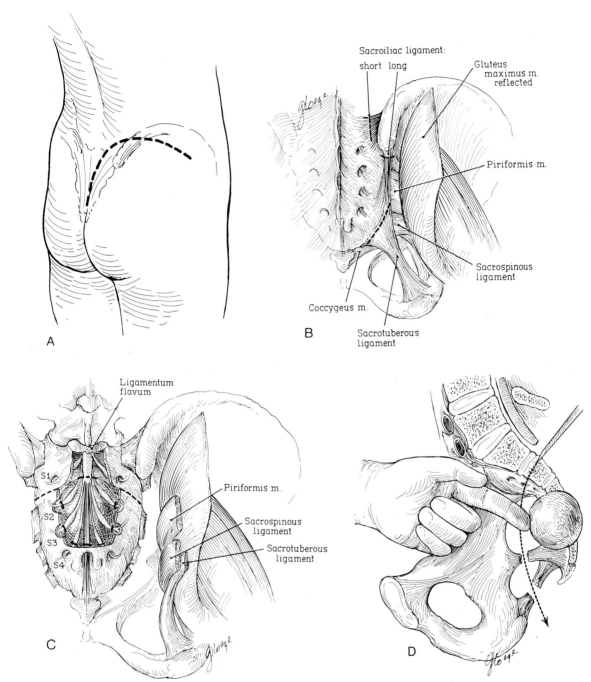

FIGURE 21–17. *A,* Skin incision for sacral resection with patient in lateral position. The invasion is begun in midline at level of the sacrococcygeal junction and is extended upward in the midline and laterally above the iliac crest approximately 2 inches lateral to the posterior superior iliac spine. *B,* The muscular and ligamentous attachments of the sacrum are shown; the gluteus maximus has been retracted laterally. The sacroiliac, sacrospinous, and sacrococcygeal ligaments will be divided in the course of the dissection. The coccygeus and piriformis muscles can be divided at their origin. *C,* Shown are the sacral nerve roots seen from the posterior approaches after sacral laminectomy. The tumor can be seen bulging beneath sacral roots. The S1 nerves are carefully preserved, and a watertight closure of the dura is performed. All other nerve roots are clipped and divided at their exit from the dura. *D,* The surgeon performing the abdominal portion delineates the extent of the tumor with his finger, selects the level of sacral resection, and protects intraabdominal structures such as the ureters and iliac vessels. (*A* from Huth JF, Dawson EG, Eilber FR: Abdominosacral resection for malignant tumors of the sacrum. Am J Surg 148(1):157–161, 1984, with permission.)

through the anterior cortical wall of the sacrum. The anterior wounds are then closed with drains.

For the next phase of the operation, the patient is turned prone, and the posterior incision is begun by a midline incision that will involve an L5 laminectomy as well as the development of flaps laterally (Fig. 21–

21). Both iliac crests on either side should be exposed, and the upper portion of the gluteus maximus should be separated subperiosteally from the iliac crests posteriorly. The gluteus maximus muscle is transected away from the sacrum, and the underlying piriformis muscle is also cut. The superior and infe-

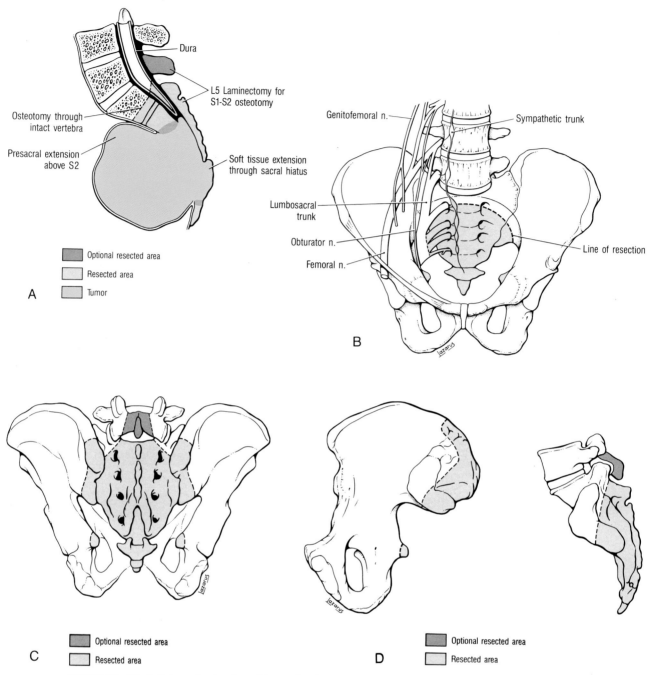

FIGURE 21–18. *A,* Schematic drawing of large chordoma showing soft tissue extension above level of bone involvement. Shaded area indicates resection necessary for such large tumors. *B–D,* Line diagrams illustrating extent of sacral amputation necessary for large tumor. Note line of osteotomy extends through canals of S1 nerves (*B*) and posteriorly includes portions of the ischial spine and part of iliac wing. Following amputation. two thirds of the sacroiliac joints and ligaments remain intact. (Modified from Stener.)

rior gluteal vessels, which exit through the sciatic notch, are divided and ligated; however, an attempt must be made to preserve the superior nerve, which innervates the gluteus medius and minimus. Three ligaments have to be cut: the sacrotuberous ligament, the sacrospinous ligament, and the anococcygeal ligament. Depending on the upper level of the chordoma, the sacrospinalis muscles are transected, and a laminectomy of L5 is performed (Fig. 21–22 and 21–23). The S1 nerve roots are then traced outward, and the dural sac below this level is carefully dissected free. If the S2 nerve roots have to be preserved, then

the transection should continue through the dura at this point, and all holes in the dura closed primarily. Once the dural sac has been ligated, the osteotomy continues through the anterior portion, that is, the posterior longitudinal ligament, and should continue laterally to include a portion of the greater wing of the ilium. The sacral osteotomy can then be performed obliquely, with more of the S1 vertebra being preserved anteriorly rather than posteriorly (Fig. 21–24). The osteotomy laterally through the iliac crest should begin 1.5 cm posterior to the sagittal plane of the tip of the transverse process. This osteotomy

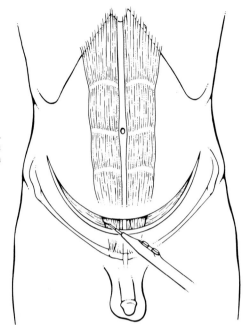

FIGURE 21–19. Technique of sacral amputation. Using a large semicircular incision, the tendon of the rectus abdominis is transected and the abdominal wall cut through on both sides along the lateral border of the aponeurotic sheath. (Modified from Stener.)

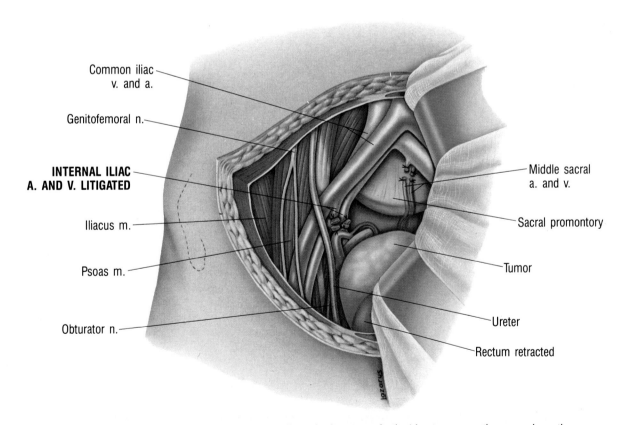

Common iliac v. and a.

Genitofemoral n.

INTERNAL ILIAC A. AND V. LITIGATED

Iliacus m.

Psoas m.

Obturator n.

Middle sacral a. and v.

Sacral promontory

Tumor

Ureter

Rectum retracted

FIGURE 21–20. The anterior parietal peritoneum is pushed away on both sides to expose the area where the common iliac vessels branch. The internal iliac artery and veins are suture ligated. The dissection proceeds medially under the posterior parietal peritoneum, with both dissections meeting behind the rectum over the promontory.

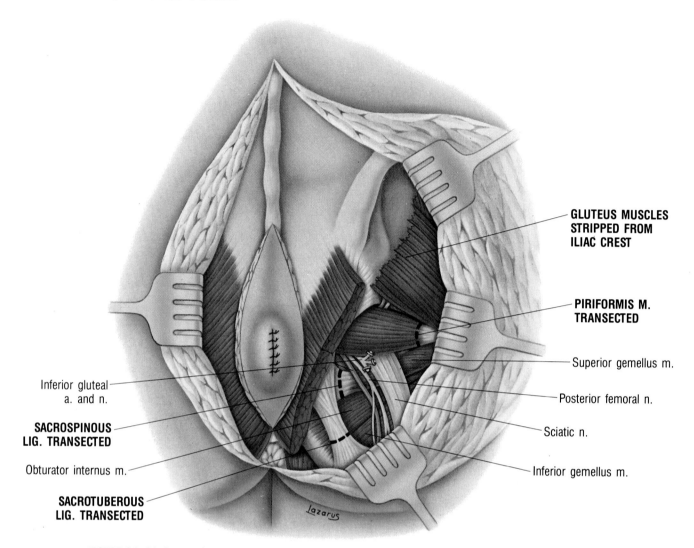

GLUTEUS MUSCLES
STRIPPED FROM
ILIAC CREST

PIRIFORMIS M.
TRANSECTED

Superior gemellus m.

Posterior femoral n.

Sciatic n.

Inferior gemellus m.

Inferior gluteal
a. and n.

SACROSPINOUS
LIG. TRANSECTED

Obturator internus m.

SACROTUBEROUS
LIG. TRANSECTED

lazarus

FIGURE 21–21. During the posterior phase, a flap of skin and subcutaneous tissue is raised, but the posterior biopsy site is included in the resected specimen. Both gluteus muscles are stripped from the iliac crest and the piriformis muscle is transected at its musculotendinous junction. The sacrotuberous and sacrospinous ligaments are released.

should be performed with an examining finger anteriorly guiding the osteotome. Once the bone has been transected, the sacral contributions to the sciatic nerve should be cut and a specimen can be removed. Hemostasis is then secured, and the operation is closed by suturing the skin flaps at the midline, with a large drain at the lower end. A compression dressing is then applied.

For chordomas arising in the vertebral body, it is important to remember that they may extend into the paraspinal tissues as well as extradurally. In the past, laminectomy and tumor resection from a posterior approach were useful in relieving cord compression and reducing pain, but recurrences occurred within the first two years in all those who had such limited resections. Although long-term survival has been reported in isolated cases, it is clear that successful treatment by surgery takes an anterior approach to the spine and that, following tumor resection, stability of the spine should be ensured as well. A variety of techniques are now available which allow complete excision of the vertebra including its

lateral elements (subtotal spondylectomy) using an anterior approach. If the tumor is thought to involve the anterior and the posterior elements, staged spondylectomy is advocated. Although the margins of the tumor may be close, we believe that by careful resection of all gross tumor it is possible to achieve complete resection of most chordomas involving the vertebral body.

For chordomas arising in the base of the skull and the clivus, a significant portion of tumor is anterior to the C1-C2 vertebral body. A transoral or transcervical approach may provide access to chordomas arising within this region, but we favor the extensive exposure afforded by the transmandibular median glossotomy for tumors arising from the C1-C2 region. Although results reported for vertebral chordomas are inferior to those for lesions of the sacrum, we believe that this statistic reflects the fact that incomplete excision was carried out in the majority of such patients.

Apart from resection of tumor, it is possible to complete repeat operations to prolong symptomatic

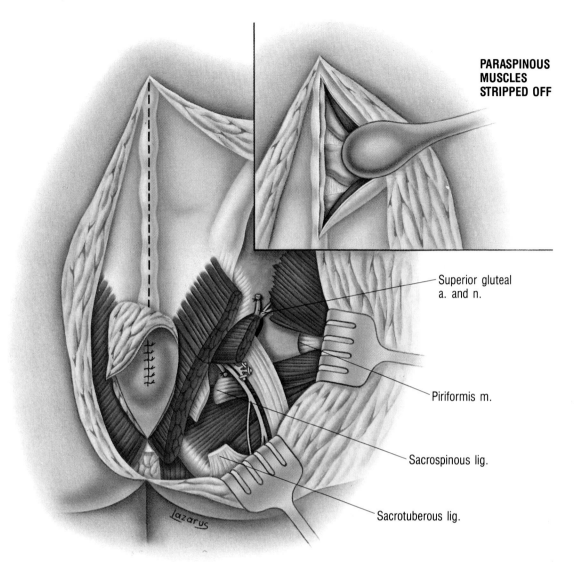

PARASPINOUS MUSCLES STRIPPED OFF

Superior gluteal a. and n.

Piriformis m.

Sacrospinous lig.

Sacrotuberous lig.

FIGURE 21–22. A midline incision is made over the lumbosacral level, and the paraspinous muscles are stripped laterally or transected.

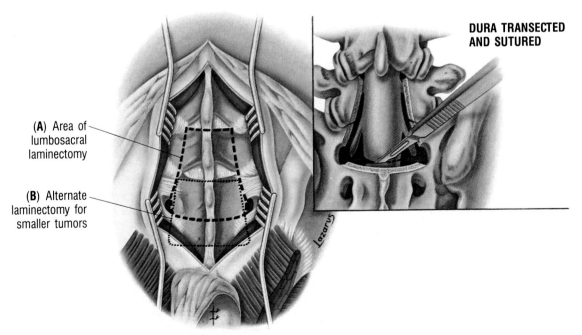

DURA TRANSECTED AND SUTURED

(A) Area of lumbosacral laminectomy

(B) Alternate laminectomy for smaller tumors

FIGURE 21–23. A lumbosacral laminectomy is performed with rongeurs, and the extent of the bone removal is outlined by dotted lines. The dural sac is mobilized and divided just below the S1 nerve roots as shown in the insert.

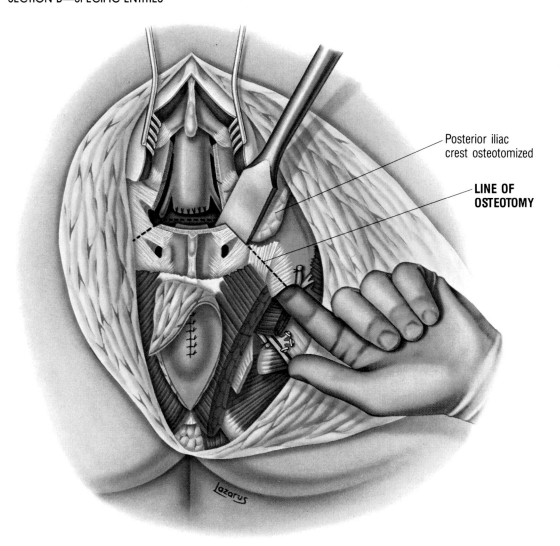

Posterior iliac
crest osteotomized

**LINE OF
OSTEOTOMY**

Lazarus

FIGURE 21–24. Once the dural sac has been ligated, the line of osteotomy is outlined. The osteotomy is guided by a finger, which palpates the previously outlined anterior cortical cut made from the anterior approach.

control both in patients with chordomas at the base of the skull and in those with tumors at other sites.

Radiation Therapy

The majority of patients referred for radiation after treatment are those who have undergone either biopsy or subtotal resection. Although chordoma is not very responsive to radiation, there may still be a role for this modality as palliative treatment for subjective control of pain and neurologic deficit.[33, 57, 60, 62, 65, 71, 83] In an extensive review of the literature, Cummings found no difference in survival between those who had undergone prior biopsy only and those who had subtotal resection prior to radiation therapy.[11] Since the response rate of chordoma tissue to radiation is slow, the actual response of the tumor mass may be difficult to measure. In Cummings' series of 24 patients, the 5-year survival rate was 65 per cent and the 10-year survival rate was 28 per cent. Pearlman and Friedman had suggested that

more beneficial responses were likely to be obtained at doses above 6000 to 8000 cGy.[57] As a result, the tendency had been for most radiation therapists to recommend doses in excess of 5000 cGy for sacral lesions. However, no dose-response rates were found by Cummings in the recent radiation therapy literature, and the value of such high doses of radiation must be balanced against the potential for delayed radiation effects, complications from subsequent surgery, as well as the small possibility of a radiation-related sarcoma.

Since chordoma seems to respond to high dose rates, Suit and colleagues have suggested that an increased response might be seen by combining both photon and high energy proton-beam therapy.[77] This combination improves the dose distribution compared with more conventional external beam therapy. High doses can therefore be delivered to critical areas such as the base of the skull and the cervical spine, with the reduced risk of necrosis of the central nervous system. Initial results with such techniques have been excellent and are reported elsewhere.

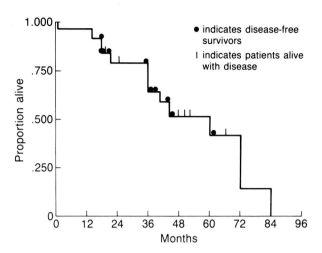

FIGURE 21–25. Kaplan-Meier survival curve showing median survival of 5 years in more recent series of 34 patients. One third of surviving patients are currently free of disease. Circles indicate disease-free survivors; tick marks, survivors with disease.

Chemotherapy

There has been no concerted effort to treat patients with this tumor via chemotherapy regimens, since the majority are referred for treatment only after maximum radiation therapy has been given or for treatment of metastatic disease. Reports in the literature have suggested occasional subjective and objective responses to chemotherapy. Razis and associates reported the response of a single patient with a recurrent chordoma of the cervical spine to 2 mg intravenous vincristine given weekly.[61] The response lasted four months, but the drug was discontinued because of toxicity. In our initial series, 14 patients received single agent or combination therapy, but there were no responses apart from two patients who obtained subjective relief of pain.

Combination chemotherapy using sarcoma regimens has been reported in the more recent literature in a number of patients. Protocols include CyVADIC (cyclophosphamide, vincristine, Adriamycin, imidazole carboxamide [dacarbazine]) combination chemotherapy, and other protocols using cyclophosphamide, Adriamycin, methotrexate, and cisplatin combinations. None of these drug combinations have produced important amounts of tumor regression.

In our more recent series, seven patients were treated with combination chemotherapy using the most effective Adriamycin-containing sarcoma regimens. No major response was noted. In patients with sarcomatous elements, it may be worthwhile using Adriamycin-cisplatin combination chemotherapy or ifosfamide.

Results of Treatment

The median survival reported in the literature is approximately 5 years for sacral lesions and varies from 20 to 40 per cent at the 10-year level. Nevertheless, very few patients (less than 10 per cent) have been free of disease, although these data may be changing. The survival of patients with both clival lesions and vertebral lesions has generally been poor, with median survival less than 5 years and very few long-term survivors. However, the presence of chon-droid differentiation of the tumor may markedly improve the survival because of its more indolent course. Cummings has suggested that no major improvement in survival has been made over the years. However, in our view, the majority of patients diagnosed at present have smaller lesions both in the sacrum and the true vertebrae. It is clear, therefore, that curative resection can be performed in the majority and should be the goal of surgical treatment. Since these tumors are rare, initial treatment has often been performed by a surgeon with little experience with the lesion. An inadequate initial attempt at resection has cut through the plane of the tumor, resulting in tumor contamination of the surgical field. With advances in diagnosis, we believe that the true disease-free interval (Fig. 21–25) should be 50 per cent if surgery is carried out by those experienced in the management of these rare tumors.

REFERENCES

1. Abenoza P, Sibley RK: Chordoma—an immunohistologic study. Hum Pathol 17:744–747, 1986.
2. Amendola BE: CNS chordoma. Radiology 158:839–843, 1986.
3. Ariel IM, Verdu C: Chordoma: An analysis of twenty cases treated over a twenty-year span. J Surg Oncol 7:27–44, 1975.
4. Batsakis JG, Kittleson AC: Chordomas: Otolaryngologic presentation and diagnosis. Arch Otolaryngol 78:168–175, 1963.
5. Belza MG, Urich H: Chordoma and malignant fibrous histiocytoma: Evidence for transformation. Cancer 58:1082–1087, 1986.
6. Boyle TM, Frank HG: The management of nasopharyngeal chordoma by repeated radiation. J Laryngol 80:533–535, 1966.
7. Chambers PW, Schwinn CP: Chordoma: A clinicopathologic study of metastases. Am J Clin Pathol 72:765–776, 1979.
8. Congdon CC: Proliferative lesions resembling chordoma following puncture of the nucleus pulposus in rabbits. J Natl Cancer Inst 12:893–907, 1952.
9. Congdon CC: Benign and malignant chordomas. A clinico-anatomical study of twenty-two cases. Am J Pathol 20:793–822, 1952.
10. Crawford T: The staining reactions of chordoma. J Clin Pathol 11:110–113, 1958.
11. Cummings BJ, Hodson DI, Bush RS: Chordoma: The results of megavoltage radiation therapy. Int J Radiat Oncol Biol Phys 9:633–642, 1983.

12. Cummings BJ, Esses S, Harwood ARL: The treatment of chordoma. Cancer Treat Rev 9:299–311, 1982.

13. Dahlin DC, McCarty CS: Chordoma. A study of fifty-nine cases. Cancer 5:1170–1178, 1952.

14. Eriksson B, Gutenberg B, Kindblom LG: Chordoma. A clinico-pathologic and prognostic study of a Swedish national series. Acta Orthop Scand 52:49–58, 1952.

15. Faust DB, Gilmore HR Jr, Mudgett CS: Chordoma: A review of the literature with report of a sacrococcygeal case. Ann Intern Med 21:678–698, 1944.

16. Firooznia H, Pinto RS, Lin JP, Baruch HH, Zawsner J: Chordoma: Radiologic evaluation of twenty cases. AJR 127:797–805, 1976.

17. Fonti E, Venturini G: Contribution to the knowledge of notochord neoplasms. Riv Anat Path Oncol 17:317–396, 1960.

18. Friedman I, Harrison DFN, Bird ES: The fine structure of chordoma with particular reference to the physaliphorous cell. J Clin Pathol 15:116–125, 1962.

19. Fu YS, Pritchett PS, Young HF: Tissue culture study of a sacrococcygeal chordoma with further ultrastructural study. Acta Neuropathol 23:223–225, 1975.

20. Gray SW, Singhabhandha B, Smith RA, Skandalabis JE: Sacrococcygeal chordoma: Report of a case and review of the literature. Surgery 78:573–582, 1975.

21. Halpern J, Kopolovic J, Catane R: Malignant fibrous histiocytoma within a recurrent chordoma: A light microscopic and immunohistochemical study. Am J Clin Pathol 82:728–743, 1984.

22. Harwick RD, Miller AS: Craniocervical chordoma. Am J Surg 138:512–516, 1979.

23. Heaton JM, Turner DR: Reflections on notochordal differentiation arising from a study of chordoma. Histopathology 9:543–550, 1985.

24. Heffelfinger MJ, Dahlin DC, McCarty CS, Beabout JW: Chordomas and cartilaginous tumors at the skull base. Cancer 23:410–420, 1973.

25. Higinbotham NL, Phillips RF, Farr HW, et al: Chordoma: Thirty-five year study at Memorial Hospital. Cancer 20:1841–1850, 1967.

26. Ho KL: Ecchordosis physaliphor and chordoma: A comparative ultrastructural study. Clin Neuropath 4:77–86, 1985.

27. Horowitz T: The human notochord. A study of its development and regression. Variations and pathologic derivatives. Chordoma. Indianapolis, Limited Private Printing, 1977.

28. Horten B, Montague SR: In vitro characteristics of a sacrococcygeal chordoma maintained in tissue and organ culture systems. Acta Neuropathol 35:13–25, 1976.

29. Hsieh CK, Hsieh HH: Roentgenologic study of sacro-coccygeal chordoma. Radiology 27:101–108, 1936.

30. Hudson TM, Galcerran M: Radiology of sacrococcygeal chordoma: Difficulties in detecting soft tissue extension. Clin Orthop 175:237–242, 1983.

31. Huth JF, Dawson EG, Eilber ER: Abdominal sacral resection for malignant tumors of the sacrum. Am J Surg 48:157–161, 1984.

32. Huvos AG: Bone Tumors: Diagnosis, Treatment, and Prognosis. Philadelphia, W. B. Saunders Co., 1979.

33. Kaiser TE, Pritchard DJ, Unni KK: Clinico-pathologic study of sacro-coccygeal chordoma. Cancer 54:2574–2578, 1984.

34. Kamrin RP, Potanos JN, Pool JL: An evaluation of the diagnosis and treatment of chordoma. J Neurol Neurosurg Psych 27:257–265, 1964.

35. Karakousis CP, Park JJ, Fleminger R, Friedman M: Chordomas: Diagnosis and management. Am Surg 47:497–501, 1981.

36. Kendall BE, Lee BCP: Cranial chordomas. Br J Radiol 50:687–698, 1977; Progr Neurol Surg 6:380–434, 1975.

37. Kindblom LG, Angervall L: Histochemical characterization of mucosubstances in bone and soft tissue tumors. Cancer 36:985–994, 1975.

38. Knechtges TC: Sacrococcygeal chordoma with sarcomatous features (spindle cell metaplasia). Am J Clin Pathol 53:612–616, 1970.

39. Krol G, Sundaresan N, Deck MDF: Computed tomography of axial chordomas. J Comput Asst Tomogr 7:286–289, 1983.

40. Localio SA, Eng K, Ranson JH: Abdomino-sacral approach for retro-rectal tumors. Ann Surg 191:555–559, 1980.

41. Mabrey RE: Chordoma: A study of 150 cases. Am J Cancer 25:501–517, 1935.

42. McCarty CS, Waugh JM, Mayo CW, Conventry MB: The surgical treatment of presacral tumor: A combined problem. Proc Staff Meet Mayo Clinic 27:73–84, 1952.

43. Makek M, Leu HJ: Malignant fibrous histiocytoma arising within a recurrent chordoma. Case report and electron microscopic findings. Virchows Arch (Path Anat) 397:241–250, 1982.

44. Mapstone TB, Kaufmann B, Ratcheson RA: Intradural chordoma without bone involvement. J Neurosurg 59:535–537, 1983.

45. Mayer K, Pentlow KS, Marcove RC, et al: Sulfur 35 therapy for chondrosarcoma and chordoma. In Spencer RP (ed): Therapy in Nuclear Medicine. New York, Grune & Stratton, 1978, pp 185–192.

46. Miettinen M, Lehto VP, Dahl D, et al: Differential diagnosis of chordoma, chondroid and ependymal tumors as aided by anti-intermediary filament antibodies. Am J Pathol 112:160–169, 1983.

47. Miettinen M, Lehto VP, Virtanen I: Malignant fibrous histiocytoma within a recurrent chordoma. A light microscopic, electron microscopic and immunohistochemical study. Am J Clin Pathol 82:738–743, 1984.

48. Miettinen M, Lehto VP, Dahl D, Virtanen I: Ecchordosis physaliphor and chordoma: A comparative ultrastructural study. Clin Neuropathol 4:77–86, 1985.

49. Miller TR, Mackenzie A, Randell HT, Tigner SP: Hemicorporectomy. Surgery 59:988–993, 1966.

50. Mindell ER: Chordoma. J Bone Joint Surg 63A:501–505, 1981.

51. Muller H: Ueber das Vorkommen von Resten der Chorda-dorsalis bei Menschen nach der Gebunt und uber ihr Verhaltniss zu den Gallert-geschwulsten am Clivus. Zeschrf Rat Med 2:202–229, 1858.

52. Murad TM, Murthy MSN: Ultrastructure of a chordoma. Cancer 25:1203–1215, 1970.

53. Murali R, Rovit RL, Benjamin MV: Chordoma of the cervical spine. Neurosurgery 9:253–256, 1981.

54. Nakamura J, Becker LE, Mark A: S100 protein in human chordoma and human and rabbit notochord. Arch Pathol Lab Med 107:118–120, 1983.

55. Paavolainen P, Teppo L: Chordoma in Finland. Acta Orthop Scand 47:46–51, 1976.

56. Pardo-Mindan FS, Guillen FJ, Villas C, Vazquez JJ: A comparative ultrastructural study of chondrosarcoma, chondroid sarcoma and chordoma. Cancer 47:2611–2619, 1981.

57. Pearlman AW, Friedman M: Radical radiation therapy of chordoma. Am J Roentgenol Radiat Ther Nucl Med 108:333–341, 1970.

58. Penzin KH, Pushparaj N: Non-epithelial tumors of the nasal cavity, paranasal sinuses, and nasopharynx chordomas. Cancer 57:784–796, 1986.

59. Poppen JL, King AB: Chordomas: Experience with thirteen cases. J Neurosurg 9:139–163, 1952.

60. Raffel C, Wright DC, Gutin PH, Wilson CB: Cranial chordomas: Clinical presentation and results of operative and radiation therapy in twenty-six patients. Neurosurgery 17:703–710, 1985.

61. Razis DV, Tsatsoronis A, Kyriazides I, Triantafyllon D: Chordoma of the cervical spine treated with vincristine sulfate. J Med 7:1709–1711, 1981.

62. Reddy ER, Mansfield CM, Hartman GV: Chordoma. Int J Radiol Oncol Biol Phys 7:1709–1711, 1981.

63. Ribbert H: Ueber die ecchondrosis physali-fora sphenooccipitalis. Zentralbl Allg Pathol 5:457–461, 1894.

64. Ribbert H: Ueber die experimentelle Erzeugung einer Ecchordosis physalifora. Verh Dtsch Longr Inn Med 13:455–464, 1895.

65. Rich TA, Schiller A, Suit HD, Mankin JH: Clinical and pathologic review of 48 cases of chordoma. Cancer 56:182–187, 1985.

66. Richter HJ, Batsakis JG, Boles R: Chordoma: Nasopharyngeal presentation and atypical long survival. Ann Otol 84:327–332, 1975.

67. Rosenthal DI, Scott JA, Mankin HJ, et al: Sacrococcygeal chordomas: Magnetic resonance imaging and computed tomography. AJR 145:143–147, 1985.
68. Salisbury JR, Isaacson PB: Demonstration of cytokeratins and an epithelial membrane antigen in chordoma and human fetal notochord. Am J Surg Pathol 9:791–797, 1985.
69. Saunders WM, Chen GTY, Austin-Seymour M, et al: Precision high dose radiotherapy. II. Helium ion treatment of tumors adjacent to critical central nervous structures. Int J Radiat Oncol Biol Phys 11:1339–1347, 1985.
70. Saunders WM, Castro JR, Chen GTY, et al: Early results of ion beam radiation therapy for sacral chordoma. J Neurosurg 64:243–247, 1986.
71. Saxton JP: Chordoma. Int J Radiat Oncol Biol Phys 7:913–915, 1981.
72. Sennett EJ: Chordoma: Its roentgen diagnostic aspects and its response to roentgen therapy. Am J Roentgenol 69:613–622, 1953.
73. Smith J, Ludwig RL, Marcove RC: Clinical radiologic features of chordoma. Skeletal Radiol 16:37–44, 1987.
74. Spjut JH, Luse SA: Chordoma: An electron microscopic study. Cancer 17:643–656, 1964.
75. Stener B, Gunterberg B: High amputation of the sacrum for extirpation of tumors: Principles and technique. Spine 3:351–366, 1978.
76. Stevenson GC, Stoney RJ, Perkins RK, Admas JE: A transcervical approach to the ventral surface of the brain stem for removal of a clivus chordoma. J Neurosurg 24:544–551, 1966.
77. Suit HD, Goitein M, Munzenrider J, et al: Definitive radiation therapy for chordoma and chondrosarcoma of the base of the skull and cervical spine. J Neurosurg 50:377–385, 1982.
78. Sundaresan N, Galicich JH, Chu FCH, Huvos AG: Spinal chordomas. J Neurosurg 50:312–319, 1979.
79. Sundaresan N: Spinal chordomas. *In* Wilkins RH, Rengacharry SS (eds): Textbook of Neurosurgery. Vol I. New York, McGraw-Hill, 1985, pp 1069–1075.
80. Sundaresan N: Chordomas. Clin Orthop 204:135–142, 1986.
81. Sundaresan N, Huvos AG, Krol G, Brennan MB: Spinal chordoma: Results of surgical treatment. Arch Surg 122:1478–1482, 1987.
82. Sundaresan N, Krol G, DiGiacinto GV, Hughes JEO: Total spondylectomy for malignant tumors of the spine. J Clin Oncol 7:1485–1491, 1989.
83. Tewfik HH, McGinnis WL, Nordstrom DG, Latourette HB: Chordoma: Evaluation of clinical behavior and treatment modalities. Int J Radiol Oncol Biol Phys 2:959–962, 1977.
84. Ulich TR, Mirra JM: Ecchordosis physaliphora vertebralis. Clin Orthop 163:282–289, 1982.
85. Utne JR, Pugh DG: The roentgenologic aspects of chordoma. Am J Roentgenol 74:593–608, 1955.
86. Valderana E, Lipper S, Kahn L, Marc J: Chondroid chordoma. Electron microscopic study of two cases. Am J Surg Pathol 7:625–632, 1983.
87. Virchow R: Untersuchungen uber die Entwickelung des Schadelgrundes im gesunden und krankhaften Zustande und uber den Einfluss der selben auf Schadelform, Gesichtsbildung und Gehirnbau. Berlin, G. Reimer, 1857, p 128.
88. Volpe R, Mazabrund A: A clinicopathologic review of 25 cases of chordoma: A pleomorphic and metastatic neoplasm. Am J Surg Pathol 7:161–170, 1983.
89. Vries JD, Oldhoff J, Hadders HN: Cryosurgical treatment of sacrococcygeal chordoma: Report of 4 cases. Cancer 58:2348–2354, 1986.
90. Wellinger CL: Rachidial chordoma (I, II, III)—Review of the literature since 1960. Rev Rhum Mal Osteoartic 42:109–116, 195–204, 287–295, 1975.
91. Willis RA: Pathology of Tumors. 4th ed. Philadelphia, F. A. Davis Co., 1967.
92. Windle-Taylor PC: Cervical chordoma: Report of a case and the technique of transoral removal. Br J Surg 64:438–441, 1977.
93. Wold LE, Laws ER Jr: Cranial chordomas in children and young adults. J Neurosurg 59:1043–1047, 1983.
94. Wood EH Jr, Himadi GM: Chordomas: A roentgenologic study of sixteen cases previously unreported. Radiology 54:706–716, 1950.
95. Wright D: Nasopharyngeal and cervical chordoma—some aspects of their development and treatment. J Laryngol Otol 81:1337–1355, 1967.
96. Wyatt RB, Schochet SS Jr, McCormick WF: Ecchordosis physalifora. An electron microscopic study. J Neurosurg 34:672–677, 1971.
97. Zoltan L, Fenyes I: Stereotactic diagnosis and radioactive treatment in a case of spheno-occipital chordoma. J Neurosurg 17:888–900, 1960.

22

DISORDERS OF THE SPINE RELATED TO PLASMA CELL DYSCRASIAS

SANFORD KEMPIN and NARAYAN SUNDARESAN

INTRODUCTION

Although all lymphocytic neoplasias may invade the bone, it is the peculiar nature of malignancies of the most mature B cell, the immunoglobulin-secreting cell, for bone destruction to dominate the clinical presentation. These disorders are collectively known as the plasma cell dyscrasias and include a broad spectrum of disease presentations (Table 22–1), some of which manifest significant bone destruction[43, 54, 65–67, 119, 132] and others in which bone destruction is minimal or absent.[19, 44, 69, 89, 96, 116] This property is not unique to B cells, since certain rare T-cell disorders may also manifest this tendency to bone destruction.

The unique clinical presentations of the lymphocytic neoplasias are derived from their phenotypic and ultimately genotypic properties. The B-cell maturational pathway is shown in Figure 22–1. Examples of lymphocytic neoplasias in which bone destruction may occur as a primary phenomenon or with secondary invasion include acute lymphocytic leukemia,[95, 131] large cell lymphomas,[106] T-cell leukemia/lymphoma (HTLV-1 associated),[130] and the plasma cell disorders. These latter disorders can be divided into two major categories: those in which bone involvement is rare or absent, such as benign monoclonal gammopathy and Waldenström's macroglobulinemia (IgM monoclonal gammopathy),[69] IgE myeloma,[89, 96] and alpha heavy chain disease;[116] and those in which bone lesions are major clinicopathologic manifestations. These latter disorders, the subject of this review, include solitary plasmacytomas without apparent bone marrow involvement (solitary plasmacytoma of bone—SPB) and those destructive lesions that represent contiguous spread of a primary bone marrow disease, multiple myeloma. Not infrequently extramedullary plasmacytomas may metastasize to bone marrow, and the two disorders then become indistinguishable.

SOLITARY PLASMACYTOMAS OF BONE

Plasmacytomas are tumors composed of malignant plasma cells. When not a part of a systemic bone marrow disease (multiple myeloma), they present either as a solitary lesion in bone (SPB) or at other extramedullary sites (EMP), most commonly the upper airway passages, gastrointestinal tract, lymph nodes, and spleen.[132] Occasionally, more than one bone lesion may be present in the absence of bone marrow involvement. SPBs and EMPs may be secretory or nonsecretory and are occasionally associated with light chain urinary excretion (Bence-Jones proteinuria). Shaw[117] and Cutler and colleagues[32] were the first to describe solitary plasmacytomas of bone and long survival with surgical resection.

These tumors represent about 3 per cent of plasma cell neoplasms.[62] The disorder is more common in men (3:1) and is seen most frequently in those over the age of 50.[132] The frequency of various bone locations as the site of solitary plasmacytomas is shown in Table 22–2.[3, 8, 24, 31, 42, 79, 86, 133] The spine is the initial site of presentation in approximately 25 to 50 per cent of cases,[8, 132] with the thoracic vertebrae representing nearly one half of the reported cases.[36] Occasionally, the intervertebral disc is the site of occurrence.[37]

Diagnosis

Histologically, these lesions consist of well to poorly differentiated plasma cells, with most lesions containing the entire spectrum of plasma cell maturation (Fig. 22–2). The cytoplasm is basophilic, and the nucleus is eccentric with pyknotic chromatin ("clock face"). Nucleoli are observed, particularly in plasmablasts. Lesions may be classified as predominantly well differentiated or poorly differentiated. Amyloid has occasionally been observed in blood vessels and interstitium,[86, 132] although systemic amyloidosis has only rarely been reported.[86] Immunohistochemical studies of a series of solitary plasmacytomas of bone demonstrated IgG but no other heavy chain in the cytoplasm. Light chain analysis demonstrated a kappa to lambda ratio of approximately 1:1.[86] Woodruff and coworkers[133] reported on a series of 12 patients

TABLE 22–1. PLASMA CELL DYSCRASIAS

Disorders	Bone Destruction	References
Benign monoclonal gammopathy	Absent	43
Waldenström's macroglobulinemia	Absent	43
Solitary plasmacytoma	Present (localized)	132
Multiple plasmacytomas	Present	132
Multiple myelomas		
IgG	Present	67
IgA	Present	67
IgD	Present	54, 66
IgE	Rare	69, 89, 96
Light chain disease	Present	65, 119
Heavy chain disease		
α-heavy chain	Absent	116
γ-heavy chain	Rare	44, 116
μ-heavy chain	Rare	19

with SPB, of which one patient was found to have an IgA serum paraprotein and one, urinary lambda chains (2 of 12 = 16 per cent). A higher incidence of paraproteinemia was found by Meis and associates;[86] 77 per cent of SPB patients in this series subsequently demonstrated a monoclonal protein, although only 8 of 17 were detected at diagnosis (47 per cent). A similar frequency of paraprotein secretion was described by Bataille and colleagues,[8] with 6 of 18 (30 per cent) demonstrating a paraprotein (IgG kappa = 3; IgG lambda = 1; kappa light chain = 2). Wiltshaw[132] reported that 7 of 11 patients at initial presentation were found to have increases in the immunoglobulin fraction as a single narrow band (immunoelectrophoretic studies not reported). A further three patients developed a paraprotein after dissemination (total: 10 of 11 patients).

Radiographically, the lesions are predominantly osteolytic and have been described as either multicystic (multilobular "soap bubble" lesions) seen predominantly in the long bones, ilium, and mandible or sharply demarcated destructive lesions.[99] These latter are seen predominantly in the spine[132] (Fig. 22–3A–B). Occasional osteosclerotic lesions have been reported.[8, 93, 105, 112, 113] Bone scintigraphy may be normal or may show reduced uptake[108] in spite of evidence of destruction on x-ray.[113] Purely lytic lesions are likely to be negative by radionuclide scanning.[128] Computed tomography (CT) scanning and magnetic resonance imaging (MRI) have been used to diagnose vertebral lesions[49, 76] (Fig. 22–3C–E). Spinal angiography is frequently used to evaluate tumor neovascularity and to identify spinal cord blood supply (Fig. 22–3F). Plasmacytomas are hypervascular tumors and frequently invade the adventitia of the vertebral artery, especially lesions involving the cervical spine (Fig. 22–4). Thus, presurgical embolization may be required to obliterate tumor blood supply prior to surgery.

The pathogenesis of these neoplasms is not known. They may arise from plasma cells already in bone structures, although lymphatic nodules are not generally found in bone, and thus they are unlikely to arise de novo. Their origin from circulating lympho-

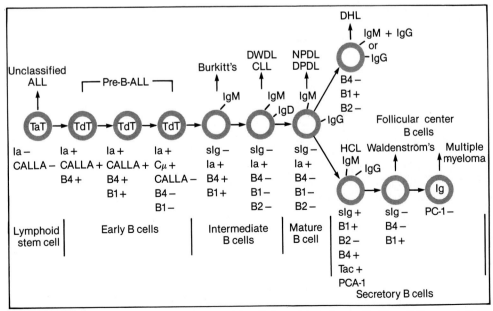

Figure 22–1. Phenotypic correlation of B-cell neoplasia. (Adapted from Longo D, Klima P, Korsmyer S: ABCO Educational Booklet, 1966.)

TABLE 22–2. LOCATION OF SOLITARY PLASMACYTOMAS OF BONE

Author (Ref.)	No. Pts.	S	R	H/F	ST/C/SC	IL/IS/SA	C-V	T-V	L-V
Woodruff et al. (133)	12	—	4	1	3	1	—	2	1
Corwin et al. (31)	12	—	2	2	1	4	—	3	—
Bataille et al. (8)	18	—	2	1	3	1	1	6	4
Bacci et al.* (3)	15	—	—	—	—	—	2	8	5
Loftus et al.* (79)	6	—	—	—	—	—	—	1	5
Feldman et al.* (42)	11	—	—	—	—	1	—	5	5
Meis et al. (86)	22	2	4	2	5	3	—	4	2
Chak et al. (24)	20	2	2	—	1	6	—	8	1

*Series reporting only spinal plasmacytomas.
S = skull; R = ribs; H/F = humerus/femur; ST/C/SC = sternum/clavicle/scapula; IL/IS/SA = ilium/ischium/sacrum; C-V = cervical vertebrae; T-V = thoracic vertebrae; L-V = lumbar vertebrae.

cytes and clonogenic plasma cells appears possible, although it is difficult to understand the solitary nature of some plasmacytomas by this route. More likely, local spread from bone marrow lymphoid nodules in close proximity to a still undefined localized bone lesion is the origin of the plasmacytoma. The vast majority (83 per cent in Wiltshaw's series) of primary osseous plasmacytomas occur in bones with active hematopoiesis, suggesting a contiguous spread from the marrow cavity. The high incidence of eventual generalized dissemination gives some credence to this concept. The etiology of these neoplasms is not known. Associations of plasmacytomas with prior injury to bone may be the basic underlying etiology. There is no known association with prior radiation; however, exposure to asbestos has been linked to the appearance of lymphoid and plasma cell malignancies.[60] Infection, if chronic, could conceivably set up a nidus for lymphocyte and plasma cell proliferation.[4]

The initial presenting symptom in SPB in almost all patients is pain, the distribution of which depends upon the location of the lesion. The mean duration of pain prior to diagnosis in the series of Bataille and colleagues[8] was 6 months. Spinal solitary plasmacytomas may involve the cord or nerve root, with subsequent pain in a radicular distribution,[42] and occasionally paraplegia.[3] In one series, nearly 25 per cent of patients with spinal SPB underwent laminectomy because of neurologic involvement. In addition to pain, the secretion of a paraprotein may result in a variety of clinical syndromes, including coagulation abnormalities, hyperviscosity, renal failure, and amyloidosis. In general, the level of paraprotein is considerably less in SPB than in multiple myeloma, and these syndromes are uncommon. An unusual paraneoplastic syndrome has been associated with an osteosclerotic tumor of the thoracic vertebrae consisting of polyneuropathy, skin hyperpigmentation, edema, and hypertrichosis.[55]

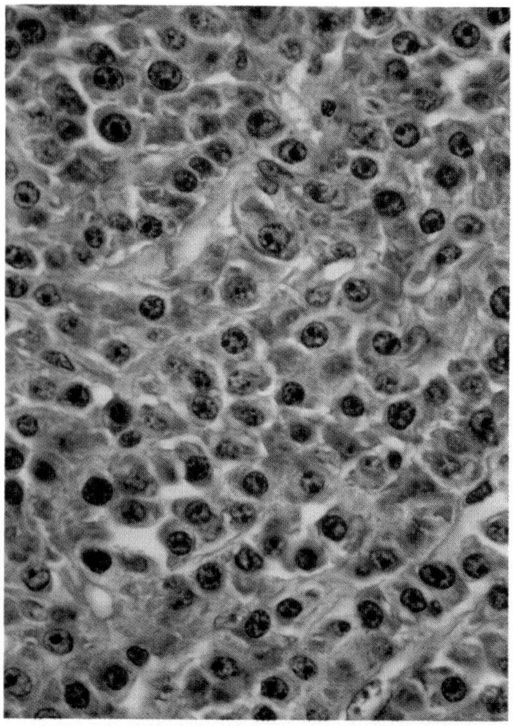

The differential diagnosis of osteolytic bone lesions includes prostate cancer[82] and breast cancer.[113] The diagnosis of SPB can be made by needle biopsy.[115] Care must be taken with this procedure in view of a reported episode of massive bleeding related to the biopsy.[109] For spine plasmacytomas, myelography is recommended to determine the extent, if any, of epidural compression. Once the diagnosis of a solitary plasmacytoma of bone is made, a search for systemic disease is undertaken. A complete skeletal survey and bone scan are necessary to determine the solitary nature of the lesion. A bone marrow aspiration and biopsy are performed. Serum and urinary (24-hour concentrated specimen) paraprotein studies should be performed. The presence of a paraprotein does not necessarily mean that the disease is systemic in nature. The level can be followed to document eradication of the disease as well as recurrence or persistence of a foci of plasma cells.

Treatment

Once staging confirms the presence of a spinal SPB, radiation therapy may be considered the treatment of choice for minimally involved vertebrae. The dose of radiation should be at least 3500 cGy,[88, 126] a dose which in one study was found to be associated with no local recurrences for SPB of the spine.[88] Once enough bone destruction has occurred to result in destabilization (Fig. 22–5), and pain or a neurologic deficit has occurred, resection of tumor and a stabilization procedure should be carried out

Figure 22–2. Plasmacytoma by light microscopy.

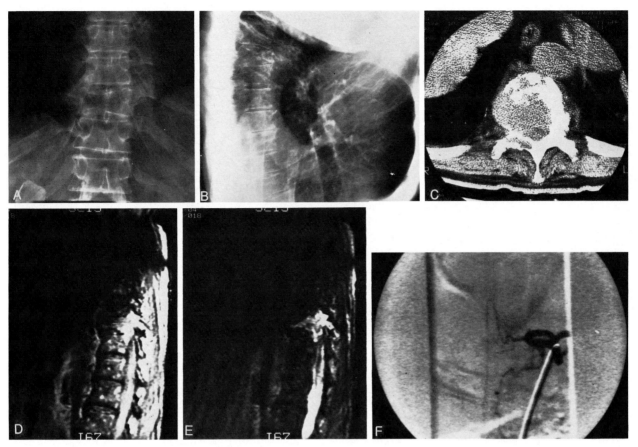

Figure 22–3. *A,* Multilobular plasmacytoma demonstrating a lytic defect of T9. *B,* Large lytic defect of T9 vertebral body demonstrating a wedge compression fracture. *C,* CT scan of T9 showing replacement of vertebral body by plasmacytoma. *D,* MRI scan (T1-weighted image) showing abnormal signal in T9 body. *E,* MRI scan (T2-weighted image) in same patient showing subarachnoid space and a paraspinal soft tissue mass. *F,* Spinal arteriogram demonstrates anterior spinal artery arising from the left T9 vascular pedicle.

promptly (Fig. 22–6). This returns the patient promptly to functional status, and further therapy, either radiotherapy or chemotherapy, can then be undertaken.

Several reviews have addressed the role of surgery for these tumors, and numerous techniques, both with anterior and posterior vertebral approaches, have been utilized.[27, 41, 59, 74, 78, 80, 81, 97, 98, 122] If the lesion has not been completely resected, postoperative radiation to a total of 3500 cGy must be given. The

role of postoperative radiation and adjuvant chemotherapy in the absence of gross residual disease and the role of chemotherapy after radiation therapy have not been rigorously tested. However, for those patients in whom a high risk for dissemination is likely to be present in spite of apparent complete resection, the use of systemic adjuvant therapy is recommended. Examples of such patients include those with soft tissue extension, cellular immaturity, and older patients. Since Bataille and coworkers[8]

Figure 22–4. *A,* CT scan of cervical spine, axial section, showing soft tissue tumor with bone destruction extending to the foramen transversorium. *B,* Left vertebral arteriogram demonstrating irregularities along the C3-C4 segment indicating tumor invasion of the adventitia.

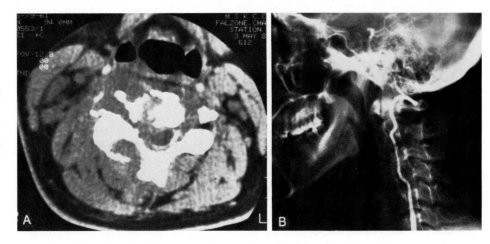

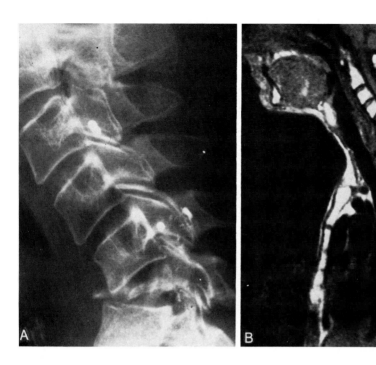

Figure 22–5. *A,* Compression fracture with subluxation of C6 vertebra. This finding should prompt consideration of surgical stabilization in addition to radiation. *B,* T1-weighted image shows abnormal signal in C7 body with extension into posterior elements.

found spinal disease itself to have a poorer prognosis than other sites of SPB, one might consider all patients with spinal SPB at risk for recurrence and dissemination and apply adjuvant chemotherapy. Unfortunately, chronic alkylating agent therapy is associated with some risk of leukemia,[61, 72] and it would be necessary in a randomized study to prove its ultimate benefit. Disappearance of a paraprotein after therapy should be documented, and its recurrence or appearance after therapy signifies residual disease or dissemination.[23, 36, 94]

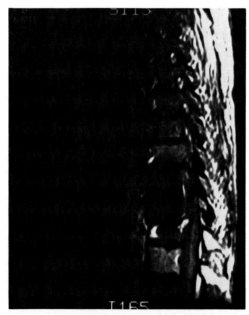

Figure 22–6. Postoperative MRI showing resection of T9 tumor and replacement of resected segment with methyl methacrylate. (Same patient shown in Figure 22–3.)

Prognosis

The evolution of surgically removed and/or radiated solitary plasmacytomas of the spine will depend upon the completeness of staging for systemic disease at initial presentation, as well as various recognized prognostic factors. Soft tissue extension appears to be a poor prognostic factor, with 5 of 8 patients (60 per cent) in one study developing multiple myeloma. Multiple plasmacytomas are harbingers of systemic disease, although survival is better than for multiple myeloma.[62, 132] Both prominence of nucleoli and cellular immaturity (poorly differentiated plasma cells) of SPB are significantly related to the development of multiple myeloma.[86] The presence of either a serum or urine paraprotein has been documented in 50 per cent of patients in one series;[31] however, its presence does not necessarily suggest dissemination into multiple myeloma, since only one quarter of patients (25 per cent) in one series developed this complication. Bataille and colleagues[8] found older age, spinal involvement, and persistence of a monoclonal protein to be poor prognostic factors for the subsequent development of dissemination. The prognosis for patients presenting with paraplegia may be quite satisfactory after aggressive surgical and radiotherapeutic approaches.[36, 58, 68, 85, 134] The occurrence of a second isolated plasmacytoma after therapy is occasionally compatible with long-term disease-free survival and cure without dissemination into multiple myeloma.

The results of treatment of plasmacytomas of the spine are outlined in Table 22–3. Bacci and co-workers[3] reported on 15 patients. Therapy included radiation therapy alone (11 patients), surgery and radiation therapy (4 patients), and systemic chemotherapy (3 patients). One half of the patients devel-

TABLE 22–3. RESULTS OF THERAPY OF PLASMACYTOMAS OF THE SPINE

Author (Ref.)	No. Pts.	Therapy	NED/MM	Time to MM Mean (Range) (Yrs)
Bacci et al. (3)	15	XRT, SURG, CTH	7/8	3.5 (1–8)
Loftus et al. (79)	6	SURG	3/3	
Feldman et al. (42)	11	XRT, CTH, (SURG)	7/4	8 (1–20)
Chak et al. (24)	9	XRT, SURG	2/7	

XRT = radiotherapy alone; SURG = surgery; CTH = chemotherapy; NED = no evidence of disease; MM = multiple myelomas.

oped multiple myeloma from 1 to 8 years (mean 3.5 years) after initial diagnosis. Loftus and associates[79] reported on a series of six patients with isolated plasmacytoma of the lower thoracic and lumbar regions. Bone marrow studies and protein electrophoresis were not performed in all patients. All patients underwent laminectomy and spinal fusion (autologous bone and Harrington rods). One half of the patients ultimately developed systemic disease. Feldman and colleagues[42] reported on 11 cases of solitary plasmacytoma of the spine, of which four developed metastatic plasmacytoma, three having developed medullary disease after 1, 4, and 20 years. These patients received radiation therapy and chemotherapy. The degree of initial surgical resection was not stated. Chak and coworkers[24] reported on a series of 20 patients with solitary plasmacytoma of bone, of whom nine presented with spine disease (45 per cent). These lesions were predominantly thoracic (8 of 9). The patients were initially treated with surgical resection (partial) followed by radiotherapy (3000 to 6000 cGy). Multiple myeloma evolved from 7 of 9 solitary plasmacytomas and was responsible for death in four patients. In this series two patients have not developed multiple myeloma. Therefore, in most patients described in the literature with solitary plasmacytoma of the spine, the condition has ultimately progressed into multiple myeloma,[3, 8] as opposed to peripheral lesions, for which the incidence is considerably less.[3] Therefore, systemic chemotherapy is warranted in this group of patients after local therapy has been applied. The type and duration of this therapy, however, should be determined by clinical trials.

MULTIPLE MYELOMA

Involvement of the spine in multiple myeloma is always present but not always symptomatic. As a systemic disorder beginning initially in the bone marrow and spreading outward to the bone surrounding the marrow cavity and to other bone structures, soft tissues, organs, and blood (leukemia phase), multiple myeloma may be considered the most osteophilic of all lymphoproliferative diseases and the one in which bone involvement and subsequent destruction are the predominant clinical manifestations of the disease.

Multiple myeloma is a disease of adult life, with an incidence ranging from 2.0 to 3.1 per 100,000.[71, 85] Only rarely have pediatric cases been reported.[50, 101] The sex incidence in males and females is equal.[67]

The median age at presentation is 62 years.[67] Multiple myeloma appears to be a more frequent manifestation of lymphoproliferative disease in blacks than in whites, with an incidence in one series of 2.1 per 100,000 whites and of 4.0 per 100,000 blacks.[85] The age at which myeloma appears in blacks is younger than in whites, and a higher frequency of thoracolumbar fractures and solitary plasmacytomas was found in one study.[118]

Diagnosis

The disorder begins as a neoplastic proliferation of plasma cells in areas of hematopoietically active bone marrow (vertebrae, ribs, skull, pelvis, sternum). The formed tumors erode adjacent bone structures and osteolytic lesions arise. The bone resorption can be observed microscopically, demonstrating prominent osteoclast activity in areas of resorption but few if any plasma cells in direct contact with bone structures. An osteoclast activating factor (OAF) has been demonstrated in short-term bone marrow culture.[91] The extent of skeletal metastases appears to be correlated with production of OAF by myeloma cells[40] and may be dependent on endogenous prostaglandin (PGE) synthesis.[16] Recent evidence suggests that tumor necrosis factor (TNF) and lymphotoxin play significant roles.[15] Grossly, the marrow is replaced by small grayish-pink soft nodules (less than 1 cm), with intervening normal bone marrow. Histologically, the nodules consist of plasma cells of relatively uniform size. The cytoplasm is intensely basophilic with the nucleus having the typical "cart wheel" appearance. Multinucleate large and bizarre-looking plasma cells may occasionally be noted. A more diffuse infiltration may result in generalized bone rarefaction or osteoporosis.[114] Occasionally, multiple myeloma demonstrating numerous lytic lesions in a single vertebral body may mimic osteoporosis and, therefore, should be considered in the differential diagnosis of osteoporotic compression fractures (Fig. 22–7).

The pathophysiology of multiple myeloma is directly related to the presence of the myeloma cells in the bone marrow, their direct proximity to bone, as well as their proliferative and secretory capacity. The result of bone marrow replacement by myeloma cells is most often anemia, not an uncommon presenting symptom.[63, 67] Most often the anemia is normochromic and normocytic; however, macrocytosis and occasionally megaloblastosis may be present.[53] Red blood cell autoagglutination (rouleaux formation) is commonly observed. Patients may present with neu-

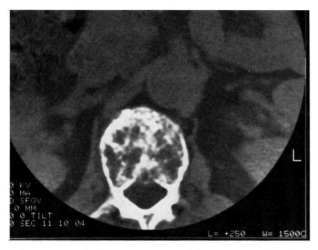

Figure 22–7. Axial CT scan of L2 showing multiple lytic lesions in the body, which can be confused with osteoporosis.

TABLE 22–4. TYPES OF MONOCLONAL PROTEINS PRODUCED BY MYELOMA CELLS

TYPE OF PROTEIN	% PATIENTS
IgG	52
IgA	21
IgM	2
IgD	<0.01
IgE	
Light chain secretion (κ or λ) only	11
Heavy chain secretion (γ, α, μ) only	<1
Two or more monoclonal proteins	0.5
No monoclonal protein in serum or urine	1

From Pruzanski W, Ogryzlo MA: Abnormal proteinuria in malignant diseases. Adv Clin Chem 13:355, 1970.

tropenia and thrombocytopenia; the incidence of these latter two complications is approximately 16 and 13 per cent, respectively.[67] The expansion of the tumors within the marrow cavity will result in pain, a common presenting symptom. As the tumors expand further, bone destruction with hypercalcemia and fractures occur. Hypercalcemia is present in 30 per cent of patients at diagnosis, and during the course of the illness may be present in as many as two thirds of the patients.[12] Occasionally, calcium-binding paraproteins may protect against the clinical manifestations of hypercalcemia.[57] The secretion of a monoclonal paraprotein can be documented in almost all patients, with IgG-secreting myelomas the most common[102] (Table 22–4). The presenting clinical features of the disorder and their relationship to the immunochemical class are shown in Table 22–5, taken from a review by Hobbs.[51] An increased plasma volume with reduction in hemoglobin concentration,[114] pseudohyponatremia and reduced anion gap,[92] and a hyperviscosity syndrome[103] may all result. Impaired hemostasis due to interference in blood coagulation is commonly observed[100] and is related to interference in fibrin polymerization,[26, 34] occasional inhibitors of clotting factors (particularly Factor VIII),[47] accelerated clearance of clotting factors,[18, 45] and platelet function abnormalities.[100] Impaired renal function is related to the tubular damage induced by immunoglobulin light chain metabolism (particularly lambda) by renal tubular cells with subsequent tubular cast formation[35] as well as to hypercalciuria and nephrocalcinosis, hyperuricosuria, and plasma cell infiltration of the kidneys.

The diagnosis of multiple myeloma is not difficult if symptoms are present. In general, such patients will complain of skeletal pain and a decreased performance status related to anemia, renal failure, or infections. Radiographs of painful regions will often disclose osteolytic lesions, and a skeletal survey will demonstrate multiple osteolytic lesions throughout the skeleton. Other malignant neoplasms may mimic the skeletal findings (breast cancer, prostate cancer, renal cancer, and other malignant lymphomas).[107] A complete blood count will demonstrate anemia, and a blood smear examination is likely to demonstrate rouleaux formation and occasional plasmacytoid lymphocytes and plasma cells. A biochemical profile will demonstrate an elevated globulin fraction and increased BUN and creatinine if renal impairment is present, hypercalcemia (30 per cent at diagnosis), and hyperuricemia. The alkaline phosphatase is frequently normal or only slightly elevated. Metabolic bone disease such as hyperparathyroidism may mimic some of the findings such as bone destruction, hypercalcemia, and renal dysfunction, but the bone marrow findings are normal and the protein studies

TABLE 22–5. CLINICAL FEATURES AT THE TIME OF DIAGNOSIS IN 212 PATIENTS WITH MYELOMATOSIS OF DIFFERENT CLASSES

CLINICAL FEATURE	CLASS			κ^2 TESTS	
	γG	γA	BJ	Classes Compared	Significance
No. of patients	112	54	40		
Mean serum level M-protein (g/100/ml)	4.3	2.8	±	γG:γA	p <0.001
Mean doubling time of M-protein (months)	10.1	6.3	3.4	γG:γA:BJ	p <0.02
Lytic bone lesions (per cent)	55	65	78	γG:BJ	p <0.02
Hypercalcemia (per cent)	33	59	62	γG:γA + BJ	p <0.001
Serum urea > 79 mg/100 ml (per cent)	16	17	33	γG + γA:BJ	p <0.02
Normal immunoglobulins < 20 mean normal (per cent)	68	30	19	γG:γA + BJ	p <0.001
Hospital admissions because of infection* (per cent)	60	33	20	γG:γA + BJ	p <0.005
Detected amyloidosis† (per cent)	0.5	7	10		

*In 48 γG, 21 γA, 20 BJ myelomata followed up to 3 years.

†In 228 γG, 102 γA, 94 BJ myelomata.

From Hobbs JR: Immunochemical classes of myelomatosis. Including data from a therapeutic trial conducted by a medical research council working party. Br J Haematol 16:599–606, 1969.

TABLE 22–6. MYELOMA STAGING SYSTEM

STAGE	CRITERIA	MEASURED MYELOMA CELL MASS (cells × 10¹²/m²)

I	All of the following:
	1. Hemoglobin value >10g/100 ml
	2. Serum calcium value normal (<12 mg/100 ml)
	3. On roentgenogram, normal bone structure (scale 0) or solitary bone plasmacytoma only
	4. Low M-component production rates
	  a. IgG value < 5 g/100 ml
	  b. IgA value < 3 g/100 ml
	  c. Urine light chain M-component on electrophoresis < 4 g/24 hrs
		<0.6 (low)

II	Fitting neither Stage I nor Stage III	0.6–1.20 (intermediate)

III	One or more of the following:
	1. Hemoglobin value < 8.5g /100 ml
	2. Serum calcium value > 12g /100 ml
	3. Advanced lytic bone lesions (scale 3)
	4. High M-component production rates
	  a. IgG value > 7 g/100 ml
	  b. IgA value > 5 g/100 ml
	  c. Urine light chain M-component on electrophoresis > 12 g/24 hrs	

Subclassification:
  A = Relatively normal renal function (serum creatinine value < 2.0 mg/100 ml).
  B = Abnormal renal function (serum creatinine value > 2.0 mg/100 ml).

From Durie BJM, Salmon SE: A clinical staging system for multiple myeloma. Correlation of measured cell mass with presenting clinical features, response to treatment, and survival. Cancer 36:842–854, 1975.

demonstrate no monoclonal proteins. A bone marrow study demonstrates increased numbers of plasma cells, many of which are large and atypical with binucleate forms. In general, greater than 30 per cent of the nucleated marrow elements are plasma cells. Occasionally, a lesser percentage may be present, but their atypia satisfies the criteria for multiple myeloma. The differential diagnosis of marrow plasmacytosis includes chronic infections, liver disease, and other neoplasms. Serum protein electrophoresis and immunoelectrophoresis are necessary to determine the presence of the abnormal protein and to define its class. Urine should be concentrated and screened as well for the presence of light chains. A β_2 microglobulin level is obtained as a prognostic factor and followed during therapy.[7] Once the patient is completely evaluated and the diagnosis established, the patient is staged according to the Myeloma Staging System[39] (Table 22–6). The classification is based upon the tumor load as manifested by various clinical parameters, including hemoglobin value, serum calcium, bone radiographs, level of M-component, and renal function. Prognostic factors that indicate an aggressive course include certain immunoglobulin classes,[52, 84] proteinuria greater than 40 mg/dl,[39, 104] a serum albumin less than 3 g/dl,[39, 104] poor performance status,[21] and excessive weight loss.[110] The influence of neurologic deficit, particularly related to spinal disease, has not been specifically examined as a prognostic factor, although a large measure of the performance status is related to this problem.

Treatment

The treatment of multiple myeloma must take into account the systemic nature of the disease, its metabolic complications, and the almost universal destruction of the skeleton, with pain as the predominant clinical manifestation and neurologic deficit as its major morbidity. Treatment of patients with Stage I disease in the absence of clinical symptoms is controversial because the time of evolution into symptomatic disease may be quite prolonged. There are no studies that demonstrate an advantage to treating the disease at diagnosis versus waiting until symptoms arise.[70] Unfortunately, the first clinical manifestation may be epidural compression and neurologic compromise. It is not known if early therapy may prevent this complication. Once symptoms arise and it is clear that the disease is progressing, treatment is instituted with specific antineoplastic agents, radiation therapy, and therapy of complications. Alkylating agents remain the predominant chemotherapy agents used and include cyclophosphamide,[64] melphalan,[14] and BCNU and CCNU.[30] Cyclophosphamide and melphalan appear equally effective, with a higher response rate than nitrosoureas.[30, 90] Both cyclophosphamide and melphalan do not appear to demonstrate cross-resistance.[11] Prednisone is an active agent both causing regression of the myeloma mass[2] and controlling hypercalcemia and proteinuria and improving myelosuppression.[13] The combination of melphalan and prednisone appears superior to either alone.[1] More recent combinations include multiple alkylating agents and vincristine,[73] alkylating agents and adriamycin,[111] and even more recently infusional therapy.[6] Although it would appear from results cited that more aggressive combination programs appear more effective, particularly for patients in an advanced stage (Stage III), this is not universally accepted.[10] High dose melphalan therapy with autologous bone marrow rescue has recently been reported and may become the treatment of choice in younger patients.[5] Interferon is an active agent in myeloma,[29, 87] and it has now been combined with chemotherapy.[127] Although significant progress has been made using chemotherapy and biologic therapy, the disease remains incurable by these methods. Bone marrow transplantation for younger patients remains a valid option.[46]

Radiation therapy when used judiciously with chemotherapy represents an important therapeutic tool, particularly for the palliative therapy of painful bone lesions and neurologic syndromes related to tumor compression of central and peripheral nervous system structures. Myelosuppression and subsequent decrease in chemotherapy tolerance (the mainstay of therapy) should limit the use of this modality to specific disease-related complications. Painful extremity lesions can be treated over a short period of time (3 to 5 days) with total doses of 500 to 1500 cGy. More proximal lesions, such as in ribs or vertebrae, may be treated with even a single dose of 800 cGy. Paraspinal lesions generally are more resistant, and dosages of 3000 cGy over several weeks will need to be administered.[9] Radiation therapy has occasionally been used in the form of total body irradiation, but results have only been palliative.[129] Other widefield techniques have been used for resistant disease, particularly with intractable pain syndromes, and include half body (both upper and lower)[56] as well as whole bone marrow irradiation.[25] Lack of response to radiotherapy suggests the presence of pathologic fractures needing orthopedic intervention.

Although every bone in the body may be involved in the myelomatous process, it is the spine that tends to dominate the clinical course of this disease, because of both its support function as well as its protective function with respect to the central and peripheral nervous system. The most common symptom of spine involvement is pain, as it is the most common presenting symptom in myeloma. In one study 87 per cent of patients with myeloma presented with back pain,[125] and in another 75 per cent presented with pain from multiple bone sites.[83] The quality of pain is described as sharp or lancinating and is frequently radiating in type. The pain may be related to bone destruction with subsequent collapse of the vertebrae as well as nerve root compression. Spinal cord compression may be present in as many as 10 per cent

of patients during the course of their disease.[17, 20, 22] Since pain is often the presenting symptom of what may ultimately lead to cord compression and paraparesis, the initial work-up of this symptom must include a careful neurologic examination. Radiographic studies should include complete spine films (generally performed as part of the initial diagnostic evaluation) as well as computed axial tomographic studies. This latter study is particularly useful in determining the degree of myelomatous involvement and destruction of the vertebral body and pedicles, extraosseous spread of the tumor, and cause of spinal cord compression (tumor, collapsed vertebrae, or both).[48, 120] A myelogram is performed if there is any evidence of neurologic deficit.

Prognosis

Once the appropriate diagnosis of the cause of the pain and/or neurologic deficit is made, the most appropriate local therapy (either surgery, radiotherapy, or both) is quickly applied in addition to systemic therapy. Surgery plays an important role in the plasma cell disorders with spinal involvement with respect to both diagnosis and therapy. Multiple myeloma rarely presents as an isolated lytic lesion of the vertebral column, and diagnosis is generally made by bone marrow examination. The role, therefore, of surgery, in multiple myeloma is more a therapeutic one. Spine involvement with myeloma represents a particularly difficult surgical problem. The general condition of the patient may be quite poor with infections, renal failure, and hypercalcemia. Hemostatic abnormalities make surgical approaches to the spine particularly hazardous. However, when pain

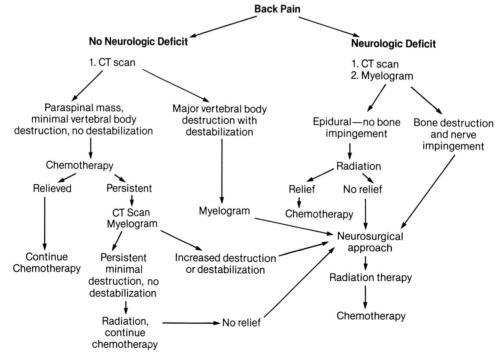

Figure 22–8. Therapeutic decision tree for spinal involvement in multiple myeloma and solitary plasmacytoma.

and neurologic deficit are caused by vertebral body destruction and collapse, surgery will be necessary to decompress the spinal cord and nerve roots. Vertebral body resection and stabilization by a variety of techniques are often necessary in order to relieve symptoms and prevent paraplegia. The extent of vertebral resection will depend upon the radiologic investigations that determine the extent of involvement, the degree of vertebral destruction, and technical factors related to local anatomic structures. A variety of techniques have been developed with respect to both surgical approaches[23, 28, 75, 80, 122] and techniques of stabilization after resection.[28, 59, 75, 77, 78, 81, 98, 121–124]

Figure 22–8 outlines in schematic form the workup of a patient with myeloma and back pain and a therapeutic decision tree. In the absence of a neurologic deficit, an anatomic localization of the cause of the pain is necessary. This can be accomplished by a CT scan. If a paraspinal mass or vertebral destruction without destabilization is present, chemotherapy is begun. An orthopedic or back support will be useful, since collapse of vertebral tissue may ensue once the myelomatous tissue is destroyed and until new bone forms. If symptoms are not relieved or worsen, a repeat CT scan and myelogram are performed. If no vertebral destabilization is present or epidural compression is diagnosed, radiotherapy is given and chemotherapy continued. If symptoms continue or worsen, a neurosurgical approach will be necessary. The presence of a neurologic deficit at diagnosis demands an aggressive diagnostic and therapeutic approach to prevent further nerve damage or subsequent paraparesis or paraplegia. Once the CT scan and myelogram define the extent of the disease, a number of surgical approaches, resection, and stabilization techniques are available. Radiotherapy will be necessary after these surgical techniques, because rarely can all tumor be removed and the reported results appear to show a better result with a combined modality approach,[33, 38] although this concept has not been rigorously tested in a clinical trial.

REFERENCES

1. Alexanian R, Bonnet J, Gehan E, et al: Combination chemotherapy for multiple myeloma. Cancer 30:382–389, 1972.
2. Alexanian R, Yap BS, Bodey GP: Prednisone pulse therapy for refractory myeloma. Blood 62:572–577, 1983.
3. Bacci G, Savini R, Calderoni P, et al: Solitary plasmacytoma of the vertebral column. A report of 15 cases. Tumori 68:271–275, 1982.
4. Baitz T, Kyle RA: Solitary myeloma in chronic osteomyelitis. Arch Intern Med 113:872, 1964.
5. Barlogie B, Hall R, Zander A, et al: High-dose melphalan with autologous bone marrow transplantation for multiple myeloma. Blood 67:1298–1301, 1986.
6. Barlogie B, Smith L, Alexanian R: Effective treatment of advanced multiple myeloma refractory to alkylating agents. N Engl J Med 310:1353–1356, 1984.
7. Bataille R, Durie BGM, Grenier J: Serum beta₂ microglobulin and survival duration in multiple myeloma: A simple reliable marker for staging. Br J Haematol 55:439–447, 1983.
8. Bataille R, Sany J: Solitary myeloma: Clinical and prognostic features of a review of 114 cases. Cancer 48:845–851, 1981.
9. Benson WJ, Scarffe JH, Todd IDH, et al: Spinal-cord compression in myeloma. Br Med J 1:1541–1544, 1979.
10. Bergsagel DE: Editorial: Progress in the treatment of plasma cell myeloma? J Clin Oncol 1:510–512, 1983.
11. Bergsagel DE, Cowan DH, Hasselback R: Plasma cell myeloma: Response of melphalan-resistant patients to high-dose, intermittent cyclophosphamide. Can Med Assoc J 107:851–855, 1972.
12. Bergsagel DE, Griffith KM, Haut A, Stuckey WF Jr: The treatment of plasma cell myeloma. Adv Cancer Res 10:311–359, 1967.
13. Bergsagel DE, Rider WD: Plasma cell neoplasms. In DeVita VT, Hellman S, Rosenberg SA (eds): Cancer: Principles and Practice of Oncology. Philadelphia, J.B. Lippincott Co., 1985, p 1767.
14. Bergsagel DE, Sprague CC, Austin C, Griffith KM: Evaluation of new chemotherapeutic agents in the treatment of multiple myeloma. IV. L-phenylalanine mustard (NSC-8806). Cancer Chemother Rep 21:87–99, 1962.
15. Bertolini DR, Nedwin GE, Bringman TS, et al: Stimulation of bone resorption and inhibition of bone formation in vitro by human tumor necrosis factors. Nature 319:516–518, 1986.
16. Bockman RS: Lymphokine mediated bone resorption requires prostaglandin synthesis. In Prostaglandin and Cancer: First International Conference. New York, Alan R. Liss, 1982, pp 555–559.
17. Brenner B, Carter A, Tatarsky I, et al: Incidence, prognostic significance and therapeutic modalities of central nervous system involvement in multiple myeloma. Acta Haematol (Basel) 68:77–83, 1982.
18. Brody JI, Haidar ME, Rossman RE: A hemorrhagic syndrome in Waldenström's macroglobulinemia secondary to immunoadsorption of factor VIII. Recovery after splenectomy. N Engl J Med 300:408–410, 1979.
19. Brouet JC, Seligmann M, Danon F, et al: U-chain diseases. Report of two new cases. Arch Intern Med 139:672–674, 1979.
20. Bruckman JE, Bloomer WD: Management of spinal cord compression. Semin Oncol 5:135–140, 1978.
21. Carbone PP, Kellerhouse LE, Gehan EA: Plasmacytic myeloma. A study of the relationship of survival to various clinical manifestations and anomalous protein type in 112 patients. Am J Med 42:937–948, 1967.
22. Carmacho J, Arnalich F, Anciones B, et al: The spectrum of neurological manifestations in myeloma. Medicine 16:597–611, 1985.
23. Carter PM, Rushman RW: Solitary plasmacytoma of the clavicle. Proc R Soc Med 67:1097–1098, 1974.
24. Chak LY, Cox RS, Bostwick DG, Hoppe RT: Solitary plasmacytoma of bone: Treatment, progression and survival. J Clin Oncol 5:1811–1815, 1987.
25. Coleman M, Saletan S, Wolf D, et al: Whole bone marrow irradiation for the treatment of multiple myeloma. Cancer 49:1328–1333, 1982.
26. Coleman M, Vigliano EM, Weksler ME, Nachman RL: Inhibition of fibrin monomer polymerization by lambda myeloma globulins. Blood 39:210–223, 1972.
27. Colyer RA: Surgical stabilization of pathological neoplastic fractures. Curr Probl Cancer 10:117–168, 1986.
28. Conley FK, Britt RH, Hanbery JW, Silverberg GD: Anterior fibular strut graft in neoplastic disease of the cervical spine. J Neurosurg 51:677–684, 1979.
29. Constanzi JJ, Cooper MR, Scarffe JH, et al: Phase II study of recombinant alpha-2 interferon in resistant multiple myeloma. J Clin Oncol 3:654–659, 1985.
30. Cornwell GG III, Pajak TF, Kochwa S, et al: Comparison of oral melphalan, CCNU and BCNU with and without vincristine and prednisone in the treatment of multiple myeloma. Cancer 50:1669–1675, 1982.
31. Corwin J, Lindberg RD: Solitary plasmacytoma of bone vs. extramedullary plasmacytoma and their relationship to multiple myeloma. Cancer 43:1007–1013, 1979.
32. Cutler M, Buschke F, Cantril ST: The course of single

myeloma of bone: A report of 20 cases. Surg Gynecol Obstet 62:918–932, 1936.

33. Dahlstrom U, Jarpe S, Lundstrom FD: Paraplegia in myelomatosis—a study of 20 cases. Acta Med Scand 205:173–178, 1979.

34. Davey FR, Gordon GB, Boral LI, Gottlieb AJ: Gammaglobulin inhibition of fibrin clot formation. Ann Clin Lab Sci 6:72–77, 1976.

35. Defronzo RA, Cooke CR, Wright JR, Humphrey RL: Renal function in patients with multiple myeloma. Medicine 57:151–166, 1978.

36. Delauche-Cavallier MC, Laredo JD, Wybier M, et al: Solitary plasmacytoma of the spine. Long-term clinical course. Cancer 61:1707–1714, 1988.

37. Demirel T: Root compression syndrome S1, simulated by a circumscribed plasmacytoma in the intervertebral disc. Neurosurg Rev 4:37–39, 1981.

38. Desproges-Gotteron R, Treves R, Loubet R, et al: Spinal cord compression caused by malignant non-Hodgkins lymphoma. Sem Hop Paris 54:704–712, 1978.

39. Durie BGM, Salmon SE: A clinical staging system for multiple myeloma. Correlation of measured cell mass with presenting clinical features, response to treatment, and survival. Cancer 36:842–854, 1975.

40. Durie BGM, Salmon SE, Mundy GR: Multiple myeloma: Clinical staging and role of osteoclast activating factor in localized bone loss. *In* JE Horton, TM Tarpley, WF Davis (eds): Mechanisms of Localized Bone Loss. Calcif Tissue Abstr (Special Suppl) 1978, pp 319–329.

41. Faccioli F, Luna J, Bricolo A: One-stage decompression and stabilization in the treatment of spinal tumors. J Neurosurg Sci 29:199–205, 1985.

42. Feldman JL, Guedri M, Ohana N, et al: Solitary plasmacytoma of the spine. Ann Med Interne (Paris) 135:259–264, 1984.

43. Fishkin BG, Orloff N, Scaduto LE, et al: IgE multiple myeloma: A report of the third case. Blood 39:361–367, 1972.

44. Frangione B, Franklin EC: Heavy chain diseases: Clinical features and molecular significance of the disordered immunoglobulin structure. Semin Hematol 10:53–64, 1973.

45. Furie B, Greene E, Furie BC: Syndrome of acquired factor X deficiency and systemic amyloidosis. In vivo studies of the metabolic fate of factor X. N Engl J Med 297:81–85, 1977.

46. Gahrton G, Tura S, Flesch M: Bone marrow transplantation in multiple myeloma: Report from the European Cooperative Group for Bone Marrow Transplantation. Blood 69:1262–1264, 1987.

47. Glueck HE, Hong RA: A circulating anticoagulant in IA-multiple myeloma: Its modification by penicillin. J Clin Invest 44:1866–1881, 1965.

48. Helms CA, Genant HK: Computed tomography in the early detection of skeletal involvement with multiple myeloma. JAMA 248:2886–2887, 1982.

49. Helms CA, Vogler JB III, Genant HK: Characteristic CT manifestations of uncommon spinal disorders. Orthop Clin North Am 16:445–459, 1985.

50. Hewell GM, Alexanian R: Multiple myeloma in young persons. Ann Intern Med 84:441–443, 1976.

51. Hobbs JR: Immunochemical classes of myelomatosis. Including data from a therapeutic trial conducted by a medical research council working party. Br J Haematol 16:599–606, 1969.

52. Hobbs JR: Growth rates and responses to treatment in human myelomatosis. Br J Haematol 16:607–617, 1969.

53. Hoffbrand AV, Hobbs JR, Kremenchuzky S, Mollin DL: Incidence and pathogenesis of megaloblastic erythropoiesis in multiple myeloma. J Clin Pathol 20:699–705, 1967.

54. Ioachim NJ, McKenna PJ, Halperin I, Chung FJ: IgD myeloma: Immunology and ultrastructure. Ann Clin Lab Sci 8:209–218, 1978.

55. Iwashita H, Ohnishi A, Asada M, et al: Polyneuropathy, skin hyperpigmentation, edema, and hypertrichosis in localized osteosclerotic myeloma. Neurology 27:675–681, 1977.

56. Jaffe JP, Bosch A, Raich PC: Sequential hemi-body radiotherapy in advanced multiple myeloma. Cancer 43:124–128, 1979.

57. Jaffe JP, Mosher DF: Calcium binding by a myeloma protein. Am J Med 67:343–346, 1979.

58. Jameson RM: Prolonged survival in paraplegia due to metastatic spinal tumours. Lancet 1:1209–1211, 1976.

59. Jelsma RK, Kirsch PT: The treatment of malignancy of a vertebral body. Surg Neurol 13:189–195, 1980.

60. Kagan E, Jacobson R, et al: Lymphoid and plasma cell malignancies: Asbestos-related disorders of long latency. Am J Clin Pathol 80:14–20, 1983.

61. Karchmer RK, Amare M, Larsen WE, et al: Alkylating agents as leukemogens in multiple myeloma. Cancer 33:1103–1107, 1974.

62. Knowling MA, Harwood AR, Bergsagel DE: Comparison of extramedullary plasmacytomas with solitary and multiple plasma cell tumours of bone. J Clin Oncol 1:255–262, 1983.

63. Kopp WL, MacKinney AA Jr, Wasson G: Blood volume and hematocrit value in macroglobulinemia and myeloma. Arch Intern Med 123:394–396, 1969.

64. Korst DR, Clifford GO, Fowler WM, et al: Multiple myeloma. II. Analysis of cyclophosphamide therapy in 165 patients. JAMA 189:758–762, 1964.

65. Kozura M, Benoki H, Sugimoto H, et al: A case of lambda type tetramer Bence-Jones proteinemia. Acta Haematol (Basel) 57:359–365, 1977.

66. Kubat R, Svehla F, Horacek J: A case of IgD plasmacytoma with unusual neurological symptoms. Folia Haematol (Leipz) 104:366–375, 1977.

67. Kyle RA: Multiple myeloma: Review of 869 cases. Mayo Clin Proc 50:29, 1975.

68. Kyle RA, Elveback LR: Management and prognosis in multiple myeloma. Mayo Clin Proc 51:751–760, 1976.

69. Kyle RA, Garton JP: The spectrum of IgM monoclonal gammopathy in 430 cases. Mayo Clin Proc 62:719–731, 1987.

70. Kyle RA, Greipp PR: Smoldering multiple myeloma. N Engl J Med 302:1347–1349, 1980.

71. Kyle RA, Nobrega FT, Kurland LT: Multiple myeloma in Ohmsted County, Minnesota, 1940S–1964S. Blood 33:739–745, 1969.

72. Kyle RA, Pierre RV, Bayrd ED: Multiple myeloma and acute myelomonocytic leukemia. Report of four cases possibly related to Melphalan. N Engl J Med 283:1121–1125, 1970.

73. Lee BJ, Sahakian G, Clarkson BD, Krakoff IH: Combination chemotherapy of multiple myeloma with alkeran, cytoxan, vincristine, prednisone, and BCNU. Cancer 33:533–538, 1974.

74. Lesoin F, Bonneterre J, Lesoin A, Jomin M: Neurologic manifestations of spinal plasmacytomas. Neurochirurgie 28:401–407, 1982.

75. Lesoin F, Jomin M, Pellerin P, et al: Transclival transcervical approach to the upper cervical spine and clivus. Acta Neurochir (Wien) 80:100–104, 1986.

76. Lingg G, Miller RP, Fischedick AR, et al: Diagnostic possibilities of computer tomography in spinal and paraspinal space occupying lesions. Rontgenblatter 38:207–212, 1985.

77. Lipson SJ, Hammerschlag SB: Atlantoaxial arthrodesis in the presence of posterior spondyloschisis (bifid arch) of the atlas. A report of three cases and an evaluation of alternative wiring techniques by computerized tomography. Spine 9:65–69, 1984.

78. Lobosky JM, Kitchon PW, McDonnell DE: Transthoracic anterolateral decompression for thoracic spinal lesions. Neurosurgery 14:26–30, 1984.

79. Loftus CM, Michelsen CB, Rapoport F, Antunes JL: Management of plasmacytomas of the spine. Neurosurgery 13:30–36, 1983.

80. Louis R, Casanova J, Baffert M: Surgical techniques in tumors of the spine. Rev Chir Orthop 62:57–70, 1976.

81. Lucantani D, Galzio R, Zenobii M, et al: Spinal cord compression by solitary plasmacytoma. J Neurosurg Sci 27:125–127, 1983.

82. Maharaj B, Kalideen JM, Leary WP, Pudifin DJ: Carcinoma of the prostate with multiple osteolytic metastasis simulating multiple myeloma. A case report. S Afr Med J 70:227–228, 1986.

83. Malpas JS: General management of myeloma. *In* Delamore

IW (ed): Multiple Myeloma and Other Paraproteinemias. Edinburgh, Churchill Livingstone, 1986, p 339.

84. McIntyre OR, Acute Leukemia Group B: Correlation of abnormal immunoglobulin with clinical features of myeloma. Arch Intern Med 135:46–52, 1975.

85. McPhedran P, Heath CW Jr, Garcia J: Multiple myeloma incidence in metropolitan Atlanta, Georgia: Racial and seasonal variations. Blood 39:866–873, 1972.

86. Meis JM, Butler JJ, Osborne BM, Ordonez NG: Solitary plasmacytomas of bone and extramedullary plasmacytomas. A clinicopathologic and immunohistochemical study. Cancer 59:1474–1485, 1987.

87. Mellstedt H, Bjorkholm M, Johannson B, et al: Interferon therapy in myelomatosis. Lancet 1:245–247, 1979.

88. Mill WB, Griffith R: The role of radiation therapy in the management of plasma cell tumors. Cancer 45:647–652, 1980.

89. Mills RJ, Fahie-Wilson MN, Carter PM, Hobbs JR: IgE myelomatosis. Clin Exp Immunol 23:228–232, 1976.

90. MRC Working Party for Therapeutic Trials in Leukaemia. Myelomatosis: Comparison of melphalan and cyclophosphamide therapy. Br Med J 1:640–641, 1971.

91. Mundy GR, Raisz LG, Cooper RA, et al: Evidence for the secretion of an osteoclast stimulating factor in myeloma. N Engl J Med 291:1041–1046, 1974.

92. Murray T, Long W, Narins RG: Multiple myeloma and the anion gap. N Engl J Med 292:574–575, 1975.

93. Mustoe TA, Fried MP, Goodman ML, et al: Osteosclerotic plasmacytoma of maxillary bone (orbital floor). J Laryngol Otol 98:929–938, 1984.

94. Myer JE, Schulz MD: "Solitary" myeloma of bone. A review of 12 cases. Cancer 34:438–440, 1974.

95. Nies BA, Kundel DW, Thomas LB, Freireich EJ: Leukopenia, bone pain, and bone necrosis in patients with acute leukemia. A clinicopathologic complex. Ann Intern Med 62:698–705, 1965.

96. Ogawa M, Kochwa S, Smith C, et al: Clinical aspects of IgE myeloma. N Engl J Med 281:1217–1220, 1969.

97. Onimus M, Schraub S, Bertin D, et al: Treatment of secondary cancer of the spine. Rev Clin Orthop 71:473–482, 1985.

98. Panjabi MM, Goel VK, Clark CR, et al: Biomechanical study of cervical spine stabilization with methylmethacrylate. Spine 10:198–203, 1985.

99. Paul LW, Pohle EA: Solitary myeloma of bone. A review of the roentgenologic features, with a report of four additional cases. Radiology 35:651–666, 1940.

100. Perkins HA, MacKenzie MR, Fudenberg HH: Hemostatic defects in dysproteinemias. Blood 35:695–707, 1970.

101. Porter FS Jr: Multiple myeloma in a child. J Pediatr 62:602–604, 1963.

102. Pruzanski W, Ogryzlo MA: Abnormal proteinuria in malignant diseases. Adv Clin Chem 13:335–382, 1970.

103. Pruzanski W, Watt JG: Serum viscosity and hyperviscosity syndrome in IgG multiple myeloma. Report on 10 patients and a review of the literature. Ann Intern Med 77:853–860, 1972.

104. Report of the Medical Research Council's Working Party for Therapeutic Trials in Leukemia. Report on the first myelomatosis trial. Part I: Analysis of presenting features of prognostic significance. Br J Haematol 24:123–139, 1973.

105. Roberts M, Rinaudo PA, Vilinskas J, Owens G: Solitary sclerosing plasma cell myeloma of the spine. Case report. J Neurosurg 40:125–129, 1974.

106. Rosenberg SA, Diamond HD, Jaslowitz B, Craver LF: Lymphosarcoma: A review of 1269 cases. Medicine 40:31–84, 1961.

107. Rossi JF, Bataille R, Chappard D, et al: B cell malignancies presenting with unusual bone involvement and mimicking multiple myeloma. Study of nine cases. Am J Med 83:10–16, 1987.

108. Rossleigh MA, Smith J, Yeh SD: Scintigraphic features of primary sacral tumors. J Nucl Med 27:627–630, 1986.

109. Rubins J, Quazi R, Woll JE: Massive bleeding after biopsy of plasmacytoma. Report of two cases. J Bone Joint Surg 62:138–140, 1980.

110. Salmon SE, Durie BGM: Cellular kinetics in multiple myeloma. A new approach to staging and treatment. Arch Intern Med 135:131–138, 1975.

111. Salmon SE, Haut A, Bonnet JD, et al: Alternating combination chemotherapy and levamisole improves survival in multiple myeloma: A Southwest Oncology Group Study. J Clin Oncol 1:453–461, 1983.

112. Sartoris DJ, Pate D, Haghighi P, et al: Plasma cell sclerosis of bone: A spectrum of disease. J Can Assoc Radiol 37:25–34, 1986.

113. Savage D, Garrett TJ: Multiple myeloma masquerading as metastatic breast cancer. Cancer 57:923–924, 1986.

114. Schajowicz F: Marrow tumors. In Schajowicz F (ed): Tumors and Tumorlike Lesions of Bone and Joints. New York, Springer-Verlag, 1981, pp 243–302.

115. Schajowicz F, Hokama J: Aspiration (puncture or needle) biopsy in bone lesions. Recent Results Cancer Res 54:139–144, 1976.

116. Seligmann M, Mihaesco E, Preud'homme JL, et al: Heavy chain diseases: Current findings and concepts. Immunol Rev 48:145–167, 1979.

117. Shaw AFB: A case of plasma cell myeloma. J Pathol Bacteriol 26:125–126, 1923.

118. Shulman G, Jacobson RJ: Immunocytoma in black and white South Africans. Trop Geogr Med 32:112–117, 1980.

119. Shustik C, Bergsagel DE, Pruzanski W: κ and λ light chain disease: Survival rates and clinical manifestations. Blood 48:41–51, 1976.

120. Solomon A, Rahamani R, Seligsohn U, Ben-Artzi F: Multiple myeloma: Early vertebral involvement assessed by computerized tomography. Skeletal Radiol 11:258–261, 1984.

121. Sundaresan N, Galicich JH, Lane JM, Greenberg HS: Treatment of odontoid fractures in cancer patients. J Neurosurg 54:187–192, 1981.

122. Sundaresan N, Galicich JH, Lane JM: Harrington rod stabilization for pathological fractures of the spine. J Neurosurg 60:282–286, 1984.

123. Sunder-Plassmann M: Dorsal inter and extracorporeal osteosynthesis for tumours of the thoracic vertebral bodies. Neurochirurgia (Stuttg) 23:99–105, 1980.

124. Sunder-Plassmann M: Vertral osteosynthesis for the treatment of metastatic tumours of the superior thoracic spine. Neurochirurgia (Stuttg) 23:106–111, 1980.

125. Talerman A: Clinico-pathological study of multiple myeloma in Jamaica. Br J Cancer 23:285–293, 1969.

126. Tong D, Griffin TW, Laramore GE, et al: Solitary plasmacytoma of bone and soft tissues. Radiology 135:195–198, 1980.

127. Tribalto M, Mandelli F, Cantonetti M, et al: Recombinant alpha 2b interferon as post maintenance therapy for responding multiple myeloma. Clinical results of a multicentric trial. New Trends Ther Leuk Lymph 2:61, 1987.

128. Valat JP, Eveleigh MC, Fouquet B, Born P: Bone scintigraphy in multiple myeloma. Rev Rhum Mal Osteoartic 52:707–711, 1975.

129. Von Scheefe C: Light chain myeloma with features of adult Fanconi syndrome. Six years remission with one course of melphalan. Acta Med Scand 199:533, 1976.

130. Wachsman W, Golde DW, Chen ISY: HTLV and human leukemia: Perspectives 1986. Semin Hematol 23:245–256, 1986.

131. Willson JKV: The bone lesions of childhood leukemia. A survey of 140 cases. Radiology 72:672–681, 1959.

132. Wiltshaw E: The natural history of extramedullary plasmacytoma and its relation to solitary myeloma of bone and myelomatosis. Medicine 55:217–238, 1976.

133. Woodruff RK, Malpas JS, White FE: Solitary Plasmacytoma. II. Solitary plasmacytoma of bone. Cancer 43:2344–2347, 1979.

134. Yentis I: The so-called solitary plasmacytoma of bone. J Fac Radiol 8:132–144, 1956.

TUMORS OF THE NERVE SHEATH INVOLVING THE SPINE

DONALD SMITH and HENRY H. SCHMIDER

INTRODUCTION

As axons exit the central nervous system (CNS) they are ensheathed by Schwann cells, perineural cells, and epineural and endoneural fibrocytes (fibroblasts). Arachnoidal cells, which loosely envelop nerve roots as they course intrathecally, are not classically considered to be a part of the nerve sheath. The histogenesis and nomenclature of the tumors arising from these ensheathing elements have long been a matter of dispute. Both Schwann cells and perineural cells are of neural crest derivation and were thought to be the tumor-forming element in Schwannomas and neurofibromas, respectively. However, there is now a large body of evidence founded on ultrastructural studies and tissue culture work supporting the Schwann cell as the common progenitor of both schwannomas and neurofibromas.[25, 30, 37] As a result, there is a growing tendency to drop the distinction between schwannomas and neurofibromas and to refer instead to a single group of "nerve sheath tumors." This terminology is sometimes confusing because there are a small number of tumors arising within the nerve sheath that do not share this histogenetic identity. Examples of such exceptions are nerve root lipomas and neuronal precursor tumors arising in the dorsal foot ganglion. In addition, there is a diverse group of tumors that may involve the spinal nerve and osseous spine by local extension or by metastasis from a remote site.

BENIGN NERVE SHEATH TUMORS

The majority of schwannomas are benign solitary tumors. Initially the affected nerve is expanded in a fusiform fashion; with continued growth, however, the tumor begins to erupt through the nerve's fascicular structure, creating an eccentric mass. Particularly favored sites of tumor formation are the vestibular branch of the eighth cranial nerve and the sensory roots of spinal nerves. Tumors in the latter occur principally as intradural extramedullary lesions. A minority of spinal schwannomas (13 per cent) have both intra- and extradural components, giving rise to "dumbbell tumors," which grow into the neural foramen and the paravertebral tissues.

Schwannomas are characterized by two distinctive patterns of histologic organization. The Antoni A pattern consists of a dense population of elongate bipolar cells with spindly nuclei and poorly defined cytoplasmic borders. Collagen and reticulin fibers are abundant in the extracellular matrix. Nuclei tend to be arranged in parallel arrays alternating with zones of pale eosinophilic cytoplasm in a distinctive fashion termed "palisading." Antoni B regions are less densely populated, and the cells are stellate-shaped with coarse processes. These are loosely arranged in bundles and cords that lack the tight organization of the Antoni A pattern. Microcystic changes are common, and no palisading is observed. Although occasional multinucleated giant cells and proliferative vascular changes and areas of thrombosis may be present, these features lack a malignant connotation in themselves. Antoni A and Antoni B regions intermingle extensively, but the tumor is mostly devoid of axons and functional neural tissue. Lipid-laden foam cells are also characteristically seen (Fig. 23–1).

The word neurofibroma is used to designate a related tumor with somewhat different gross and histologic character. These lesions are less well encapsulated than are schwannomas and may not offer a discrete, dissectable mass. The parent nerves are often diffusely swollen and indistinctly marginated from the tumor, which itself is often coursed through by functional axons. They are most commonly found in cutaneous and deep peripheral nerves, and solitary spinal neurofibromas are said to be rare. Indeed, this tumor is only occasionally encountered outside the context of von Recklinghausen's disease. Histologically, neurofibromas are characterized by spindly bipolar cells arranged in twisting cords; the extracellular matrix is rich in both collagen and mucopolysaccharides. The presence of the latter is an additional feature distinguishing neurofibromas from schwannomas. Neurofibromas lack the ordered architecture of the Antoni A regions and more closely

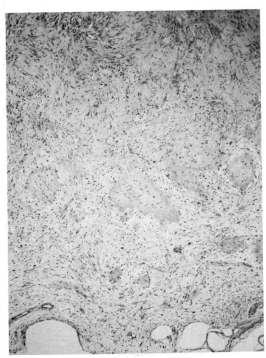

FIGURE 23–1. A schwannoma with a biphasic pattern of Antoni A and B. The Antoni A consists of spindle cells in tightly arranged bundles with their nuclei lying parallel to each other. The Antoni B configuration is that of loosely arranged spindle or stellate cells without a parallel pattern of the nuclei (H & E ×60).

resemble the Antoni B pattern, and it is sometimes difficult to differentiate neurofibromas from schwannomas, which are dominated by an Antoni B component. Both types of tumors usually stain positively for S-100 protein, an immunocytochemical marker indicative of neural crest derivation. They are slow growing, and in the absence of von Recklinghausen's disease malignant transformation is rare.[2, 25]

Schwannomas and neurofibromas together comprise one third of primary spinal cord tumors and show a predeliction for the thoracic spine over the lumbar and cervical spine. These tumors are well encapsulated and are occasionally cystic. Patients with either a benign spinal schwannoma or a neurofibroma typically present with radicular dysfunction in the distribution of the affected root, which may in all ways mimic the radiculopathies associated with a herniated intervertebral disc and degenerative spondylotic disease. If the early symptoms should go unrecognized or unattended, tumor progression will eventuate in compression of the spinal cord or cauda equina with its characteristic clinical features. Pedicular widening or erosion, vertebral scalloping, or foraminal expansion on standard roentgenographs may suggest the presence of such a tumor. The interpretation of such radiographic changes in the presence of von Recklinghausen's disease must be cautious, however, since the spine may develop dysplastically in this condition, and the same abnormalities together with kyphoscoliosis may be observed in the absence of a mass lesion. Definitive evaluation requires computed tomography (CT)–myelography or magnetic resonance imaging (MRI) scanning.

The surgical treatment typically consists of fully exposing the tumor's intraspinal, foraminal, and extraspinal extension through a laminectomy with facetectomy. The involved root, if not of crucial importance, may be sacrificed. In the case of an important nerve involved by a schwannoma, it may be possible to preserve function and dissect the tumor away from the nerve's fascicles with microsurgical technique and intraoperative electrophysiologic monitoring. An intradural exploration is mandatory to ensure the completeness of the resection, and this may necessitate a dural grafting procedure depending on the degree of proximal involvement. Tumors with significant extraspinal extension into the neck, chest, or retroperitoneum may require combined or staged procedures to effect a total cure. It is generally safest to resect the intraspinal component first to reduce the possibility of spinal cord injury, which may attend manipulation of the extraspinal component during the surgical dissection. The remaining extraspinal portion can then be removed using lateral or enterolateral exposures in the cervical spine; in the thoracic region, depending on tumor size and level, transthoracic or costotransverse approaches are available; and in the lumbar spine, a retroperitoneal approach is useful. Complete resection of intrasacral lesions may necessitate a posterior sacral laminectomy combined with an anterior transabdominal approach. The spine is seldom rendered unstable either by the tumor or by the surgical resection thereof, and internal fixation and bony fusion are seldom required Long-term results are excellent, with a cure being obtained in upwards of 90 per cent of patients. Symptomatic recurrence of incompletely resected lesions is slow to occur and lends itself to reoperation. There is no role for radiotherapy except possibly in the patient too infirm to withstand operation. In this circumstance, a diagnosis could be established by needle biopsy, and external radiation therapy could then be recommended on the basis of the apparent modest response to this modality observed in acoustic neuromas.

NEUROFIBROMATOSIS

The presence of multiple schwannomas is virtually diagnostic of neurofibromatosis. These tumors differ from solitary schwannomas in that they less often offer a discrete dissectable mass. The involved nerves are often diffusely swollen, with indistinct margination from the tumor. Two distinct forms of neurofibromatosis have been identified. These are separate genetic entities caused by different genes or different alleles of the same gene. Both forms of this disease show autosomal dominant transmission and high penetrance. If a person possesses the genetic defect, some characteristic of the condition is therefore usually expressed. In the case of classic von Recklinghausen's neurofibromatosis (VRNF = NR1), the penetrance is nearly 100 per cent, but the expression is variable and the diagnosis can be difficult. The most common manifestations are the multiple cutaneous or subcutaneous neurofibromas that are pathognomonic of the disease. Café au lait (CAL) spots occur due to the abnormally large melanosomes (macromelanosomes) in the skin, this being another phenotypic abnormality within cell series derived from neural crest. Lisch nodule of the iris is a hamartomatous lesion that may be present particularly in postpubertal patients. Other abnormalities that may be associated with VRNF include kyphoscoliosis (2 per cent) and pheochromocytoma (1 per cent).

Bilateral acoustic neurofibromatosis (BANF = NFII) is the other form of neurofibromatosis. The VRNF gene is located on the long arm of chromosome 17, whereas the inherited defect in BANF is in a gene on chromosome 22. Both VRNF and BANF are associated with multiple spinal neurofibromas, most commonly orginating on their dorsal root ganglia. Multiple spinal and intracranial meningiomas can occur in either form of neurofibromatosis, along with astrocytomas of the spinal cord, brain stem, and cerebrum.

The formation of a tumor through loss or inactivation of a suppressor gene has been demonstrated in retinoblastoma and is suggested by recent studies in neuroblastoma. It is possible that in the case of BANF the long arm of chromosome 22 contains a tumor suppression gene that is important in the growth control of cells of neural crest origin. A benign tumor forms when a deletion or mutation occurs involving the normal copy of the gene. Chromosomal abnormalities are multiplied in the case of malignant tumors, and these neoplasms often demonstrate extra copies of genes or entire chromosomes. Whereas sporadic neurofibromas are almost always benign, it is estimated that there is a 3 to 30 per cent chance of malignant transformation in the context of von Recklinghausen's disease.

PIGMENTED NERVE SHEATH TUMORS

Melanocytic cells may normally be found with the leptomeninges at the base of the brain and about the spinal cord. Particularly large and confluent aggregation of such cells results in melanosis of the leptomeninges. These cells are of neural crest derivation and may have arrested at these sites in the course of their migration with cutaneous ectoderm. They are the likely cells of origin for very rare primary pigmented tumors of the CNS, melanocytomas, and malignant melanomas. They may also be the cells responsible for pigmentation within the occasional reported examples of melanotic meningioma and schwannoma.

Pigmented tumors of the nerve sheath are extraordinarily rare. As of 1974, only 19 cases had been recorded in the world's literature. The majority of these tumors were peripherally located, benign, and unassociated with von Recklinghausen's disease. Mandybur reported a benign pigmented nerve sheath tumor arising intraspinally in association with a dorsal root ganglion and with extraforaminal extension into the chest.[33] Histologically the tumor was composed of nerve sheath elements resembling a

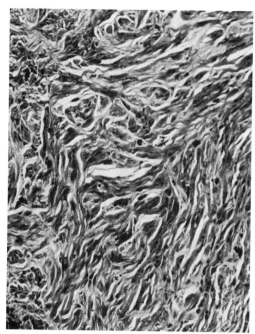

FIGURE 23–2. The rare pigmented schwannoma has features of a typical schwannoma with melanin-laden spindle cells (H & E × 200).

plexiform neurofibroma intermingled with an Antoni A pattern. Melanin contained within the tumor cells was of a peripheral type. The histogenesis of these tumors remains obscure.

MALIGNANT NERVE SHEATH TUMORS

The classification of malignant tumors of the nerve sheath has been as arcane as has that of their benign counterparts. There is a parallel tendency to drop the distinction between malignant schwannoma, malignant neurofibroma, and neurofibrosarcoma, and instead to refer to a group of malignant nerve sheath tumors. These tend to occur either in association with neurofibromatosis or within the field of previous therapeutic irradiation to a large degree. Diagnostic criteria are based on microscopic, gross, and clinical features.[12] Histologically, these tumors are characterized by hypercellularity, pleomorphism, nuclear atypia, pseudopalisading, vascular proliferative changes, multinucleated giant cells, frequent mitoses, and areas of necrosis. The cells may be arrayed as fascicles of spindly cells or organized in a herringbone or epithelioid pattern. Staining for S-100 protein is frequently negative. Divergent differentiation toward rhabdomyosarcoma, chondrosarcoma, and osteosarcoma is not uncommon. At an ultrastructural level, branching cytoplasmic processes that may contain microtubules or microfilaments may be seen. Often there is a coexisting component of benign nerve sheath tumor. From a histologic standpoint the differential diagnosis would include fibrosarcoma, malignant fibrous histiocytoma, leiomyosarcoma, and synovial sarcoma. The diagnosis of malignant nerve sheath tumor is strongly supported by the finding of the tumor origin within a nerve or an adjacent nerve sheath tumor or by the presence of neurofibromatosis (Fig. 23–3).

Malignant nerve sheath tumors are extremely dangerous tumors with low survival rates. They seem to behave in similarly aggressive fashion regardless of their individual histologic character. Attempts at grading of malignant nerve sheath tumors have not been rewarding for this reason.[19] Although sometimes giving the appearance of being well encapsulated grossly, local invasion of surrounding tissues is the rule. As with other soft tissue sarcomas, there is a tendency to advance locally along fascial planes of least resistance and thus to extend axially within the substance of the parent nerve trunk.[4, 46, 49] This propensity results in early involvement of the CNS with tumors proximally situated within or adjacent to the spine. It is this characteristic and the inability to obtain an adequate margin of resection that restrict the surgical management of these tumors to diagnosis and debulking procedures, except in the case of some extremity and truncal lesions. Blood-borne metastases, especially to the lungs, are common and are the frequent proximate cause of death. The best treatment results have been realized in distal extremity lesions with limb amputation, which is able to achieve a wide margin of resection. Nonetheless, the 5-year survival in this group is only 40 per cent. Survival with truncal lesions is much less. Other features that adversely affect prognosis are the presence of neurofibromatosis, tumor size greater than 5 cm, and the inability to achieve gross total resection.[19]

Although a variety of chemotherapeutic agents including methotrexate, vincristine, doxorubicin, cyclophosphamide, and cisplatin have been employed against malignant schwannomas and neurofibrosarcomas, these tumors have shown little response to

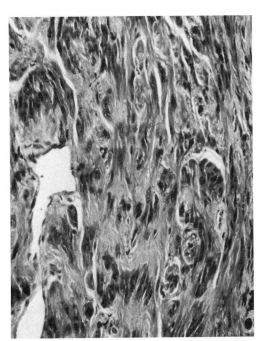

FIGURE 23–3. A malignant nerve sheath tumor with pleomorphic and hyperchromatic nuclei and prominent vascular structures. Some of the spindle cells have their nuclei arranged in parallel with other cells (H & E ×250).

this modality. The results of both pre- and postoperative external beam irradiation and brachytherapy are similarly discouraging.[46] In those patients in whom surgical decompression is warranted for palliative purposes, concomitant spinal reconstruction is frequently required to ensure clinical stability. Harrington or Luque rods together with a biologic or prosthetic fusion are frequently useful for this purpose. In general, we favor methyl methacrylate over bony fusion in these circumstances because of the immediate stability it provides, because graft incorporation may be compromised by radiation effect or chemotherapy, and because local tumor control is frequently incomplete. The primary site is radiated postoperatively with 5000 to 6000 cGy by convention, although there are few data to support the efficacy of treatment.[24, 40] Although there is a possibility of distant intra- and extraaxial spread within the CNS and remote relapse, the role of total craniospinal irradiation is unknown. Furthermore, there are few data to support the use of either systemic or intrathecally administered chemotherapy at this time. Survival in the individual case reports and small series is usually in the range of several months to a year, which is in agreement with our experience.[12, 27]

CASE 1

MCHV reported a case of multiple spinal and extraspinal neurofibroma that formed a massive tumor encasing the brachial plexus and extending into the spinal canal. The patient had undergone wide cervical laminectomy elsewhere for intraspinal neurofibroma and had subsequently developed severe swan-neck deformity and attendant myelopathy. These were partially corrected in traction; then the patient underwent anterior multilevel corpectomy with strut grafting and was maintained in halo postoperatively until solid fusion was obtained. Surgical exposure was complicated by a huge neurofibroma that overlay the spine ventrally. Subsequently the patient developed rue monoparesis and a rapidly expanding neck mass that was explored and was subtotally excised, with the finding of a malignant neurofibroma. The patient was treated with external radiation therapy (Figs. 23–4 through 23–6).

RADIATION-INDUCED MALIGNANT NERVE SHEATH TUMORS

The potential oncogenic effect of therapeutically administered irradiation was recognized by Cahan in 1948,[7] and criteria for the diagnosis of radiation-induced malignancies were proposed. Osteosarcomas, neurofibrosarcomas, and malignant schwannomas are the tumors most often associated with this phenomenon. In particular, Hodgkin's lymphoma, breast cancer, and cervical cancer are malignancies in which therapeutic irradiation figures prominently in treatment and in which cure or very extended survival is now possible. It is in this group of patients and in those irradiated for benign conditions that the bulk of radiation-induced malignancies occur. The exact risk in any individual patient is unknown, but it has been estimated that there is approximately

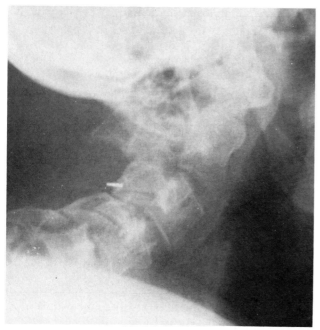

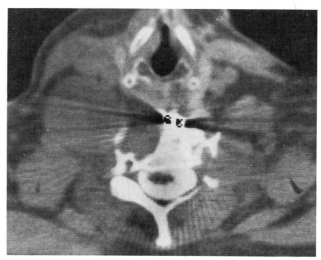

FIGURE 23–6. Case 1. Two years later the patient presented with a malignant neurofibroma originating in the brachial plexus on the right and shown here invading the anterior element of C6.

FIGURE 23–4. Case 1. Swan-neck deformity at C5-C6 two years after extensive cervical laminectomy for spinal neurofibroma.

1 per cent cumulative risk of such a development after 8 years' survival from Hodgkin's disease. On the other hand, there is a mean latent interval of 10 years to the time of occurrence of the second malignancy. The minimum radiation dosage capable of inducing these malignancies is unknown, but it could be as low as 1000 cGy.[52] Radiation-induced malignancies of the nerve sheath behave as treacherously as do those malignant nerve sheath tumors that arise in the context of neurofibromatosis.

Approximately 30 per cent of such radiation-induced malignancies arise in relation to the axial skeleton, and Sundaresan has recently reviewed an experience in the treatment of 13 such patients. Seven of the 13 tumors were either fibrosarcomas, malignant schwannomas, or spindle cell sarcomas; the remainder were osteosarcomas. The mean survival in this group was only 8 months despite aggressive surgery, brachytherapy, and chemotherapy.

CASE 2

Tampa General Hospital treated a man with malignant schwannoma arising in the lumbar plexus. This was locally resected twice with proximal amputation of the L2 root at the level of the neural foramen and "negative" tumor margin. The patient experienced further recurrence in the cauda equina, which was decompressed and debulked, and died 10 months from first diagnosis with seeding of entire neuraxis and at least two intraparenchymal mets (Figs. 23–7 and 23–8).

OTHER TUMORS INVOLVING THE NERVE SHEATH

There exists a wide variety of primary and secondary neoplasms arising within or involving the spinal nerves which may mimic nerve sheath tumors and raise parallel management concerns. Primary tumors of the spinal nerve arising in other than nerve sheath elements would seem to be extraordinarily rare, but may include lipomas (reported thus far in peripheral nerves, e.g., median)[45] and neuronal cell tumors originating in the dorsal root ganglion. A much more common problem is that of compression of the spinal roots and cord structures by local expansion of tumors arising in a metastasis to the vertebral column or paraspinal soft tissues. Whereas these tumors are usually malignant, this is not always the case (Fig. 23–9).

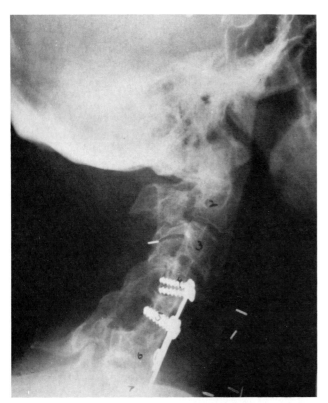

FIGURE 23–5. Case 1. Appearance of same patient after closed reduction and anterior cervical fusion with plate and screw fixation.

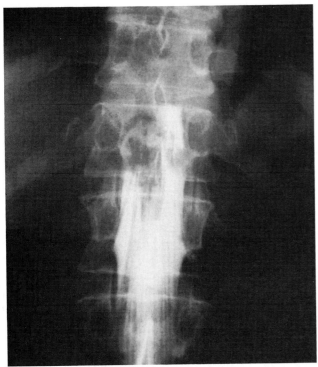

FIGURE 23–7. Case 2. Intra- and extramedullary metastasis at T12 level from a malignant schwannoma arising in the right lumbar plexus.

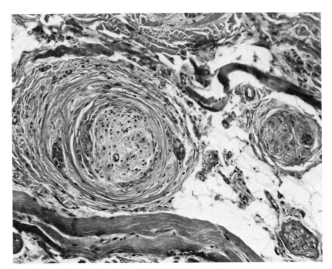

FIGURE 23–9. A metastatic squamous cell carcinoma invading nerve sheaths. Tumor cells are the dark islands embedded in the nerve fiber (H & E ×175).

Of particular neuropathologic interest is the group of tumors of neural crest derivation that originate in tissues of the sympathetic and paraganglionic systems. The ganglia of both these systems are distributed paraaxially in close relation to the spine, which may then be involved by their local growth and expansion. Neuroblastoma is a primitive tumor arising from neural crest stem cells. It is highly aggressive in its local growth characteristics and also frequently gives rise to remote metastases. It is principally a tumor of infancy and childhood which arises from undifferentiated neural crest cells commonly found in the adrenal or sympathetic ganglia. This tumor appears to represent an arrest in normal differentiation of these cells. Occasionally the tumor will undergo spontaneous maturation into a benign tumor (Fig. 23–10).

The study of neuroblastoma has yielded important insights into the molecular genetics of CNS neoplasia. One member of the the *myc* family of oncogenes, *n-myc*, was discovered by virtue of its amplification in

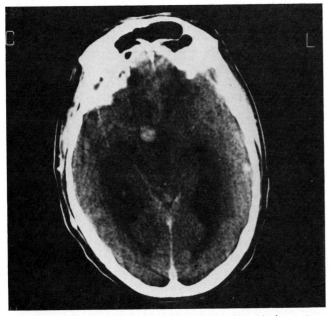

FIGURE 23–8. Case 2. Hydrocephalus and periventricular metastasis from seeding of the craniospinal axis with malignant schwannoma.

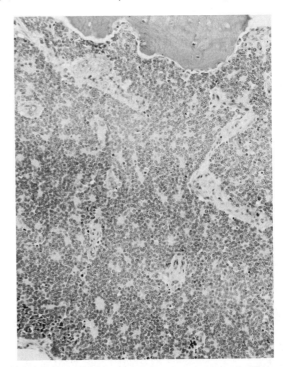

FIGURE 23–10. A low power view of neuroblastoma illustrating sheets of small round cells, some of which are arranged about an oval space forming a rosette pattern. Such rosettes are formed by neuroblasts aggregated about neurofibrils simulating a vascular space. Such a finding is often characteristic of a neuroblastoma. At the top of the picture is a portion of cortical bone (H & E ×160).

human neuroblastoma. This example of gene amplification is demonstrated in human neuroblastoma by direct counting of the number of oncogenes in fresh biopsy specimens from previously untreated patients. In some cases it is possible to identify hundreds of thousands of copies of the amplified gene. It can be presumed that one cloning of these genes resulted in overexpression of the normal gene products and the subsequent transformation of the affected sympathetic nerve cells. A direct relationship can often be demonstrated between the extent of gene amplification and the subsequent biologic aggressiveness of these tumors. The *n-ras* gene has also been implicated in the pathogenesis of neuroblastoma. The *n-ras* gene differs from its nontransforming cellular homologue by a single nucleotide point mutation in the amino acids adjacent to the binding site of *ras* proteins which has caused glycine to be replaced by valine in the protooncogene. The malignant transformation of a normal cell is probably not a single-step process but may require the cooperative interaction of oncogenes belonging to different gene families. For example, *n-myc* is able to cooperate with *ras* oncogene to transform embryonic fibroblasts, whereas neither of these genes by itself is sufficient to produce tumorigenesis.[38]

Because of their propensity to arise paraaxially and expand locally, neuroblastomas may invade the neural foramen to create a dumbbell tumor and cause cord compression. Laminectomy for diagnosis and resection of the intraspinal component followed by extraspinal resection for tumor debulking is the usual treatment.[29] This may then be followed by radiation and chemotherapy depending on the age of the patient and the stage of the disease.

Ganglioneuromas are rare benign tumors com-

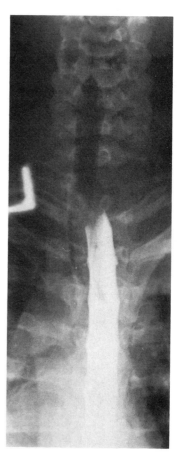

FIGURE 23–12. Case 3. Myelography of the same patient showing a complete block at T1-T2 with displacement of the spinal cord leftward.

posed of mature neurons, Schwann cells, and axonal processes. They typically present in children and young adults. Favored locations are the posterior mediastinum and retroperitoneum, although they may also arise in spinal ganglia and thereby mimic dumbbell tumors. This tumor may represent a matured form of neuroblastoma and has been reported in association with neurofibromatosis.[3, 4] Ganglioneuroblastoma is a tumor with histologic characteristics intermediate between those of neuroblastoma and ganglioneuroma; its biologic behavior is more akin to that of neuroblastoma, however.

Tumors of the paraganglionic system include pheochromocytomas, carotid body tumors (chemodectoma), jugulotympanic paragangliomas (glomus jugulare tumors), and the rarer aorticopulmonary and aorticosympathetic paragangliomas. They are generally well-differentiated tumors, with only a minority (7 to 10 per cent) behaving in a malignant fashion to give rise to distant metastases. Pheochromocytomas are the most common of the paragangliomas; 70 to 90 per cent are localized in the adrenal medulla, although they may also arise at ectopic locations throughout the paraganglionic system. They are recognized clinically by their excessive catecholamine secretion, which may produce hypertension, headache, palpitations, and other signs of adrenergic excess. Spinal involvement is fortunately infrequent.

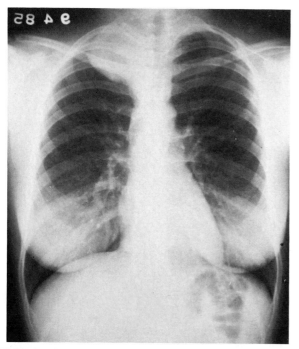

FIGURE 23–11. Case 3. A 19-year-old woman presents with a myelopathy and a right apical lung mass with extensive destructive changes in C7 and T1 on chest x-ray.

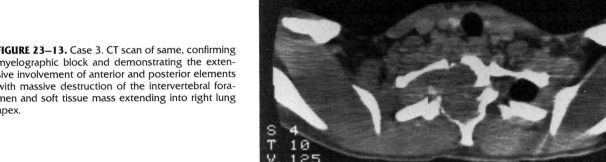

FIGURE 23–13. Case 3. CT scan of same, confirming myelographic block and demonstrating the extensive involvement of anterior and posterior elements with massive destruction of the intervertebral foramen and soft tissue mass extending into right lung apex.

The remaining paragangliomas are named according to their anatomic region of origin and are less consistently associated with endocrinologic activity. The principal neoplastic element appears to be the chief cell, although generally the tumor reproduces quite faithfully the histology of the normal gland, and mitotic figures are rare. Most are slow-growing lesions, although a minority will behave in a frankly malignant fashion with extreme local aggressiveness and distant metastases. Local growth even in the typical tumors may result in spinal involvement in consequence of their paraaxial location and their ability to become vascular. These tend to be extremely vascular lesions, and the surgeon will be well advised to obtain an angiogram preoperatively and to consider embolization if this is technically feasible. Surgical excision is the only known curative therapy. Local recurrence is anticipated following incomplete resection. Opinion is divided about the efficacy of radiation therapy in these tumors. One recent report has suggested a modest response to chemotherapy with Adriamycin and cisplatin.

CASE 3

At MCHV a 20-year-old female with misdiagnosed radicular symptoms for two years developed myelopathy and was found on plain films to have a destructive lesion in C7-T1 with an associated large pleurally based mass. The patient was operated on in several stages for debulking and stabilization, but there was incomplete resection and profound blood loss. Although there was no embolization, good angiograms were available (Figs. 23–11 through 23–14).

Locally arising sarcomas or carcinomas may also involve neural structures through contiguous growth along perineural planes.[3, 4, 17] Primary tumors of the osseous skeleton, such as chordoma, chondrosarcoma, osteosarcoma, and so forth, are taken up elsewhere in this volume. Pulmonary apex tumors (Pancoast tumor), carcinoma of the breast, and retroperitoneal tumors are particularly likely to invade nerve sheaths and the spinal canal. Treatment will be dictated by the nature of the primary tumor, the burden of systemic disease, the degree of control achieved at the primary site, and the types of treatments already employed. The same guidelines that govern the treatment of spinal epidural metastases would seem equally appropriate here. In certain instances (e.g., lymphoma), radiation alone might be indicated, whereas in others (such as foraminal invasion by a contiguous lung carcinoma) aggressive multimodality therapy with surgical resection and spinal reconstruction, external radiation therapy, and systemic chemotherapy would be warranted.[16]

REFERENCES

1. Abernathey CD, Onofrio BM, Scheithauer B, et al: Surgical management of giant sacral schwannomas. J Neurosurg 65:286–295, 1986.
2. Arseni C, Dumitrescu L, Constantinescu A: Neurinomas of the trigeminal nerves. Surg Neurol 4:497–503, 1975.
3. Ballantyne AJ, McCarten AB, Ibanez ML: The extension of cancer of the head and neck through peripheral nerves. Am J Surg 106:651–667, 1963.
4. Barber JR, Coventry MB, McDonald JR: The spread of soft-tissue sarcomata of the extremities along peripheral-nerve trunks. J Bone Joint Surg 39A:5324–5340, 1957.

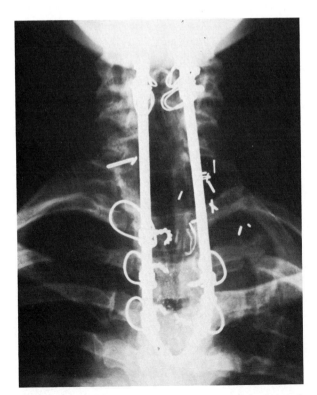

FIGURE 23–14. Case 3. Internal fixation of cervicothoracic junction with segmentally secured rods and posterior fusion.

5. Bird CC, Willis RA: The histogenesis of pigmented neurofi-bromas. J Pathol 97:631–637, 1968.

6. Black P: Spinal metastasis: Current status and recommended guidelines for management. Neurosurgery 5-726–746, 1979.

7. Cahan WG, Woodard HQ, Higinbotham NL, et al: Sarcoma arising in irradiated bone. Cancer 1:3–29, 1948.

8. Christensen C: Malignant melanocytic schwannoma: A case report. Acta Chir Scand 152:385–386, 1986.

9. Cravioto H: Studies on the normal ultrastructural of periph-eral nerve: Axis cylinders, Schwann cells, myelin. Bull Los Angeles Neurol Soc 30:169–190, 1965.

10. Cravioto H: The ultrastructure of acoustic nerve tumors. Acta Neuropathol (Berl) 12:116–140, 1969.

11. Cravioto H, Lockwood R: The behavior of acoustic neuroma in tissue culture. Acta Neuropathol (Berl) 12:141–157, 1969.

12. D'Agostino AN, Soule EJ, Miller RH: Primary malignant neoplasms of nerves (malignant neurilemmomas) in patients without manifestations of multiple neurofibromatosis (von Recklinghausen's disease). Cancer 16:1003–1027, 1963.

13. Das Gupta TK: Tumors of the peripheral nerves. Clin Neu-rosurg 25:574–590, 1977.

14. Das Gupta TK, Brasfield RD: Solitary malignant schwannoma. Ann Surg 171:419, 1970.

15. Das Gupta TK, Brasfield RD, Strong EW, Jajdu SI: Benign solitary schwannomas (neurilemmomas). Cancer 24:355–366, 1969.

16. Dewald RL, Bridwell KH, Prodromas C, Rodts MF: Recon-structive spinal surgery as palliation for metastatic malig-nancies of the spine. Spine 10(1):21–26, 1985.

17. Dodd GD, Dolan PA, Ballantyne AJ, et al: The dissemination of tumors of the head and neck via the cranial nerves. Radiol Clin North Am 8:445–461, 1970.

18. Ducatman BS, Scheithauer BW: Post radiation neurofibrosar-coma. Cancer 51:1028–1033, 1983.

19. Ducatman BS, Scheithauer BW, Pipgras DG, et al: Malignant peripheral nerve sheath tumors. Cancer 57:2006–2021, 1986.

20. Feigin I: The nerve sheath tumor, solitary and in von Reck-linghausen's disease: A unitary mesenchymal concept. Acta Neuropathol (Berl) 17:188–200, 1971.

21. Feigin I, Cohen M: Maturation and anaplasia in neuronal tumors of the peripheral nervous system with observations on the glia-like tissues in ganglioneuroblastoma. J Neuro-pathol Exp Neurol 36:748–763, 1977.

22. Ghosh BC, Ghosh L, Huvos AG, Fortner J: Malignant schwan-noma: A clinicopathological study. Cancer 31:184, 1973.

23. Greenberg R, Rosenthal I, Falk GS: Electron microscopy of human tumors secreting catecholamines: Correlation with biochemical data. J Neuropathol Exp Neurol 28:475–500, 1969.

24. Handler SD, Canalis RF, Jenkins HA, Weiss AJ: Management of brachial plexus tumors. Arch Otolaryngol 103:653–657, 1977.

25. Harkin JC, Reed RJ: Tumors of the Peripheral Nervous System. Washington, DC, Armed Forces Institute of Pa-thology, 1968.

26. Herrera GH, Pinto de Morees H: Neurogenic sarcomas in patients with neurofibromatosis. Virchows Arch 403:361–376, 1984.

27. Hutcherson RW, Jenkins HA, Canalis FR, et al: Neurogenic sarcoma of the head and neck. Arch Otolaryngol 105:267–270, 1979.

28. Huvos AG, Woodard HQ, Cahan WG, et al: Post irradiation osteosarcoma of bone and soft tissues: A clinicopathological study of 66 patients. Cancer 55:1244–1255, 1985.

29. King D, Goodman J, Hawk T, et al: Dumbbell neuroblastoma in children. Arch Surg 110:888–891, 1975.

30. Kramer W: Tumors of nerves. *In* Vinken PJ, Bruyn GW (eds): Handbook of Clinical Neurology. Amsterdam, North Hol-land Publishing, 1970, pp 412–512.

31. Levy WJ, Latchaw J, Hahn JF, et al: Spinal neurofibromas: A report of 66 cases and a comparison with meningiomas. Neurosurgery 18:331–334, 1986.

32. Lodding P, Kindblom LG, Angervall L: Epithelioid malignant schwannoma. Virchows Arch 409:433–451, 1986.

33. Mandybur TI: Melanotic nerve sheath tumors. J Neurosurg 41:187–192, 1974.

34. Matsuno H, Schimoda T, Kakimoto S, et al: Histopathologic and immunohistochemical study of malignant tumors of peripheral nerve sheath (malignant schwannoma). Cancer 56:2269–2279, 1985.

35. Mickalites CJ, Rappaport I: Perineural invasion by squamous-cell carcinoma of the lower lip: Review of the literature and report of a case. Oral Surg 46:74–78, 1978.

36. Richards JL, Matolo NM: Malignant schwannoma: Report of a case mimicking lumbar disc disease. Am Surg 45:49–51, 1979.

37. Rubinstein LJ: Tumors of the cranial and spinal nerve roots. *In* Tumors of the Central Nervous System. Washington, DC, Armed Forces Institute of Pathology, 1972, pp 205–214.

38. Schmidek HH: The molecular genetics of nervous system tumors. J Neurosurg 67:1–16, 1987.

39. Schneider SJ, Blacklock JB, Bruner JM: Melanoma arising in a spinal nerve root: Case report. J Neurosurg 67:923–927, 1987.

40. Snyder M, Batzdorf U, Sparks FC: Unusual malignant tumors involving the brachial plexus: A report of two cases. Am Surg 45:42–48, 1979.

41. Sorenson SA, Mulvihill JJ, Nilsen A: Long term follow up of von Recklinghausen's neurofibromatosis. N Engl J Med 314(16):1010–1015, 1986.

42. Sundaresan N, Bains M, McCormack P: Surgical treatment of spinal cord compression in patients with lung cancer. Neu-rosurgery 16:350–356, 1985.

43. Sundaresan N, Galicich JH, Bains MB, et al: Vertebral body resection in the treatment of cancer involving the spine. Cancer 53:1393–1396, 1984.

44. Sundaresan N, Huvos AG, Krol G, et al: Postirradiation sarcoma involving the spine. Neurosurgery 18:721–724, 1986.

45. Terzis JK, Daniel RK, Williams HB, Spencer PS: Benign fatty tumors of the peripheral nerves. Ann Plast Surg 1:193–216, 1978.

46. Vieta JO, Pack GT: Malignant neurilemmomas of peripheral nerves. Am J Surg 82:416–431, 1951.

47. Weatherby RP, Dahlin DC, Ivins JC: Postirradiation sarcoma of bone. Mayo Clinic Proc 56:294–306, 1981.

48. Weiner MA, Harris MB, Siegel RB, Klein G: Ganglioneuroma and acute lymphoblastic leukemia in association with neu-rofibromatosis. Am J Dis Child 136:1090–1091, 1982.

49. White HR: Survival in malignant schwannoma: An 18-year study. Cancer 27:720–729, 1971.

50. Woodruff MM, Chernik NL, Smith MC, et al: Peripheral nerve tumors with rhabdomyosarcomatous differentiation. Cancer 32:426, 1973.

51. Youmans JR, Ishida WY: Tumors of peripheral and sympa-thetic nerves. *In* Youmans JR (ed): Neurological Surgery. 2nd Ed. Philadelphia, WB Saunders Co., 1982, pp 3299–3315.

52. Yoshizawa Y, Kusama T, Orimoto K: Search on the lowest irradiation dose from literature on radiation induced bone tumors. Nippon Acta Radiol 37:63–72, 1977.

EWING'S TUMOR OF THE SPINE

JOHN K. BRADWAY and DOUGLAS J. PRITCHARD

INTRODUCTION

Ewing's sarcoma of bone was described in 1921 by James Ewing.[3] It accounts for approximately 6 per cent of all malignant primary bone tumors[1] and, since its description, has received considerable attention in the literature. Ewing's sarcoma of the spine, as a subgroup of Ewing's sarcoma in all locations, has received relatively little attention. Although spinal locations of Ewing's sarcoma are included in several studies,[1, 2, 4, 12, 14] the lesion is usually grouped with those in other axial locations or with pelvic lesions and is not analyzed separately. This chapter focuses on a relatively unusual location for this tumor and on the features that identify it as a separate subgroup among all Ewing's sarcomas. Data accumulated at the Mayo Clinic on 35 patients with Ewing's sarcoma of the spine form the basis for these observations.

INCIDENCE

Through 1983, Dahlin and Unni[1] recorded 402 cases of Ewing's tumor in all locations. During this same time period, 33 patients had an osseous spinal location as the primary site, which represents slightly more than 8 per cent of all Ewing's sarcomas seen at our institution. Ewing's sarcoma of the spine represents only about 0.5 per cent of all primary malignant tumors of bone.

DIAGNOSIS

Clinical Findings

Ewing's sarcoma of the spine has a distinct predilection for males, as do Ewing's sarcomas in other locations.[1, 4, 8, 10, 11, 14] The ages of the patients are also similar to those of patients with Ewing's sarcomas in other locations, averaging 16.5 years and ranging from 7 to 45 years. In the latest series, 88 per cent of the patients were 20 years old and younger.

More than half of the tumors occurred in the sacrum, with the lumbar region second in frequency.

Two patients had lesions in the thoracic spinal column, and one patient had a cervical tumor.

The average time from the onset of symptoms to diagnosis was 8 months (range, 1 to 31 months). This is different from that seen with other locations of this tumor, in which diagnosis is usually made within 2 or 3 months from the onset of symptoms.[10] However, a recent series on osteosarcoma of the spinal column[13] reported an interval similar to what we found. This similarity may be due to the difficulty in interpreting spinal radiographs, especially around the sacrum, and because a mass in the spinal column is not so easily seen as one in an extremity (Fig. 24–1). The most frequent symptom in Ewing's sarcoma of the spinal column, regardless of the location, was pain near the tumor. Pain was present in 34 (97 per cent) of the 35 patients. Other common symptoms—and symptoms unique to spinal locations because of the proximity of the tumor to the spinal cord and nerve roots—included leg pain in 78 per cent, weakness or gait difficulties in 52 per cent, sensory changes in 33 per cent, and urinary or bowel problems in 30 per cent.

Physical examination revealed localized tenderness in 60 per cent of the patients. Motor weakness was documented in more than half of the patients, and sensory deficits were noted in about 40 per cent. A distinct cauda equina syndrome or radiculopathy was present in one third of the group. Fever occurred in less than one fourth of the patients. A palpable mass was evident in only eight patients (23 per cent) and usually was discovered on rectal examination in patients with sacral lesions. Patients with tumors in other spinal locations seldom had a palpable mass.

Laboratory Results

Results of laboratory tests were generally nonspecific. In our series, of the patients who had these tests, 41 per cent had an elevated erythrocyte sedimentation rate, 23 per cent had an elevated alkaline phosphatase level, and 19 per cent had anemia. The laboratory results did not seem to correlate with overall survival, and laboratory findings were not particularly helpful in making a diagnosis.

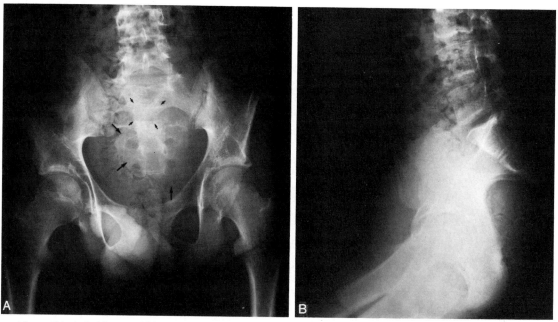

Figure 24–1. A 15-year-old boy had a two-year history of left buttock pain (which extended to ipsilateral leg) and difficulty initiating micturition. Initial anteroposterior (A) and lateral (B) roentgenograms demonstrate subtle, mixed sclerotic and lytic lesion of sacrum (A) with large presacral soft tissue mass (A and B).

Roentgenographic Findings

In most of the cases, the roentgenogram showed a lytic destructive lesion with some sclerosis surrounding the lytic area. Plain radiographs often revealed little in comparison with that provided by computed tomographic (CT) scans. CT scans, with contrast enhancement, are the most helpful study in determining the three-dimensional extent of the tumor (Figs. 24–1 and 24–2). Myelography continues to have a role when there is a neurologic deficit by further delineating the most proximal site of the obstruction of the soft tissue mass and any subsequent neural obstruction. The role of magnetic resonance imaging (MRI) is evolving, and its precise indications in the study of this tumor have not yet been delineated.

Pathologic Findings

When tissue specimens are adequate, the correct pathologic diagnosis is not difficult to make. Grossly, the tissue has the appearance of a soft mucinous gray-white tumor. Ewing's tumor occasionally appears purulent, being semiliquid in nature.[1, 10] This semiliquid nature was not characteristic of the specimens in our series. The vast majority of the spinal lesions have a definite semisolid or gelatinous consistency, and the gross appearance of the solid masses has been similar to that of Ewing's sarcoma in other skeletal locations. The tumor is generally gray-white to blue and is somewhat translucent. Additionally and also somewhat unique to tumors in spinal locations has been the gross appearance of a very red, vascular, friable tissue that forms a large part of the tumor. In virtually every case, the tumor in spinal

locations has been noted to bleed freely and often excessively, and in some circumstances the bleeding has been difficult to control. The histopathology of spinal specimens is that of a highly cellular tumor

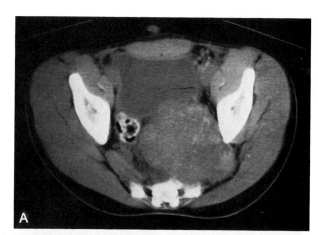

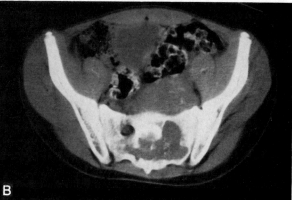

Figure 24–2. Pretreatment CT scans strikingly demonstrate lytic lesion in left wing of upper sacral elements and huge soft tissue mass anterior to sacrum, which engulfs sciatic nerve.

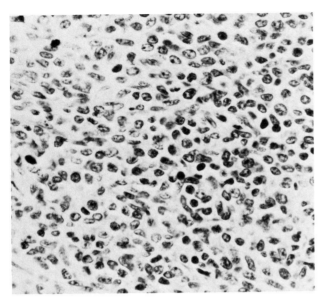

Figure 24–3. Ewing's sarcoma composed of sheets of small round to oval cells with clear cytoplasm (H & E, ×400).

with features identical to those of Ewing's tumors in other skeletal locations.[1, 10]

These features include sheets of small round to oval cells that are generally larger than lymphocytes with a clear scant amount of cytoplasm and round to oval nuclei. Mitoses are not abundant and nucleoli are not prominent. There are often foci of necrosis, and viable cells aggregate about small vessels, producing a pseudorosette pattern. The tumor cells infiltrate between bone trabeculae and often extend into the cortical vascular channels and periosseous soft tissues (Fig. 24–3).

Various staining techniques are useful in distinguishing between Ewing's sarcoma and other round cell tumors. Ewing's sarcoma cells are positive for glycogen when stained with periodic acid-Schiff (PAS) and treated with diastase. Reticulin silver stains indicate whole islands of cells surrounded by the reticulin meshwork rather than investing individual cells, as seen in lymphomas. There are no specific immunoperoxidase stains for Ewing's sarcoma; how-

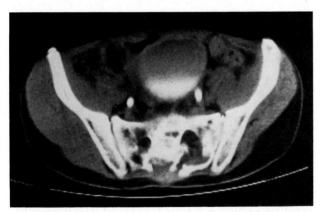

Figure 24–4. CT scan after L5 to S2 laminectomy with subtotal resection, 5000 cGy of local irradiation, and four-agent chemotherapy. Size of tumor has decreased dramatically. Patient survives at 17-month follow-up and is considered to be in remission without evidence of metastatic disease.

ever, such techniques are useful because they may be specific for other round cell tumors.

TREATMENT

As for Ewing's tumors elsewhere in the skeleton, the role of surgical excision is still evolving. Recent series have suggested that surgical ablation is beneficial as part of a combined regimen of surgery, radiation, and chemotherapy.[2, 5, 8, 9, 11, 12, 14] Excision, however, is often more challenging for spinal Ewing's tumor than for Ewing's tumor in a long bone. Because of the proximity of the spinal cord, peripheral nerves, and major vessels and the complex anatomic geometry of the vertebrae, total resection of the tumor is rarely a consideration (Fig. 24–2). The frequent presence of a soft tissue mass compounds the problems of surgical management. In most patients, even subtotal resection is, at best, difficult. These considerations explain why an attempt at total resection was made in only one of the patients in our series. The excised tumor in this patient had microscopically positive margins, but the patient is alive and disease-free 12 years after the original diagnosis. Of the other 18 patients in our series who were treated since 1970, 9 had decompressive laminectomy and partial debulking and 9 had biopsy only (generally through a single-level hemilaminectomy), which again testifies to the difficulty in surgical management of tumors in the spinal column.

Because of the obvious limitations in excising the tumor and achieving adequate margins, patients must be treated with adjunctive therapy. Recent published series have documented a role for chemotherapy in the treatment of Ewing's sarcoma in all locations.[2, 6, 8, 11, 12, 14] Radiation therapy, generally in the range of 4000 to 6000 cGy, is also currently recommended adjunctive therapy and is of benefit[8, 14] (Fig. 24–4).

At our institution since 1970, patients with Ewing's sarcoma of the spinal column were given a standard treatment protocol that involved postoperative radiation and four-agent chemotherapy (cyclophosphamide, doxorubicin, actinomycin D, and vincristine). Generally, radiation was administered in localized fields to the primary tumor site and subsequently to the same area or other areas if recurrence or metastasis developed. Response to therapy varies among patients and is dependent on several variables, including extent of disease.

PROGNOSIS

For purposes of survival, patients in our series were considered in two groups. Those treated before 1970 received various therapies, most often radiation and occasionally some nonprotocol chemotherapeutic regimens. Because our earliest patient was seen in 1935, when treatment was not as sophisticated as it is today, this early experience may provide some insight as to the natural history of the disease.

The average survival of the 16 patients treated before 1970 was 15 months (range, 5 to 45 months). There were no 5-year survivors in this group of patients. Although data from the early records tended to be less detailed than the later records, the demographic features were not different.

The 19 patients treated since 1970 have had an increase in survival, although the increase is a modest one (Table 24–1). Thirteen patients died of their diseases, having survived an average of 33 months; only one patient survived more than 5 years. Of the six remaining patients in this group, four are still alive at intervals ranging from 14 to 28 months, and two are still alive more than 5 years after diagnosis.

Patients who underwent partial debulking of the tumor did not have appreciably longer survival than those who had biopsy only. However, patients who underwent partial debulking often had more extensive neurologic dysfunction at the time of presentation. Thus, the average survival in the two treatment groups may reflect other factors, such as extent of disease. The location of the tumor in the spinal column (sacral or lumbar) did not affect survival appreciably, although all patients who survived more than 5 years (two are still alive) had tumors of the sacrum. If only the patients treated since 1970 are considered, the overall 5-year survival is 20 per cent for those with primary osseous Ewing's sarcoma of the spinal column.

Metastasis most commonly involved the lungs or other locations in the spinal column. Other common locations for spread of tumor were ribs, lymph nodes, brain, and abdominal viscera. Local recurrence was a less common indication of disease progression.

Osseous involvement of the spinal column in Ewing's tumor should be differentiated from involvement in paraspinal extraosseous locations. A recent study from our institution cited a 5-year survival rate of 40 per cent for 16 patients with Ewing's sarcoma of the spinal column.[14] However, that study did not distinguish between skeletal and extraskeletal involvement. Tumors that originate in extraskeletal paraspinal locations are often amenable to more complete excisional procedures.

Four patients from the previous series had such tumors. All four underwent total or near-total (microscopic margins positive only) resection of the soft tissue mass, along with additional radiation (three patients) and chemotherapy (four patients). All four patients are presently alive at more than 5 years (average 7.25) and are disease-free. Intraspinal Ewing's tumor without bone involvement is also possible, but these patients in our experience have a course similar to that of patients with lesions of vertebral origin. Thus, the prognosis seems to be better for patients with soft tissue Ewing's tumors that are amenable to total resection.

CONCLUSION

Ewing's sarcoma of the spine is an uncommon but highly lethal tumor. Demographically, the patient characteristics are similar to those of patients with Ewing's sarcoma in other locations. However, the time from the onset of symptoms to diagnosis is longer, and the presentation often is more dramatic because of a high incidence of neurologic problems associated with spinal location.

Although the number of patients in the series is small, it seems that complete removal of the tumor is justified wherever possible because of the poor prognosis. In a recent experience from the Intergroup Ewing's Sarcoma Study (IESS 1),[2] which considered only pelvic locations of the tumor (sacrum included), 28 per cent of 46 patients undergoing biopsy alone had local recurrence, compared with 18 per cent of 11 patients undergoing complete resection. In this same group, among patients with Ewing's sarcoma of the sacrum, 30 per cent developed local recurrence of tumor after biopsy alone, while no patients developed recurrence after incomplete (one patient) or complete (two patients) surgical resection. The value of partial debulking compared with complete resection of tumor is currently under investigation in IESS 2. Because of the intimate association with vital neurologic structures, the selection of surgical procedure must be tempered by considerations of the anticipated deficit. The sacral location may be best suited for excisional procedures.

Adjunctive therapy seems to improve survival, but the degree of improvement is not as well documented as it is when Ewing's sarcoma involves other locations. The results of one series[8] suggest that tumors of the spinal column are controlled with radiation and chemotherapy. However, the length of follow-up was not specified other than to indicate that it was at least one year. Other studies with longer follow-up, including our present series, suggest no such optimism for overall control of disease and survival in patients with spinal Ewing's sarcoma.[2, 5, 7, 11, 14] Additional studies are needed in order to address this question.

TABLE 24–1. DATA ON 19 PATIENTS (SEEN SINCE 1970) WITH EWING'S SARCOMA OF SPINE

CASE	SEX AND AGE (YR)	LOCATION OF LESION	DURATION OF SYMPTOMS (MO)*	STATUS
1	F, 19	Sacrum	7	Died, 20 mo
2	M, 17	Sacrum	10	Died, 23 mo
3	F, 20	Sacrum	31	Died, 58 mo
4	F, 12	Sacrum	19	Died, 22 mo
5	F, 45	Lumbar	1	Died, 20 mo
6	M, 12	Sacrum	5	Died, 63 mo
7	F, 19	Sacrum	4	Alive, 120+ mo
8	M, 24	Lumbar	. . .	Died, 31 mo
9	M, 34	Sacrum	10	Died, 51 mo
10	F, 10	Sacrum	2	Alive, 68+ mo
11	M, 16	Lumbar	3	Died, 26 mo
12	M, 17	Sacrum	2	Died, 16 mo
13	M, 7	Lumbar	9	Died, 58 mo
14	M, 18	Sacrum	6	Died, 34 mo
15	M, 20	Sacrum	4	Died, 9 mo
16	F, 17	Sacrum	2	Alive, 28 mo
17	M, 12	Sacrum	8	Alive, 14 mo
18	M, 15	Sacrum	24	Alive, 15 mo
19	M, 12	Sacrum	2	Alive, 20 mo

*Before diagnosis.

REFERENCES

1. Dahlin D, Unni KK: Bone Tumors. 4th ed. Springfield, IL, Charles C Thomas, 1986, pp 322–336.
2. Evans R, Nesbit M, Askin F, et al: Local recurrence, rate and sites of metastases, and time to relapse as a function of treatment regimen, size of primary and surgical history in 62 patients presenting with non-metastatic Ewing's sarcoma of the pelvic bones. Int J Radiat Oncol Biol Phys 11:129–136, 1985.
3. Ewing J: Diffuse endothelioma of bone. Proc NY Pathol Soc 21:17–22, 1921.
4. Falk S, Alpert M: Five-year survival of patients with Ewing's sarcoma. Surg Gynecol Obstet 124:319–324, 1967.
5. Gehan EA, Nesbit ME Jr, Burgert EO Jr, et al: Prognostic factors in children with Ewing's sarcoma. Natl Cancer Inst Monogr 56:273–278, 1981.
6. Glaubiger DL, Makuch R, Schwarz J, et al: Determination of prognostic factors and their influence on therapeutic results in patients with Ewing's sarcoma. Cancer 45:2213–2219, 1980.
7. Glaubiger DL, Makuch RW, Schwarz J: Influence of prognostic factors on survival in Ewing's sarcoma. Natl Cancer Inst Monogr 56:285–288, 1981.
8. Perez CA, Tefft M, Nesbit ME Jr, et al: Radiation therapy in the multimodal management of Ewing's sarcoma of bone: Report of the Intergroup Ewing's Sarcoma Study, Natl Cancer Inst Monogr 56:263–271, 1981.
9. Pritchard DJ: Surgical experience in the management of Ewing's sarcoma of bone. Natl Cancer Inst Monogr 56:169–171, 1981.
10. Pritchard DJ: Bone tumors. Part I. Small cell tumors of bone. Instr Course Lect 33:26–39, 1984.
11. Rosen G, Caparros B, Nirenberg A, et al: Ewing's sarcoma: Ten-year experience with adjuvant chemotherapy. Cancer 47:2204–2213, 1981.
12. Rosen G, Wollner N, Tan C, et al: Disease-free survival in children with Ewing's sarcoma treated with radiation therapy and adjuvant four-drug sequential chemotherapy. Cancer 33:384–393, 1974.
13. Shives TC, Dahlin DC, Sim FH, et al: Osteosarcoma of the spine. J Bone Joint Surg (Am) 68:660–668, 1986.
14. Wilkins RM, Pritchard DJ, Burgert EO Jr, Unni KK: Ewing's sarcoma of bone. Experience with 140 patients. Cancer: 58:2551–2555, 1986.

POSTRADIATION SARCOMAS INVOLVING THE SPINE

NARAYAN SUNDARESAN, DANIEL I. ROSENTHAL,
ALAN L. SCHILLER, and GEORGE KROL

INTRODUCTION

The development of a second malignancy resulting from intensive therapy is a well-recognized complication of cancer treatment.[7, 14, 25] Sarcomas arising within the field of radiation portals represent an important example of radiation oncogenesis. These tumors originate from either bone or soft tissue, and the clinical presentation may often mimic recurrence of the original tumor.[11, 16, 21, 22, 28–31] Some believe that the incidence of second malignancies is increasing. This is presumably because of more effective therapy (and presumed curability) of some tumors such as Hodgkin's disease and breast cancer, increasing both the period and the population at risk.

The earliest report of bone sarcomas complicating external radiation therapy appeared in 1922, when Beck noted the appearance of three cases of "pleomorphic spindle cell sarcoma" in bone following irradiation of tuberculous arthritis.[4] Shortly thereafter, Martland and Humphries noted the development of osteosarcoma of the jaw related to the use of radioactive radium-226 in dial painters, who had the habit of holding or pointing their brushes in the mouth.[26] In 1945, Hatcher reviewed 24 cases of sarcomas in irradiated bone and reported the first case of sarcoma developing in normal bone following treatment of a nonosseous condition.[15] In 1948, Cahan and colleagues reviewed the data on radiation-induced neoplasms and reported an additional 11 cases of such secondary tumors. He then proposed criteria for their diagnosis which are still largely valid today: (1) there must be microscopic or roentgenographic evidence of the benign nature of the initial lesion; (2) irradiation must have been given, and the sarcoma must arise in the area included within the therapeutic beam; (3) a relatively long interval must elapse before the appearance of the bone sarcoma; and (4) all sarcomas must be proved histologically. Since his original report, numerous investigators have described sarcomas arising both in irradiated normal bone and following treatment of benign bone neoplasms such as osteoblastoma or giant cell tumor.[8, 9, 18, 39] Cahan's strict criteria have been loosened to include secondary sarcomas related to radiation for malignant bone tumors such as Ewing's sarcoma.[12, 37] Although a latent period of five years is usual, bona fide cases have been reported after shorter intervals. The actual risk of radiation oncogenesis is unknown since it may persist indefinitely throughout the lifetime of the individual; recently Weatherby and coworkers reported a case of radiation sarcoma that occurred 55 years after treatment of the original tumor.[41]

Prompt recognition and early surgical treatment are important, since these tumors grow rapidly and respond poorly to conventional radiation and chemotherapy. Although all portions of the skeletal system may be involved, tumors involving the axial skeleton pose special problems in management. Frequently, the precise site of origin (from either bone or juxtaspinal soft tissue) may not be evident. Over an eight-year period, 15 patients with this complication of cancer therapy involving the spine were encountered by the authors, the majority of whom underwent treatment for this complication at Memorial Sloan-Kettering Cancer Center; a portion of this material has been previously reported.[38]

CLINICAL MATERIAL

Fifteen patients with secondary sarcomas involving the spine were seen by the authors at Memorial Sloan-Kettering Cancer Center and St. Lukes/Roosevelt Hospital Center, New York, between the years 1978 and 1985. Indications for radiation therapy included nonosseous malignancies in 13 patients and benign thymic enlargement in one. The remaining patient had received two courses of radiation therapy for a sacral chordoma. There were nine females and six males, with ages ranging from 18 to 65 (median 46) years at the time of initial radiation. The primary cancer for which treatment was given included Hodgkin's disease (5), breast (2), cervix (2), ovary (1), testes (1), lung (1), non-Hodgkin's lymphoma (1), and chordoma (1). The latent period to the development of the second malignancy varied from 6 to 30 years, with a median of 10 years.

Data on the original radiation treatments were available through contact with the radiation therapist, except in one patient. This patient, who had received an unknown amount of radiation therapy in childhood for "benign enlargement of the thymus," then developed another well-recognized sequela of neck radiation[32, 35]—papillary carcinoma of the thyroid—which was successfully treated. This was followed several years later by a sarcoma of the cervical spine. The remaining patients had received radiation dosages ranging from 2800 to 7600 cGy using conventional fractionation. Three patients had received treatment in the 1950s using orthovoltage equipment, while more recently treated patients had received therapy using the Cobalt 60 unit or the linear accelerator. One patient with carcinoma of the cervix had received an intracavitary insertion of cesium-137 in addition to external radiation therapy.

The clinical presentation varied with the location of the tumor. All patients reported steadily worsening back pain, which was associated with a radicular component in eight. Four patients noted a rapidly enlarging posterior paraspinal mass that was more than 10 cm in diameter. Associated skin and subcutaneous changes suggestive of prior radiation (including telangiectasia, atrophy, and fibrosis) were noted in five patients. The tumor was located in the cervical spine in one patient, in the thoracic region in seven patients, in thoracolumbar segments in two patients, and in the sacrum in five patients.

The plain radiographic findings were generally nonspecific; lytic destruction of the spine with little reactive sclerosis was the most common radiologic finding. These destructive changes were more apparent within the vertebral body than in the posterior elements, and the distinction between radiation osteitis and malignancy could be difficult from plain films. Calcification was seen in one patient with a paraspinal soft tissue mass. The most valuable diagnostic test was the computed tomography (CT) scan, which revealed extensive soft tissue tumor in addition to bone destruction. These soft tissue masses were generally located either antero- or posterolateral to the spinal canal. In two patients, the intrathoracic extension of tumor was so large that involvement of the spine was not suspected at the time of initial radiologic evaluation. Myelography revealed epidural extension of tumor in nine patients. Angiography was carried out in one patient, revealing vascular invasion of the subclavian artery.

TREATMENT AND RESULTS

Prior to referral eight patients had undergone treatment. Two patients had undergone biopsy only, three had undergone decompressive laminectomy because of the presumptive diagnosis of disc herniation, and two others had undergone attempted partial resection of the paraspinal tumor. One patient had undergone emergency decompression for spinal cord compression. Major tumor resection was attempted in only 10 patients, with no surgery being possible in three patients, and the remaining two undergoing limited debulking of their tumor by intralesional curettage. Following tumor resection, an attempt was made to treat residual disease with the use of brachytherapy, that is, with temporary implants of iridium-192. Since the majority had already received radiation dosages approaching spinal cord tolerance, external radiation therapy was thought feasible. Eight patients received chemotherapy in varying combinations; the agents used included methotrexate, doxorubicin (Adriamycin), cisplatin, cyclophosphamide, and vincristine. In one patient, chemotherapy was given by intraarterial perfusion of the internal hypogastric artery.

The overall median survival was eight months, with only three patients (20 per cent) surviving two years. These patients had undergone extended resection as well as brachytherapy. Five of the six patients who underwent both extensive resection and brachytherapy were believed to have adequate local control of the tumor, but eventually distant metastases were noted; thus no patient was cured of disease.

DISCUSSION

Fortunately, radiation-related sarcomas are rare. Over a 60-year period, 78 cases of bone sarcomas were reported from the Mayo Clinic,[41] and over a similar time period (1921 to 1983) Huvos reviewed the clinical and pathologic features of 66 cases of postradiation osteosarcomas at Memorial Sloan-Kettering Cancer Center.[19] Thus close to 40 per cent of postradiation sarcomas reported in the literature represent the experience of two institutions alone.

In most reported series, sarcomas have been classified based on tissue of origin (bone versus soft tissue), histology (osteosarcoma versus other spindle cell tumors), or the primary cancer for which treatment was instituted.[1, 3, 6, 7, 10, 11, 13, 16, 17, 20, 21, 33, 34, 36, 37] Of these, up to 30 per cent arise in or around the axial skeleton. Regardless of histology, malignant tumors arising around the axial skeleton have a poor prognosis, with no cures reported in the literature; whereas 5-year survival rates of 20 per cent are seen in peripheral tumors following radical resection. In this and other series, another contributing factor to the poor results was the delay in clinical diagnosis, which was often thought to be disc disease, frequently resulting in the wrong surgical approach being chosen for decompression.

It is important to remember that the three most common primary neoplasms for which the spine is included in the radiation portal are Hodgkin's disease, breast cancer, and cervix cancer. In patients treated for these neoplasms, the appearance of late onset of spinal pain or neurologic symptoms following clinical remission of the original cancer should prompt appropriate radiologic evaluation including both CT scans and myelography. In the differential diagnosis, it is important to consider late-onset metastases, but this distinction cannot often be made on radiographic grounds alone. Open biopsy is frequently indicated to rule out a second primary neoplasm, if the radiographic appearances suggest a tumor. The proper surgical approach should then be chosen for tumor resection. Decompressive laminectomy is rarely of value and frequently results in loss of stability of the spine. More extensive surgical exposures that allow adequate tumor resection should be used, and immediate reconstruction of the spine performed. Our limited data indicate that local control can best be achieved by maximal tumor resection in combination with brachytherapy.

Histologic examination of all 15 cases in this series confirmed the presence of highly malignant sarcomas, consistent with other series. The majority of postradiation sarcomas are either osteosarcomas, malignant fibrous histiocytomas, or spindle cell sarcomas with extremely high mitotic rates. Frequently, the histologic distinction between spindle cell sarcomas and neurogenic malignant schwannomas cannot be

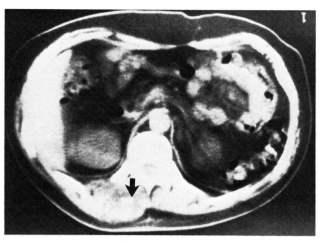

FIGURE 25–2. Paraspinal tumor mass on left side (*arrow*) with speckled calcification in patient with Hodgkin's disease who had received radiotherapy to spine. Biopsy revealed mesenchymal chondrosarcoma. Treatment included wide resection and implantation with radioactive seeds.

made on light microscopy. Neurogenic tumors may demonstrate gland-like areas or other foci of mesodermal differentiation, with those showing areas of rhabdomyoblasts being called "Triton" tumors.[42] The use of electron microscopy as well as immunoperoxidase studies may be helpful in such patients, although the overall prognosis is similar.

Precise data with regard to the risk of radiation oncogenesis as a function of total radiation dose are not available. Epidemiologic studies have focused on absorbed doses in the low range (under 100 cGy) in long-term atomic bomb survivors and on intermediate dose ranges (150 to 500 cGy) used either in experimental animals or for treatment of benign conditions in the past such as ankylosing spondylitis, but the most important clinical studies are those that have resulted from the use of dosages in the therapeutic range (3000 cGy and above). Kim and associates noted that a minimum dose of 3000 cGy was used in most patients[21] but that the lower limit may be variable, with cases having been reported even after 1000 cGy.[43] The actual risk of developing postradiation sarcomas is unknown; the best estimates for the risk of developing a second malignancy have focused on long-term follow-up of patients with Hodgkin's disease. Halperin estimated the probability of developing bone sarcoma to be 0.9 per cent at 5 years after follow-up of Hodgkin's disease.[14] In a larger study, Tucker recently evaluated the risk of second cancers in 1507 patients with Hodgkin's disease and found that 83 second cancers occurred more than one year after follow-up (relative risk 5.2).[40] After 10 years, the risk of a second neoplasm was approximately 10 per cent. Although the risk of leukemia plateaued by this time, the risk of solid tumors had increased over time. At the end of 15 years, there was a 17.6 per cent cumulative risk, representing a six-fold excess risk of second cancer.[40] Similar findings were noted by Kushner, who studied 320 patients with childhood Hodgkin's disease; of 254 patients, 12 second malignancies were noted, representing a cumulative risk of 18.7 per cent at 15

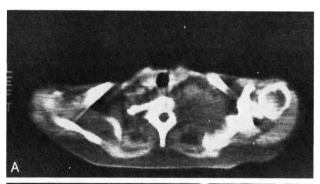

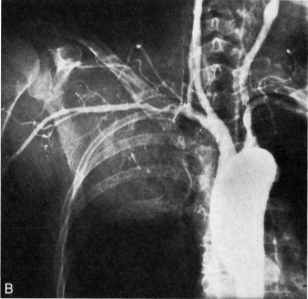

FIGURE 25–1. *A,* Axial CT scan showing destruction of transverse processes and spine in a 56-year-old patient who had received radiotherapy for breast cancer. Biopsy revealed high-grade spindle cell sarcoma. *B,* Arteriogram in same patient reveals extensive neovascularity and narrowing of left subclavian artery due to tumor invasion.

years. Bone sarcomas predominated during the first decade after treatment, and the cumulative probability was 5.5 per cent at 10 years.[24]

A number of variables are thought to affect the final malignant transformation: genetic constitution, age at exposure, interaction with other carcinogens (i.e., chemotherapy), as well as biologic modifiers during the long latent period.[22] The best example of bone sarcomas resulting from interaction of radiation and genetic mechanisms is in patients with hereditary retinoblastoma; Abramson and others have demonstrated that the cumulative risk of a second bone cancer after radiation therapy of hereditary retinoblastoma may approach 15 per cent at 20 years.[1, 23]

It has been assumed that the use of orthovoltage equipment represented an increased hazard because a correspondingly higher proportion of the delivered energy was absorbed by bone. Weatherby noted no decline in the incidence of postradiation sarcomas following the use of megavoltage equipment, but no cases were encountered following treatment with linear accelerators. Three patients in this series had undergone treatment with the linear accelerator, and

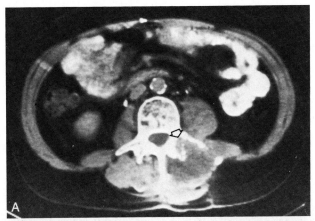

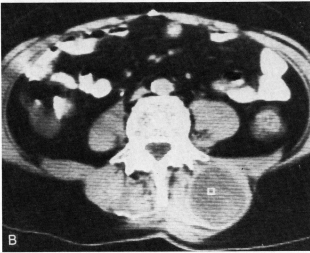

FIGURE 25–3. *A*, Paraspinal tumor (*arrow*) with destruction of the spine in patient with Hodgkin's disease who had received radiotherapy. Biopsy revealed osteosarcoma with predominant soft tissue component. *B*, Following several courses of chemotherapy, marked reduction in soft tissue component was seen. Surgical resection with implantation of radioactive seeds in the residual tumor was carried out.

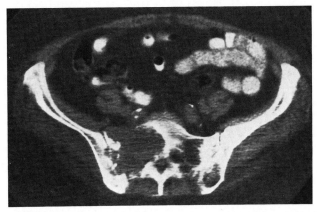

FIGURE 25–4. Destructive tumor of sacrum in patient who had received radiotherapy for cancer of the cervix. Patient presented with L5-S1 radiculopathy, and biopsy revealed malignant fibrous histiocytoma.

it therefore appears that the risk of radiation sarcomas cannot be eliminated merely by using sophisticated photon energy sources.

A more important clinical consideration is the fact that approximately two thirds of the patients in Weatherby's series and 36 per cent in Huvos' series had received radiation for benign osseous tumors or for tumorlike conditions of the spine. These lesions included giant cell tumors, aneurysmal bone cysts, fibrous dysplasia, chondromas, osteoblastomas, as well as bone cysts.[19, 41] In the current series, one patient with a sacral chordoma received two separate courses of radiation therapy, resulting in the development of a malignant fibrous histiocytoma and the eventual demise of the patient from disseminated metastases. No evidence of residual chordoma was found at autopsy. Halpern has reported a similar case,[13] and our experience suggests that radiation of a sacral chordoma occasionally results in transformation of the tumor into a spindle cell tumor at the time of recurrence. While radiation therapy is generally indicated for palliation or following incomplete resection of chordoma, there is little evidence in the literature to support the use of radiation therapy for benign tumors of the spine following incomplete resection, and the incidence of malignant transformation may be directly linked to the use of radiation therapy, especially in giant cell tumor of bone.[8, 9] With the development of anterior surgical approaches to all levels of the spine, we recommend that the majority of benign tumors involving the spine should be treated by surgery alone, since the risk of postradiation carcinogenesis represents an important consideration in long-term survivors.

REFERENCES

1. Abramson DH, Ellsworth RM, Kitchin FD, Tung G: Second nonocular tumors in retinoblastoma survivors; are they radiation induced? Ophthalmology 91:1351–1355, 1984.
2. Arlen M, Higinbotham NL, Huvos AG, et al: Radiation induced sarcoma of bone. Cancer 28:1087–1099, 1971.
3. Arsenau JC, Sponzo RW, Levine LD: Non-lymphomatous malignant tumors complicating Hodgkin's disease: Possible

association with intensive therapy. N Engl J Med 287:1119–1122, 1972.

4. Beck A: Zur Frage des Röntgensarkoms, zugleich ein Beitrag zur Pathogenese des Sarkoms. Muench Med Wochenschr 69:623–625, 1922.

5. Cahan WG, Woodard HQ, Higinbotham NL, et al: Sarcoma arising in irradiated bone. Cancer 1:3–29, 1948.

6. Canellos GP: Second malignancies complicating Hodgkin's disease. Lancet 1:1294, 1975.

7. Coleman CN: Secondary neoplasms in patients treated for cancer: Etiology and perspective. Radiat Res 92:188–200, 1982.

8. Dahlin DC, Cupps RE, Johnson EW Jr: Giant cell tumor: A study of 195 cases. Cancer 25:1061–1070, 1970.

9. Dorfman HD: Malignant transformation of benign bone lesions. Proc Natl Cancer Conf 7:901–913, 1973.

10. Ducatman BS, Scheithauer BW: Post-radiation neurofibrosarcoma. Cancer 51:1028–1033, 1983.

11. Ferguson DJ, Sutton HG, Dawson PJ: Late effects of adjuvant radiotherapy for breast cancer. Cancer 54:2319–2323, 1984.

12. Greene MH, Glaubiger DL, Mead GD, Fraumeni JF Jr: Subsequent cancer in patients with Ewing's sarcoma. Cancer Treat Rep 63:2043–2046, 1979.

13. Halpern J, Kopolovic J, Catane R: Malignant fibrous histiocytoma developing in irradiated sacral chordoma. Cancer 53:2661–2662, 1984.

14. Halperin EC, Greenberg MS, Suit HD: Sarcoma of bone and soft tissues following treatment of Hodgkin's disease. Cancer 53:232–236, 1984.

15. Hatcher CH: The development of sarcoma in bone subjected to roentgen or radium irradiation. J Bone Joint Surg 27:179–195, 1945.

16. Hatfield PM, Schulz MD: Post irradiation sarcoma: Including 5 cases after X-ray therapy of breast carcinoma. Radiology 96:593–602, 1970.

17. Huvos AG: Primary malignant fibrous histiocytoma of bone: Clinico-pathologic study of 18 patients. NY State J Med 76:552–559, 1976.

18. Huvos AG: Bone Tumors: Diagnosis, Treatment and Prognosis. Philadelphia, W. B. Saunders, 1979, pp 116–126.

19. Huvos AG, Woodard HQ, Cahan WG, et al: Post radiation osteosarcoma of bone and soft tissues: A clinicopathological study of 66 patients. Cancer 55:1244–1255, 1985.

20. Kim JH, Chu FC, Woodard HQ, et al: Radiation induced soft tissue sarcoma and bone sarcoma Radiology 129:501–508, 1978.

21. Kim JH, Chu FC, Woodard HQ, Huvos AG: Radiation induced sarcomas of bone following therapeutic radiation. Int J Radiat Oncol Biol Phys 9:107–110, 1983.

22. Kohn HI, Foy RJ: Radiation carcinogenesis. N Engl J Med 310:504–509, 1984.

23. Koten JW, DerKinderen DJ, Den Otter W: Bone sarcomas linked to radiotherapy and chemotherapy in children. N Engl J Med 318:581–582, 1988.

24. Kushner BH, Zauber A, Tan CTC: Second malignancies after childhood Hodgkin's disease. The Memorial Sloan-Kettering Cancer Center Experience. Cancer 62:1364–1370, 1988.

25. Li FP, Cassady JR, Jaffe N: Risk of second tumors in survivors of childhood cancer. Cancer 35:1230–1235, 1975.

26. Martland HS, Humphries RE: Osteogenic sarcoma in dial painters using luminous paint. Arch Pathol 7:406–417, 1929.

27. Meadows AT, Strong LC, Li FP: Bone sarcoma as a second malignant neoplasm in children: Influence of radiation and genetic predisposition. Cancer 46:2603–2606, 1980.

28. Mindell ER, Shah NK, Webster JH: Post radiation sarcoma of bone and soft tissues. Orthop Clin North Am 8:821–834, 1977.

29. Peimer CA, Yuan HA, Sagerman RH: Post radiation chondrosarcoma: A case report. J Bone Joint Surg (Am) 58:1033–1036, 1976.

30. Phillips TL, Sheline GE: Bone sarcomas following radiation therapy. Radiology 81:992–996, 1963.

31. Sabanas AO, Dahlin DC, Childs DS Jr, Ivins JC: Post radiation sarcoma of bone. Cancer 9:528–542, 1956.

32. Saenger EL, Silverman FN, Sterling TD, Turner ME: Neoplasia following therapeutic irradiation for benign conditions in childhood. Radiology 74:889–904, 1960.

33. Sagerman RH, Cassady JR, Tretter P, Ellsworth RM: Radiation induced neoplasia following external beam therapy for children with retinoblastoma. Am J Roentgenol 105:529–535, 1969.

34. Schomberg PL, Evans RG, Banks PM, et al: Second malignant lesions after therapy for Hodgkin's disease. Mayo Clin Proc 59:493–497, 1984.

35. Shore-Freedman E, Abrahams C, Recant W, Schneider AB: Neurilemomas and salivary gland tumors of the head and neck following childhood irradiation. Cancer 51:2159–2163, 1983.

36. Smith J, O'Connell RS, Huvos AG, Woodard HQ: Hodgkin's disease complicated by radiation sarcoma in bone. Br J Radiol 53:314–334, 1980.

37. Strong LC, Herson J, Osborne BM, Sutow WW: Risk of radiation related subsequent malignant tumors in survivors of Ewing's sarcoma. J Nat Cancer Inst 62:1401–1406, 1979.

38. Sundaresan N, Huvos AG, Krol G, Cahan W: Post-radiation sarcomas involving the spine. Neurosurgery 18:721–724, 1986.

39. Tillotson C, Rosenburg A, Gebhardt M, Rosenthal DI: Post-radiation multicentric osteosarcoma. Cancer 62:67–71, 1981.

40. Tucker MA, Coleman CN, Cox RS, et al: Risk of second cancers after treatment of Hodgkin's disease. N Engl J Med 318:76–81, 1988.

41. Weatherby RP, Dahlin DC, Ivins JC: Post radiation sarcoma of bone. Mayo Clin Proc 56:294–306, 1981.

42. Woodruff JM, Chernik NL, Smith MC, et al: Peripheral nerve tumors with rhabdomyosarcomatous differentiation (malignant "Triton" tumors). Cancer 37:426–439, 1973.

43. Yoshizawa Y, Kusama T, Morimoto K: Search for the lowest irradiation doses from literature on radiation induced bone tumor. Nippon Acta Radiol 37:63–72, 1977.

SURGICAL MANAGEMENT OF SUPERIOR SULCUS TUMORS

NARAYAN SUNDARESAN, VED P. SACHDEV,
GEORGE KROL, and WALTER WICHERN

INTRODUCTION

The American Cancer Society[1] estimates that approximately 150,000 new cases of lung cancer were diagnosed in the United States in 1990; data from other Western countries indicate a similar incidence. The age-adjusted cancer death rate for lung cancer has doubled every 15 years; it is now the leading cause of cancer deaths in men and is soon expected to be the leading cause in women as well. The five-year survival rate is approximately 10 per cent because more than 70 per cent of patients have regional or metastatic disease at initial presentation. Since the presence of metastatic disease precludes attempts at cure by resection of the primary tumor, it is evident that systemic approaches are indicated in many patients with lung cancer. However, approximately 5 per cent of lung cancers involve the chest wall and spine by direct extension and remain localized at the time of diagnosis (Fig. 26–1). Of these, Pancoast (superior sulcus) tumors deserve special consideration in this textbook; their clinical presentation frequently results in neurologic symptoms,[28] and involvement of the spine is a frequent cause of recurrent or progressive disease.[45] In patients who have failed local treatment, severe pain from brachial plexopathy or postradiation fibrosis is common; frequently, pain is of multifactorial origin and results from recurrent tumor, radiation, or surgery. In addition, signs of brachial plexopathy are frequently harbingers of spinal cord compression.[21, 25]

The earliest case in the English literature of a superior sulcus tumor is probably the patient reported by E.S. Hare in 1838.[11] The case reported was a 40-year-old patient who presented with pain, tingling, and numbness along the course of the left ulnar nerve. On examination, a small tumor in the "inferior triangular space" was noted which was associated with a constricted pupil and ptosis of the left eye. The patient became rapidly paraplegic and died. At autopsy, he had a tumor involving the lung, which extended to the brachial plexus and invaded the spinal cord through the intervertebral foramina of the eighth cervical nerve and first thoracic nerve. In addition, the carotid artery, sympathetic chain, and vagus nerves were completely enmeshed by tumor.

Although several others have since reported the association of tumors of the apical pleura with the clinical presentation, the classic papers by Pancoast[33, 34] clearly established the syndrome as a clinical entity. In 1924, H.K. Pancoast, a radiologist, called attention to the importance of careful radiologic evaluation of apical chest tumors and described three patients with the tumor. In 1932, he published a paper entitled "Superior Pulmonary Sulcus Tumor" in which he reported four more patients and defined the tumor as occurring at a definite location at the thoracic inlet "characterized by pain around the shoulder and down the inner side of the arm, and often the ulnar side of the forearm, wasting of muscles of the hand, Horner's syndrome, and signs of dullness in the apex of the chest." The roentgenographic appearance was that of a small circumscribed shadow in the apex of the lung, owing to displacement and destruction of the posterior portions of one or more ribs and of the adjacent articular and transverse processes, including a little of the sides of the bodies of one or more vertebrae. He erroneously believed that the tumor arose from embryonic epithelial rests of the branchial clefts which formed an abnormal sulcus in the lung, thus giving the tumor its name. It was Tobias in 1932 who provided a detailed description of the clinical syndrome in five cases, termed it the "apico-costo-vertebral syndrome," and correctly attributed its cause to primary lung cancer.[50] By 1946, Herbut and Watson[14] had collected 134 cases of the Pancoast syndrome from the literature and added an additional 17 cases. Only 12 of these 17 cases were due to lung cancer; the others were due to cancers of the thyroid, larynx, and mesothelioma and from Hodgkin's disease.

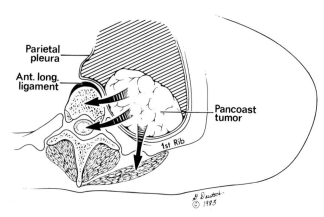

Figure 26—1. Line drawing showing patterns of local invasion by superior sulcus tumors. Note that invasion of the spinal cord may result from bone involvement as well as from perineural invasion through the intercostal nerves and brachial plexus.

In his classic paper, Pancoast believed that the tumor was uniformly fatal, with no favorable response to radiotherapy, and concluded that its location precluded surgical excision. Over the next two decades, attempts at surgical ablation of the lesion with or without radiation therapy failed to improve on his prediction.[53] Although there have been isolated reports of cures of superior sulcus tumors either by surgical resection combined with external radiation[8, 10] or by the use of interstitial implants,[6] the median survival remained less than a year during this time.[13] It was the pioneering work of Paulson and Hilaris over the last two decades that finally provided a framework for a systemic approach to this tumor.[15–19, 35–39, 41] Paulson advocated a course of preoperative radiation therapy followed by en bloc resection of the tumor, the involved chest wall, the lung, and a portion of the lower brachial plexus. Hilaris combined this technique with the use of either permanent or temporary implants of radioactive seeds, thus extending the indications for operation to those with even more advanced tumors. Although a significant proportion of patients benefit from therapy, with 25 to 33 per cent being cured of localized tumors, more than half the patients fail locally with recurrent disease.[2, 24, 40, 46, 51] In such patients, unrelenting pain from brachial plexopathy and ultimate cord compression remains a major cause of morbidity, and the management of plexopathy in superior sulcus tumors is a major problem in pain management.[4, 20, 21, 42, 45, 47, 48, 52]

INCIDENCE AND CLINICAL PRESENTATION

The annual incidence is estimated to be from one to four cases per 100,000 male population in the United States, similar to that in other Western countries. Carcinomas of the superior pulmonary sulcus account for between 2 and 5 per cent of all lung cancers.[5] The average age at diagnosis ranges from 50 to 60 years in surgical series but is between 60 and 70 years in those patients treated by external radiation therapy alone.[5, 7, 27, 30] The male:female ratio is 9:1, and curiously more than 70 per cent of reported cases have been on the right side. There is no explanation for this occurrence other than the fact that the right lung composes 55 per cent of the total lung volume. Analysis of the histologic types shows that out of a total of 453 cases, 216 (47.7 per cent) were epidermoid cancers, 99 (21.8 per cent) were adenocarcinomas, and 87 (19.2 per cent) were anaplastic large cell carcinomas. Apart from these histologic subtypes, 21 (4.6 per cent) were small cell cancers, 4 (1 per cent) were mixed tumors, and 26 (5.7 per cent) were not classified.[5]

Clinically, the majority of patients (90 per cent) present with pain in the shoulder or in the interscapular region. In very early cases when the tumor is confined to lung tissue, no pain may be reported; in such patients, these tumors are discovered following a routine work-up or if the patients present with other symptoms. When the tumor involves the visceral pleura, referred pain usually develops; this may be the shoulder for tumors at the level of the first thoracic vertebra (T1), or the interscapular region for tumors adjacent to the second thoracic vertebra (T2). At this time, the patient may not be able to locate the pain exactly, and there may be no local tenderness on palpation. When the tumor involves the periosteum of bone, pain becomes more intense and local tenderness may be evident. In view of the nonspecific nature of the initial pain, the clinical diagnosis is frequently mistaken for cervical arthritis, bursitis, thoracic outlet syndrome, or peripheral nerve entrapment. As a result, the median duration of pain prior to correct diagnosis is 6 months; in exceptional cases pain has been present for several years.[21, 28]

Involvement of the brachial plexus and lower intercostal nerves usually results from direct perineural invasion and is clinically characterized by paresthesias (numbness, burning, tingling) along the corresponding dermatome; this may involve the interscapular or anterior chest region (T3), the axilla (T2), or the ulnar aspect of the hand (C8-T1). Involvement of the inferior cervical sympathetic (stellate) ganglion results in a classic Horner's syndrome, with drooping of the upper eyelid, enophthalmos, miosis, and loss of sweating on the affected side. Although the reported incidence of Horner's syndrome has varied from 20 to 62 per cent in the literature, we have noted a much higher incidence (90 per cent) in our patients[45, 46] because subtle signs of pupillary inequality and ptosis were carefully looked for.

Sensory paresthesias along the C8-T1 distribution represents the earliest clinical manifestation of brachial plexopathy. In more advanced cases of invasion of the brachial plexus, motor weakness of the intrinsic hand muscles and wrist extensors will be noted. When clinical signs of brachial plexopathy (weakness) are seen, epidural invasion may already be present. Tumor extension in such cases results from two mechanisms: direct perineural invasion as well as destruction of the spine. In our experience, 20 to 50 per cent of patients with superior sulcus tumors present with cord compression or develop it during the course of their disease. In patients who have undergone treatment, escalating pain and plexopathy generally indicate recurrent tumor from treatment failure. On physical examination, the presence or absence of weight loss should be noted. Careful palpation of the supraclavicular region should be performed to exclude adenopathy; in our experience, supraclavicular masses may represent the actual tumor itself with displacement of the brachial plexus in front of it. The presence of hoarseness (indicating recurrent laryngeal nerve involvement) and distended veins (from superior vena caval obstruction) should also be looked for. Pulmonary symptoms are seen in less than 15 per cent of patients, but the presence of these symptoms should be noted.

RADIOLOGIC INVESTIGATION

The initial evaluation of all patients suspected of having a superior sulcus tumor should be routine radiography of the chest (Fig. 26–2). However, routine chest x-rays do not always disclose an apical density that is typical of the tumor. In 20 per cent of patients, the chest findings may be nonspecific and may be interpreted as apical fibrosis or old granulomatous disease.[13] In earlier series, radiographic evidence of bone destruction was noted in approximately half the patients, with rib destruction being the major feature. In 10 to 20 per cent of patients, both ribs and vertebrae may be involved at initial presentation. Whereas the use of apical lordotic views has been recommended in the past, we believe that all suspected cases of this tumor should undergo computed tomography (CT) scans of the apical chest and brachial plexus. This is especially important in evaluating a C8-T1 radiculopathy in patients with a long smoking history. Cervical osteoarthritis, bursitis, musculoskeletal spasm, and tardy ulnar palsy are all syndromes that have been mistakenly diagnosed in these patients on the basis of limited radiologic evaluation. With CT scans, it is possible to precisely delineate the extent of tumor, destruction of the ribs, or portions of the vertebrae, as well as involvement of the brachial plexus with a single technique.

Previously, all superior sulcus tumors were considered T3 lesions by virtue of involvement of the parietal pleura. More recently, the American Joint Committee for Staging of Cancer has further subdivided these tumors according to whether the spine is involved.[31] T3 lesions are those with varying degrees of rib destruction but an uninvolved spine; T4 lesions are those in which the vertebra is involved (Fig. 26–3) and are considered inoperable. Our recent data (using magnetic resonance imaging [MRI]) suggest that early spine invasion is a feature in approximately 20 per cent of patients with superior sulcus tumors at initial presentation, and this should not necessarily preclude an attempt at local cure.

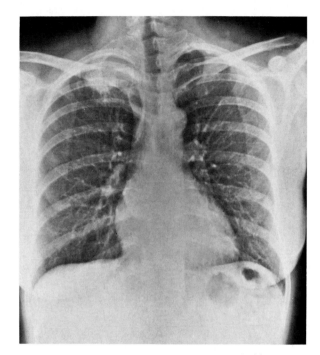

Figure 26–2. Chest radiograph demonstrating apical lung mass, a typical finding in large superior sulcus tumors.

In addition to CT scans, we recommend the use of myelography to evaluate the epidural space. Early epidural spread may be identified in 20 to 30 per cent of patients and is radiologically characterized by a nodular thickening of the C8 or T1 roots at their entrance into the spinal cord. In patients with larger tumors, the anteromedial relationships should be noted in determining operability. Here, the tumor is adjacent to the trachea and may invade the subclavian artery on the right side or the aortic arch on the left. Even in its early stages, it is intimately related to the subclavian artery and its branches, especially the vertebral artery (Figs. 26–4 through 26–6). We have occasionally used angiography to evaluate the relationship of tumor to the subclavian artery but have found it of limited value. With the introduction of MRI, it is now possible to replace all these tests with a single examination that provides a multiplanar outline of the tumor, its relationship to the brachial plexus, the spinal cord, and the adjacent major vessels. With CT scanning, it is also possible to radiologically stage the tumor and to ensure that it is localized by scanning through the mediastinum, abdomen, and adrenals. The adrenals frequently represent occult sites of metastasis. Repeat CT scanning following operation, as well as serial CT scanning throughout the course of the patient's illness, is also used to provide an accurate assessment of the tumor site in the first year following surgery when the risk of local recurrence is extremely high.

If CT scans of the chest demonstrate mediastinal node enlargement (nodes larger than 1 cm) or evidence of direct mediastinal invasion, some advocate mediastinoscopy to confirm the findings; no patient should be denied operative resection on the basis of CT findings alone, since the false-positive rate can be as high as 30 per cent.

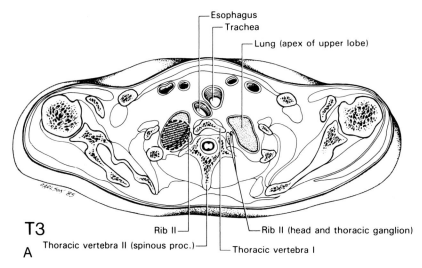

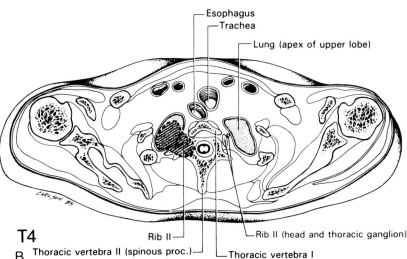

Figure 26–3. Current American Joint Committee staging system subdivides superior sulcus carcinoma into T3 (*A*) or T4 (*B*) lesions based on invasion of the vertebra. Although T4 lesions are considered inoperable for cure, palliative resection is often indicated to prevent or treat spinal cord compression.

TREATMENT

In all patients, the tissue diagnosis of non–small cell cancer should be established by percutaneous needle biopsy of the tumor either under fluoroscopy or by CT guidance. While the use of a Tru-cut needle allows a larger specimen to be sampled, it is far easier and more comfortable to confirm the diagnosis by cytologic examination of cells aspirated through a smaller 22-gauge needle. In patients presenting with a supraclavicular mass, an open biopsy can be performed. In many patients, the presumed supraclavicular adenopathy actually represents the superior pole of the tumor with the displaced brachial plexus, which is potentially vulnerable to injury during biopsy. Bronchoscopy is not routinely recommended because of the peripheral location of the tumor; even with fiberoptic techniques, a positive yield is seen in only 30 per cent of patients. We recommend performing bronchoscopy only if a large upper lobe tumor is present or if there are associated symptoms (e.g., hemoptysis, bronchial obstruction). Bronchoscopy is also recommended if there is radiologic evidence of mediastinal enlargement.

The value of proper preoperative staging has been emphasized by several authors,[2, 43] but the precise role of extensive radiologic evaluation (CT of the abdomen and brain and radionuclide bone scans) in all patients has yet to be clarified. Our philosophy has been that in patients with good performance status, normal screening profiles, and absence of systemic complaints, such tests should be performed on an individual basis or the potential initial treatment planned.

Following confirmation of non–small cell carcinoma, several different treatment options exist: preoperative radiation followed by surgery, external radiation alone, surgery followed by radiation, or the use of neoadjuvant chemotherapy prior to surgery (Fig. 26–7). Each of these treatment strategies has its proponents,[2, 3, 9, 15, 17, 19, 22, 24, 26, 29, 35, 38, 30, 40, 49, 51] but we believe that different treatment strategies may be applicable in subsets of patients.

The widely accepted standard treatment is to use a course of external radiation therapy to the primary tumor, the supraclavicular area, and the mediastinum for a period of three to four weeks (Fig. 26–8). Although Paulson recommended a total dose of 3000

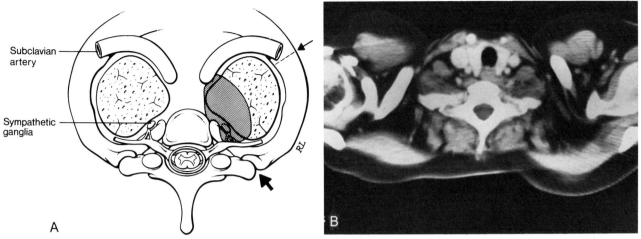

Figure 26–4.

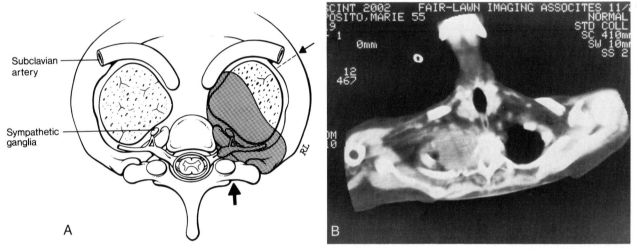

Figure 26–5.

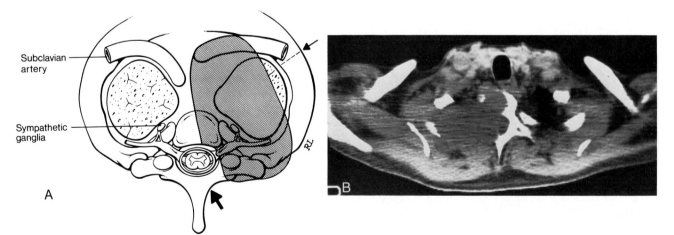

Figure 26–6.

Figures 26–4 through 26–6. Line diagrams illustrating various patterns of local extension at time of presentation, with corresponding CT scans. In small tumors (Fig. 26–4) resection can often be accomplished without preoperative radiation. For larger tumors, depicted in Figures 26–5 and 26–6, radiation therapy has generally been advocated for palliation; current data indicate that doses in excess of 5000 cGy may be required for local control. Our experience indicates that advanced tumors such as that depicted in Figure 26–6B probably benefit from de novo surgery followed by external RT.

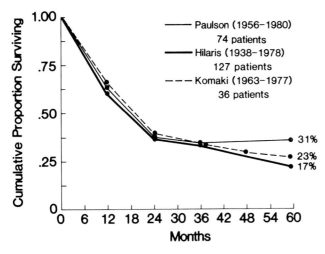

Figure 26–7. Survival curves from three large series resulting from various methods of treatment: preoperative RT and resection (Paulson), preoperative RT followed by resection and/or brachytherapy (Hilaris), and external RT alone (Komaki). These data suggest that patient selection may be largely responsible for differences in long-term results, with two-year survival rates being comparable in all series.

cGy in 10 fractions over two weeks, most radiation oncologists favor a more conventional fractionation (200 cGy/day) for a total dose of 4000 to 4400 cGy in 20 fractions over four weeks. This is tolerated better by the patients, with a lower incidence of esophagitis and skin reactions. Following the course of external radiation therapy, patients are reevaluated and thoracotomy is recommended if the tumor is still localized.

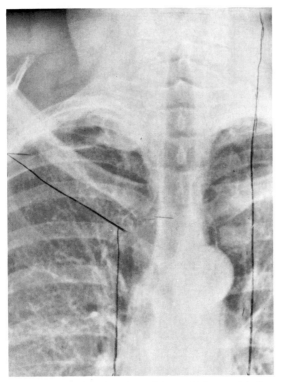

Figure 26–8. Chest radiograph outlining radiation portals for preoperative RT to tumor. Since the spinal cord lies within the RT portal, shielding of the spinal cord is necessary after 4000 cGy.

The basic goals of surgery are en bloc resection of the tumor, the involved lung and chest wall, and the spine through a standard posterolateral thoracotomy. Operation should also include a mediastinal node dissection for therapeutic and prognostic reasons. In the majority, the defect following resection rarely requires reconstruction because the scapula provides an adequate cover. In patients in whom the tumor is found to be unresectable, permanent implantation with iodine-125 seeds may be performed. The technique of implantation requires adequate surgical exposure to allow access to the tumor from within the rib cage as well as through the intercostal spaces. It is thus necessary to detach the lung apex from the thoracic inlet to enable the brachytherapist access to the paraspinal and thoracic inlet. Permanent implants with radioactive iodine-125 may then be positioned within the tumor itself. In patients in whom all gross tumor has been removed, after-loading catheters for temporary implants with iridium-192 are used to boost the local dose to the tumor bed.[17] These catheters are placed in the region of the tumor, and are then brought out and fixed to the skin.

Postoperatively, iridium-192 sources are introduced through these catheters and left in place for three to four days, after which both the catheters and the sources are removed. These implants allow another 3000 to 4000 cGy to be delivered locally to the tumor without compromise of the spinal cord. If these techniques, which require an expert brachytherapist, are not available, it may be possible to deliver additional local radiation using computerized dosimetric planning. In patients in whom mediastinal nodes are found to be involved, postoperative radiation therapy to the mediastinum has been recommended.[40]

Technique of En Bloc Resection

For extended resections of the chest wall and spine, proper preoperative evaluation of the patient is important. This should include routine pulmonary function tests, including determination of arterial blood gases. If reversible chronic obstructive disease is present, preoperative bronchodilator therapy may be helpful. Surgery is generally performed within three to six weeks if preoperative radiation therapy is used. We prefer to use a combined neurosurgical and thoracic team in most patients. Operation is performed with the patient in the lateral position under general endotracheal anesthesia using double lumen tubes. A long parascapular incision is made starting just above the spine of the scapula and extending around the tip of the scapula to end in the anterior axillary line (Fig. 26–9). Using cautery, the skin incision is deepened through the fascia and the muscles, and the trapezius, levator scapulae, and rhomboid muscles are detached from the medial margin of the scapula. A portion of the trapezius muscle must be left attached to the scapula so that it does not become completely detached from the spine.

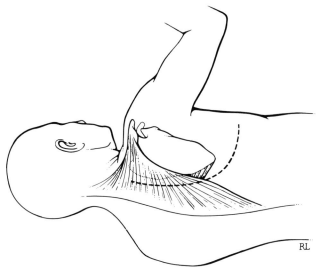

Figure 26–9. Posterolateral thoracotomy incision used for superior sulcus tumors; arm should be draped to allow it free movement and displacement.

Inferiorly, the latissimus and pectoralis major muscles are cut in the plane of the incision. The serratus posterior muscle is divided at its insertion to the upper ribs, and the paraspinal muscles are retracted medially. Using blunt dissection underneath the scapula, the apex of the thoracic cage is exposed outside the chest cavity.

Thoracic Phase

The chest cavity is generally entered through an incision in the fourth or fifth interspace to determine resectability (Fig. 26–10) and to document whether intrathoracic spread of the tumor has occurred. When the tumor is deemed resectable, the chest cavity is reentered through the third or fourth interspace, and the first three ribs along with the intercostal and neurovascular bundles are divided anteriorly with rib shears (Fig. 26–11). By traction with

Kocher clamps attached to the sectioned ribs, the posterior costotransverse articulations are identified. The transverse processes of the corresponding vertebra are then bitten off with Adson rongeurs or detached with a high speed power drill (Fig. 26–12), while the intercostal nerves are carefully isolated and clipped at the neural foramina. By placing the chest wall under tension and pulling inferiorly, resection proceeds superiorly to the first rib, which is cut at its costochondral junction. Since the first rib is horizontal, it should be dissected with extreme care in the subperiosteal plane prior to section to avoid injury to the brachial plexus and subclavian vessels superior to it. When the chest wall is mobilized and freed, segmental or wedge resection of the lung may be performed to facilitate exposure. During the maneuver, the neurosurgical team assists with the posterior portion of the chest wall resection (costotransversectomy) and by mobilizing the heads of the ribs completely from their articulations to the transverse processes and vertebral bodies in a caudocranial direction. All bleeding vessels are controlled with the bipolar current and vascular clips. Occasionally, bleeding from the intervertebral foramina may be profuse and may require the use of Gelfoam and Avitene pledgets. The first thoracic nerve root is routinely divided at two separate points: one near the intervertebral foramina, and one at a second level more distally at its attachment to the brachial plexus (Fig. 26–13). This dissection is crucial to the operation and is performed using magnification and microdissection. Lobular tongues of tumor are frequently seen both anterior and posterior to the lower cord of the brachial plexus and should be carefully dissected and removed. We make every effort to preserve the eighth cervical nerve root by careful microdissection of tumor from its perineurium. In patients with extensive brachial plexopathy, the lower and middle trunks of the brachial plexus may be involved by tumor, and there may be no discernible plane for dissection. In such cases, we have chosen not to resect the plexus but have relied on permanent implants to achieve control of the tumor. During this phase, the

Figure 26–10. The chest is entered through the fourth interspace to determine overall resectability; if pleural implants, lung metastases, or unresectable lymph nodes are seen, palliative implants with iodine-125 seeds may be indicated. The scapula is retracted and the posterior chest wall is mobilized by identification and section of the scalene muscles.

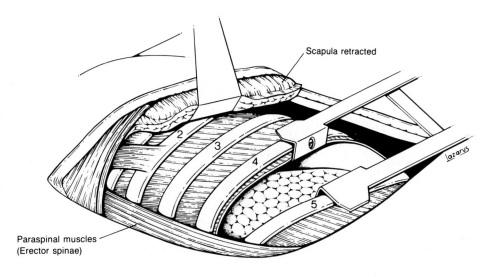

Scapula retracted

Paraspinal muscles
(Erector spinae)

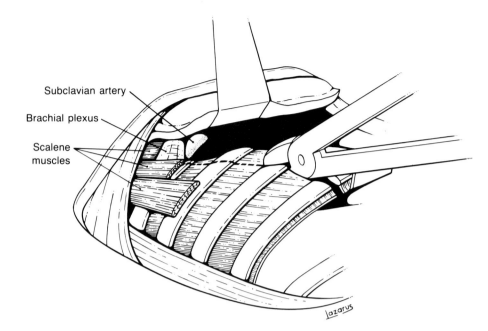

Subclavian artery

Brachial plexus

Scalene muscles

Figure 26–11. The chest wall is resected anteriorly to remove the upper three or four ribs; the first rib has a horizontal inclination and should be resected with care because the brachial plexus lies above it. The thoracic surgeon then performs a segmentectomy or wedge resection of the lung to free the tumor from the lung.

neurosurgical team helps mobilize the tumor medially from the vertebral body.

Superiorly and medially, the tumor involves the stellate ganglion, and this is included in the resection with the main tumor mass. Mobilization of the tumor from the subclavian artery often necessitates meticulous dissection in its adventitial tissue plane, and bleeding may be encountered from its branches, including the costocervical trunk and the vertebral artery. In some patients, there is frank invasion of the subclavian artery. Although Paulson has suggested resection and repair of the artery, we believe that the prognosis in such patients is poor and have relied on implantation instead.

In patients without invasion of the vertebra, the tumor is elevated in the plane of its pseudocapsule posteriorly and separated from the front of the vertebra. When the spine is minimally involved, we remove a portion of the vertebral body along with the tumor by drilling out portions of the vertebral bodies to obtain a satisfactory margin. When there is overt involvement of the spine or epidural extension of tumor, the entire vertebral body (frequently both T1 and T2) are removed together with discs above and below. This allows access to the epidural space for tumor resection. Posteriorly, the exposure is enhanced by performing a small hemilaminectomy. Reconstruction of the resected segments is carried out with methyl methacrylate and Steinmann pins (Fig. 26–15) using techniques we have previously described.[44, 46]

Once the main mass of tumor is removed, bleeding

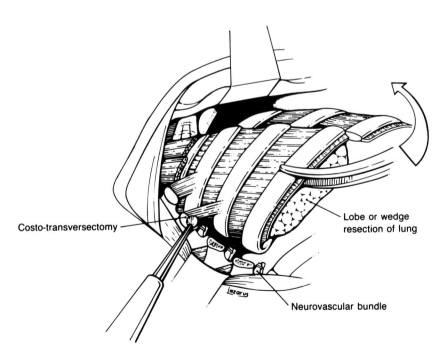

Costo-transversectomy

Lobe or wedge resection of lung

Neurovascular bundle

Figure 26–12. The neurosurgical team next performs a costotransversectomy with either a high speed drill or Adson rongeurs while traction is exerted on the chest wall with a Kocher clamp. In more advanced cases, a small hemilaminectomy may be necessary.

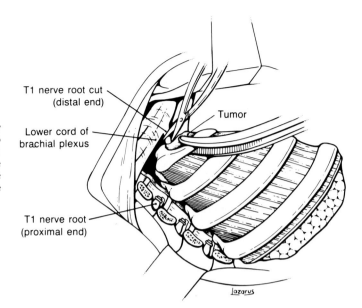

Figure 26–13. The individual nerve roots should be carefully ligated and clipped close to the intervertebral foramina to prevent CSF leakage into the chest postoperatively. The T1 nerve root has to be sectioned at two places: once at the intervertebral foramina, and again more distally as it enters the brachial plexus. The tumor needs to be dissected free from the rest of the brachial plexus by careful microdissection.

is controlled with local application of Avitene and use of bipolar current. The procedure is then turned over to the thoracic surgeon, who completes a standard upper lobectomy or segmental resection (if it has not already been completed). A mediastinal node dissection is also carried out. At this stage, the brachytherapist is called to evaluate the resection site for possible permanent or temporary implants. Pleural drainage is established by means of chest tubes both anteriorly and posteriorly, and hemostasis is achieved in the chest cavity. Closure of the thoracotomy then proceeds by careful reapproximation of the muscle layers, subcutaneous tissues, and skin.

Complications and Postoperative Management

Patients are generally kept on assisted ventilation for 12 to 18 hours after surgery and are nursed in

intensive care. The chest tube drainage is closely monitored, but patients are allowed to ambulate by the second day. Permanent deficits resulting from the section of the C8-T1 nerve roots result in an ulnar nerve deficit, and a Horner's syndrome invariably results from resection of the stellate ganglion.

Although seemingly extensive, the mortality rate from this operation is surprisingly low. In Paulson's series, two operative deaths occurred with a mortality rate of less than 5 per cent. Similarly in our series, the mortality rate was less than 5 per cent, and no deaths were encountered in our recent series of 30 patients.[46] Occasionally, persistent cerebrospinal fluid (CSF) leak may occur from resection of the nerve roots, leading to profuse prolonged drainage from the chest tubes. This can usually be managed conservatively by chest tube drainage. If this does not succeed, a lumbar spinal drain should be placed; only

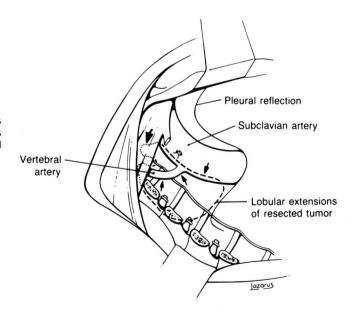

Figure 26–14. The tumor insinuates itself by lobular extensions around the plexus, vertebral body, sympathetic chain, as well as the subclavian artery. Branches of the subclavian or vertebral artery may be directly invaded by tumor but can be sacrificed.

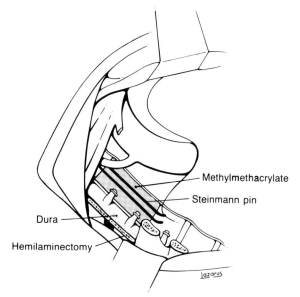

Figure 26–15. In those cases with spine invasion, resection of the upper two thoracic vertebrae may be necessary; stabilization is then performed with methyl methacrylate and Steinmann pins. At this point, the brachytherapist is consulted for the purposes of supplementing the tumor bed with after-loading catheters. Closure of the chest wall and thoracotomy incision are performed in layers with pleural drainage.

rarely is direct operative repair of the torn dura necessary.

In patients who require postoperative radiation (generally because of disease noted microscopically in the mediastinal nodes), such treatment is delivered on an outpatient basis.

Results of Treatment

In Tables 26–1 and 26–2, the long-term results of treatment in the major recent series are presented. As shown, the proportion of patients who undergo treatment are not always specified and selection criteria have varied considerably, making comparison between the various modes of therapy impossible. With current surgical techniques and postoperative management, operative mortality in selected patients should be less than 3 per cent.

In Paulson's series, 120 patients with superior sulcus tumors were seen through 1980. Of these, 33

TABLE 26–1. LOCOREGIONAL TREATMENT FAILURES IN REPORTED SERIES

Series and Year	No. Patients	Local Failures (%)
Paulson 1982	67	?
Komaki 1981	36	53
Houtte 1984	31	45
Devine 1986	50	70
Sundaresan 1987	30	30
Hilaris 1987	128	33

were considered inoperable because of the presence of distant metastases, local extent of tumor, or age. Of the 75 patients (63 per cent) who were operated upon, only one was judged unresectable because of multiple intrathoracic metastases. Thus, resection was completed in 74 patients (98 percent), with an operative mortality rate of 2.7 per cent. The actuarial survival rates were 31 per cent at 5 years, 26 per cent at 10 years, and 22 per cent at 15 years for patients who underwent operation. In patients with hilar or mediastinal node involvement, no patient survived two years. If there was no nodal involvement, the median survival was 5 years, and one third of the patients lived 10 years.

At Memorial Sloan-Kettering Cancer Center, Hilaris and Martini reviewed data of 170 patients treated over a 40-year period from 1938 to 1978.[19] All patients had proven histologic or cytologic evidence of cancer. Of these, 43 patients (25 per cent) were not treated by surgery because of advanced disease or unrelated medical problems and received external radiation therapy alone. One hundred and twenty-seven patients underwent surgery combined with external radiation and/or interstitial radiation. Of these, 66 patients received preoperative external radiation and 61 patients did not. Resectability rate was twice as high with the use of preoperative radiation, that is, 21 per cent compared with 10 per cent without it. Of the 127 patients who underwent thoracotomy, the 30-day operative mortality was 3 per cent. More recently, Hilaris has updated the series, including 129 patients who underwent thoracotomy from 1960 to 1982. In this study, the five-year survival was 25 per cent.[17] The most important prognostic variables were the presence or absence of involved mediastinal nodes, the use of preoperative radiation, and histology. Using a multivariate regression model, the probability of five-year survival

TABLE 26–2. REPORTED RESULTS OF TREATMENT

Series and Year	No. Patients	Inclusion Criteria	Percentage Treated	5-Year Survival
Paulson 1982	120	Localized	62	31
Hilaris & Martini 1982	170	Localized	75	17
Komaki 1981	36	Localized	—	23
Houtte 1984	31	Localized	—	23
Devine 1986	66	"Curative"	76	13
Sundaresan 1987	30	All	100	*
Hilaris 1987	129	Localized	—	25

*Insufficient follow-up.

ranged from 34 per cent in those with negative nodes who received preoperative radiation therapy, to 21 per cent for those with negative nodes who did not receive such preoperative RT. Similarly, survival of patients with positive nodes ranged from 15 per cent if preoperative RT was used, to 8 per cent if it was not. Unfortunately, patients who received preoperative RT were treated more recently in the series, and thus they do not truly represent a concurrent control group.

Since various other studies recommend preoperative RT, it is important to examine the reasoning behind this strategy, which is not generally recommended for lung cancers with chest wall invasion below the level of the upper thoracic vertebra.[22, 32] In Paulson's early experience, the exact anatomic extent of tumor could not be accurately determined since only plain radiography was available. He further stated that when preoperative RT was used, a well-demarcated pseudocapsule was found, allowing the tumor dissection to be carried close to the margin without risk of systemic dissemination. Whether preoperative RT improves the probability of resection is debatable, since we have noted that the major cause for failure to complete resection is invasion of major vessels or extensive invasion of the brachial plexus. We have further shown that resectability can be improved with the use of a neurosurgical-thoracic team, and that spine invasion is not necessarily a contraindication to gross total resection.[46] Indeed, in those patients with spine invasion at initial presentation, we have noted that it is technically easier to operate on patients who have not had previous operation.

It is important to recognize that the clinical and radiologic spectrum of superior sulcus tumors varies considerably, from small tumors without bone involvement to larger tumors with rib destruction alone, and extensive tumors with spine and neural invasion. The prognosis is clearly poorer for larger tumors, which are more likely to be associated with nodal involvement. In such patients, local control for palliation of pain and prevention of cord compression may represent important therapeutic goals. More recently, Komaki and colleagues and Van Houtte and associates have suggested that external radiation therapy alone can produce results comparable to combined modality treatment.[24, 51] They suggest that the concept that radiation therapy is ineffective in controlling the tumor locally is erroneous and is based on historic radiation dosages that were insufficient in both field size and intensity. They believe that with the use of sophisticated megavoltage radiation to higher doses (6000 cGy in 6 to 6½ weeks), results comparable to operation can be obtained. In our series, patients were often referred after tumor progression had been noted, despite having received more than 5000 cGy. Histologically viable tumor was noted in the resected specimens, and this is especially true when the tumor involves bone. Since the spinal cord must be shielded after 4000 cGy to prevent radiation myelopathy, this poses a major obstacle to obtaining local control in advanced tumors by external radiation alone.

A number of important prognostic variables have been noted to affect survival. These include the absence of metastatic disease, scalene or mediastinal node involvement, absence of extensive local invasion, as well as histology—with adenocarcinoma having a better prognosis than squamous or large cell carcinoma.[2, 17, 29, 38, 40, 43, 51] There is general consensus that obtaining local control is critical, since it is the major determinant of survival in the first year. The proportion of patients who fail locally ranges from 30 to 70 per cent, with the majority suffering from unremittent pain from brachial plexus involvement. We have found that local control also correlates well with tumor extension at initial presentation, and thus patients with overt clinical brachial plexopathy are less likely to have local tumor control. To improve this, we believe efforts must be made to diagnose these tumors when they are smaller and more amenable to resection. Of those who fail with distant metastases, the brain represents the predominant site of involvement, with frequencies ranging from 10 to 34 per cent.[23, 46] As a result, Komaki has suggested that results can be further improved by prophylactic radiation therapy to the brain. The value of such an approach should be balanced against the potential morbidity of whole brain radiation in long-term survivors, which may result in delayed morbidity from radiation leukoencephalopathy.

The management of pain resulting from recurrent tumor or from radiation is yet another important aspect of treatment of superior sulcus tumors.[4, 20, 21, 42, 47, 48, 52] In the majority, brachial plexus pain implies tumor recurrence rather than pain from radiation. It is important to evaluate these patients by CT scans and myelography, since approximately 30 per cent have insidious epidural extension of tumor.[25] Brachial plexopathy from recurrent tumor is particularly difficult to control, even with the use of narcotics, because it is often associated with a deafferentation component. Traditional methods of pain control when systemic narcotic therapy is ineffective include the use of intrathecal or epidural drug delivery systems (Infusaid pump), or the use of local neurolytic blocks, although the development of tolerance is a problem. In patients in whom such measures are unsuccessful, cordotomy is indicated. The highest levels are obtained with the use of percutaneous techniques, and reported success rates range from 30 to 50 per cent.[4, 20, 48] It is our impression that there is a general reluctance to use this invaluable procedure in this country, with the resulting loss of technical skills and a higher rate of failure than that reported in Europe.[20]

Because the use of radiation therapy to improve resection rates and improve survival in locally advanced cases has apparently reached its zenith, there is considerable interest in the use of newer approaches, especially combination chemotherapy, to improve current treatment. Over the past five years, a number of combination chemotherapy regimens using cisplatin have had the highest and most impressive response rates (exceeding 50 per cent), but their overall impact on survival is disappointing. The use of these drugs prior to resection is intriguing, since it allows for in vivo determination of the tumor response to the agents used. A notable concern has been the potential pulmonary toxicity of mitomycin, but the use of short courses and concomitant steroid administration may make this unlikely.[26] Although the approach is conceptually attractive, its role in the management of this tumor has yet to be established. It is clear, however, that multimodality approaches using the combination of surgery, radiation, and chemotherapy represent the most fruitful areas for investigation in the next few years.

REFERENCES

1. American Cancer Society: Facts and Figures, 1990.
2. Anderson TM, Moy PM, Holmes EC: Factors affecting survival in superior sulcus tumors. J Clin Oncol 4:1598–1603, 1986.
3. Attar S, Miller JE, Satterfield J: Pancoast's tumor: Irradiation or surgery. Ann Thorac Surg 28:570–586, 1979.
4. Batzdorf K, Brechner VL: Management of pain associated with the Pancoast syndrome. Am J Surg 137:638–646, 1979.
5. Berrino F: Epidemiology of superior pulmonary sulcus syndrome (Pancoast syndrome). In Bonica JJ, Ventafridda V, Pagni CA (eds): Advances in Pain Research and Therapy. Vol 4. New York, Raven Press, 1982, pp 15–21.
6. Binkley JS: Role of surgery and interstitial radon therapy in cancer of the superior sulcus of the lung. Acta Un Int Cancer 6:1200–1203, 1950.
7. Bretz G, Lott S, El-Mahdi, Hazra T: The response of superior sulcus tumors to radiation therapy. Radiology 96:145–150, 1970.
8. Chardak WM, MacCallum JD: Pancoast's tumor; five year survival without recurrence of metastases following radical resection and post operative radiation. J Thorac Surg 31:535–542, 1958.
9. Devine JW, Mendenhall WM, Million RR, Carmichael MJ: Carcinoma of the superior pulmonary sulcus treated with surgery and/or radiation therapy. Cancer 57:941–943, 1986.
10. Fry WA, Carpenter JWJ, Adams WE: Superior sulcus tumor with 14 year survival. Arch Surg 94:142–145, 1967.
11. Hare ES: Tumor involving certain nerves. London Medical Gazette 23:16–18, 1838.
12. Heelan RT, Bains MS, Yeh S: Medical imaging in lung cancer. Surg Clin North Am 67:1015–1023, 1987.
13. Hepper NGG, Herdkovic T, Witten DM, et al: Thoracic inlet tumors. Ann Intern Med 64:949–989, 1966.
14. Herbut PA, Watson JS: Tumors of the thoracic inlet producing the Pancoast syndrome. Arch Pathol 42:88–103, 1946.
15. Hilaris BS, Martini N, Liskow A, et al: Superior sulcus lung cancer: A 35 year experience. Int J Radiat Oncol Biol Phys 5:54, 1979.
16. Hilaris BS, Martini N, Luomanen RJK, Beattie EJ: The value of preoperative radiation therapy in apical cancer of the lung. Surg Clin North Am 54:831–840, 1974.
17. Hilaris BS, Martini N, Wong GY, Nori D: Treatment of superior sulcus tumor (Pancoast). Surg Clin North Am 67:965–977, 1987.
18. Hilaris BS, Luomanen RK, Beattie EJ: Integrated irradiation and surgery in the treatment of apical lung cancer. Cancer 27:1369–1373, 1971.
19. Hilaris BS, Martini N: Multimodality therapy of superior sulcus tumors. In Bonica JJ, Ventafridda V, Pagni CA (eds): Advances in Pain Research and Therapy. Vol 4. New York, Raven Press, 1982, pp 113–122.
20. Ischia S, Ischia A, Luzzani A, et al: Results up to death in the treatment of persistent cervico-thoracic (Pancoast) and thoracic malignant pain by unilateral percutaneous cervical cordotomy. Pain 21:339–355, 1985.
21. Kanner RM, Martini N, Foley KM: Incidence of pain and other clinical manifestations of superior pulmonary sulcus (Pancoast) tumors. In Bonica JJ, Ventafridda V, Pagni CA (eds): Advances in Pain Research and Therapy. Vol 4. New York, Raven Press, 1982, pp 27–39.
22. Kirsh MM, Dickerman R, Fayos J: The value of chest wall resection in the treatment of superior sulcus tumors of the lung. Ann Thorac Surg 15:339–346, 1973.
23. Komaki K, Derus SB, Perez-Tamayo C, et al: Brain metastases in patients with superior sulcus tumors. Cancer 59:1649–1653, 1987.
24. Komaki R, Roh J, Cox JD, Lopes da Conceicao A: Superior sulcus tumors: Results of irradiation in 36 patients. Cancer 48:1563–1568, 1981.
25. Kori S, Foley KM, Posner JB: Brachial plexus lesions in patients with cancer: 100 cases. Neurology 31:45–50, 1981.
26. Kris MG, Gralla RJ, Martini N, et al: Preoperative and adjuvant chemotherapy in locally advanced non-small cell cancer. Surg Clin North Am 67:1051–1059, 1987.
27. Mantell BS: Superior sulcus (Pancoast) tumors: Results of radiotherapy. Br J Dis Chest 67:315–318, 1973.
28. Martini N: General clinical manifestations of superior pulmonary sulcus carcinoma. In: Bonica JJ, Ventafridda V, Pagni CA (eds): Advances in Pain Research and Therapy. Vol 4. New York, Raven Press, 1982, pp 23–25.
29. Miller JI, Mansour KA, Hatcher CR Jr: Carcinoma of the superior pulmonary sulcus. Ann Thorac Surg 28:44–47, 1979.
30. Morris RW, Abadir R: Pancoast tumor: The value of high dose radiotherapy. Radiology 132:717–719, 1979.
31. Mountain C: A new international staging system for cancer. Chest 89:225–233, 1986.
32. Pairolero PC, Trastek VF, Payne WS: Treatment of bronchogenic carcinoma with chest wall invasion. Surg Clin North Am 67:959–967, 1987.
33. Pancoast HK: Superior pulmonary sulcus tumor. JAMA 99:1391–1396, 1932.
34. Pancoast HK: Importance of careful roentgen-ray investigation of apical chest tumors. JAMA 83:1407–1411, 1924.
35. Paulson DL: The importance of defining location and staging of superior pulmonary sulcus tumors. Ann Thorac Surg 15:549–551, 1973.
36. Paulson DL: Carcinomas in the superior pulmonary sulcus. J Thorac Cardiovasc Surg 70:1095–1104, 1975.
37. Paulson DL: Extended resection of bronchogenic carcinoma in the superior pulmonary sulcus. Surg Rounds 1:10–21, 1980.
38. Paulson DL: Combined preoperative irradiation and extended resection for carcinoma in the superior pulmonary sulcus. In Bonica JJ, Ventafridda V, Pagni CA (eds): Advances in Pain Research and Therapy. Vol 4. New York, Raven Press, 1982, pp 47–63.
40. Shahian DM, Neptune WB, Ellis RH: Pancoast tumors: Improved survival with preoperative and post-operative radiotherapy. Ann Thorac Surg 43:32–38, 1987.
41. Shaw RR, Paulson DL, Kee JL Jr: Treatment of the superior sulcus tumor by irradiation followed by resection. Ann Surg 154:29–40, 1961.
42. Sindou M, Lapras C: Neurosurgical treatment of pain in the Pancoast-Tobias syndrome: Selective posterior rhizotomy and open anterolateral C2 cordotomy. In Bonica JJ, Ventafridda V, Pagni CA (eds): Advances in Pain Research and Therapy. Vol 4. New York, Raven Press, 1982, pp 199–206.
43. Stanford W, Barnes RP, Tucker AR: Influence of staging in superior sulcus (Pancoast) tumors of the lung. Ann Thorac Surg 29:406–409, 1980.

44. Sundaresan N, Galicich JH, Lane JM, et al: Treatment of neoplastic epidural cord compression by vertebral body resection and stabilization. J Neurosurg 63:676–684, 1985.

45. Sundaresan N, Foley KM, Hilaris BS, Martini N: Neurological complications of superior sulcus tumors. Proc Am Soc Clin Oncol 4:189, 1985.

46. Sundaresan N, Hilaris BS, Martini N: The combined neuro-surgical-thoracic management of superior sulcus tumors. J Clin Oncol 5:1739–1745, 1987.

47. Sundaresan N, DiGiacinto GV: Antitumor and antinociceptive approaches for pain control. Med Clin North Am 71:329–348, 1987.

48. Sweet WH, Poletti CE, Umansky F: Neurosurgical techniques to control the pain of superior sulcus and other tumors in this region. *In* Bonica JJ, Ventafridda V, Pagni CA (eds): Advances in Pain Research and Therapy. Vol 4. New York, Raven Press, 1982, pp 211–233.

49. Takita H, Regal AM, Antkowiak JG, et al: Chemotherapy followed by lung resection in inoperable non–small lung carcinomas due to locally far advanced disease. Cancer 57:630–635, 1986.

50. Tobias JW: Syndrome apico-costo-vertebral dolorosa por tumour, apexiamo. Su valor diagnostico en el cancer primitivo pulmonar. Rev Med Lat Am 17:1522–1666, 1932.

51. Van Houtte P, MacLennan I, Poulter C, Rubin P: External radiation in the management of superior sulcus tumor. Cancer 54:223–227, 1984.

52. Ventafridda V, Conno FD, Fothi C: Cervical percutaneous cordotomy. *In* Bonica JJ, Ventafridda V, Pagni CA (eds): Advances in Pain Research and Therapy. Vol 4. New York, Raven Press, 1982, pp 185–198.

53. Walker JE: Superior sulcus pulmonary tumor (Pancoast syndrome). J Med Assoc Gazette 35:364–365, 1946.

SPECIAL CONSIDERATIONS IN SURGERY OF PEDIATRIC SPINE TUMORS

TADANORI TOMITA

INTRODUCTION

Spinal tumors, either primary or secondary, are relatively uncommon in childhood. The clinical presentation and management of such tumors in children differ in several ways from those in adults. First, difficulties in verbal communication with infants and young children may result in delay in early detection; second, the histologic spectrum of these tumors is different from the adult counterpart; third, management of these tumors should take into consideration the ongoing development of the central nervous system and spine during growth. This chapter is based on the author's experience with 33 spinal and/or spinal extradural tumors occurring in the pediatric age group (Table 27–1). These include tumors that are located either in the intradural space or the subarachnoid space. Dysraphic states such as lipoma and dermoid and neurenteric cysts are excluded.

General Considerations

The most common presenting symptom of spinal tumors is pain in the back with or without a referred component. Pain is often expressed in a nonverbal fashion.[25] Young children may express pain by being irritable or cranky and may hold or point to the site of pain. Referred pain may draw attention away from the original site of the lesion. For instance, referred pain in the abdomen has led to the misdiagnosis of "acute abdomen," and one patient in this series erroneously underwent an exploratory laparotomy. Changes in urinary habits due to the development of a neurogenic bladder may be missed or completely ignored in a young child. In infants or toddlers, urinary incontinence is not easily detectable. Weakness of the extremities may be subtle, but shuffling or foot drop in toddlers or older children is a presenting symptom that often draws parental attention. A stiff neck or head tilt may be the sole presenting symptom of tumors located in the cervical region. Painless or painful scoliosis may be found in association with tumors located in the thoracic or lumbar spine.

Examination of infants or young children requires special skills, patience, wisdom, and good instincts.[28] The neurologic examination should be carefully conducted. Among the cranial nerve examinations, a Horner's syndrome should be looked for and documented. Motor weakness, changes in reflex (hypo- or hyperreflexia, pathologic reflex), muscle atrophy, sphincter involvement, sensory changes, and positive straight leg raising should be carefully tested. Sensory examination using pins may frighten the young child and should be deferred to the end. Examination of the back is important and should include attention to tenderness, mobility and stiffness of the spine, the presence of a mass or fullness, as well as the presence of scoliosis or kyphosis. All patients should be examined undressed. Abdominal examination may disclose a palpable mass or distended bladder.

Investigations

Careful examination of plain x-rays of the spine is the first step in the radiologic evaluation of a spinal

TABLE 27–1. SPINE TUMORS IN CHILDHOOD

HISTOLOGY	INCIDENCE
Neuroblastoma	7
Osteosarcoma	5
Ganglioneuroma	4
Neurofibroma	3
Undifferentiated sarcoma	3
Ewing's sarcoma	2
Aneurysmal bone cyst	2
Lymphoma	2
Osteoblastoma	1
Wilms' tumor	1
Benign teratoma	1
Malignant germ cell tumor	1
Meningioma	1
Total	33

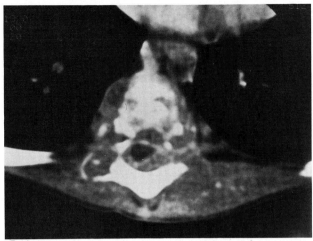

FIGURE 27–1. CT scan of upper thoracic region after intravenous contrast material administration, showing destructive lesions of the spinal body and lateral masses along with intraspinal and paraspinal soft tissue tumor. The spinal dura is enhanced. Paravertebral mass biopsy showed a histiocytic lymphoma.

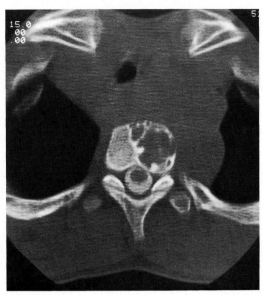

FIGURE 27–2. CT scan after metrizamide myelography, showing a lytic expansile lesion of the thoracic spinal body and a large posterior mediastinum mass. The histology of the tumor was benign neurofibroma.

lesion. The following radiographic signs should be scrutinized, as they may suggest a possible spinal tumor[31, 33, 38]: (1) changes in the spinal curvature (scoliosis, kyphosis, lordosis); (2) changes in the bony trabeculae (lytic, blastic, destructive, expansile); (3) the presence of a paravertebral mass and altered paraspinal contour; and (4) a widened interpediculate distance.

Computed tomography (CT) scans of the spine are now performed with increasing frequency. If adequate CT scans are available, the patient may not require further invasive studies (Fig. 27–1). Currently available CT scanners can generally detect osseous changes with as much clarity as tomography. They also demonstrate the presence of paraspinal masses, extensions of soft tissue into the spinal canal, and abnormal calcification. However, myelography is often required to demonstrate more detailed pathologic changes within the spinal canal. Newly available water-soluble contrast material (such as metrizamide) cause fewer side effects in myelographic procedures and are recommended.

If a lumbosacral lesion is suspected, lumbar puncture should be avoided because a dry tap may result and the procedure carries the risk of causing hemorrhage in the tumor. In such situations and in other cases with a complete block, a high cervical puncture is required for the completion of myelography. Cervical (C1–C2) puncture can be done safely even in the neonatal period. The patient is usually well sedated with a combination of chloral hydrate (50 mg/ kg), Nembutal (2 mg/kg), and Nubain (0.15 mg/kg). The cervical puncture is performed under fluoroscopic guidance with the patient in a strict recumbent position. Under fluoroscopy, the needle is advanced into the posterior subarachnoid space of C1–C2. At the same time, cerebrospinal fluid (CSF) is aspirated for cytologic evaluation. We routinely perform CT-myelography shortly after injection of the contrast material into the subarachnoid space. This imaging

not only discloses the extent of the spinal cord compression, but also provides the information in terms of associated osseous changes and paraspinal extensions of the tumor (Figs. 27–2 and 27–3). Plain myelography may not necessarily outline these details.

If radiographic evidence of a high grade block is found, with or without a neurologic deficit, dexamethasone therapy should be initiated. We use doses of dexamethasone empirically—10 mg in infancy and 20 mg in children—which are given as intravenous boli, followed by 2 to 4 mg of dexamethasone every 6 hours. While awaiting surgical decompression, two patients in our series with complete block deteriorated rapidly after metrizamide myelography, despite

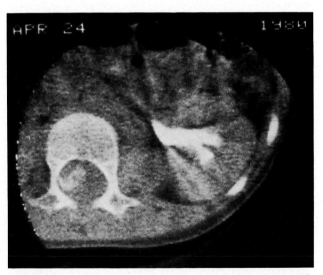

FIGURE 27–3. CT scan of the lumbar region after metrizamide myelography and intravenous contrast material infusion, showing a ganglioneuroblastoma of intra- and extraspinal extension.

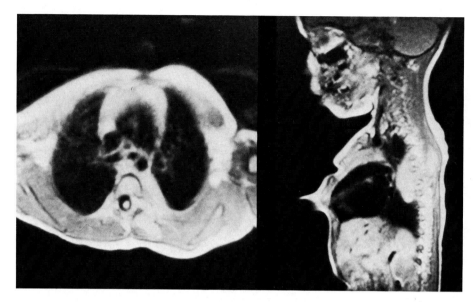

FIGURE 27–4. Magnetic resonance image (transverse section [*left*] and sagittal section [*right*]), showing increased signal areas in the paraspinal, intraspinal, and posterior mediastinum spaces. The spinal cord is displaced by the epidural tumor. The histology of the tumor was a neuroblastoma.

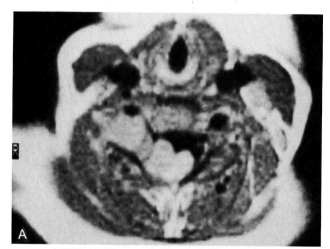

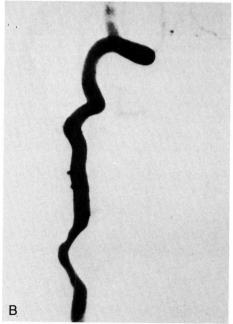

FIGURE 27–5. Magnetic resonance image (*A*) of the midcervical region shows a dumbbell-shaped meningioma of subdural, epidural, and extraspinal extension through the transverse foramen. A subtraction vertebral angiogram (lateral projection) (*B*) shows a segmental displacement of the vertebral artery by the tumor in the transverse foramen.

the use of a fine needle for the lumbar puncture and care being taken to avoid a sudden escape of CSF. Thus, close clinical observation is important after myelography has demonstrated a total block. If the patient deteriorates, emergency decompression is necessary.

Further advances in medical technology have brought magnetic resonance imaging (MRI) into daily practice in the United States, and its value is still being established. The MRI scan gives a multidimensional view and a clearer anatomic image of soft tissue, including the spinal cord, to disclose the degree of extension of the tumor mass (Fig. 27–4). Osseous changes, however, are not always appreciated by currently available MRIs; therefore CT scans, particularly with bone windows, may be needed as a supplement to the MRI. The combination of MRI and CT scans will probably further diminish the frequency of myelographic examination in the future. However, these studies do not allow the cytologic examination of CSF, which still requires a lumbar puncture.

Another invasive study, angiography, may be needed when one suspects a vascular tumor of the spine. Tumors that involve the transverse foramina of the cervical spine should be evaluated by angiography to determine their relationship to the vertebral arteries (Fig. 27–5). For thoracic lesions, spinal angiography is carried out through the respective intercostal arteries and, for lumbar lesions, through the respective lumbar arteries. The angiogram may suggest the malignant nature of spine lesions by showing extensive pathologic neovasculature, arteriovenous shunts, and blood pools; early venous filling during the arteriolar phase; and a tumor blush with a poorly defined outline of the tumor.[62] Angiography may be used in conjunction with embolization prior to vascular tumor resection for intraarterial chemotherapy for malignant spine tumors.

SURGICAL CONSIDERATIONS

The goals of surgery for pediatric spine tumors are (1) decompression of the spinal cord and nerves; (2) relief of pain; (3) possible total resection of the tumor and affected osseous structures; and (4) reconstruction or maintenance of spine alignment. Careful preoperative evaluation of the tumor dictates the surgical approach to be used. If extensive spine resections are performed in children, post surgical kyphosis and instability may pose clinical problems later in the course of management. Post laminectomy deformities have been extensively reported in the literature.[11, 21, 57, 64, 65] Usually they occur in young children who undergo multilevel laminectomies, especially in the cervical and cervicothoracic regions. Yasuoka and colleagues reported that spinal deformity occurred in all children following cervical laminectomy, in 36 per cent following thoracic laminectomy and in 8 per cent with lumbar laminectomy. The most common postlaminectomy deformity in the

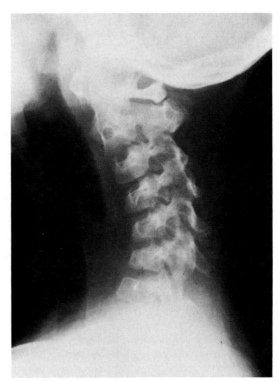

FIGURE 27–6. Preoperative cervical spine radiograph (lateral projection) of a 7-year-old girl with a cervical cord astrocytoma. Note the swan-neck deformity without osseous abnormalities.

cervical spine is kyphosis, which gives rise to the so-called swan-neck deformity. Upper thoracic laminectomies often result in both kyphosis and scoliosis. These spinal deformities after multilevel laminectomies may be attributed either to facet removal or to postlaminectomy irradiation. However, these complications may occur with no irradiation and even when facets are preserved. Yasuoka postulated that the deformity may be due to wedging of the cartilaginous portion of the vertebral body, and to the viscoelasticity of ligaments in children.[65] Occasionally, the swan-neck deformity may be present prior to laminectomy (Fig. 27–6), possibly from denervation of the paravertebral muscle resulting in muscle imbalance. Extensive paravertebral muscle dissection during operation may cause further denervation.

This theory is supported by the fact that such deformity may not always be prevented by the application of a brace or jacket.[11, 57] The paravertebral muscles are important. A permanent physiologic curvature of the spine, away from the gestational C-shaped curvature in lateral profile, occurs through the pull of the paravertebral muscle and the prolonged effects of erect posture during childhood and adolescence.[2]

Laminotomy

In order to prevent postlaminectomy deformities of the spine, Raimondi and coworkers proposed that the posterior elements be replaced after careful removal en bloc.[45] He termed this procedure "laminotomy." The advantage of laminotomy is the reconstruction of the posterior arches of the spine, which restores anatomic integrity and immediate fusion of the spine. This procedure requires experience and the use of high speed drills, but it can be done safely without intraoperative compression upon the underlying spinal cord. The indications and rationale for this procedure have been described in detail previously.[45]

At the laminotomy, the patient is placed in a prone position. Care should be undertaken to avoid pressure upon the abdomen by application of rolls of towels under the chest cage and iliac crests. Cervical laminotomies are done with the head positioned by either a head holder or Mayfield three-tong pins. Excess flexion and extension should be avoided, as the former causes further disruption of the facet joints intraoperatively, and the latter makes it difficult to enter the interlaminal spaces. The spinous processes are exposed through the midline incision, extending from one full spinal level above through one full spinal level below the planned extent of the laminotomy. Paravertebral muscles are stripped off from the laminae and spinous processes by a sharp dissection technique. The depth of the laminae from the skin in infants and young children is very shallow when compared with that of adults. The use of electrocautery during dissection should be minimized, as it may produce thermal damage to the paravertebral muscles, the posterior arches, and the capsular ligaments. The muscle dissection should extend laterally to the articular facets of the respective spinal levels, and trauma to the capsular ligament and joint should be carefully prevented.

Once the desired levels are exposed, a laminotomy incision is made using a high speed drill along a line medial to the facets (Fig. 27–7). The osteotomy should be bevelled so that the replaced laminotomy flap does not sink and stays in position after replacement. The surgeon should be able to feel the depth of osteotomy at the laminotomy by the burr of the high speed drill. The superior portion of the lamina is slightly thicker than the inferior portion. Small bony bridges in the laminotomy groove may be broken by wedging a small dissector and twisting it. Once incisions are carried out bilaterally at the desired lamina, the interspinous ligaments to be removed below and above the spine are cut. Then the yellow ligaments at these levels are incised horizontally up to the laminotomy site. The spinal process of the lowermost spine may require partial resection in order to enter the interspinous space above. The lowermost laminotomy flap is elevated, following which the yellow ligament is incised at the laminotomy groove. This incision of the yellow ligaments is continued rostrally from one lamina to another on either side. Subsequently, the multilevel laminotomy is completed, and the laminae are removed en bloc, connected to each other by the yellow and interspinous ligaments (Fig. 27–8).

After the intraspinal procedure has been completed, the laminotomy flaps are replaced. Corre-

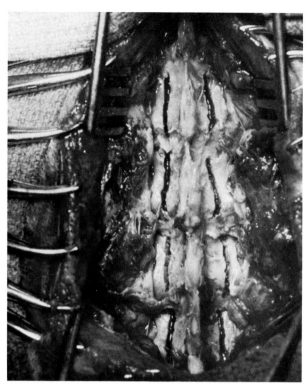

FIGURE 27–7. Operative photograph of laminotomy procedure. Bilateral laminae of four spinal levels are osteotomized.

sponding small drill holes are made in the flap and at the laminotomy site. It may be difficult to bring in a pneumatic air drill and to place drill holes at the laminotomy site, and therefore the author prefers to use towel clamps to make holes. As there is always some bone loss during the drilling process, a gap is present between the laminotomy edge and the bone flap. The laminotomy flap must therefore be cen-

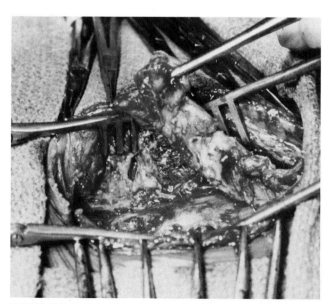

FIGURE 27–8. Operative photograph of laminotomy procedure. The laminotomy flap of four spinal levels is lifted. Each resected lamina is connected to each other by the intact yellow ligaments and interspinous ligaments.

tered and secured in its anatomic position by non-absorbable sutures placed through the drill holes. The gap is filled by bone dust to facilitate fusion. It is also important to sew the individual interspinous ligaments and supraspinous ligaments and to keep the laminotomy flap elevated in order to avoid future compression of the cord by bony callus.

Postoperatively, the patient needs external immobilization. The author prefers to place the patient with a wire-frame cervical collar (Hallmark, Arcadia, CA) after a cervical laminotomy. However, if the patient demonstrated preoperative swan-neck deformity, the temporary application of a halo vest is indicated. For lumbar or thoracic laminotomy, a molded body jacket is applied. These are used for 2 to 3 months, until the laminotomy flaps and soft tissues are healed.

Although anatomic reconstruction of spine is achieved by the laminotomy method, postoperative spinal deformities cannot be avoided in all cases. Laminotomy flaps afford a reroofing of the spinal canal. Each replaced lamina is connected to the other by the yellow ligaments but is not secured to the intact laminae above and below. Thus, longitudinal fixation of the laminotomy flap is not sufficient to prevent progressive kyphosis caused by the existing denervation of posterior cervical muscles. The author once treated a patient with progressive swan-neck deformity after a four-level cervical laminotomy (C3-C6) by posterior wiring, using No. 2 silk ligature between the C2 and C7 laminae. This procedure successfully reduced and prevented further swan-neck deformity. A more definitive treatment of the postlaminectomy cervical deformity is anterior cervical fusion using autologous bone such as tibial bone graft.[11, 65] Anterior fusions are generally more effective with regard to future accessibility to the operative site than are posterior fusions. Complications of the laminotomy procedure include depression of the lamina flap into the spinal canal (Fig. 27–9) and the lack of an acoustic window for postoperative evaluation using ultrasonography.

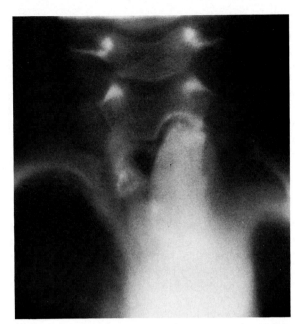

FIGURE 27–10. Cervicothoracic spinal tomogram after vertebrectomy and reconstruction using tibial bone graft and methyl methacrylate.

Vertebral Body Resection

If the vertebral body is involved exclusively by tumor, vertebral body resection may be indicated.[51, 52, 55] Through a laminotomy or costotransverse resection, the posterolateral portion of the vertebral body is accessible, and partial vertebral body resection is possible. When more radical resection of the vertebral body and reconstruction of the body with bone graft are needed, the procedures are better performed by means of anterior or anterolateral approaches. Through these approaches, the paravertebral and intraspinal tumor ventral to the spinal cord can be resected simultaneously. The involved bodies along with the intervertebral discs above and below are removed by high speed drills and curettage. The structural integrity of the spine is essential to its stability. Spinal stability is achieved by bone graft from the tibia rather than the iliac crest,[11] as the former bone graft is more solid in pediatrics. Bone grafts that are simply placed into position may dislodge, so they should be secured in place by the application of methyl methacrylate and Steinmann pins (Fig. 27–10). The spine in a young child may develop further kyphosis as the patient grows, even after the use of autologous bone grafts which lack a growth center. However, bone grafts are far superior for fusion and replacement of the resected vertebrae in childhood in comparison to the adult spine, which can only be stabilized by methyl methacrylate.

PRIMARY VERTEBRAL TUMORS

Aneurysmal Bone Cyst

Aneurysmal bone cysts are lesions consisting of anastomosing cavernous spaces usually filled with

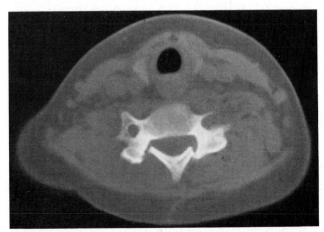

FIGURE 27–9. CT scan of cervical region after cervical laminotomy procedure. Note the depressed laminotomy flap, causing spinal stenosis and spinal cord compression.

blood. They are neither vascular aneurysms nor true bone cysts. The common age of patients presenting with aneurysmal bone cysts is 5 to 20 years, and females are more commonly affected than males. These lesions can occur throughout the spinal column, but the lumbar region and the posterior elements of the spine are frequent sites of occurrence. Radiologically, a lytic expanding lesion is the typical finding for an aneurysmal bone cyst, but on occasion a collapsed vertebral body may be noted. This lesion is often extremely vascular, although this feature may be more apparent pathologically than angiographically.

The lining of the cyst cavity is composed of fleshy, rubbery, pink-red vascular tissue. Focal gritty areas are also present. The vascular areas are the source of intraoperative bleeding, and such tissue may invade the surrounding soft tissues.

Microscopically an aneurysmal bone cyst consists of benign fibrous tissue, large vascular spaces, and long delicate spicules of woven or lamellar bone which support the lining tissue. The large cyst-like spaces seen grossly are not lined by any specific cell population but rather represent areas of hemorrhage and/or exudation of serum. Osteoclast-type giant cells are commonly seen adjacent to the hemorrhage and in the pools of blood (Fig. 27–11).

Since the above description is nonspecific, the diagnosis of aneurysmal bone cyst is really one of exclusion. Lesions that may undergo hemorrhage and cyst-like formation must be ruled out histologically before arriving at the diagnosis of aneurysmal bone cyst. In the spine these include giant cell tumor, osteosarcoma, osteoblastoma, and fibrous dysplasia.

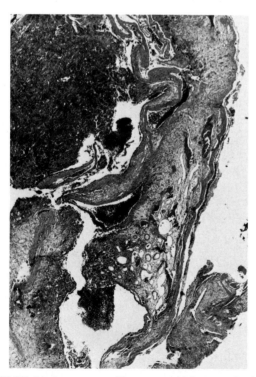

FIGURE 27–11. An aneurysmal bone cyst with large pools of blood and walls of fibrous tissue and bone spicules (H & E ×20).

Profuse intraoperative hemorrhage can be controlled by rapid removal of the cyst wall lining. The treatment of choice is the complete resection of the affected portion of the spine, which should lead to cure of the disease. After incomplete resection or curettage, the recurrence rate is reportedly 25 per cent; however, risk of recurrence lessens with age.[26, 59] The value of radiotherapy is limited; in one series, irradiation without surgery was associated with poor results in half of the patients.[9] More importantly, empiric radiation therapy should be condemned because of the adverse effect upon the child's developing spine and spinal cord. In addition, both radiation myelopathy and radiation-induced sarcomas have been reported following treatment of some benign lesions.[42, 59]

Osteoblastoma and Osteoid Osteoma

Osteoblastomas and osteoid osteomas are benign tumors composed of a vascular stroma, abundant osteoblasts, and osteoid tissue (see Chapter 13). About half the cases of osteoblastomas occur in the vertebrae, and osteoblastoma is the only bone tumor that favors the spinal column.[49] A common site is the base of the transverse process, and the lumbar spine is the most common segment involved.[5, 32] Vertebral body involvement is rare.[43]

Spinal pain with scoliosis is the cardinal symptom, and about 25 per cent of cases occur in childhood.[16, 49] These tumors are well known to cause marked spinal stiffness and painful scoliosis. Excision of the lesions usually ensures complete resolution of the scoliosis.[46] Radiographic and CT features of these lesions (Fig. 27–12) are discussed in Chapter 13.

Since these tumors often involve the pedicle and transverse process, a surgical approach allowing direct access to the pedicle without entering the spinal canal or jeopardizing spinal stability was proposed by Kirwan and colleagues.[32] Through a long midline incision along the back, the soft tissue of the side of the lesion is stripped as far laterally as the tip of the transverse process. The soft tissue attachment to the anterior surface of the transverse process is cleared with blunt dissection, and then the transverse process is excised. Subsequently, the pedicular lesion is easily accessed. By Kirwan's approach, the junction of the apophyseal joint and the pars interarticularis are preserved after resection of the pedicle, and spinal stability is maintained. The only disadvantage is a wide skin incision that is necessary to access the tip of the transverse process in older patients. However, in young children, the less bulky soft tissue in the paravertebral region requires a skin incision of shorter length. On occasion these tumors may be very vascular on angiography.[5] For tumors involving both anterior and posterior elements, a staged operation or combined anteroposterior approach may be required.[63]

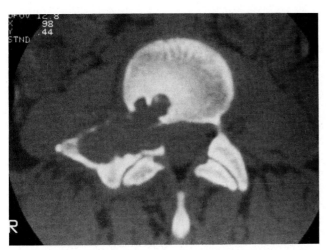

FIGURE 27–12. CT scan of lumbar osteoblastoma without contrast enhancement. Note an expansile lesion affecting the lateral mass and posterolateral portion of the spinal body.

Giant Cell Tumors

Giant cell tumors occur less frequently in the pediatric population than do osteoblastomas and aneurysmal bone cysts.[14, 16, 17, 48, 54] This tumor is composed of a highly vascularized network with numerous mutinucleated giant cells. Its radiographic and pathologic features have been described in Chapters 18 and 19.

Eosinophilic Granuloma

Eosinophilic granuloma is the most benign form of histiocytosis and is thus not a true neoplasm. The lesion consists of an abnormal proliferation of lipid-containing histiocytes of the reticuloendothelial system. Eosinophilic granulomas often affect young children or adolescents and are more common in males.[53] Compared with other variants of histiocytosis, eosinophilic granulomas rarely involve the viscera. However, spinal eosinophilic granulomas may affect multiple spinal levels.[49] They often present with localized pain but rarely with neurologic deficits. The thoracic and lumbar spine are common sites, and granulomas nearly invariably affect the body of the vertebrae. Involvement of the pedicles and the lateral, posterior segments are rare even in advanced cases. The degree of compression collapse is dependent upon the extent of involvement of the vertebral body; in younger children, most of the affected vertebral body shows a rapid collapse, resulting in a completely flattened "vertebra plana." Sometimes the disease evolves so gradually and painlessly that the diagnosis of vertebra plana is made on radiographic examination. In older children and adolescents, relatively smaller areas are affected, which may cause a wedge-shaped deformity or a punched-out lytic lesion. The adjacent intervertebral disc spaces are well maintained, and a paravertebral soft tissue mass is generally absent.[39]

The macroscopic findings of eosinophilic granu-loma are those of soft yellow and focally hemorrhagic tissue. Microscopically, sheets of benign histiocytes with folded or creased nuclei are the most populous and diagnostic cells (Fig. 27–13). Scattered foci of eosinophils are usually prominent, as well as lymphocytes, plasma cells, and leukocytes. Foci of necrosis are common, as are scattered osteoclast-like giant cells. Lipid-laden macrophages ("foamy cells") may also be present. There is no reliable histologic way to distinguish between eosinophilic granuloma and other forms of histiocytosis. The differential diagnosis of acute osteomyelitis or even Hodgkin's disease must be entertained on histologic grounds. The former is sometimes very difficult to distinguish from eosinophilic granuloma. However, infections are usually associated with abundant necrotic bone spicules, fewer histiocytes, and the absence of S-100 protein when examined with immunoperoxidase methods. The histiocytes of eosinophilic granuloma usually produce this protein. Also, electron microscopy is very helpful because histiocytes of eosinophilic granuloma have characteristic cytoplasmic tennis racket–shaped bodies, called Birbeck granules, which are not present in osteomyelitis. Hodgkin's disease is diagnosed by the presence of Reed-Sternberg cells, and the histiocytic component does not produce S-100 protein.

Eosinophilic granuloma is usually a self-limited disease and may heal spontaneously[23, 39] (Fig. 27–14). Greenfield classified three phases of spinal eosinophilic granulomas.[23] The earliest is a destructive lesion in the center of the vertebral body, followed by collapse or wedge-shaped deformity of the vertebral body. The final phase is a regenerative one, in which the vertebral body regains height to a certain degree. This spontaneous reconstitution of vertebral height is attributed to the sparing of areas of enchondral ossification.[50] The potential for regeneration is greater in younger patients, and reconstitution of vertebral height may be observed regardless of the mode of treatment. Selmon reported six patients

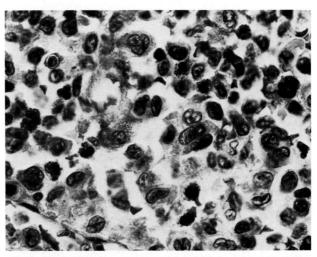

FIGURE 27–13. Eosinophilic granuloma with sheets of benign histiocytes. The nuclei are bean-shaped and folded. Scattered eosinophils and lymphocytes are present (H & E ×440).

FIGURE 27–14. Spine radiograph (*A*) of a 4-year-old male showing collapsed L3 spinal body due to an eosinophilic granuloma. Nearly full spontaneous reconstitution of L3 vertebra is evident 3 years later (*B*).

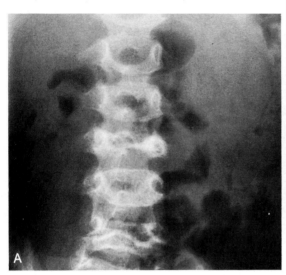

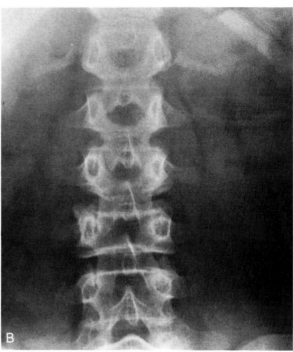

with spinal lesions, all of whom healed spontaneously without surgical intervention or radiation therapy.[50] The need for vertebral biopsy may be questioned in typical cases. However, whereas eosinophilic granuloma is the most frequent cause of vertebral plana in children, malignant lesions of the spine may also result in a similar radiologic picture (Figs. 27–15 and 27–16). Therefore, tissue diagnosis by needle biopsy is appropriate to rule out the possibility of malig-

nancy. Care should be taken to save some tissue for electron microscopy.

Once eosinophilic granuloma is diagnosed by simple biopsy or curettage, no further surgical de-

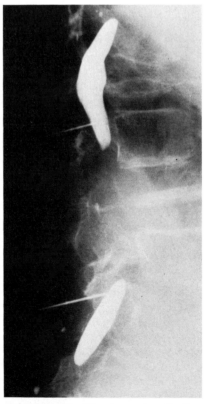

FIGURE 27–16. Myelogram of lumbar region of a 9-year-old male with history of osteogenic sarcoma. There are two collapsed spinal bodies of L1 and L3 due to the metastatic osteogenic sarcoma. Note a myelographic complete block.

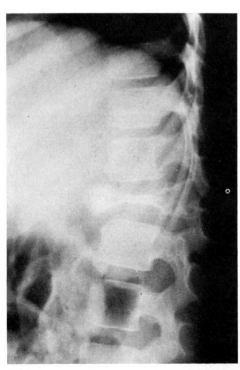

FIGURE 27–15. Spine radiograph of a 5-year-old child showing a collapsed L2 vertebral body due to a metastatic neuroblastoma.

compression is needed unless progressive neurologic and/or radiographic deterioration is encountered. The most effective treatment is bed rest during the acute stages of pain, followed by external immobilization by means of a body jacket for thoracolumbar lesions or wire-frame collars for cervical lesions. Pain usually subsides rapidly with simple bed rest. External immobilization may be required for up to one year. Even advanced cases of vertebra plana rarely result in cord compression, nor do they produce complete block on myelography.[22] If neural compression (particularly progressive) is noted, some recommend applying low dose (1200 cGy) irradiation, which may be effective and justified in such circumstances.[22]

Osteogenic Sarcoma

Primary osteogenic sarcomas arising in the spine are rare. Only 0.85 to 2 per cent of osteogenic sarcomas occur in the vertebral column[7] (Fig. 27–17). Most osteogenic sarcomas of the spine in the pediatric population are metastatic in nature, resulting from blood-borne metastasis from other sites or from irradiation or malignant transformation of preexisting benign tumors. Osteosarcoma is often seen in the pediatric population.[29, 41, 47] However, the radiographic, pathologic, and clinical features of osteogenic sarcoma are discussed in Chapter 14.

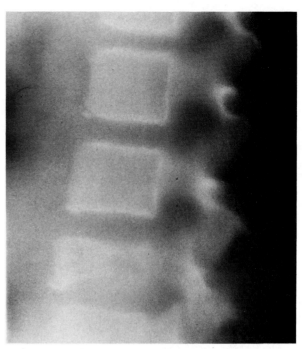

FIGURE 27–18. Spine tomogram showing a partially collapsed vertebral body with irregular density of the lumbar region due to a primary Ewing's sarcoma.

Ewing's Sarcoma

Ewing's sarcoma is a tumor composed of small, round cells resembling neuroblastomas, rhabdomyosarcomas, and non-Hodgkin's lymphomas (Fig. 27–18). Approximately 84 per cent of malignant round cell tumors of the bone are Ewing's sarcoma.[6] The origin of the Ewing's sarcoma cell is unknown. The common age for Ewing's sarcoma is the second decade of life, and it is uncommon below five years of age. Chapter 24 deals with the diagnostic and clinical features of the disease.

If the neurologic signs are absent or stable, Ewing's sarcoma may be treated by a combination of local radiation and chemotherapy. Patients with neurologic symptoms and radiographic evidence of cord compression may be treated by chemotherapy alone with good neurologic recovery.[27] Extensive paraspinal Ewing's sarcoma may be treated with chemotherapy alone to reduce the size of the mass, which allows a safe, less mutilating surgical resection.[40, 56] Currently, many authors advocate delaying irradiation until several cycles of chemotherapy are completed.[58] Since the vertebral body fuses to the pedicle at the neurocentral synchondrosis by age seven, this approach in treating younger patients may well be justified.

Neuroblastoma and Ganglioneuroblastoma

Neuroblastomas are the most common systemic malignant tumors in infancy. Approximately 50 per

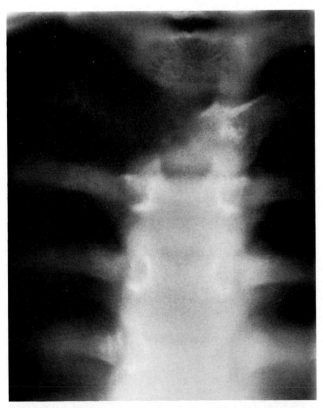

FIGURE 27–17. Spine tomogram showing a destructive lesion due to a primary osteogenic sarcoma of vertebral body and lateral mass of T3.

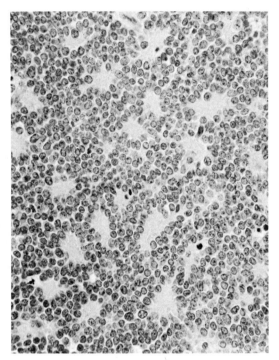

FIGURE 27–19. A neuroblastoma with a prominent rosette pattern formed by tumor cells surrounding a focus of neurofibrils (H & E ×320).

cent of neuroblastomas are diagnosed during the first two years of life, and over two thirds are diagnosed during the first five years of life. Neuroblastomas are most common among paravertebral mass lesions in infants and children.[31] As opposed to central neuroblastomas, paraspinal neuroblastomas (cervical, mediastinal, retroperitoneal, and presacral) originate from neural crest cells, which give rise to the sympathetic ganglia and adrenal medulla. They often produce catecholamine. Typically, neuroblastomas are composed of small round cells with rosette formation (Fig. 27–19). Ganglioneuroblastoma contains a variable degree of cellular differentiation from ganglion cells and is clinically categorized as neuroblastoma.

Distinguishing between neuroblastoma and Ewing's sarcoma on purely histologic grounds depends upon electron microscopy and immunoperoxidase staining methods. Therefore, when entertaining the diagnosis of so-called round cell lesions—lymphoma-leukemia, Ewing's sarcoma, neuroblastoma, rhabdomyosarcoma, eosinophilic granuloma, metastatic carcinoma—care should be taken to have enough tissue for these most important studies.

Neuroblastoma arising from paravertebral ganglia has a tendency to grow through the intervertebral foramen, causing a dumbbell-shaped mass to invade and destroy the spinal body. Dumbbell-type neuroblastoma comprise 6 to 14 per cent of neuroblastomas, but only 1 to 6 per cent of these present with neurologic symptoms.[30, 61] Radiographic examination may show paravertebral mass, widening of intervertebral foramen, and erosion of the body or pedicles and, occasionally, of the adjacent ribs. The intraspinal

component of dumbbell neuroblastoma can be demonstrated by myelography but is better appreciated with myelography CT or MRI scan. The dumbbell neuroblastoma should be detected and treated in an early stage, as the majority of patients with dumbbell neuroblastoma have an excellent chance of survival if diagnosed early (Stage 3 or less).[30, 61] Mediastinal neuroblastomas have a better prognosis than do retroperitoneal neuroblastomas.[10, 18]

All patients with paraspinal masses should be evaluated by CT or MRI scan to rule out intraspinal extension, despite lack of neurologic signs. Stage I neuroblastomas, which are confined to a single organ of origin, are managed by surgical therapy alone. Stage II neuroblastomas undergo operative resection but often show small portions of tumor that extend into the intervertebral foramina.

The treatment of choice for these dumbbell tumors is an attempt at complete surgical excision. Approaches combining hemilaminectomy with thoracotomy or laparotomy, with the patient in the lateral position, are used for patients with no or stable neurologic deficits. A small, tongue-like extension through the intervertebral foramen may be resected by thoracotomy without the need for laminectomy. However, if the neurologic deficit is progressive, surgical decompression should be carried out. This can be followed by staged excision of the paraspinal portion of the tumor. Postoperative irradiation is required and is effective in Stage II neuroblastomas.[35] More recent reports suggest that systemic chemotherapy may be effective and should be the primary choice of treatment for the stable or asymptomatic child.[27] This approach results in rapid regression of the peridural tumor in a high proportion of patients

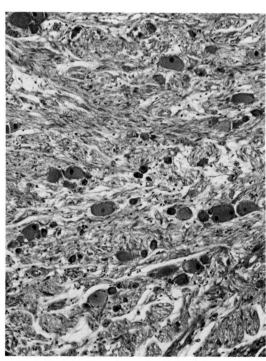

FIGURE 27–20. A ganglioneuroma with prominent mature large ganglion cells and Schwann cells (H & E ×125).

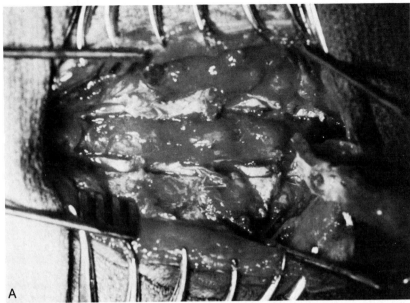

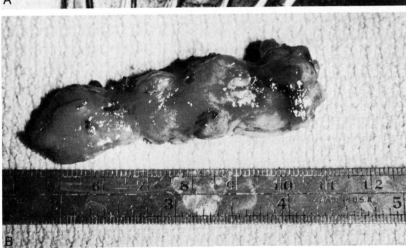

FIGURE 27–21. Operative photograph of a four-level lumbar laminotomy. There is a large ganglioneuroma occupying the spinal epidural space (*A*). The resected ganglioneuroma (*B*) shows multiple indentations by the laminae.

and may avoid the need for surgical intervention or irradiation. These patients should be closely observed neurologically, since neural decompression by surgery may be needed if the tumor does not respond. Young children with neurologic deficits frequently respond to aggressive treatment, including laminectomy and irradiation. Full neurologic recovery from complete paralysis has been reported.[30, 61] Occasionally, spontaneous remission or maturation of neuroblastomas to benign ganglioneuroma occurs in young infants, but tumor progression may occur despite the presence of a large area of maturation in the neoplasms.[4]

Ganglioneuroma is the benign counterpart of neuroblastoma and is composed of fibroblasts, collagen and Schwann cells, with collections of mature ganglion cells (Fig. 27–20). Pure ganglioneuroma is relatively rare in comparison with neuroblastoma and ganglioneuroblastoma (the ratio was 1:14 in one series).[10] Paravertebral ganglioneuromas tend to grow into the spinal canal through enlarged vertebral foramina and on occasion may be located exclusively intraspinally.[34] Surgical resection is the treatment of choice, and a combination of anterior and posterior approaches may be required. These tumors are well delineated but may extend several spinal levels epidurally (Fig. 27–21). All gross tumor should be excised and examined pathologically, since in some cases the intraspinal portion may be a benign ganglioneuroma, but the paravertebral component may contain ganglioneuroblastoma, or vice versa.[44]

METASTASES

The rarity of carcinoma in childhood is the major reason for the relatively infrequent occurrence of metastases to the spine.[8, 13] Tomita and colleagues reported that there were only two children among 78 patients of all ages with spinal epidural metastases with complete block.[60] Between 6 and 14 per cent of spinal or spinal cord tumors in children represent blood-borne metastases.[15, 28] Sarcomas are responsible for one half to two thirds of all metastatic tumors in children, followed by neuroblastoma and lymphoma-leukemia.[13, 24] In the author's experience with 13 spinal metastases in childhood, the most common histologic type was osteosarcoma (five cases), followed by undifferentiated sarcoma (three cases), and Ewing's sarcoma (two cases). Eleven of these 13 cases were known to have had previously treated sites of cancer.

As the pathologic distribution in our series and others indicates, a great majority of metastatic spinal malignancies in childhood are radioresistant sarcomas. Surgical decompression affords a more prompt and reliable relief of pressure on the spinal cord, unless the tumor is known to be radiosensitive, for example, lymphomas or leukemia. Recovery is much more complete and dramatic in younger children than in adult counterparts, and therefore severely paraparetic patients should be given the maximum potential for cure. Total eradication of tumor may be impossible by surgery, and these patients need postoperative irradiation or chemotherapy. A more serious concern related to surgical laminectomy is the postoperative mechanical instability of the spine (fracture, fracture dislocation) when the vertebral body or facet joints are involved. An appropriate surgical approach, either anterior or posterolateral, should be chosen to resect the diseased vertebrae and then to reconstruct the resected spine with bone grafts. If the posterior approaches are used, segmental spinal instrumentation may be applied to achieve postoperative spinal stabilization, even in children.[20]

REFERENCES

1. Amacher AL, Eltomey A: Spinal osteoblastoma in children and adolescence. Child's Nerv Syst 1:29–32, 1985.
2. Angevine JB: Clinically relevant embryology of the vertebral column and spinal cord. Clin Neurosurg 20:95–113, 1973.
3. Aterman K, Schueller EF: Maturation of neuroblastoma to ganglioneuroma. Am J Dis Child 120:217–222, 1970.
4. Awari OE, Payne WS, Onofrio BM, et al: Dumbbell neurogenic tumors of the mediastinum. Diagnosis and management. Mayo Clinic Proc 53:353–358, 1978.
5. Azouz EM, Kozlowski L, Marton D, et al: Osteoid osteoma and osteoblastoma of the spine in children. Report of 22 cases with brief literature review. Pediatr Radiol 16:25–31, 1986.
6. Bacci G, Picci P, Gherlinzoni F, et al: Localized Ewing's sarcoma of bone: Ten year's experience at the Instituto Orthopedico Rizzoli in 124 cases treated with multiple therapy. Eur J Cancer Clin Oncol 21:163–173, 1985.
7. Barwick KW, Huvos AG, Smith J: Primary osteogenic sarcoma of the vertebral column. A clinicopathologic correlation of ten patients. Cancer 46:595–604, 1980.
8. Baten M, Vanucci RC: Intraspinal metastatic disease in childhood cancer. J Pediatr 90:207–212, 1977.
9. Capanna R, Albisinni U, Picci P, et al: Aneurysmal bone cyst of the spine. J Bone Joint Surg 67A:527–531, 1985.
10. Carachi R, Campbell PE, Kent M: Thoracic neural crest tumors. A clinical review. Cancer 41:949–954, 1983.
11. Cattel HS, Clark GL: Cervical kyphosis and instability following multiple laminectomies in children. J Bone Joint Surg 49A:713–720, 1967.
12. Charnoff SK: Radiology notes. Case 1. Mt Sinai J Med 52:133–135, 1985.
13. Ch'ien LT, Kalwinsky DK, Peterson G, et al: Metastatic epidural tumors in children. Med Pediatr Oncol 10:455–462, 1982.
14. Cohen DM, Dahlin DC, MacCarty CS: Vertebral giant-cell tumor and variants. Cancer 17:461–472, 1964.
15. DeSousa AL, Kalsbeck JE, Mealey J Jr, et al: Intraspinal tumors in children. A review of 81 cases. J Neurosurg 51:437–445, 1979.
16. DiLorenzo N, Spallone A, Nolletti A, Nardi P: Giant cell tumors of the spine. A clinical study of six cases with emphasis on the radiological features, treatment and follow-up. Neurosurgery 6:29–34, 1980.
17. Eftenekhari F, Wallace S, Chuang VP, et al: Intraarterial management of giant cell tumors of the spine in children. Pediatr Radiol 12:289–293, 1982.
18. Filler RM, Traggis DG, Jaffe N, Vawter GF: Favorable outlook with mediastinal neuroblastoma. J Pediatr Surg 7:136–143, 1972.
19. Fink LH, Meriwether MW: Primary epidural Ewing's sarcoma presenting as a lumbar disc protrusion. Case report. J Neurosurg 51:120–123, 1979.
20. Flatley TJ: Spinal instability due to malignant disease. Treatment by segmental spinal stabilization. J Bone Joint Surg 66A:47–52, 1984.
21. Fraser RD, Paterson DC, Simpson DA: Orthopaedic aspects of spinal tumors in children. J Bone Joint Surg 59B:143–151, 1977.
22. Green NE, Robertson WE, Kilroy AW: Eosinophilic granuloma of the spine with associated neural deficit. J Bone Joint Surg 62A:1198–1202, 1980.
23. Greenfield GB: Radiology of Bone Diseases. Philadelphia, J.B. Lippincott, 1980, pp 464–472.
24. Haft H, Ransohoff J, Carter S: Spinal cord tumors in children. Pediatrics 23:1152–1159, 1959.
25. Hahn YS, McLone DG: Pain in children with spinal cord tumors. Child's Brain 11:36–46, 1984.
26. Hay M, Paterson D, Taylor TKF: Aneurysmal bone cysts of the spine. J Bone Joint Surg 60B:406–411, 1978.
27. Hayes FA, Thompson EI, Hvizdala E, et al: Chemotherapy as an alternative to laminectomy and radiation in the management of epidural tumor. J Pediatr 104:221–224, 1984.
28. Hendrick EB: Spinal cord tumors in children. In Youmans JR (ed): Neurological Surgery. Philadelphia, W.B. Saunders Co., 1982, pp 3215–3221.
29. Jaffe N, Robertson R, Takaue Y, et al: Control of primary osteosarcoma with chemotherapy. Cancer 56:461–466, 1985.
30. King D, Goodman J, Hawk T, et al: Dumbbell neuroblastomas in children. Arch Surg 110:888–891, 1975.
31. Kirks DR, Berger PE, Fitz CR, Harwood-Nash DC: Myelography in the evaluation of paravertebral mass lesions in infants and children. Radiology 119:603–608, 1976.
32. Kirwan EO, Hutton PA, Pozo JL, Ransford AO: Osteoid osteoma and benign osteoblastoma of the spine. Clinical presentation and treatment. J Bone Joint Surg 66B:21–26, 1984.
33. Kozlowski K, Beluffi G, Masel J, et al: Primary vertebral tumours in children. Report of 20 cases with brief literature review. Pediatr Radiol 14:129–139, 1984.
34. Ljung F, Helin I, Stromblad LG: Ganglioneuroma with an uncommon location in a six-year-old girl. Acta Paediatr Scand 73:411–413, 1984.
35. McGuire WA, Simmons D, Grosfield JL, Baehner RL: Stage II neuroblastoma: Does adjuvant irradiation contribute to cure? Med Pediatr Oncol 13:117–121, 1985.
36. McLeod RA, Dahlin DC, Beabout JW: The spectrum of osteoblastoma. Am J Roentgenol 126:321–335, 1976.
37. Modic MT, Masaryk T, Paushter D: Magnetic resonance imaging of the spine. Radiol Clin North Am 24:229–245, 1986.
38. Naidich TP, Doundoulakis SH, Poznanski AK: Intraspinal masses: Efficacy of plain spine radiograph. Pediatr Neurosci 12:10–17, 1986.
39. Nesbit ME, Kieffer B, D'Angio GJ: Reconstitution of vertebral height in histiocytosis: A long-term follow-up. J Bone Joint Surg 51A:1360–1368, 1969.
40. Oberlin O: The response to initial chemotherapy as a prognostic factor in localized Ewing's sarcoma. Eur J Cancer Clin Oncol 21:463–467, 1985.
41. Ogihara Y, Skiguchi K, Tsuruta T: Osteogenic sarcoma of the fourth thoracic vertebra. Long-term survival by chemotherapy. Cancer 53:2615–2618, 1984.

42. Palmer JJ: Radiation myelopathy. Brain 95:109–122, 1972.
43. Pettine KA, Klassen RA: Osteoid-osteoma and osteoblastoma of the spine. J Bone Joint Surg 68A:354–361, 1986.
44. Punt J, Pritchard J, Pincott JR, Till K: Neuroblastoma: A review of 21 cases presenting with spinal cord compression. Cancer 45:3095–3101, 1980.
45. Raimondi AJ, Gutierrez FA, DiRocco C: Laminotomy and total reconstruction of the posterior spinal arch for spinal canal surgery in childhood. J Neurosurg 45:555–560, 1976.
46. Ransford AO, Poso JL, Hutton PA, Kirwan EO: The behavior pattern of the scoliosis associated with osteoid osteoma or osteoblastoma of the spine. J Bone Joint Surg 66B:16–20, 1984.
47. Rosen G, Caparros B, Huvos AG, et al: Preoperative chemotherapy for osteogenic sarcoma: Selection of postoperative adjuvant chemotherapy based on the response of the primary tumor to preoperative chemotherapy. Cancer 49:1221–1230, 1982.
48. Savini R, Gherlinzoni F, Morandi M, et al: Surgical treatment of giant-cell tumor of the spine. The experience at the Institute Orthopedico Rizzoli. J Bone Joint Surg 65A:1283–1289, 1983.
49. Savini R, Giunti A, Boriani S: Benign and malignant spinal tumors. In Bradford DS, Hensinger RN (eds): The Pediatric Spine. Stuttgart, Georg Thieme Verlag, 1985, pp 131–154.
50. Seimon LP: Eosinophilic granuloma of the spine. J Pediatr Orthop 1:371–376, 1981.
51. Siegal T, Siegal T, Robin G, et al: Anterior decompression of the spine for metastatic epidural cord compression: A promising avenue of therapy? Ann Neurol 11:28–34, 1982.
52. Siegal T, Tiqva P, Siegal T: Vertebral body resection for epidural compression by malignant tumors. J Bone Joint Surg 67A:375–382, 1985.
53. Silberstein MJ, Sundaram M, Akbarnia B, et al: Eosinophilic granuloma of the spine. Orthopedics 8:264, 267–274, 1985.
54. Stener B, Johnsen OE: Complete removal of three vertebrae for giant-cell tumor. J Bone Joint Surg 53B:278–287, 1971.
55. Sundaresan N, Galicich JH, Bains MS, et al: Vertebral body resection in the treatment of cancer involving the spine. Cancer 53:1393–1396, 1984.
56. Sundaresan N, Rosen G, Fortner JG, et al: Preoperative chemotherapy and surgical resection in the management of posterior paraspinal tumors. Report of three cases. J Neurosurg 58:446–450, 1983.
57. Tachdjian MO, Matson DD: Orthopaedic aspects of intraspinal tumors in infants and children. J Bone Joint Surg 47A:223–248, 1965.
58. Thomas PR: The management of Ewing's sarcoma: Role of radiotherapy in local tumor control. Cancer Treat Rep 68:703–710, 1984.
59. Tillman BP, Dahlin DC, Lipscomb PR, Stewart JR: Aneurysmal bone cyst: An analysis of ninety-five cases. Mayo Clinic Proc 43:478–495, 1968.
60. Tomita T, Galicich JH, Sundaresan N: Radiation therapy for spinal epidural metastases with complete block. Acta Radiol Oncol 22:135–143, 1983.
61. Traggis DG, Tiller RM, Druckman H, et al: Prognosis for children with neuroblastoma presenting with paralysis. J Pediatr Surg 12:419–425, 1977.
62. Voight K, Hoogland PH, Stoeter P, Djindjian R: Diagnostic value and limitation of selective spinal angiography in different lesions of the vertebral bones. Radiol Clin 47:73–90, 1978.
63. Weatherley CR, Jaffray D, O'Brien JP: Radical excision of an osteoblastoma of the cervical spine. A combined anterior and posterior approach. J Bone Joint Surg 68:325–328, 1986.
64. Yasuoka S, Peterson HA, MacCarty CS: Incidence of spinal column deformity after multilevel laminectomy in children and adults. J Neurosurg 57:441–445, 1982.
65. Yasuoka S, Peterson HA, Laws ER Jr, MacCarty CS: Pathogenesis and prophylaxis of postlaminectomy deformity of the spine after multiple level laminectomy: Difference between children and adults. Neurosurgery 9:145–152, 1981.

NEUROLOGIC COMPROMISE DUE TO SPINAL TUMORS

TALI SIEGAL AND TZONY SIEGAL

The management of spinal column neoplasms that cause neurologic deficit has been the subject of debate for many years. Most of the available information relates to metastatic tumors of the spine, since vertebral metastases are a common occurrence in contrast to primary spinal tumors, which are rare. The last two decades have witnessed significant shifts in therapeutic approaches, ranging from urgent laminectomy, to a combination of laminectomy and radiotherapy, to nonsurgical treatment by radiotherapy alone. More recently, attention has been directed to radiotherapy[6, 11, 16, 17, 37, 44] and/or anterior surgical decompression[19, 33, 34, 38] as preferred treatment modalities. Some attempts have been made to compare various management methods, but the absence of satisfactory, controlled trials still leaves no clear consensus.[2, 6, 11, 13, 14, 16, 17, 24, 37, 44] A synopsis of the current knowledge and concepts related to various therapeutic measures and prognostic factors is presented.

The diagnosis of cord compression requires evidence of a high degree, greater than 80 per cent, extradural myelographic block or its equivalent magnetic resonance imaging. The management of extradural metastases that partially obliterate the spinal canal (to less than 60 per cent) will not be considered in this chapter.

INCIDENCE

Nearly 5 per cent of patients with systemic cancer develop spinal extradural metastases,[3, 14] and nearly 20 per cent of the patients with vertebral column involvement will develop spinal cord compression.[32] In large series, the three most frequent types of primary tumors spreading to the spine and extradural space are bronchogenic carcinoma, breast carcinoma, and lymphoma.[6] The origin of metastases cannot be identified in 9 per cent of the cases. Although spinal metastases generally occur in patients with known malignancy, in 8 per cent of the patients who present with spinal cord compression this is the initial symptom of cancer.[6, 16]

TUMOR LOCATION

The involvement of any area of the spine by metastatic deposits corresponds roughly to the number of vertebrae contained therein. Thus, the thoracic spine is involved in about 60 per cent of the cases.[6, 16] A large majority of tumors are localized to one or two vertebral segments, but in 17 per cent of the patients two or more sites may show evidence of epidural compression at some time during the course of the disease.[6, 16, 17]

When a neoplasm invades the spinal canal, it is usually restricted to the extradural space, with variable involvement of the anterior (ventral) compartment, the lateral gutters, the posterior compartment, or any combination of these sites. However, the majority of epidural tumors (85 per cent) arise in a vertebral body, invade the epidural space anteriorly, and remain largely anterior to the spinal cord.[1, 3, 16, 39] The location of the extradural tumor has important surgical implications. A compressing tumor in the posterior extradural compartment is easily accessible by laminectomy, whereas the accessibility of a ventral mass by this approach is largely limited and requires an anterior or anterolateral approach. The location of the tumor within the spinal canal can usually be inferred from spinal x-ray studies. However, accurate definition of the compressive mass as either posterior, lateral, cuff, or anterior usually requires the combination of myelography and computer tomography (CT). Magnetic resonance imaging (MRI) studies, where available, may constitute an excellent noninvasive alternative procedure for the pretreatment investigation.

SYMPTOMS AND SIGNS

The onset of symptoms of spinal cord or nerve root compression may be acute or insidious. The duration of symptoms varies widely before diagnosis. Pain is usually the initial symptom (in 96 per cent of cases), preceding other symptoms by five days to two years (median seven weeks).[6, 16, 17] The pain can be localized close to the site of the lesion or can be radicular. Radicular pain results from compression or infiltration of the nerve roots at the affected level.[6] By the time of diagnosis, neurologic signs are common[6, 16] and include various degrees of muscle weakness (in 76 per cent of the cases), bladder and bowel dysfunction (in more than 50 per cent), and sensory symptoms (in about 50 per cent). It is important to note that nearly half of the severely affected patients will develop a complete deficit (no residual cord function) after diagnosis and before undergoing any treatment. Twenty-eight per cent of the paraparetic patients become paraplegic in less than 24 hours as a function of time elapsed before treatment.[2] Therefore, it seems critical to treat patients with cord compression as soon as possible.

PATHOPHYSIOLOGY

The pathophysiologic mechanisms involved in neoplastic cord compression were investigated in experimental animal tumor models.[20–22, 41] The expanding extradural tumor causes early obstruction of the spinal epidural venous plexus and enhances production of a vasogenic type of edema. The edema involves initially the white matter and eventually the gray matter in the late stage of compression. In the end stage, the spinal cord blood flow decreases rapidly at the site of compression. Ischemia may play the final deleterious role, leading to irreversible loss of function if the compression is not rapidly alleviated. The spinal cord can adjust to gradual compression over a period of weeks or months but is unable to tolerate rapid compression, such as that caused by rapidly growing malignant tumors. In such cases it is not uncommon for the spinal cord tolerance to be reached within a matter of hours or days after the onset of the first symptoms. This results in rapid development of paralysis below the level of compression.

SURVIVAL AND SPINAL CORD COMPRESSION

Neoplastic spinal cord compression usually occurs in patients with metastatic systemic cancer. In spite of the overall grim prognosis of the basic disease, treatment is warranted in many cases[6] and is aimed at preserving or restoring spinal cord function (ambulation and continence) or at alleviating intractable pain. Spinal cord compression in itself is generally not fatal (except in the upper portion of the cervical spine). Depending upon the natural history of the systemic malignancy, patients may survive for extended periods: 30 per cent may be expected to survive beyond a year and, rarely, as long as four to nine years.[4, 42] Patients with widespead metastatic disease have a more limited life expectancy of a few months.[5, 26, 34]

The overall effect of successful treatment on survival is not clear. Some investigators have suggested that treatment of spinal cord compression is unlikely to prolong survival.[8, 42] However, three separate studies[4, 8, 39] have shown improved survival in patients responding to treatment. It appears that effective treatment is associated with improved survival, but the precise significance of this association is uncertain, since non–treatment related factors (e.g., tumor histology) can also influence both the ability to walk and the expected survival.

FACTORS INFLUENCING RECOVERY OF FUNCTION

Some factors have been considered important determinants of functional prognosis in patients with spinal neoplasms, including tumor biology, pretreatment neurologic status, progression rate of symptoms, location of tumor within the spinal canal, and therapy employed.[2, 6, 8, 14, 18, 42, 44]

Tumor Biology

Cell Type

The biologic activity of the primary neoplasm determines both systemic and local aggressiveness, which are represented, respectively, by posttreatment survival rate and the rate of therapy success.[2, 8] Patients with myeloma, lymphoma, Ewing's sarcoma, neuroblastoma, or carcinoma of the breast have a favorable prognosis for recovery of function.[2, 6, 16, 17] The outlook for patients with metastatic bronchogenic carcinoma is generally poor. However, exceptions to these results make it difficult to prognosticate in individual cases. In general, high tumor radiosensitivity is significantly related to a favorable prognosis, and the contrary is true for radioresistant tumors. It also appears that the tumor cell type has a greater importance in determining outcome than does the type of treatment. This is suggested by a critical review of the results of management obtained by radiotherapy and laminectomy plus radiotherapy.[2, 6, 16, 17]

Response to High Dose Dexamethasone

The use of steroids in the treatment of spinal cord compression is widely accepted.[2, 6, 16, 17, 25, 29, 33, 34] The scientific basis for steroid use stems from animal models of spinal cord compression, in which reduction of spinal cord edema and delayed onset of paraplegia were observed following treatment with dexamethasone.[20, 40, 41] Greenberg and coworkers[17] recommended the use of high dose steroids based on their experience of rapid relief of symptoms in some patients receiving initial doses of 100 mg of dexamethasone. However, they were unable to demonstrate a superior outcome in comparison to their historic group who had received lower doses of steroids.[16] Several other reports have noted a dramatic resolution of symptoms following treatment with steroids alone.[9, 10, 25, 29] The response to dexamethasone was considered to have a prognostic value in one series of spinal metastases.[25] However, steroid-related improvement was closely related to the type of tumor and probably represented a direct oncolytic effect,[29] as in lymphomas and leukemias. Therefore, the response to dexamethasone has no proven intrinsic prognostic value.

Pretreatment Neurologic Status

The results obtained by radiotherapy and by laminectomy plus radiotherapy relate to neurologic status at the time of treatment. There is a positive correlation between the pretreatment motor status and the functional outcome[2, 6, 14, 16]: 70 per cent of the patients who can walk at the time of diagnosis retain that ability after treatment, 35 per cent of those who are initially paraparetic become ambulatory, and only 5 to 7 per cent (range, 0 to 25 per cent) of paraplegic patients regain the ability to walk. These success rates show no significant difference between the two modalities of management when the proportion of tumors with favorable histology is comparable.[2, 14] The success rate achieved by all therapies in paraplegic patients[2] is different, depending on whether the patient has complete functional cord transection or whether there is preservation of some neurologic function. The fact that only 2 per cent of the former patients recovered the ability to walk after treatment, as compared with 20 per cent of the latter, indicates the strong prognostic significance of residual neurologic function. Complete paraplegia carries a bad functional prognosis regardless of the mode of therapy employed. The results of treatment emphasize the value of early diagnosis and treatment, and therefore it is discouraging that only 25 per cent of the patients are diagnosed while still being able to walk.[6, 14, 16, 17, 33, 34]

Progression Rate of Symptoms

It has been claimed that rapid onset and progression of neurologic symptoms are associated with a worse prognosis when compared with gradual onset and slow progression.[8, 16, 36] It has also been stated that the outlook for recovery is worse if bladder function is also impaired. However, these results should be analyzed in relation to completeness of spinal cord damage. If this is taken into account, then in patients with rapidly developing symptoms (less than 24 hours) the neurologic grade itself has a greater influence on prognosis than has the symptom progression rate.[2] Twenty per cent of paraparetic patients whose deficit evolved in less than 24 hours recovered, compared with no paraplegic patients.[2, 8, 16]

The rapidity of neurologic deterioration may be related to other prognostic variables, such as tumor cell type or tumor topography within the spinal canal. In one series[36] in which metastases of lung and prostatic carcinoma caused paraparesis, the proportion of cases presenting with a sudden deficit (developing within a few hours) was 15 per cent and 14 per cent, respectively. These findings indicate that two lesions with significantly different surgical prognosis (22 per cent and 49 per cent success rates with laminectomy for lung and prostate, respectively) produce a similar symptom progression rate. Unfortunately, the current available information related to tumor topography and the rate of progression of symptoms is rather contradictory,[2, 8, 16, 36] and a definite relationship cannot be established. It seems that the rapidity of neurologic deterioration is unrelated to other prognostic variables, and that the progression rate of symptoms should not be given intrinsic prognostic value unless further controlled studies indicate the contrary. On the other hand, the residual cord function should be taken into consideration in a rapidly evolving deficit as an important prognostic variable. Once paraplegia has set in, the duration of paralysis does have a prognostic significance, although recovery has been reported even after long periods of time (four to eight weeks).[19, 28, 33, 34]

Location of Tumor Within the Spinal Canal

It has been claimed that there is a positive correlation between the location of the extradural metastatic deposit and the response to surgical treatment.[8, 12, 18] Furthermore, some authors stated that vertebral collapse reduced the chances of neurologic recovery.[8, 14] However, it should be emphasized that these statements are based on success rates obtained by laminectomy performed in ventrally located tumors. Following laminectomy, only 9 to 16 per cent of patients with ventral tumor masses maintained ambulation, and these figures are considerably less than the overall rates of 30 to 50 per cent ambulation for patients with tumors located posterolaterally.[2, 14, 18]

When the epidural tumor is situated anterior to the spinal cord, the accessibility of the tumor to surgical removal by laminectomy is limited. Accordingly, an alternative approach to the spine by way of an anterolateral route has recently been reported.[19, 33, 34, 38] The anterior approach yielded favorable results: 70 to 80 per cent of the patients regained or maintained ambulation. In only one study was the surgical approach for decompression carefully selected according to tumor topography in the spinal canal.[34] The success rate for the ventrally located tumors was 80 per cent when decompressed by an anterior approach, but was only 39 per cent for the posteriorly located tumors decompressed by laminectomy. Although the figure for posterior compartment tumors seems inferior, the results should not be considered discouraging, since only 8 per cent of the patients with posterior compression were ambulatory at presentation.

We conclude that the currently available information presents no clear evidence that tumor position within the spinal canal carries an intrinsic prognostic factor. However, it is important to realize that all the available studies are nonrandomized, and that noncomparable variables may affect final outcome. Until such studies are carried out, it is suggested that treatment endeavors be aimed at rapid and efficient decompression if surgery is selected as the preferred modality of treatment.

Therapy Used

The retrospective analysis of different series of spinal metastases shows that the rate of favorable responses obtained by either radiotherapy or laminectomy plus radiotherapy is overall the same with posttreatment ambulation rates of 46 per cent and 40 per cent, respectively.[2, 6, 7, 14, 16, 44] Because cure is usually beyond expectation, palliation is generally accepted as a reasonable goal in the management of patients with spinal metastases. Preservation or restoration of neurologic function—ambulation and bladder control—are the criteria of successful therapy. Pain relief is also an important, but secondary, goal. Since treatment of malignant cord compression can rarely be curative in its own right, it emphasizes the importance of considering not only the success rates but also the treatment effect on the quality of further survival of the entire group.[14] When the limited success rate of laminectomy was critically reviewed, it was balanced by an almost equal rate of adverse neurologic effects. Thus, when combined with the other nonneurologic complications and mortality, the role of laminectomy as the first-line therapy for malignant cord compression has been questioned.[2, 6, 14, 16, 34, 44] There is little doubt that radiotherapy supported by steroids can give comparable results[16, 17] and that patients treated by radiotherapy can deteriorate neurologically in the same way as surgical patients. However, they are spared the other adverse effects of surgery. Reviewing patients treated by primary radiotherapy or by laminectomy with radiotherapy, approximately 25 per cent of ambulant patients on presentation will deteriorate neurologically. Similarly, of those paraparetic before therapy, about 20 per cent will get worse.[6, 14, 16, 17, 34, 44] However, patients who do deteriorate following radiotherapy could still undergo surgery as a treatment option at an early stage in their deterioration.

Based on the above, some trends have emerged regarding surgical indications. It has been recommended that surgery be reserved for (1) cases in which the nature of spinal cord compression is unknown; (2) cases in which there is spinal instability or bone collapse into the spinal canal; (3) cases with reactivation of a spinal lesion which cannot receive additional radiotherapy; (4) cases with tumors known to be radioresistant; and (5) cases presenting further clinical deterioration while on radiotherapy. These guidelines for surgery may have to be modified in response to new clinical experience with anterior decompression[19, 33, 34, 38] and research data in the future. It should be emphasized here that anterior decompression was carried along the recommended guidelines for surgical intervention, yielding encouraging results with 79 to 80 per cent ambulation rates. In one series,[34] one third of the anteriorly decompressed patients received no combination of postsurgical radiotherapy, since they faced their second episode of cord compression and had already eliminated any option for further irradiation. It is interesting that the rate of success in this group was similar to that obtained in the other patients. It is not yet clear whether anterior decompression should be recommended as the primary modality of therapy in cord compression, and it should be critically examined in a controlled prospective study. In the case of radiosensitive neoplasm such as lymphomas, Ewing's sarcoma, neuroblastoma, seminoma, and myeloma, radiotherapy is most clearly indicated as the primary modality of therapy for cord compression. The success rate with radiotherapy varies between 44 per cent and 83 per cent, with a pooled improvement rate of 60 per cent.[2, 15, 16, 25, 27, 28, 31, 34, 35, 43]

Choice of Treatment

Recent trends in the management of malignant epidural cord compression are outlined here.

RADIOTHERAPY AS THE FIRST-LINE THERAPY

Radiotherapy is most clearly indicated for radiosensitive tumors, but it may well also be the primary therapy for moderately radiosensitive tumors, such as breast carcinoma. In the latter group (relatively radiosensitive tumors), the need for surgical intervention should be critically reviewed for each patient. We have no doubt that in stable patients who are ambulatory or paraparetic on presentation, radiotherapy should be tried out first. However, in severely paraparetic patients surgical decompression should be considered. This is based on the knowledge that the use of radiotherapy implies a delay in the reduction of spinal cord damage. In a group of 16 patients harboring lymphomas and other radiosensitive tumors who were extracted from different series,[27, 31, 35] improvement owing to radiotherapy, which occurred in 83 per cent of the cases, began 5.6 days (mean) after the initiation of therapy. Thus, when using radiotherapy, one may expect 28 per cent of severely paraparetic patients to become paraplegic within 24 hours of treatment.[2] Moreover, the 25 per cent favorable response rate obtained in this type of patient with any form of therapy[8, 12, 28, 36] will decrease to 17 per cent with the use of radiotherapy.[2] That this group of patients may benefit from surgery is further supported by the high rate of ambulation obtained in this unfavorable prognostic group by anterior decompression of the spine.[33, 34] If surgery is contraindicated, radiotherapy should be employed. This means that patients with a poor general medical status, patients with multiple myelographic blocks, and those with long-standing paraplegia will be offered radiation therapy only.

The indication for radiotherapy is less clear for tumors generally regarded as radioresistant; even here, however, radiotherapy should be tried as a primary modality if the patient's neurologic deficit is not severe and if the rate of progression of the deficit is such that there would be time to resort to surgical decompression should radiotherapy fail. In situations in which surgical decompression is used as the primary modality of therapy, postoperative radiation should generally be employed in the hope that this may help eradicate or suppress residual tumor as well as contribute to pain relief.

INDICATIONS FOR SURGICAL INTERVENTION

It is usually recommended to reserve surgery for the following situations.

Diagnosis in Doubt. When the etiology of the spinal lesion is in doubt, surgical decompression is advisable to establish a tissue diagnosis and to achieve rapid decompression. The source of the primary tumor cannot be identified in 9 per cent of cases of spinal metastases,[6] and in an additional 8 per cent spinal involvement is the initial presentation of cancer.[16] Thus, up to 17 per cent of the patients may require surgical intervention by this indication.

Previous Radiation Exposure. When radiotherapy cannot be used, surgical decompression is indicated as the primary therapeutic modality. This applies even in highly radiosensitive tumors due to the risk of exceeding spinal cord tolerance by adding further irradiation. Surgery is warranted for relapse occurring months or even years after a successful previous treatment in hope of preserving neurologic function.

Radioresistant Tumors. When dealing with a radioresistant tumor, decompressive surgery might be considered as the primary mode of therapy. Postoperative radiotherapy is administered hopefully to retard tumor regrowth. However, this indication is not generally accepted and sometimes, especially in neurologically stable patients, radiotherapy may be tried first.

Neurologic Deterioration During Radiotherapy. Neurologic deterioration that occurs during radiotherapy of a relatively radiosensitive tumor should prompt early consideration of surgical decompression. The decline in neurologic function may reflect radioresistancy, progressive spinal instability, or bone compression secondary to vertebral collapse. All these may be most effectively treated by spinal decompression and stabilization.

There has been concern that radiation therapy may result in neurologic deterioration, presumably by inducing radiation edema in the tumor, spinal cord, or both.[23] Experimental studies do not support the concept of radiation edema.[30] Therefore, it is most likely that neurologic deterioration that occurs during the course of radiotherapy suggests its failure, and serious consideration should be given to surgery as an alternative treatment.

Spinal Instability or Bone Compression. Not every case of instability requires surgical intervention. If the tumor is radiosensitive, a course of radiotherapy not infrequently results in satisfactory settling and pain relief over a period of weeks or months. However, when spinal instability endangers spinal cord or nerve root function, or when a pathologic fracture produces direct compression on the neural structures, surgical decompression and stabilization are essential.

Instability is present whenever one of the following situations arises before or during surgery: (1) a bone loss of more than 50 per cent of the width of the vertebral body, (2) a bone loss extending over two or more vertebrae, or (3) the presence of additional involvement of the posterior elements at the same level. The instability is augmented by any combination of the above. The vertebral bodies, when destroyed by tumor, will collapse into a localized kyphosis, which is associated with increasing pain and eventual neural deficit. The loss in the height of the vertebrae results in a relative laxity and redundancy in the surrounding soft tissues. This is the essential mechanism of segmental instability. The goal of instrumentation is to obtain a firmly stable spine, but also to correct local deformity and to replace destroyed or excised structures (vertebral bodies or posterior elements). To achieve these aims, any instrumentation, whether anterior or posterior, must satisfy two main requirements—distraction and fixation. Gradual distraction is intended to cause optimal tension in the spinal and paraspinal soft tissues (ligaments, joint capsules, muscles), taking out the slack that accompanies vertebral compression. It may also correct local kyphosis, restore lost vertebral height, and lessen compression at the level of the intervertebral foramina. The resulting compressive forces on a vertebral body replacement will enhance its stability and diminish the chances of dislodgement.[33] When the spine is approached posteriorly, double Harrington distraction rods, if coupled with sublaminar wiring, provide a firm and solid internal fixation system with instant spinal stability. No external appliances (braces, jackets, and so forth) are required, and early mobilization of patients is possible.

THE ISSUE OF BONE GRAFTING

The advisability of bone grafting to achieve bony arthrodesis is a matter of debate. Orthopedic surgeons have traditionally regarded bone grafting as an integral part of spine fusion with internal fixation. This is because experience has shown that single or even double Harrington rods may break, especially in young and active people, if solid bony arthrodesis of the spine has not been obtained. However, the great majority of patients with primary or metastatic spinal deposits are not young, and with the advent of segmental instrumentation, rod breakage is a rare occurrence. In many cases, activity is restricted by some neurologic deficit, by pain, or by less-than-optimal medical status. The median survival of patients with spinal cord compression is 12 to 18 months.[4, 5, 26, 34, 42] It is therefore reasonable to assume that in these conditions the internal fixation alone will provide durable spinal stability.

There are additional arguments against bone autografting: (1) it requires a separate incision with an increase in operating time and in morbidity in patients with active disease, (2) the iliac bone graft may be microscopically involved with tumor, and (3) the bone graft incorporation may be inhibited by radiotherapy. Furthermore, if bone autografts are employed, the time required for spinal arthrodesis to occur is about 6 months and to mature, 6 more months. When one resorts to bank bone (allografts), the required time is longer, especially if postoperative irradiation is scheduled. Therefore, the main indication for adding iliac cancellous bone grafts is a benign or slow-growing tumor (osteoblastoma, giant cell tumor, aneurysmal bone cyst, and so forth) in children and young adults.

Complications of Therapy

RADIOTHERAPY

Most papers dealing with radiotherapy alone do not comment on complications of therapy or mortality. There has been concern that radiation edema may bring about neurologic deterioration.[23] However, it is still unclear whether such edema accumulates in the irradiated spinal cord.[30] In any case, most patients are protected with high doses of dexamethasone.[6, 16, 17, 34]

Death in the first month following radiotherapy is likely to be due to primary disease: in one series, 70 per cent of the patients considered severely ill at the time of diagnosis of spinal cord compression died within 30 days after diagnosis.[34]

SURGICAL COMPLICATIONS

Mortality. The incidence of death within the first month after decompressive laminectomy ranges from 3 to 14 per cent, with an average mortality rate of 9 per cent.[6, 14, 16, 17, 34] Surgical mortality rate after vertebral body resection falls within the same range and does not exceed the rate reported for laminectomy.[19, 33, 34, 38]

Morbidity. The risk of neurologic deterioration as a result of surgery is a major concern in patients who present while still able to walk. Worsening of neurologic status occurred in 7 to 26 per cent of an unselective group of patients after decompressive laminectomy, with an overall mean of 12 per cent.[6, 14] In a group of patients with posterior compartment epidural tumors who underwent laminectomy, neurologic deterioration occurred in 20 per cent as a direct result of the operation.[34] Although the vertebral body resection procedure seems to be more formidable, neurologic worsening is a rare complication, seen in only 2 to 4 per cent of the patients.[19, 33, 34, 38]

NONNEUROLOGIC COMPLICATIONS. In patients undergoing laminectomy combined with radiotherapy, nonneurologic complications include wound infection, dehiscence, spinal epidural hematoma, CSF leak, and spinal instability. The frequency of these complications ranges from 8 to 42 per cent, with a mean of 11 per cent.[6, 14] Only a few authors specifically mentioned the problem of instability,[8, 16] reporting its occurrence in about 9 per cent of the cases. The incidence of nonneurologic complications in vertebral body resection is similar to the reported rate in laminectomies. However, the operation and instrumentation techniques require considerable expertise. The anterior approach to the spine may subject the patient to a variety of potentially serious complications, such as severe bleeding, damage to the adjacent vital organs, infection, and poor healing of irradiated tissues. Therefore, these procedures should be undertaken by a surgeon familiar with the anterior surgical approach to the spine and the technique of spinal instrumentation with its different options.

RECURRENT COMPRESSION

Recurrence of pain in a persistent or radicular pattern may indicate nerve root compression, infiltration by tumor, or both. Recurrence of neurologic symptoms suggests either severe instability or regrowth of the epidural tumor. In these situations, reassessment and repeat myelography are indicated. If a high degree myelographic block is present or instability is evident, decompression and additional stabilizing instrumentation are considered. Tumor recurrence usually occurs in patients with a survival longer than six months following initial therapy.

Complete excision or eradication of malignant tumors of the spinal column is difficult, perhaps impossible, even when two-stage procedures are employed. Therefore, the addition of radiotherapy is the rule, if it has not already been employed. But in spinal tumors with a low metastatic potential (chordoma, giant cell tumor of bone, and so forth), patients may live for many years in a long relapse-free interval. In this case consideration of radiotherapy is not automatic, as the delayed, undesirable side effects of this treatment modality—radiation-induced sarcoma or radiation myelopathy—must be taken into account. Radiation myelopathy is a diagnosis excluded only after repeat MRI or myelography shows no compression.

CONCLUSION

This chapter is a plea for early diagnosis and treatment of neoplastic spinal cord compression. This may be achieved in part by educating physicians to maintain a high index of suspicion, especially in patients known to harbor a neoplastic process. Future improvement in treatment outcome may be achieved mainly by early diagnosis and by use of improved surgical techniques, combined with novel biomechanical devices for vertebral body replacement and for spine stabilization.

REFERENCES

1. Arseni CN, Simionesu MD, Horwath L: Tumors of the spine. Acta Psychiatr Neurol Scand 34:398–410, 1959.
2. Barcena A, Lobato RD, Rivas JJ, et al: Spinal metastatic

disease: Analysis of factors determining functional prognosis and the choice of treatment. Neurosurgery 15:820–827, 1984.

3. Barron KD, Hirano A, Araki S, Terry RD: Experiences with metastatic neoplasms involving the spinal cord. Neurology 9:91–105, 1959.

4. Benson H, Scarffe J, Todd ID, et al: Spinal cord compression in myeloma. Br Med J 1:1541–1544, 1979.

5. Barnat JL, Greenberg ER, Barrett J: Suspected epidural compression of the spinal cord and cauda equina by metastatic carcinoma. Cancer 51:1953–1957, 1983.

6. Black P: Spinal metastases: Current status and recommended guidelines for management. Neurosurgery 5:726–746, 1979.

7. Brady LW, Antonaides J, Prasasvinichai S, et al: The treatment of metastatic disease of the nervous system by radiation therapy. In Seydel HG (ed): Tumors of the Nervous System. New York, John Wiley, 1975, pp 176–189.

8. Brice J, McKissock W: Surgical treatment of malignant extradural spinal tumors. Br Med J 2:1341–1344, 1965.

9. Canta RC: Corticosteroids for spinal metastases. Lancet 2:912, 1968.

10. Clarke P, Saunders M: Steroid-induced remission in spinal canal reticulum cell sarcoma. Report of two cases. J Neurosurg 42:346–348, 1975.

11. Cobb CA, Leavens ME, Eckles N: Indications for nonoperative treatment of spinal cord compression due to breast cancer. J Neurosurg 47:653–658, 1977.

12. Constans JP, deDivitiis E, Donzelli R, et al: Spinal metastases with neurological manifestations: A review of 600 cases. J Neurosurg 59:111–118, 1983.

13. Dunn RC Jr, Kelly WA, Wohns RN, Howe JF: Spinal epidural neoplasia: A 15-year review of the results of surgical therapy. J Neurosurg 52:47–51, 1980.

14. Findlay GFG: Adverse effects of the management of malignant spinal cord compression. J Neurol Neurosurg Psych 47:761–768, 1984.

15. Friedman M, Kim TH, Panahom AM: Spinal cord compression in malignant lymphoma: Treatment and results. Cancer 37:1485–1491, 1976.

16. Gilbert RW, Kim JH, Posner JB: Epidural spinal cord compression from metastatic tumor: Diagnosis and treatment. Ann neurol 3:40–51, 1978.

17. Greenberg HS, Kim JH, Posner JB: Epidural spinal cord compression from metastatic tumor: Results with a new treatment protocol. Ann Neurol 8:361–386, 1980.

18. Hall AJ, Mackay NNS: The results of laminectomy for compression of the cord and cauda equina by extradural malignant tumor. J Bone Joint Surg 55B:497–505, 1973.

19. Harrington KD: Anterior cord decompression and spinal stabilization for patients with metastatic lesions of the spine. J Neurosurg 61:107–117, 1984.

20. Ikeda H, Ushio Y, Hayakawa T, Mogami H: Edema and circulatory disturbance in the spinal cord compressed by epidural neoplasms in rabbits. J Neurosurg 52:203–209, 1980.

21. Ikeda H, Ushio Y, Shimizu K, et al: Experimental spinal cord compression by epidural neoplasms. Neurol Surg 6:891–898, 1978.

22. Kato M, Ushio Y, Hayakawa T, et al: Circulatory disturbance of the spinal cord with epidural neoplasm in rats. J Neurosurg 63:260–265, 1985.

23. Lawes FAE, Ham HJA: A case of Hodgkin's disease with spinal cord involvement treated by nitrogen mustard. Med J Aust 1:104–106, 1953.

24. Livingstone KE, Perrin RG: The neurosurgical management of spinal metastases causing cord and cauda equina compression. J Neurosurg 49:839–843, 1978.

25. Marshall LF, Langfitt TW: Combined therapy for metastatic extradural tumors of the spine. Cancer 40:2067–2070, 1977.

26. Martenson JA, Evans RG Jr, Lie MR, et al: Treatment outcome and complications in patients treated for malignant epidural spinal cord compression. J Neurooncol 3:77–84, 1985.

27. Mones RJ, Dozier D, Berrett A: Analysis of medical treatment of malignant extradural spinal cord tumors. Cancer 19:1842–1853, 1966.

28. Mullan J, Evans JP: Neoplastic disease in the spinal extradural space: A review of fifty cases. Arch Surg 74:900–907, 1957.

29. Posner JB, Howieson J, Cvitkovic E: "Disappearing" spinal cord compression: Oncolytic effect of glucocorticoids (and other chemotherapeutic agents) on epidural metastases. Ann Neurol 2:409–413, 1977.

30. Rubin P: Extradural spinal cord compression by tumor. Part 1: Experimental production and treatment trials. Radiology 93:1243–1248, 1969.

31. Rubin P, Mayer E, Poulter C: Extradural spinal cord compression by tumor. Part II: High daily dose experience without laminectomy. Radiology 93:1248–1260, 1969.

32. Schaberg J, Gainor BJ: A profile of metastatic carcinoma of the spine. Spine 10:19–20, 1985.

33. Siegal Tz, Siegal T: Vertebral body resection for epidural compression by malignant tumors. Results of forty-seven consecutive operative procedures. J Bone Joint Surg 67A:375–382, 1985.

34. Siegal Tz, Siegal T: Surgical decompression of anterior and posterior malignant epidural tumors compressing the spinal cord: A prospective study. Neurosurgery 17:424–432, 1985.

35. Silverberg IJ, Jacobs EM: Treatment of spinal cord compression in Hodgkin's disease. Cancer 27:308–313, 1971.

36. Smith R: An evaluation of surgical treatment for spinal cord compression due to metastatic carcinoma. J Neurosurg Psych 28:152–158, 1965.

37. Stark RJ, Henson RA, Evans SJW: Spinal metastases—A retrospective survey from a general hospital. Brain 105:189–213, 1982.

38. Sundaresan N, Galicich JH, Bains MS, et al: Vertebral body resection in the treatment of cancer involving the spine. Cancer 53:1393–1396, 1984.

39. Torma T: Malignant tumors of the spine and spinal epidural space—A study based on 250 histologically verified cases. Acta Chir Scand 225:1–138, 1957.

40. Ushio Y, Posner R, Kim J, et al: Treatment of experimental spinal cord compression caused by extradural neoplasms. J Neurosurg 47:380–390, 1977.

41. Ushio Y, Posner R, Posner JB, Shapiro WR: Experimental spinal cord compression by epidural neoplasms. Neurology 27:422–429, 1977.

42. Vieth R, Olson G: Extradural spinal metastases and their neurosurgical management. J Neurosurg 23:501–508, 1965.

43. Williams HM, Diamond HD, Craver LF, Pearsons H: Neurological Complications of Lymphomas and Leukemias. Springfield, IL, Charles C Thomas, 1959.

44. Young RF, Post EM, King GA: Treatment of spinal epidural metastases. Randomised prospective comparison of laminectomy and radiotherapy. J Neurosurg 53:741–748, 1980.

METASTATIC TUMORS OF THE SPINE

29

NARAYAN SUNDARESAN, GEORGE KROL,
GEORGE V. DIGIACINTO, AND JAMES E. O. HUGHES

INTRODUCTION

Compression of the spinal cord, cauda equina, and nerve roots is a major cause of morbidity in cancer patients. Although this text focuses mainly on the subject of primary neoplasms of the axial skeleton, metastatic tumors constitute by far the major cause of neoplastic cord compression.

The American Cancer Society estimates that approximately 950,000 Americans were diagnosed as having cancer in 1989, of whom 472,000 will die of their disease.[2] Recent data also suggest an increasing incidence and prevalence of cancer. The proportion of deaths due to cancer increased from 4 per cent in 1900, to 15 per cent in 1950, to 22 per cent in 1988; thus, cancer accounts for slightly less than one fourth of all deaths in the United States.[6, 160] There are several explanations for the increased prevalence: progress in the treatment of cancer, with approximately 40 per cent surviving five years[135]; technologic advances resulting in earlier diagnosis; as well as aging of the United States population.

In Connecticut, Feldman[46] reported that the prevalence rate for cancer was 1789 per 100,000 in males, and 2222 per 100,000 in females. Prevalence rates reflect both incidence as well as survival. Thus, although lung cancer is the most common cancer in men, its low survival rate accounts for the fact that it is the fifth most prevalent cancer. Although the overall incidence rate of cancer is higher in males, the age-adjusted prevalence rate shows an almost 25 per cent increase in women by virtue of their longer survival. The prevalence of cancer also varies considerably with age. Thus, the overall 2 per cent prevalence rate for cancer in the Connecticut population does not take into account the low prevalence of cancer in younger patients. In the age group over 70 years, approximately 12 per cent of men and 11 per cent of women had a history of cancer. In a positive sense, the high prevalence rate reflects successful treatment of a variety of tumors by current multidisciplinary approaches. Important negative consequences include problems related to disease recurrence, morbidity from therapy, development of

second neoplasms, psychosocial and economic losses due to disability, as well as difficulties in obtaining adequate health coverage for survivors of cancer.

The economic costs of treating cancer are enormous: it was estimated to be $51 billion and increasing in 1981, and accounted for 11 per cent of the total costs of illness[134]; others have estimated the total costs to be twice this amount.[160] Rising to this challenge, the National Cancer Institute has initiated a major effort in cancer control to reduce morbidity and mortality from the disease; currently the stated objective is a reduction in the mortality rate by 50 per cent in the next decade.[2]

Although spectacular advances have been achieved in some tumors, cancer mortality has largely been unaffected in some of the more common cancers, such as lung and breast cancer. In a pessimistic assessment, Bailar and Smith[6] concluded that the best single measure of progress against cancer—that is, age-adjusted mortality—actually increased over the past few decades, and suggested that previous efforts in improving treatment should be considered a qualified failure. However, if one examines age-specific death rates, a different picture emerges: cancer mortality has been declining among younger people but rising among older people. To a large extent, the dramatic rise in lung cancer has largely been responsible for the cancer mortality in those above 54 years.

Despite the remarkable accomplishments in the treatment of localized cancers, the major cause of death in most patients remains complications secondary to metastatic disease. In many patients, occult micrometastases are present at the time of primary tumor diagnosis. Tumors of divergent histologic type have varying metastatic potential related to their intrinsic histology, size, stroma, as well as a number of yet imperfectly understood biochemical mechanisms. The value of an aggressive surgical approach to metastatic disease involving the lungs, liver, and brain in selected patients has been validated by the results, which include both long disease-free intervals and a small proportion of cures.[140] However, this approach has not been thought feasible with metastases to the spine because of the relative inaccessibility

279

TABLE 29–1. ESTIMATED NEW CASES AND DEATHS FOR MAJOR SITES OF CANCER, INCLUDING INCIDENCE OF SPINE INVOLVEMENT

SITE	NO. OF CASES	DEATHS	% SPINE INVOLVEMENT
Lung	149,000	130,100	10–30
Colon-rectum	140,000	60,000	20–30
Breast	123,000	40,000	50–70
Prostate	90,000	26,100	50–80
Urinary tract	60,500	19,180	10–25
Uterus	50,000	9,700	< 10
Mouth	29,500	9,400	< 10
Blood (leukemia)	25,600	17,400	< 10
Pancreas	25,500	24,000	10–30
Skin	23,000	7,500	< 10
Ovary	19,000	11,600	< 10
Bone	2,000	1,400	10

of the tumor within the vertebral body. With the advent of newer radiologic tools such as magnetic resonance imaging (MRI) and computed tomography (CT) scans, it is now possible to diagnose spinal metastases early and to plan more effective treatment. We believe that the goal of gross total resection of tumor can be accomplished in many instances using surgical approaches and stabilization that have been developed during the past decade for the management of both trauma and tumors. In this review, we have sought to emphasize recent developments in the management of this common clinical complication of cancer, and the pertinent literature of the past decade is reviewed.

INCIDENCE AND FREQUENCY

The axial skeleton is the third most common site of metastases after lung and liver, with the majority of metastatic foci involving the lumbar spine.[8, 11, 14, 18, 60, 75] In a classic autopsy study, Barron and colleagues noted that 5 per cent of all cancer patients had epidural metastases at time of death.[8] In the more common solid tumors, the incidence of osseous metastases (and spine involvement) is considerably higher and may range from 20 to 70 per cent (Table 29–1). Unfortunately, these estimates do not define the magnitude of the clinical problem. If one extrapolates estimated cancer mortality data (169 per 100,000) and uses a conservative 5 per cent estimate for epidural metastases, this translates into an annual incidence of cancer-induced spinal cord injury of 8.5 per 100,000.[113] Thus, the calculated incidence of neoplastic paraplegia would exceed traumatic spinal cord injury (3 to 5 per 100,000).

At present, the socioeconomic impact of spinal cord injury secondary to neoplasia is much less than that of traumatic neoplasia because of the relatively high mortality (80 to 85 per cent at one year) in such patients. With increasing ability to control metastatic cancer, the economic consequences of caring for cancer-related spinal cord injury will be enormous. Another estimate for the frequency of this complication may be the actual number of patients with spinal cord compression encountered in cancer centers; Slatkin estimates that 80 to 100 patients with spinal cord compression are diagnosed each year at Memorial Hospital,[155] making it the most common central nervous complication of cancer. In most surgical series, between 10 and 40 per cent of patients have involvement of the spine at initial presentation of their malignancy.[29, 164, 165, 168] Pathologic compression fractures resulting in cord compression from an occult primary neoplasm represent a common problem encountered in neurosurgical practice; it has been estimated that occult primary neoplasms account for 7 per cent of all solid tumors seen in major centers.[47] Although virtually any neoplasm may involve the spine, the four most frequent primary sites are the breast, lung, prostate, and hematopoietic system; these sites alone may account for one half to two thirds of all causes of neoplastic cord compression in the reported literature.[22, 23, 29, 62, 85, 94, 99, 125, 136, 143, 158, 162]

In Table 29–2, the relative frequency of the various solid tumors in several large individual and pooled data from the literature is shown. In the pediatric population, the most common cause of spinal cord compression is neuroblastoma; apart from this, spinal cord compression frequently results from a variety of sarcomas and non-Hodgkin's lymphoma.[12, 26, 96, 131]

TABLE 29–2. SITES OF PRIMARY TUMOR IN PATIENTS WITH SPINAL CORD COMPRESSION

SITE	SUNDARESAN 1985 No. (%)	CONSTANS 1983 No. (%)	BRUCKMAN 1978 No. (%)	POSNER 1977 No. (%)
Lung	52 (20)	73 (12)	129 (16)	30 (13)
Breast	26 (10)	153 (26)	94 (12)	48 (20)
Unknown Primary	12 (5)	65 (11)	91 (11)	4 (2)
Lymphoma	3 (1)	38 (6)	86 (11)	26 (11)
Myeloma	8 (3)	—	68 (9)	9 (4)
Sarcoma	37 (14)	41 (7)	65 (8)	22 (9)
Prostate	11 (4)	47 (15)	52 (7)	21 (9)
Kidney	32 (12)	20 (3)	44 (6)	17 (7)
GI Tract	11 (4)	28 (5)	34 (4)	9 (4)
Thyroid	4 (2)	22 (4)	24 (3)	—
Others	61 (24)	113 (19)	116 (15)	49 (21)
Total	257	600	803	235

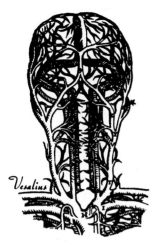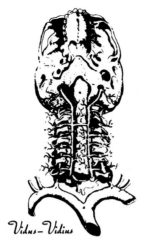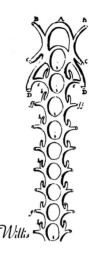

Figure 29–1. Vesalius was the first to illustrate veins leaving the spinal canal. Vidus-Vidius first illustrated the longitudinal sinus. He showed one cross connection. Willis showed the cross connections for the entire canal. (Reprinted with permission from the J.B. Lippincott Company.)

PATHOGENESIS

Many factors influence the pattern of metastases, including anatomic aspects of the vasculature draining the tumor, susceptibility of the different organs, as well as properties of the individual tumor cells.[11] The concept that vasculature plays an important role was originally demonstrated by Batson,[9] who showed retrograde flow of injected dyes toward the valveless vertebral plexuses, a mechanism that would favor retrograde tumor emboli during periods of increased abdominal pressure. This would explain the propensity of prostate cancer to spread to the lumbar spine

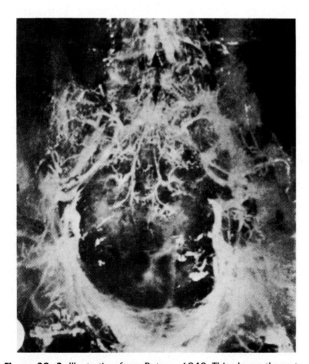

Figure 29–2. Illustration from Batson, 1940. This shows the extensive spread from an injection in the deep dorsal vein of the penis into the vertebral system. (Reproduced from Caldwell Lecture, with permission from Roentgen Ray Society.)

and of breast cancer to the thoracic spine, but does not explain the fact that bone, which receives only 5 to 10 per cent of the cardiac output, is a more frequent site for metastatic deposits than would be expected from its relative blood flow. Since the fate of tumor emboli depends also on the properties of the organ involved, the "seed and soil" hypothesis has been invoked to explain the propensity of tumor cells to involve red marrow preferentially; in addition, the microvasculature of the marrow sinusoids also promotes extravasation of tumor cells. In addition to these factors, the phenomenon of "osteotropism," whereby tumor cells selectively migrate to the target site by both chemotactic and humoral factors, may explain the selective pattern of metastases to bone from breast and prostate cancer. Supporting experimental data from the Walker rat mammary tumor indicates that products of resorbing bone (osteoclasts or matrix cells) may be chemotactic for tumor cells in vitro.

Involvement of the spine may come about in several different ways: actual replacement of the marrow by tumor cells such as myeloma, hematogenous dissemination of tumor to the vertebral body, as well as direct extension from a paraspinal focus. In some tumors, tumor extension occurs through the intervertebral foramina without bone destruction, through either the perineurium of the spinal nerves or its lymphatics. Perineurial spread frequently results in intradural extension of tumor. The fundamental cellular mechanisms of bone destruction by neoplastic cells are yet imperfectly understood and may vary from tumor to tumor.[56, 59] Apart from actual destruction, which may result in pathologic compression fractures, systemic effects may result from hypercalcemia, which is thought to be mediated from a variety of mechanisms.[16, 110] Putative indirect hormonal mechanisms that result in bone destruction include parathyroid hormone or analogues, prostaglandin E2, osteoclast-activating factor, adrenocorticotropic hormone (ACTH), calcitonin, and other substances causing vitamin-D resistance and osteomalacia.[139] Yet unexplained is the generalized osteopenia that is often noted in patients with advanced disease.

Several different theories may explain the mechanism of tumor-bone interaction, which can be classified as follows: (1) direct tumor lysis at sites of contact or by release of diffusible substances; (2) indirect mechanisms whereby tumor either blocks blood supply or produces pressure atrophy or the release of substances that activate bone cells. In a histologic study of 80 cases of metastatic lung cancer involving bone, Cramer and coworkers[33] noted that the patterns of tumor-bone interaction varied considerably with the histologic type. Osteoblastic activity was characterized by a seam of relatively eosinophilic matrix on the surface of lamellar bone covered with osteoblasts; osteoclastic activity was denoted by the presence of resorption lacunae (Howship lacunae), with or without mononucleated or multinucleated cells. Osteocytic osteolysis was suggested by the presence of enlarged osteocytic lacunae within cancellous bone. Metabolic activation was the most frequently observed pattern of tumor-bone interaction. In epidermoid cancer, metabolic activation was universal and bone remodeling was the predominant mechanism. In adenocarcinoma, the histologic patterns were more diverse, and the majority of cases were complicated by associated fracture repair. Considerable heterogeneity was seen in patients with small cell anaplastic carcinoma, characterized by a uniform lack of cellular response. Cramer concluded that both ischemic necrosis and metabolic activation of bone-lining cells were the primary mechanisms of interaction of tumor cells with bone. Experimental models of tumor-mediated osteolysis, which have been studied in a variety of animal models, include plasma cell tumors in mice, the VX2 carcinoma in rabbits, the Walker 256 carcinoma, as well as prostate carcinoma in the rat. These studies suggest that the consequences of tumor invasion include activation of both osteoblasts and osteoclasts, with osteoclastic effects predominating in the majority. Galasko and Bennett have shown that in the early phases, osteoclasts proliferate and secrete diffusible substances that enhance bone resorption, which are probably a combination of osteoclast-activating factors as well as prostaglandins.[59] These findings have been confirmed by transplantation of human tumor explants into mice, which suggests that osteoclasts play the major role in bone destruction along with possible humoral factors.[5, 115]

Histologic studies suggest that several different mechanisms may be implicated in the development of paraplegia secondary to extradural neoplasms[79, 86, 128, 184]; in the early phases, the primary event is a vasogenic edema of the white matter resulting perhaps from compression of the vertebral venous plexus. Vasodilation, with plasma exudation and edema formation, may be promoted by local production of mediators such as prostaglandins. Siegal and associates have recently demonstrated that indomethacin is effective in reducing spinal cord edema by inhibition of prostanoid formation.[151] With further growth of the tumor, a mechanical component is added until cord blood flow decreases to a critical level, following which neural function is irreversibly lost. Pathologic studies have shown little correlation between the clinically observed neurologic deficit and autopsy findings; in the majority, an edematous malacia involving the white matter is noted. Occasionally, hemorrhagic necrosis of the cord may be seen, corroborating the role of venous infarction secondary to tumor compression.[128]

CLINICAL PRESENTATION

Despite the vast variety of neoplasms that may involve the spine, the clinical syndrome is relatively uniform. Pain is noted in more than 90 per cent of patients, with a median duration of approximately eight weeks.[14, 67] The range may be extremely wide, from two weeks to more than a year prior to the onset of neurologic deficit. It is associated with a referred or radicular component in 80 to 90 per cent of patients with cervical and lumbar lesions, and in 55 per cent of patients with thoracic lesions. Pain generally results from nerve root compression, compression fractures, segmental instability, as well as direct invasion of the dura. Although the presence of back pain should alert the clinician to the diagnosis, delay in diagnosis frequently results because pain may be nonspecific or referred to other sites. This is especially true in patients who do not have a known history of cancer. Not uncommonly, radiologic studies may be focused at the wrong segmental level, and the erroneous diagnosis of musculoskeletal pain or disc disease may be made. Early diagnosis of the spinal pain due to malignancy is critical, since outcome largely depends on neurologic function before treatment.[73, 137, 144] Yet, for a variety of reasons, up to half the patients with neoplastic cord compression are nonambulatory prior to therapy, and 10 per cent are almost paraplegic, even in major centers.[168] This is even more true in the community setting, where early diagnosis remains the exception rather than the rule, with 73 per cent of patients having an interval of more than 72 hours between the onset of neurologic deficit and surgery, and the interval was greater than one week in half the patients.[144, 147]

In patients who have undergone treatment, recurrence of pain after initial therapy is indicative of recurrent tumor. In patients with paraspinal tumors, increasing brachial or lumbosacral plexopathy is a frequent harbinger of spinal cord compression. In a clinical radiographic study of 100 patients, 32 per cent of the patients presenting with increasing pain, Horner's syndrome, and weakness involving the C8-T1 roots were noted to have epidural invasion of tumor[91]; this frequently occurred in the setting of apparently normal spine x-rays. Similarly, Jaeckle and colleagues noted that tumor involvement of the lumbosacral plexus resulted from direct extension in 73 per cent and from metastases from extraabdominal neoplasms in 27 per cent. In the patients in whom myelography was performed, epidural extension was seen in 45 per cent.[81] Of the various malignancies in the pelvis, recurrences of rectal cancer with direct invasion of the sacrum and lumbar spine continue to represent a disproportionate cause of clinical morbidity, accounting for more than 50 per cent of single site recurrences.[122, 127] Pelvic recurrences also have significant implications for survival, since 90 per cent of such patients die of their cancer.

On physical examination, evidence of local tenderness along the involved spine may be evident in addition to the neurologic deficit. At present, most assessments are usually made in patients who have been treated with high dose corticosteroid therapy, and thus the initial examination may often reflect the salutary effects of steroid therapy. A careful motor and sensory examination is essential and may help the clinician plan appropriate diagnostic studies. Since ambulatory status is often taken as the objective end point of therapy, we have divided neurologic deficits into two major categories depending on whether or not patients are ambulatory. In addition to motor loss, sensory abnormalities such as numbness and paresthesias as well as signs of autonomic dysfunction may be present. The presence of autonomic dysfunction (bowel and bladder dysfunction) has been thought to portend a poor prognosis for recovery but probably reflects more advanced compression.

Based on the neurologic deficit, various grading systems have been proposed. A simple classification is based on Gilbert's paper: (I) normal muscle strength, (II) mild paraparesis, (III) moderate paraparesis, (IV) severe paraparesis or paraplegia; orthopedic surgeons are more familiar with Frankel's classification (Table 29–3). We believe it is useful to classify the various syndromes into four major categories based on the tempo of evolution of the neurologic deficit (Table 29–4). *Asymptomatic* patients with spinal involvement are generally detected during myelography performed for the evaluation of posterior mediastinal or retroperitoneal tumors—examples include neurogenic tumors of the posterior mediastinum, superior sulcus tumors, and paraspinal sarcomas. In patients with solid tumors, radionuclide bone scanning or MRI may identify spine involvement when performed as a routine staging procedure. Other patients may have *back pain* alone, with minor neurologic deficits, that is, radiculopathy. Patients presenting with neurologic deficits may be

TABLE 29–3. CLASSIFICATION OF NEUROLOGIC DEFICIT

Nonambulatory Patients
Pain only—compression fracture, unstable spine
Radiculopathy or plexopathy
Cauda equina compression
Paraparesis—mild, moderate, severe
Other causes—Brown-Séquard syndrome, ataxia, etc.

Frankel's Classification
Grade A: Complete motor and sensory loss
Grade B: Complete motor and incomplete sensory loss
Grade C: Some motor function, incomplete sensory loss
Grade D: Useful motor function, incomplete sensory loss
Grade E: Normal motor and sensory function

TABLE 29–4. SYNDROMES OF SPINAL METASTASES

Clinical Manifestations	Myelographic Finding
Asymptomatic	Varying degrees of intraspinal extension
Back pain, no deficit	Intraosseous or epidural disease
Neurologic deficit: stable on steroids	Varying degrees of epidural block
Neurologic deficit: unstable on steroids	Complete block, unstable spine

ambulatory or *nonambulatory*. We propose that neurologic deficits be classified as *stable* or *unstable* depending on their response to steroid therapy. The response to steroid therapy will also help determine the pace and necessity for emergency evaluation and treatment. Apart from the typical syndrome of spinal cord compression, which should be easily recognized in most patients with known cancer, several other presentations may also be seen. Patients may present with an atypical Brown-Séquard syndrome, with ataxia secondary to posterior column dysfunction, or with a herpetic rash along the affected dermatome. In our experience, the Brown-Séquard syndrome is seen frequently in patients with intradural invasion of tumor or others with intramedullary metastases, and it is also observed in radiation myelopathy.

RADIOLOGIC EVALUATION

Accurate radiologic assessment of the spinal segments involved, including bone and soft tissue components, as well as the extent of systemic metastases may require several studies and several days of evaluation. With the current emphasis on controlling health care costs, the clinician may be pressed into ordering tests based on risk-benefit considerations as well as cost. The pace of radiologic evaluation should be based on the urgency for treatment, and every effort should be made to obtain a definitive radiologic diagnosis. X-rays of the spine, including coned-down films, should preferably be the initial study, since abnormalities may be noted in 60 to 80 per cent of patients with clinical signs of cord compression. Classic signs of spinal metastases include vertebral collapse (Fig. 29–3), destruction of the pedicle, lytic destruction or focal osteopenia (Fig. 29–4), and malalignment of the spine. Radiologically, metastases to the spine may be classified as osteolytic, osteoblastic, or mixed, but the fundamental process in the majority is one of bone destruction by tumor, and the osteoblastic appearance merely indicates a radiologic host response.[60] Radiologically, osteoblastic metastases predominate in prostate cancer, Hodgkin's disease, occasional cervical and gastric cancers, as well as in some breast cancers.[4, 13, 25] In Constan's series, 71 per cent were classified as osteolytic, 8 per cent were purely osteoblastic, and 21 per cent were mixed.[29]

In patients with normal x-rays, the decision to

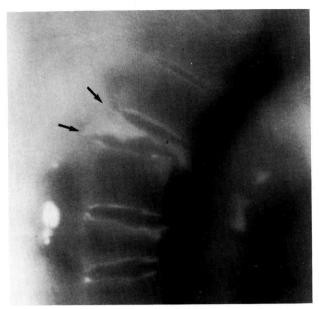

Figure 29–3. Lateral tomogram. Metastatic breast carcinoma in a 58-year-old female. There is complete collapse of T5 with protrusion into the spinal canal (*arrows*).

perform the next procedure is generally based on the evolving neurologic deficit. Patients with paraparesis generally undergo myelography. Those with pain alone may be further evaluated by MRI, CT, or radionuclide bone scan. In the past, oil-based contrast media (Pantopaque) was used for myelography to assess compromise of the spinal canal. At present, most radiologists prefer water-soluble contrast agents such as Omnipaque (iohexol) or Isovue (iopamidol). These agents are nonionic and have lower osmolarity (approximately 400 to 800 milliosmoles/liter) but contain sufficient organic iodine (180 to 370 mg/ml) to provide satisfactory radiographic visualization. Sev-

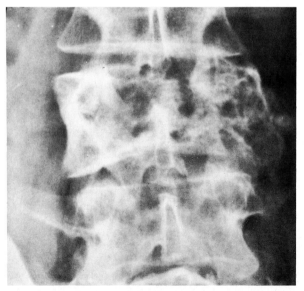

Figure 29–4. Anteroposterior radiograph. There is partial collapse of the L3 vertebra with destruction of the pedicle and vertebral body on the left side.

eral algorithmic approaches that improve the probability of detecting epidural disease have been proposed.[67, 129, 136, 137] Rodichok and others have recommended that myelography be performed in any cancer patient with back pain if either the plain x-rays are abnormal or a clear-cut radiculopathy is noted regardless of the plain x-ray findings (Fig. 29–5). Myelography is recommended in most patients with spinal metastases for several reasons: (1) it is currently the most accurate test for distinguishing intraosseous from epidural disease (Fig. 29–6); (2) discontinuous epidural blocks may be seen in 10 per cent of patients (Fig. 29–7), especially those with breast cancer, lymphoma, or prostate cancer[10, 100]; (3) other causes of spinal pain and neurologic deficits in the cancer population may be diagnosed; and (4) proper identification of epidural extension allows planning of treatment portals for radiotherapy.

If a complete block is found, the upper limits of the block should be identified. There are several different methods of demonstrating the upper level of a block, including a C1-C2 puncture, the instillation of a little air from below to force the dye past the block, or a CT scan following myelography.[50, 88, 95, 121] It is not uncommon for patients with complete block to show some degree of neurologic deterioration following lumbar puncture, and Hollis and colleagues[78] have estimated that the incidence may be as high as 14 per cent. All patients with suspected epidural extension of tumor should be treated with an intravenous bolus of dexamethasone (10 to 20 mg) either before or following myelography. This should be followed by more definitive therapy depending upon the clinical situation. Myelography is not indicated in patients with unstable spines and may be dispensed with in those in whom adequate demonstration of the subarachnoid space or tumor encroachment has been demonstrated adequately by MRI or CT scans.

The most sensitive and economical test for detecting bone metastases is scintigraphy using 99m technetium-labeled compounds[27, 61, 107]; Galasko and others have shown that 30 to 50 per cent of lesions detected by scintigraphy are not visualized by radiographs. In many newly diagnosed cancer patients, including those with pathologic compression fractures, scintigraphy allows a simple method of staging the extent of bone involvement, since 10 to 30 per cent of patients have multifocal involvement of the skeletal system. Tumor sites are shown as focal or regional areas of increased radiotracer activity, which is related to the extent and magnitude of bone repair and vascularity that occur in response to tumor invasion.

Occasionally, destructive lesions may elicit a poor response and appear photopenic on the radionuclide scan—a typical example being multiple myeloma. The major limitation of scintigraphy is its relative nonspecificity; the presence of a solitary focus should prompt careful clinical evaluation and other radiologic studies.[30] In patients who undergo surgery with metallic implants, radionuclide scans are useful in following residual tumor activity, since other studies

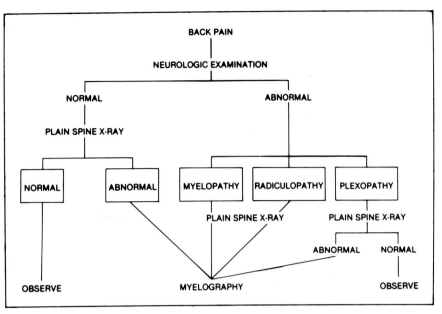

Figure 29–5. The early diagnosis of spinal epidural metastases. Patients with known or suspected cancer who have back pain, alone or with symptoms of spinal root or spinal cord injury, are evaluated initially by neurologic examination, followed by radiographic examination of the spine. Myelography is recommended in patients with spinal cord (myelopathy) or spinal root injury (radiculopathy) and in patients with roentgenographic evidence of spinal metastases at the appropriate segment. (From Rodichok LD, Harper GR, Ruckdeschel JC, et al: Early diagnosis of spinal epidural metastases. Am J Med 70:1181–1188, 1981; with permission.)

may be difficult to interpret because of the number of artifacts caused by metal and surgery. In addition, scintigraphy may be used to localize isolated "hot" spots accurately for purposes of excisional biopsy; this is clearly valuable when the x-rays appear normal. The most exciting area of development of radionuclide imaging is the identification of tumors with radionuclide-labeled antibodies; tumors that can be detected include those producing carcinoembryonic antigen (CEA) (Fig. 29–8), alpha fetoprotein, human chorionic gonadotropin, and prostatic acid phosphatase, as well as melanoma.

At the present time, CT scan is still widely used for the evaluation of paraspinal and soft tissue involvement and for the accurate staging of tumors by scanning of the chest and abdomen (Figs. 29–9, 29–10). The CT scan is particularly useful in demonstrating small areas of bone destruction and of bone and tumor impingement on the canal.[3, 41, 133, 189] Since it is

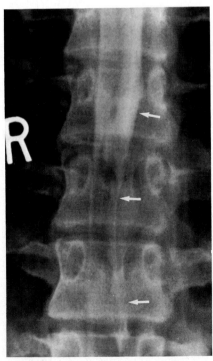

Figure 29–6. Thoracic myelogram. A 32-year-old white male with embryonal rhabdomyosarcoma and metastases to the epidural space. A long fusiform left-sided defect (*arrows*) is shown with partial obstruction of the subarachnoid space.

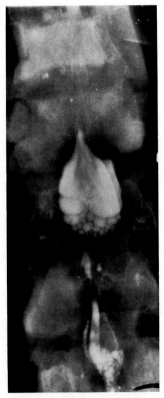

Figure 29–7. Thoracic myelogram. Complete epidural block at T12 with tapering of subarachnoid space indicating circumferential lesion.

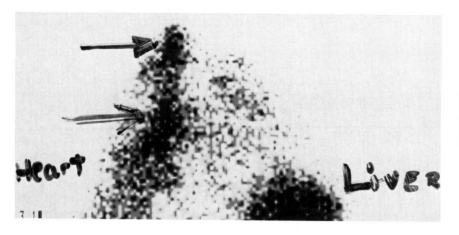

Figure 29–8. Metastases to the spine from an unknown primary tumor. Increased activity of anti-CEA–tagged antibody as shown by arrows documents recurrence in spine.

rapidly performed and noninvasive, it can be used in patients with suspected spinal instability. Osteoporosis can often be differentiated from tumor destruction when evaluating isolated wedge compression fractures.[72] The major limitations include failure to demonstrate a second discontiguous site of metastasis, missing epidural extension when the attenuation values of the tumor approach those of the spinal cord, and if the sections are too thick. The presence of significant streak artifacts from metal implants may also interfere with the assessment of tumor recurrence.

With the advent of MRI scans, another important modality for evaluating the spine is available. Major advantages of MRI include superior soft tissue and tumor contrast, demonstration of the spinal involvement in both the axial, coronal, and sagittal planes, and lack of exposure to ionizing radiation.[63, 70, 142] Early experience suggests that MRI may be superior to bone scanning in detecting marrow infiltration by tumor. Relative disadvantages include its current high cost, the logistics of obtaining studies on an emergency basis and in patients who are hemodynamically unstable, as well as the feeling of claustrophobia experienced by some patients. Unenhanced MRI is not a sensitive modality for detection of leptomeningeal metastases. Large lesions, including those resulting in complete obstruction of the canal, may be missed by this technique. Initial experience with the paramagnetic agent gadolinium-DTPA (Gd-DTPA) suggests that subarachnoid metastatic tumors enhance prominently and can be detected relatively easily against the background of nonenhanced normal nerve tissue and spinal fluid.[178] The use of this contrast agent has not significantly improved the detection of tumors affecting the epidural space, because tumors often become isointense and difficult to visualize. Contrast scans are indicated in the following situations: to distinguish disc disease from epidural tumor and to outline more accessible areas for biopsy. In the immediate postoperative period, contrast scans can also help distinguish residual tumor from postoperative changes. Sze and coworkers have noted that enhancement with Gd-DTPA may correlate with activity of the tumor, since loss of enhancement was noted with positive response to therapy.[177] We have also found that MRI is superior

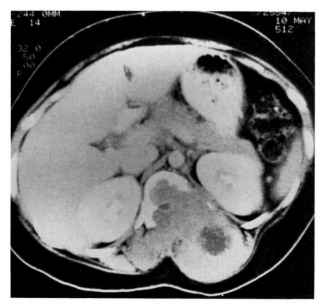

Figure 29–9. Axial CT scan. Large posterior paraspinal sarcoma with central necrosis and total obliteration of spinal canal.

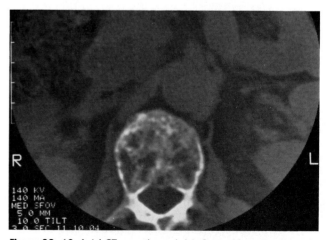

Figure 29–10. Axial CT scan through L1. Several low density areas consistent with a destructive process are identified within the vertebral body. The lesions are limited to bone without compromise of the spinal canal—typical of multiple myeloma.

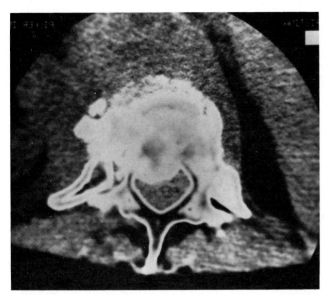

Figure 29–11. Hodgkin's lymphoma. There is bony compression of the canal at T11 level with protrusion into the spinal canal. An anterior paraspinal soft tissue mass is noted.

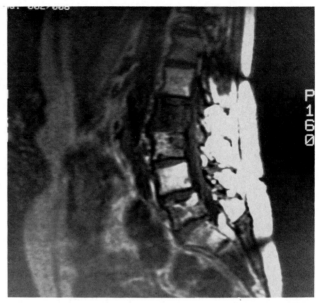

Figure 29–13. Sagittal MRI, T1-weighted image. There is total loss of signal from L2 vertebral body consistent with diffuse infiltration. Ventral epidural defect is noted at this level. Patchy areas of involvement are also present in L3, L5-S1, and S2 vertebrae.

to CT scanning in evaluating patients with metal implants and methyl methacrylate. Although several studies now cite MRI as the radiologic imaging procedure of choice, others have found that conventional myelography is comparable in demonstrating epidural disease.[70, 93]

In patients with hypervascular tumors, spinal angiography is indicated to diminish tumor vascularity, to demonstrate feeding vessels, and to determine the location of critical spinal arterial supply such as the artery of Adamkiewicz. For presurgical embolization, a variety of therapeutic agents may be used. Temporary materials (such as autologous clot, gelatin foam, and microfibrillar collagen) are easy to handle, are associated with minimal risk of permanent damage, and are used for temporary embolization until

operative resection is scheduled within several days. Permanent materials include polyvinyl alcohol foam (Ivalon) in particulate form, Silastic spheres, silicone polymers, and absolute alcohol. Particles of Ivalon

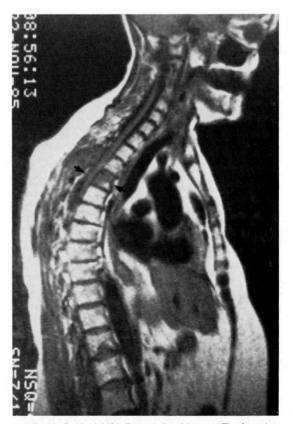

Figure 29–14. Sagittal MRI, T1-weighted image. The hypointense signal originating from the T3 vertebra is consistent with marrow replacement in this 62-year-old female with breast carcinoma.

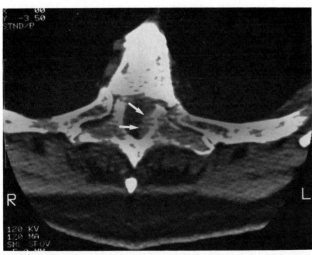

Figure 29–12. Diffuse metastases from prostate carcinoma. Axial CT scan through T5 identifies tumor involving the vertebral body and posterior elements with soft tissue mass extending into the spinal canal from the left side (*arrows*).

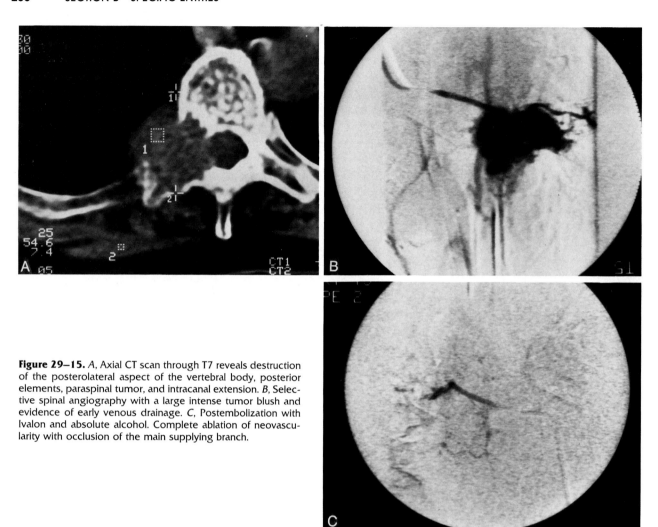

Figure 29–15. *A,* Axial CT scan through T7 reveals destruction of the posterolateral aspect of the vertebral body, posterior elements, paraspinal tumor, and intracanal extension. *B,* Selective spinal angiography with a large intense tumor blush and evidence of early venous drainage. *C,* Postembolization with Ivalon and absolute alcohol. Complete ablation of neovascularity with occlusion of the main supplying branch.

(150 to 500 microns in diameter) are mixed with solutions of warmed saline and radiographic contrast in proportion, designed to produce a liquid slurry of a concentration and viscosity appropriate to the lesion.[89] In our experience, patients with primary tumors and those with metastases from kidney, thyroid, or sarcomas have been safely embolized, with resulting lowered morbidity from intraoperative blood loss.[19, 171] In addition to Ivalon, absolute alcohol may also be used as a sclerosing agent for permanent tumor necrosis prior to surgery. Recent data suggest that the risk of neurologic deficit following selective spinal angiography is less than 2 per cent,[55] and there should be little hesitation in using it whenever indicated. Apart from embolization, the intraarterial route is often used to deliver higher concentrations of chemotherapeutically effective drugs.[122]

DIFFERENTIAL DIAGNOSIS

In evaluating the cancer patient with myelopathy or back pain, it is important to keep several entities in the differential diagnosis. Both intradural and intramedullary metastases may occur, with estimates of their frequency ranging from 2 to 5 per cent.[31,]

[112, 124] The clinical picture is characterized by a more fulminant course, early sphincteric involvement, and poor prognosis because accurate diagnosis is seldom made.[69] We have observed several instances of both extradural and intradural tumor resulting from perineural invasion, which has often been difficult to distinguish on myelography. In patients who have received prior radiation, the symptoms of radiation myelopathy may often mimic those of recurrent tumor, especially if myelography reveals a swollen cord.[66] In patients with isolated spinal abnormalities, an osteoporotic vertebra may often present as a pathologic fracture and show increased uptake on the radionuclide scan. Similarly, radiation osteitis may occur within an isolated vertebra if it is within the field of therapeutic radiation, and benign tumors of the bone or dura may mimic recurrent disease.[120, 195] It is important to evaluate patients with solitary abnormalities on bone scanning to avoid missing these treatable conditions. Benign disc disease may frequently occur in the setting of stable malignant disease and should be identified as such.[24, 65] Patients who undergo radiation therapy for osteoblastic metastases frequently develop secondary stenosis and canal encroachment that may become symptomatic. Such patients should be considered for surgical decompression, since compression by bone cannot be expected to be relieved by conservative treatment. In patients receiving prolonged steroid therapy, symptomatic cord compression may occasionally result from epidural lipomatosis[83] and may even produce paraplegia.

PRINCIPLES OF MANAGEMENT

The philosophy of management of spinal metastases has undergone considerable change in the past decade. Whereas palliation of pain and preservation of neurologic and sphincteric function clearly represent important goals of therapy, important advances in surgery of the spine as well as the development of newer forms of instrumentation have considerably expanded the role of the surgeon in the management of spinal metastases. In most patients, treatment needs to be individualized based on the general condition, extent of cancer, type of tumor, tempo and degree of neurologic deficit, and expertise available. Several studies have accurately shown the importance of prognostic factors that independently affect outcome, including the extent of neurologic deficit, its tempo of evolution, the primary cancer, the presence of a complete block on myelography, as well as response to steroid therapy.[7, 14, 179] The overall prognosis for patients with exclusively bony metastases from sites such as breast, prostate, and kidney is relatively good,[109, 145, 149, 171] whereas patients with lung cancer do poorly. In addition, the clinical course of some tumors such as thyroid cancer,[64] carcinoids, and salivary gland tumors may be so indolent that the presence of multiple bone and visceral metastases is often compatible with survival for many years. Patients with adenocarcinoma from unknown primary sites respond poorly to radiotherapy and chemotherapy,[47] and surgery offers the best prospect for local tumor control. Patients with advanced cancer and poor performance status should be treated conservatively, since they seldom respond to aggressive management. With these generalizations, it is important to consider the three major options available for initial management: chemotherapy, radiation therapy, and surgery.

Chemotherapy

There is general agreement that corticosteroid therapy (specifically dexamethasone) is clearly beneficial in patients with neoplastic cord compression. In the past, extremely high initial doses (100 mg dexamethasone) were given intravenously as a bolus,[68] with subsequent doses given four times a day. In tumors such as lymphoma, neuroblastoma, and other round cell malignancies, steroid therapy may have a beneficial effect not only by reduction of vasogenic edema, but also by a more specific oncolytic effect.[130] Recent experimental data have confirmed the beneficial effects of steroids,[36] but no advantage was seen with higher doses as compared with more conventional doses. Although many clinicians continue to use such high doses, it is important to keep in proper perspective the associated serious side effects that can arise with corticosteroid use. These include hyperglycemia, gastrointestinal bleeding, and intestinal perforation resulting from stress ulcers. When used as an intravenous bolus, dexamethasone may cause a severe burning in the genitalia; other side effects include intractable hiccoughs, psychosis, and hallucinations, especially in the postsurgical patient. Prolonged use may cause proximal weakness of the extremities (steroid myopathy), resulting in an inability to walk. In addition, too rapid tapering may result in diffuse aches and pains associated with lassitude (steroid pseudorheumatism). Steroids may also interact with other drugs (such as nonsteroidal anti-inflammatory drugs, anticonvulsants, and anticoagulants). For the surgeon, the most important side effects include failure of the surgical wound to heal and the devastating potential for superinfection in the immunologically suppressed patient.

Weissman has recently reviewed the incidence of serious complications related to steroid usage[191, 192] and noted that 51 per cent of patients developed at least one steroid-related toxicity and 19 per cent required hospital admission for diagnosis and management. Both the duration of steroid therapy and the total dose predicted toxicity, and patients with steroid toxicity had significant falls in serum albumin. Martenson has also noted a significant increase in severe steroid complications, including several cases of fatal sepsis, when dexamethasone was used for more than 40 days in patients with neoplastic cord compression.[103] Although others have suggested that the incidence of toxicity may be minimal,[185] our experience corroborates that of Weissman and Martenson, since the major complications in our series occurred in those who had received steroids for more than one month. It is therefore important to use steroids judiciously and to discontinue their use as rapidly as possible or otherwise to taper them down to the lowest possible level compatible with clinical benefit.

The use of chemotherapeutic agents to reverse hypercalcemia, the most common paraneoplastic syndrome encountered in patients with spine metastases, represents another example of nonspecific chemotherapy. Hypercalcemia is a frequent and occasionally life-threatening complication of cancer, and the spectrum of drugs used in its treatment includes glucocorticoids, calcitonin, phosphates, indomethacin, and mithramycin.[16, 17, 44, 111, 132] More recently, a variety of diphosphonates have been found that reduce serum calcium levels, and these include ethane-1-hydroxy-1,1-diphosphonate (EHDP), dicholoromethylene diphosphonate (Cl2 MDP), as well as amino-hydroxypropane diphosphonate (APD). Diphosphonates are analogues of pyrophosphate and bind to hydroxyapatite. The newer analogues may work by inhibiting bone resorption but require parenteral administration because of poor oral absorption. Of the diphosphonates, only etidronate diso-dium (Didronel) is commercially available in the United States. Warrell has recently shown that gallium nitrate, a heavy metal analogue, has shown some promise in the management of osteolytic metastases, but this drug is also available only on an experimental basis.[187]

When specific chemotherapy is available, such as those for osteosarcoma, round cell sarcomas, or germinoma, it is often possible to reduce tumor size by the use of these agents despite the presence of epidural encroachment if steroid therapy is given concomitantly. We have used this approach to reduce the size of large paraspinal tumors before attempting definitive surgery, since this allows early treatment of micrometastases and reduction in tumor size so that less mutilating procedures can be performed. In addition, the use of hormonal ablation (such as orchiectomy) can often be used with steroids in patients presenting with metastatic prostate cancer, if their neurologic deficit is stable.

External Radiation Therapy

Over the past two decades, several series have reported the beneficial effects of radiation therapy (RT) in treating spinal cord compression from a variety of solid tumors. Approximately one third to one half of the treated patients improve and are able to walk following treatment.[155] It has been shown that approximately one half of the patients who improve maintain that improvement at the end of a year. Similarly, pain relief is noted in half of the patients treated with RT, and these results also depend upon the radiosensitivity of the tumor and the patient's neurologic status. Patients with radiosensitive tumors (such as breast, prostate, or lymph) are more likely to maintain ambulatory status, as are those who were ambulatory when treatment was begun. RT continues to be the mainstay of treatment in neoplastic cord compression, since patients with advanced cancer are generally not candidates for surgery. Currently, most patients are usually treated at a dose rate of 200 cGy per day, for a total of 3000 cGy using a single posterior port whose field encompasses two segments above and below the level of involvement. This dose approaches cord tolerance in the thoracic region, and retreatment is not an option when the tumor recurs. In patients with potentially controllable disease in the lumbar segments (solitary foci from the breast), a slower, more protracted course (150 cGy/day) to a total dose of 5000 cGy may be used.

Since the results of external RT are largely unsatisfactory, more recent attempts have focused on the use of higher dose fractionation[68] or radiation sensitizers (such as mizonidazole). Obbens and coworkers recently reported a prospective trial of 83 patients using metronidazole in conjunction with a short course of high dose fractionation, consisting of 500 cGy daily for three days followed by 400 cGy daily

for three days.[116] No difference in outcome was seen, with response rates of 30 to 40 per cent for both groups. Similarly, no difference in the overall palliative index was noted by the radiation therapy oncology groups using various dose fractionation schemes; despite initial improvement rates approaching 50 to 80 per cent, the majority relapsed within six months.[182]

The major limiting factor with regard to improving cure rates by external RT alone is the limited radiation tolerance of the spinal cord. Although the risk of radiation myelopathy is negligible in patients whose life expectancy is limited, it assumes considerable importance in those patients whose prognosis is good. Dorfman and associates recently showed evidence of electrophysiologic evidence of subclinical injury to the thoracic cord in patients receiving mediastinal RT using doses ranging from 2000 to 4380 cGy for lung cancer.[40] These changes were directly related not to total dose but to the treatment time and total number of fractions used. With the use of CT planning, it is now feasible to deliver much higher doses (radiobiologic dose equivalent of 7000 to 8000 cGy) using a combination of photon beams and particles (proton or heavy particles), and this is currently used to treat chordomas and chondrosarcomas in the upper cervical spine. The advantages of particle beams include a better dose distribution with sparing of adjacent neural tissue and a relatively enhanced radiobiologic effect for heavy particles such as helium. These treatment options are available in only a few centers and are both time consuming and expensive. This limits their applicability in the cancer population. Attempts to improve local control by the use of brachytherapy (locally implanted radioactive isotopes) have met with limited success because of difficulties in treating a large volume of tumor adjacent to the cord. In selected patients in whom curative therapy is planned, these options should clearly be considered.

For the spinal surgeon, the major concern regarding the use of radiation is the problem of wound dehiscence, as well as the difficulties in obtaining successful bone union with the use of autologous grafts[57, 101]; wound-related complications are further increased when intensive chemotherapy and steroid therapy are used, as there is the potential for fatal sepsis.[45] We recently analyzed the results of decompressive laminectomy over a 5-year period in 71 patients with neoplastic cord compression treated at Memorial Sloan-Kettering Cancer Center between 1979 and 1984.[102] In this study, 25 patients underwent de novo surgery followed by RT; the remaining 46 patients were those who had undergone prior RT and who fit traditional criteria for decompressive laminectomy. Although pain relief was comparable in both groups (50 per cent), neurologic improvement was more marked in the de novo group (with 6 out of 7 nonambulatory patients regaining ambulation) compared with the previously irradiated patients (7 of 21 nonambulatory patients regaining ambulation). A statistically significant finding was the increased complication rate (36 per cent) noted in those who had undergone prior treatment, in comparison to those undergoing de novo surgery (16 per cent). The median survival in the de novo patients was 12 months, and was only 6 months in those receiving prior RT. Those who deteriorated during RT had the worst outcome: only one third of the patients improved, their 30-day mortality was 21 per cent, and only one third survived 6 months. These findings indicate that prior RT clearly increases surgical morbidity, although many other factors also contribute to the risk of poor healing in the cancer patient. Similar experiences have been noted if stabilization procedures are used.[77, 166] For this reason, we strongly advocate avoidance of midline surgical incisions in the back in patients who have received prior RT.

Surgical Approaches

The oldest approach for decompression of neoplastic cord compression is decompressive laminectomy; this is then followed by a course of postoperative RT. This midline posterior approach is technically easy and safe, allowing for tissue diagnosis but providing adequate decompression only when the tumor mass lies dorsal to the dura. Laminectomy also destabilizes the spine if the anterior and middle columns (vertebral bodies and pedicles) are destroyed by tumor and allows very little access to tumor lying

ventral to the cord. In a retrospective analysis, Gilbert and colleagues[62] compared the results of laminectomy with those of RT and concluded that laminectomy provided no extra benefit over RT and steroids alone. Similar conclusions were reached by other investigators,[14, 42, 49, 138, 158] and a small prospective study by Young and coworkers[194] reinforced the belief that there was no difference in patients treated by RT or by laminectomy. Findlay[49] reviewed the published literature on surgical decompression for neoplastic cord compression and noted that of the 1816 patients reviewed, 32 per cent, 38 per cent, and 51 per cent of the patients treated by laminectomy alone, laminectomy with RT, or by RT alone, respectively, were able to walk at the end of treatment. Approximately 20 per cent in each group experienced neurologic worsening. In addition, approximately 11 per cent of patients undergoing operation experienced perioperative complications, with a mortality of 9 per cent. It is therefore not surprising that current oncology texts[23] favor RT and steroid therapy in all patients as initial management, and relegate surgery to a purely salvage or diagnostic role. These studies ignore the fact that the only surgical procedure used as a basis for comparison was laminectomy.

Although some recent studies still advocate laminectomy,[29, 114] its current role is limited, and the nonselective application of this approach in all cases of neoplastic cord compression is condemned. Laminectomy is contraindicated when the tumor mass lies anterior to the cord, if the vertebral body is collapsed,

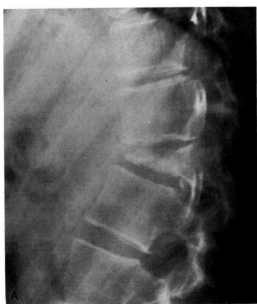
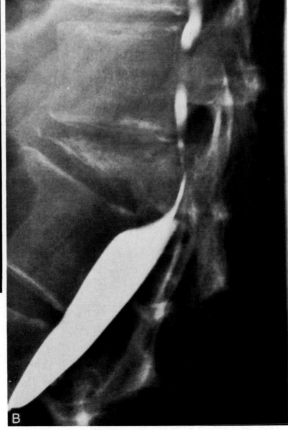

Figure 29–16. A, Postlaminectomy instability caused by wrong choice of operative procedure. B, Myelogram following laminectomy demonstrates persistent high grade block. Laminectomy is clearly contraindicated in the presence of a pathologic compression fracture, unless posterior stabilization is also planned.

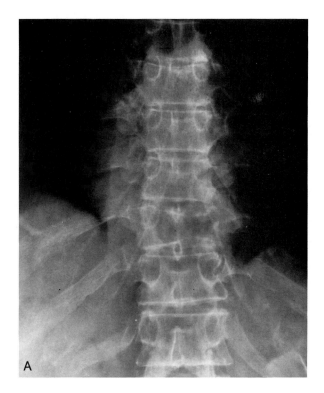

A

EVALUATION OF PATHOLOGICAL COMPRESSION FRACTURE

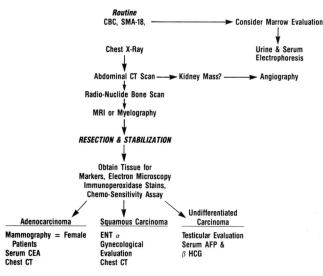

B

Figure 29–17. When a radiologically suspected pathologic compression fracture (A) is diagnosed, the work-up should proceed along the algorithm shown in (B). An abdominal CT scan as well as a radionuclide bone scan should be performed to exclude a kidney tumor. If a primary lesion cannot be identified, resection and stabilization are recommended. Tissue obtained at time of resection should be carefully examined to help identify the primary site as well as to guide therapy.

or if there is a kyphotic deformity or subluxation of one vertebra over another; the fact that it is technically easy to perform and is well tolerated by most patients does not condone its use when an alternate procedure would have been more appropriate. With the development of newer surgical approaches to the spine, there has been an associated recognition that

stability of the spine involved by neoplasia is almost as important a contributing factor in the symptomatology. There has also been a resurgence and interest in both the biomechanics of the spine and the development of sophisticated instrumentation, with the resulting growth of spinal surgery as a separate subspecialty during the past decade.[1, 37–39, 43, 48, 52, 74, 77, 84, 87, 92, 117, 126, 148, 152–154, 159, 161–176, 186, 188, 190, 193]

There are several important reasons for the surgical failures in the past, which can be summarized as follows: nonselective use of a single surgical approach, inadequate tumor resection, ineffective stabilization, poor patient selection, and intradural extension of tumor. In addition, emergency decompression carried out without adequate preoperative assessment has a much higher morbidity and likelihood of poor results. Treatment must be individualized in many patients, and a knowledge of important prognostic factors is important in the selection process. The site of primary tumor and histology, as well as the pretreatment neurologic deficit, are now accepted as the most important pretreatment variables. Aggressive surgical intervention should be reserved for patients who are ambulatory; there is little purpose in subjecting paraplegic or near-paraplegic patients to extensive operation. Patients who have rapidly evolving deficits (less than 24 hours) may have a poor outcome regardless of therapy, especially if the deficits progress on high dose steroid therapy. Patients with structural abnormalities (instability, retropulsed bone fragments, acute collapse of the vertebral body) do not respond to RT alone, since compression of the neural elements results from bone. The extent of myelographic block (complete versus incomplete) is considered an important factor, but we believe that this should not influence the decision regarding initial management. The presence of paraspinal soft tissue tumor is an adverse prognostic factor[29, 117] but is not that relevant if the operative procedure is planned to also resect the soft

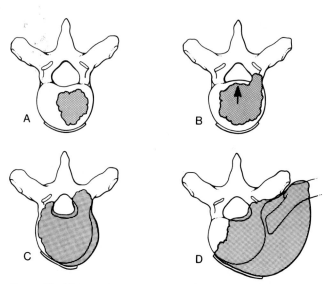

A   B

C   D

Figure 29–18. Line diagram illustrates progressive stages of tumor extension from the vertebral body; for cancer therapy, surgery is indicated when the tumor is still purely intraosseous (A).

tissue tumor. Finally, the phase in the cancer patient's illness in which treatment is undertaken is important; patients with advanced widespread disease and others who have failed previous treatment are less likely to benefit from operation. With these generalizations, we believe that RT and steroid therapy should be the initial treatment in patients with the following conditions: (1) advanced visceral metastases and poor performance status; (2) lymphoma and other round cell malignancies, such as neuroblastoma, Ewing's sarcoma, and so forth; and (3) breast and prostate cancer without structural abnormalities of the spine. In all other patients with spinal metastases, surgical evaluation is mandatory. Since the goal of therapy in any individual patient may differ, we have classified indications for surgery along five major categories.

Cancer Therapy

In patients with primary osseous neoplasms, localized paraspinal tumors with direct spine involvement, and solitary rates of relapse, effective local treatment has a major bearing on overall survival.[161, 169] Other patients presenting with pathologic compression fractures and radioresistant tumors, such as kidney cancer with limited systemic disease, also fall into this category.[171] In such patients, neither the absence of significant deficit, pain, nor epidural extension have bearing on the timing of operation. Rather the goal of operation should be maximal reduction of tumor bulk, which may require a combined anteroposterior approach.

Stabilization

A major goal of operation is the restoration or maintenance of stability of the spine. Patients with fracture-dislocations, localized kyphosis, or collapsed vertebra with retropulsion of a bone fragment may require operative decompression in conjunction with RT. In these patients, the radiosensitivity of the primary tumor has little bearing on the indication for therapy. A major subgroup of patients in this category present with "segmental instability" of the spine, commonly seen in the post-RT patient. Surgical reduction of movement across this motion segment will generally result in prompt relief of pain.

Neurologic Salvage

In patients who present with acutely evolving deficit, surgery offers the potential of neurologic palliation even though there may be little impact on overall survival. Similarly, patients who deteriorate while undergoing RT, or others who cannot receive further RT, may be relieved for several months by surgical decompression. In such patients, the goal of therapy is more limited because the surgery is performed for salvage. Since these patients have received both RT and prolonged steroid therapy, potential morbidity may be considerable, and more limited decompression by posterolateral approaches may be appropriate.

Tissue Diagnosis

With current radiologic evaluation, the need for a major procedure to document a diagnosis of malig-

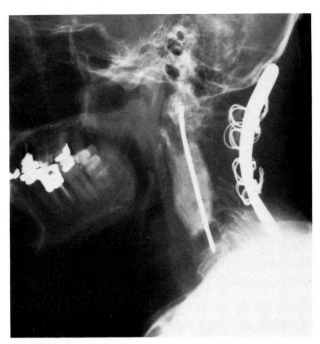

Figure 29–19. In the cervical spine, combined anterior and posterior approaches are often necessary. The anterior stabilization is generally performed with methyl methacrylate and Steinmann pins, and the posterior fixation with segmental sublaminar wiring and Luque rods contoured to conform to the cervical lordosis.

nancy should be rare. Frequently the primary site may be obvious, for example, on chest x-ray or abdominal CT, or a more accessible bony site may be visualized on radionuclide bone scan. If no site is evident, the diagnosis of malignancy can frequently be established by needle biopsy,[58] especially if a paraspinal soft tissue mass is present. The major indication for operative intervention is to differentiate benign from malignant compression, for example, disc disease versus metastatic tumor, or in the occasional intradural lesion in which distinction from a primary intraspinal tumor such as meningioma versus metastases cannot be made.

Pain Relief

In most patients, resection of tumor and restoration of stability frequently result in pain relief; exceptionally, in patients with intractable pain either from local plexus or nerve root invasion, the goal of therapy may be pain relief even though motor deficits are permanent and irreversible. Local rhizotomies, cordotomy, and resection of lesions compressing the brachial plexus fall into this category.[53, 163]

PREOPERATIVE EVALUATION AND ASSESSMENT

Many patients with spinal cord compression are referred for neurosurgical evaluation either with an evolving neurologic deficit or after a myelogram has demonstrated a complete block. This may result in a hasty decision by the surgeon to decompress the cord on an emergency basis to preserve or improve neurologic function. Although such clinical situations cannot always be avoided, emergency surgery should be considered only in those patients whose neurologic deficits are unstable or progress on steroid therapy. With an initial bolus dose (Decadron 10 to 20 mg IV) of corticosteroid therapy, most patients stabilize long enough for more complete radiologic assessment. (There is currently little rationale for the use of higher doses, such as 100 mg Decadron as used in the past.) In all patients, spinal CT scan should be performed to determine the proper operative approach.

In patients presenting with a pathologic compression fracture without a prior history of cancer, several diagnostic possibilities exist: (1) a primary cancer may be evident on chest x-rays or abdominal CT scan, or (2) no primary site is seen. Radiologic evaluation should include radionuclide bone scan, but other extensive radiologic studies looking for a primary site are not indicated. Specific laboratory tests that are indicated in the diagnosis include serum acid phosphatase, serum and urine immune electrophoresis, and CEA levels. A bone marrow examination should be performed if myeloma is suspected. If a kidney mass is seen on abdominal CT scan, angiography is clearly indicated.

Since the majority of symptomatic cord compression occurs in the thoracic segments, assessment for a possible thoracotomy should include preoperative pulmonary function tests. In patients with chronic obstructive pulmonary disease (COPD) and in others with recent respiratory compromise, therapy with Bronchosol or ultrasonic nebulizers a few days prior to operation will allow for a smoother recovery.

In patients with vascular tumors, a complete coagulogram should be performed, and adequate whole blood and blood products should be available. A final most important aspect of preoperative care is to have the patient evaluated for a custom made or prefabricated orthosis prior to operation.

CHOICE OF OPERATIVE APPROACHES

There are three basic approaches to the spine: (1) posterior approaches by laminectomy, (2) lateral approaches by transverse osteotomy, and (3) anterior approaches by vertebral body resection. Complete resection of both anterior and posterior elements is termed *spondylectomy* and requires a two-stage procedure.[176] In addition, stabilization procedures are either required in conjunction with decompression or are indicated for pain resulting from spinal instability. Prior to performing a stabilization procedure, the integrity of the neural canal and lack of significant tumor encroachment must be confirmed by myelography or MRI. The operative procedure should be based on the radiographic extent of tumor, the assessment of the patient's general condition and extent of disease, as well as the desired goal of therapy. Familiarity with all aspects of spinal surgery and the complex instrumentation systems currently

available will allow the surgeon to choose the most appropriate procedure for the patient based on these considerations.

Laminectomy

There is a growing realization that the role of laminectomy is limited, with little evidence to suggest any major clinical benefit if used indiscriminately in all patients. It is clearly *contraindicated* when the tumor lies ventral to the cord, in the presence of kyphosis, or if instability is present. Frequently neurosurgeons may be asked to perform "decompression" for neural palliation, pain relief, or tissue diagnosis; laminectomy frequently does not achieve this proposed goal of palliation unless major tumor resection is also performed. Laminectomy *is only indicated* for posteriorly placed tumors, for neural decompression and pain relief caused by secondary hypertrophic stenosis involving the facets and pedicles, and whenever intradural exploration is necessary. Currently, we believe that the major indications for laminectomy are in patients with prostate cancer and lymphoma who relapse after radiation therapy; such patients have an intact vertebral body without evidence of collapse. We also use laminectomy to complete the posterior portion of a "staged" spondylectomy; it is always combined with posterior instrumentation and bone grafting.

Posterolateral Approaches

Since laminectomy alone does not provide access to the anterior aspect of the cord, a variety of posterolateral approaches are used to enable more extensive tumor resection. In the thoracic region, this generally includes costotransversectomy, whereas in the lumbar region, removal of the facets or pedicles allows tumor within the vertebral body to be removed. Several authors have reported improvement rates of 75 per cent in pain relief and neurologic deficit in patients so treated.[21, 118, 119, 125, 148, 156] The major indications for posterolateral approaches are (1) multisegment involvement, especially if they are discontinuous, (2) radiographic demonstration of a significant lateral or posterolateral mass, (3) three-column disease, and (4) patient's inability to tolerate an anterior approach.[21] This procedure, especially in conjunction with posterior instrumentation, is clearly beneficial in patients with advanced disease. Perrin and colleagues have noted pain relief in 80 per cent, a posttreatment ambulatory rate of 65 per cent (a gain in ambulation of 28 per cent), and a mortality rate of 8 per cent in a series of 200 consecutive patients.[125] At six months, 42 per cent of the patients were walking and continent. Criteria for selecting the posterolateral approach include tumor location not only in the axial, but also in the sagittal, plane. Exposures of the upper two cervical vertebrae, cervicothoracic junction, and lumbosacral junction are not within the province of the occasional surgeon. In addition, anterior stabilization is more difficult at these levels. We would, however, caution against the use of the posterolateral approach when an anterior approach is indicated, since it does not provide adequate access for complete tumor resection.

Posterior Stabilization

As Denis has elegantly stated, the term "instability" as it relates to the spine has become a key word within the last decade, since it is often equated with a need for therapeutic internal stabilization.[37] In trauma, the accepted biomechanical model is the three-column concept of the spine. The anterior column consists of the anterior vertebral body, anterior longitudinal ligament, and annulus fibrosus; the middle column includes the posterior longitudinal ligament, posterior half of the vertebral body, and annulus; the posterior column is the posterior ligamentous complex. Spinal fractures are classified according to the mechanism of injury and involvement of the columns. A wealth of experimental data now allows a more rational approach to designing the proper internal fixation system that provides stability.[4, 39, 190, 193] In the spine involved by neoplasia, these concepts may not always be applicable, and definitions of instability are largely empiric.

Instability of the spine may be presumed if radiographic studies reveal the following: (1) translational deformity, (2) loss of vertebral height greater than 50 per cent, (3) three-column involvement, and (4) involvement of two or more vertebral bodies. In addition, segmental instability is assumed to be present when the clinical syndrome is characterized by pain aggravated by movement (in the absence of significant neural encroachment), associated with the presence of progressive collapse of the vertebral bodies or localized kyphosis on the MRI scan. There is now a general consensus that stabilization of the spine involved by malignancy has a major role in treatment—one that cannot be achieved by either chemotherapy or RT.

Although posterior stabilization is frequently performed in conjunction with decompression, it may occasionally be indicated for those in whom instability alone is the predominant problem. Patients with atlantoaxial or atlantooccipital instability from metastases to the upper cervical spine or skull base represent such examples.[167] Although our experience suggests that conservative treatment with steroids and RT while the patient is immobilized in a cervical orthosis may suffice in the majority of patients with radiosensitive tumors, the presence of persistent pain following RT is an indicator of instability and suggests the need for operative stabilization. Instability at these levels may be rotational or axial (resulting from cranial settling).

The most widely used techniques for fixation include the use of sublaminar wiring in conjunction with bone grafts or with methyl methacrylate.[28, 48, 71]

Historically, the use of wiring through the base of the spinous processes (or around it), with the incorporation of methyl methacrylate that is allowed to polymerize in situ, represents the earliest surgical efforts in spinal fixation. Whereas the use of methyl methacrylate in conjunction with sublaminar wiring is applicable in the upper cervical spine, posterior stabilization with methyl methacrylate (with or without wiring) should not be used in the thoracic or lumbar regions. Even in the cervical region, wiring of the individual spines with methyl methacrylate does not produce major resistance to axial loading, with the result that collapse of the vertebral bodies with pull-out of the wires can occur with time.

Of the various posterior instrumentation systems, the most widely used is the Harrington rod system developed for scoliosis. This system consists of either compression rods or distraction rods. The distraction rods apply axial forces through sublaminar hooks attached by means of a hub at one end and a ratchet mechanism at the other end. Spinal deformity is corrected by applying a distraction force and three-point bending and depends upon an intact anterior longitudinal ligament to prevent overdistraction. The compression system consists of thinner threaded rods, hooks, and small nuts, which allow less correction of sagittal deformities but which provide stability using a "tension band" of the posteriorly disrupted ligamentous complex. Early reports suggested that distraction instrumentation might have a useful role in the management of tumors causing pain by localized collapse, with pain relief noted in more than 75 per cent of patients.[34, 97, 166] Although still widely used for thoracolumbar fractures in trauma, there have been a number of problems related to hook displacement, increased neurologic deficits, and failures of instrumentation, such that its current role is very limited.[92, 105] From a biomechanical standpoint, the major drawback of the system is that the corrective force is applied only at the ends of the rods; thus, loosening or cutting through of the upper hooks is a potential complication. In addition, its use is limited to the lower thoracic and thoracolumbar segments; long-term results from its use in the lumbar region may result in the flat back syndrome from reversal of the lumbar lordosis.

Although the modification of the Harrington system suggested by Jacobs and associates represents a major improvement in design,[80] there is little experience with its use in tumors. Since the majority of spinal surgeons treating scoliotic deformities are now using the Cotrel-Dubousset Universal System, this system may be indicated in those cases in which Harrington distraction instrumentation was used in the past.[32, 176] The CD rods are of two types: longitudinal and transverse (DTT). The longitudinal rod used in CD instrumentation is supple, has no notches, and has diamond-shaped irregularities on its entire surface. It allows fixation of a system of vertebral hooks and screws by bolting at any level, and allows both distraction and compression. It can be prebent along its entire length to fit the physiologic curvatures

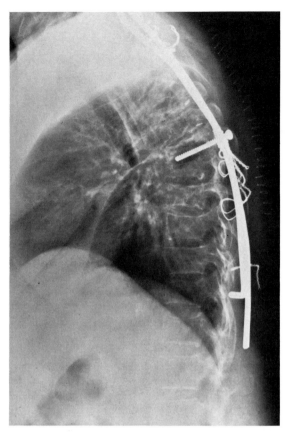

Figure 29–20. Following posterolateral decompression, extremely long segments can be stabilized with Luque L-rods at least two levels above and below the site of decompression. The distal ends are wired and crossed over one another to resist torsional stresses. A transpedicular screw has also been placed to enhance fixation.

osteoporotic vertebrae. Experimental data using axial loading suggest that it is superior to Harrington instrumentation and may be comparable to the CD system, except in resisting torsional stresses.[4, 190] We and others have found it of value either following posterolateral decompression or as a primary stabilization procedure, with improvement in pain ranging from 60 to 80 per cent.[38, 52, 77, 92, 148, 156, 157] Although some have advocated the additional use of methyl methacrylate, we have found that the additional use of acrylic in a radiated field may predispose to wound dehiscence. The major drawback is that the technique of sublaminar wiring takes a long time, with operations averaging 4 to 6 hours in length; it may occasionally be accompanied by considerable blood loss.

In Europe, posterior stabilization is generally performed by instrumentation fixed through the pedicles into the vertebral bodies, which was introduced by Roy-Camille more than 20 years ago.[39, 141] Biomechanical data suggest that pedicle fixation, by incorporating all three columns, is the most stable form of mechanical fixation; in addition, a major advantage is the limited number of motion segments that have to be incorporated.[39, 69] This is particularly useful in the patient who has undergone prior laminectomy. Although there is tremendous enthusiasm for pedicle fixators in Europe, the approach in the United States has been more guarded. The technical process of passing screws from the posterior approach through the pedicle is fraught with the possibility of nerve root and vessel injury and should therefore not be attempted by the occasional surgeon.

of the spine; by rotation of the prebent rod from the sagittal to the coronal plane, three-dimensional correction (derotation) can be achieved. In addition to the rods, it comes with a system of hooks and screws that allow fixation both at the ends and in the intermediate segment. Experience with this system in tumors is limited, and there is a substantial learning curve when one is learning to use the system.[176] It is also the most expensive of the posterior instrumentation systems.

At present, the most widely used posterior instrumentation is the Luque rod with segmental spinal fixation. It is currently available in two diameters (3/16 and 1/4 inches) and comes as a system of L-shaped, C-shaped, or retangular rods of varying lengths. For proper fixation, sublaminar wiring with 16- or 18-gauge wire three levels above and below the level of decompression is recommended. The rod can be contoured to the physiologic curvatures of the spine, which is important in the cervical, cervicothoracic, and lumbar regions. Using the Galveston technique,[1] it allows fixation across the lumbosacral junction and maintains the normal lumbar lordosis. By distributing the stresses evenly by multiple sublaminar wires, its use can be expanded to those with

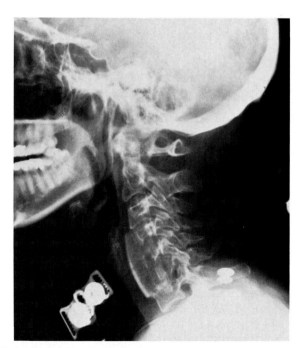

Figure 29–21. In potential long-term survivors, the vertebral bodies can be resected and replaced with an iliac strut graft as shown. We generally use a course of radiation therapy prior to using autologous grafts.

Anterolateral Approaches (Vertebral Body Resection)

In our experience, the anterior approach by vertebral body resection fulfills the basic principles of tumor surgery: it provides extensive exposure, allows for complete resection of all gross tumor, and provides adequate access for anterior stabilization. In patients with neoplasms, the importance of immediate stabilization cannot be overemphasized. Stabilization allows immediate ambulation and minimizes pulmonary and embolic complications. In view of the limited life expectancy in the cancer patient and the need for postoperative radiation therapy, we believe that polymethyl methacrylate (PMMA) is the stabilizing construct of choice and has several major advantages over bone grafts. If autologous bone grafts are used, the time required for arthrodesis may range from three to six months; in patients who have received prior RT, time for fusion may be even longer. In those who require postoperative radiation, bone grafts may not incorporate at all. Thus, bone grafts should be used primarily in patients with slowly growing primary benign tumors or with other low grade malignancies in whom RT is not being contemplated.

Polymethyl methacrylate is an acrylic polymer belonging to the polyolefin group of synthetic plastics. It is commercially available as a liquid monomer (40 ml) that is mixed with the powdered polymer (20 grams). "Curing" or self-polymerization occurs through a self-catalytic process as well as additives. During the heat of polymerization, intense heat is generated (80 to 100 degrees centigrade) for periods of 5 minutes. The orthopedic polymethyl methacrylate is impregnated by 10 per cent barium sulfate, which allows radiographic visualization. There is no bonding at the bone-cement interface, and therefore the acrylic has to be kept in place with additional instrumentation. Its strength is not adversely affected by irradiation or by the incorporation of antibiotics.[74, 183]

To prevent displacement of the construct and to enhance resistance to flexion loads, a variety of instrumentation techniques have been proposed to prevent collapse; these include the Dunn device, Kostuik-Harrington device, Kaneda implant, Knodt and Harrington distraction rods, Armstrong and A-O plates, as well as Steinmann pins.[13, 43, 84, 92, 123, 153, 165] As a substitute for acrylic, some have proposed metal or ceramic prostheses, none of which have gained general acceptance.[87, 90] The Dunn device has since been withdrawn from the market because it was associated with vascular injury, and many complex anterior distraction devices are not generally available, except for the Kaneda device, which is currently undergoing trials. Some of the drawbacks of distraction devices have been summarized by Harrington: (1) a large amount of metal has to be left outside the vertebral column, which may predispose to vessel injury; (2) the axis of distraction is lateral rather than anterior, thus limiting the correction of kyphosis; and (3) vertebral fixation is aligned at right angles to the weight-bearing axis, subjecting them to large torque stresses in the lumbar spine.[74]

Although we have experimented with a variety of distraction devices, we have found that the technique of using Steinmann pins to ensure fixation of the acrylic is satisfactory in most cases; this technique is simple, easily mastered, and requires minimal special equipment. Our experience with this anterior fixation now totals more than 200 cases, and it has been associated with a minimal incidence of complications. Although there has been concern that acrylic constructs would fail over time and a number of mechanical failures have been described by McAfee and colleagues,[105] our experience suggests that it is stable over many years. The major cause of displacement is poor technique or failure to appreciate additional posterior stability; in our experience, tumor recurrences in the adjacent vertebra is the single most important cause of recurrent failure and movement of the construct.

The anterior spine requires a variety of approaches because of the complex soft part anatomy anterior to the prevertebral space (Table 29–5). A familiarity with all approaches is important in getting adequate exposure for tumor resection. An initial considera-

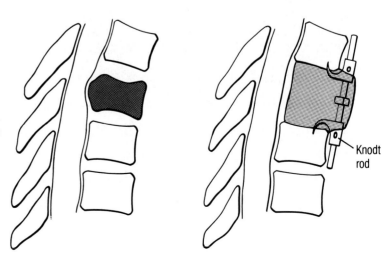

Figure 29–22. A variety of anterior distraction instrumentation is available, of which the simplest is the Knodt rod technique advocated by Harrington.

Knodt rod

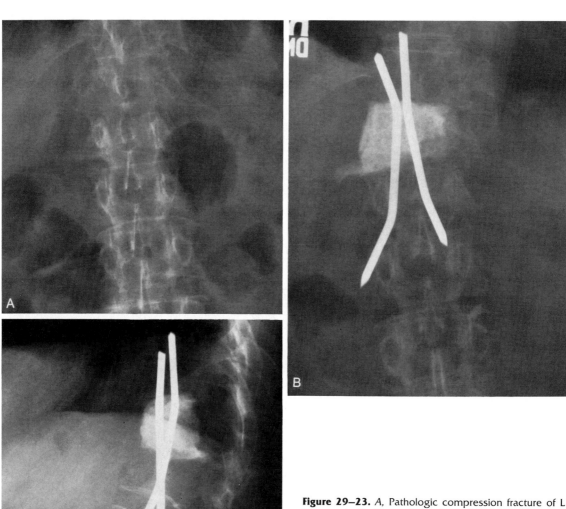

Figure 29–23. *A,* Pathologic compression fracture of L1. The most effective and simple method of stabilization is replacement of the body with methyl methacrylate and Steinmann pins as illustrated in (*B*) and (*C*).

TABLE 29–5. CLASSIFICATION OF ANTERIOR SPINAL APPROACHES

SEGMENT	LEVELS	APPROACH
Cervical	C1–C2	Transoral, transmandibular
	C3–C7	Transcervical (Cloward)
Cervicothoracic	C7–T1	Transsternal, transthoracic
Thoracic	T3–T10	Transthoracic, posterolateral thoracotomy
Thoracolumbar	T11–L1	Transthoracic, extrapleural, thoracoabdominal
Lumbar	L2–L4	Retroperitoneal
Lumbosacral	L5–S1	Transabdominal
Sacral	S2–S5	Extra- or intraabdominal, transperineal

tion is the side from which an anterolateral exposure should be performed. In the majority, the side that allows maximal tumor resection should be chosen. This can usually be ascertained by CT or MRI scan. If a CT scan is not available, then the side of increased pedicle destruction or collapse, or the symptomatic side of radiculopathy or plexopathy, probably indicates the site of tumor compression. In equivocal cases, a right-sided approach is chosen for thoracic segments, and a left-sided approach is chosen for lumbar segments. In all patients, complete tumor resection down to the dura must be accomplished; this frequently involves removal of the posterior longitudinal ligament by microdissection. Since tumor resection is carried out by intralesional curettage, recurrence is inevitable unless microscopic residual tumor can be eradicated by RT or chemotherapy. The anterior approach also allows resection of tumor posterior to the dura in the thoracic and lumbar segments, if the facets and pedicles are removed. In the cervical region, a second-stage posterior approach may be required; a second posterior approach is also indicated in potential long-term survivors if MRI scans reveal tumor posterior to the cord following anterior decompression. Following tumor resection, stabilization should be carried out. Postoperative RT may be given within a week, since the skin incision frequently lies outside the RT portal.

Lateral Osteotomy Approach

The spine may also be approached from the side by the lateral osteotomy approach, which is performed by cutting through the transverse process of the vertebra and by fracturing the osteotomized portion of the paraspinal structures anteriorly. The major indications for this procedure are in patients with superior sulcus tumors or other lung cancers with chest wall involvement, as well as in those with large paraspinous sarcomas with both anterolateral and posterolateral components. The skin incision may be oblique, as in the thoracic region, or may be T-shaped, with the shorter limbs of the T in the midline. Initially, the paraspinal tumor mass is dissected free from the lateral and anterior attachments, including the intraabdominal and intrathoracic ves-

sels; secondly, it is freed superiorly and inferiorly by resection of the chest wall or the paraspinous muscles. Finally the paraspinous muscles are cut over the transverse processes and the main mass of the tumor is fractured forward. Nerve roots are carefully isolated and clipped. If the intraspinal extensions of tumor are noted, the spinal resection should include a partial hemilaminectomy and facetectomy. No additional reconstruction is required after such lateral ostectomy procedures. Following extensive chest wall resection, extensive skeletal defects may require reconstruction with a Marlex mesh prosthesis.

Results

Patients undergoing anterior spinal surgery and stabilization procedures require monitoring in the intensive care unit because of the potential for respiratory complications in addition to the other common postoperative problems, such as ileus, venous thrombosis, and infection. Complications related to surgery may be classified into general and more specific neurologic complications. Since the cancer patient is generally more ill, has hematologic abnormalities, and is likely to be immunosuppressed from therapy, the morbidity rate from surgery is generally in the range of 10 to 15 per cent. Neurologic worsening or deficit from surgery can be seen in 10 to 20 per cent of patients treated by posterior laminectomy but in less than 5 per cent of patients treated by the anterior approach in several large series.[72, 92, 153, 162] We allow early ambulation and recommend rapid tapering of steroid therapy. In our experience, patients who have received recent radiation therapy, as well as high dose steroid therapy for more than a month, are particularly likely to develop perioperative complications. In high risk patients, we use subcutaneous heparin therapy (5000 to 10,000 units subcutaneously twice a day). A custom-fitted polyform orthosis is generally recommended for most patients.

Despite their seeming magnitude, anterolateral decompression by vertebral body resection and stabilization is well tolerated by most cancer patients. Indeed current morbidity is lower than that previously reported for laminectomy. This is attributable to two major causes: (1) this operation is more effective, and thus there are fewer deaths resulting from complications of failed treatment; and (2) patients are generally more carefully selected for the anterior procedure, whereas the posterior operation is frequently used in patients with far advanced disease. In our experience with the first 160 patients, the 30-day mortality rate was 6 per cent, and an additional 15 per cent developed surgical complications. However, the mortality rate for patients undergoing de novo operation was 4 per cent, and the morbidity was 10 per cent. No serious permanent neurologic defect was encountered, and all other complications were effectively treated without sequelae. Neurologic improvement exceeded 80 per cent, and two thirds of patients who were nonambulatory improved to the point of ambulation. In those patients with significant pain, more than 80 per cent experienced relief. In long-term survivors, the long-term ambulation rate exceeded 90 per cent at one year, although repeat anterior or posterior decompressions were necessary in 20 per cent of patients. These figures are superior to those reported for external RT and steroid therapy alone. Similar results have been noted by others, including Siegal, Harrington, and Kostuik.[74, 92, 154] The superiority of this procedure for specific tumors has been demonstrated by retrospective case comparisons for kidney and lung cancer.[161, 165, 171] We have recently completed a phase II prospective study that shows that surgery followed by RT produces ambulation rates that are far superior (90 per cent) to RT alone, with more than 90 per cent of such patients maintaining their status until death.[174] We have been able to keep many patients alive for two to five years if they have localized disease, although multiple operations (including spondylectomy) may be required in the majority. Thus, the goal of potential curability for those with primary neoplasms and solitary metastases is no longer impossible. We therefore would advocate early operation (even for purely intraosseous disease) in selected patients for solitary sites of relapse in the spine. The results currently achieved by experienced spine surgeons are so superior to those reported for external RT, that a controlled prospective trial to demonstrate the value of operation does not seem ethical unless our colleagues who advocate RT in all patients as initial treatment can produce comparable results.

REFERENCES

1. Allen BL, Ferguson RL: The Galveston technique for Luque rod instrumentation of the scoliotic spine. Spine 7:276–284, 1984.
2. American Cancer Society: Facts and Figures, 1989.
3. Anand AK, Krol G, Deck MD: Lumbosacral epidural metastases: CT evaluation and comparison with myelography. Comput Radiol 7:351–354, 1983.
4. Ashman RB, Birch JG, Bone LB, et al: Mechanical testing of spinal instrumentation. Clin Orthop Rel Res 227:113–125, 1988.
5. Aoki J, Yamamoto I, Hino M, et al: Osteoclast mediated osteolysis in bone metastases from renal cell carcinoma. Cancer 62:98–104, 1988.
6. Bailar III JC, Smith EM: Progress against cancer. N Engl J Med 314:1226–1232, 1986.
7. Barcena A, Lobato RD, Rivas JJ, et al: Spinal metastatic disease: Analysis of factors determining functional prognosis and choice of treatment. Neurosurgery 15:820–827, 1984.
8. Barron KD, Hisano A, Araki S, Terry RD: Experiences with metastatic neoplasms involving the spinal cord. Neurology 9:91–106, 1959.
9. Batson OV: The role of vertebral veins in metastatic processes. Ann Intern Med 16:38–45, 1942.
10. Bernat JL, Greenberg ER, Barrett J: Suspected epidural compression of the spinal cord and cauda equina by metastatic cancer. Cancer 51:1953–1957, 1983.
11. Berrettoni BA, Carter JR: Mechanisms of cancer metastasis to bone. J Bone Joint Surg 68(A):308–312, 1986.
12. Bever CT Jr, Koenigsberger MR, Antunes JL, Wolff JA: Epidural metastasis by Wilms' tumor. Am J Dis Child 135:644–646, 1981.
13. Black RC, Gardner VO, Armstrong GWD, et al: A contoured anterior spinal fixation plate. Clin Orthop Rel Res 227:135–142, 1988.
14. Black P: Spinal metastases: Current status and guidelines for management. Neurosurgery 5:726–746, 1979.
15. Boccardo M, Ruelle A, Mariotti E, Severi P: Spinal carcinomatous metastases. Retrospective study of 67 surgically treated cases. J Neurooncol 3:251–258, 1984.
16. Bockman RS: Hypercalcemia in malignancy. Clin Endocrinol Metab 9:317–333, 1980.
17. Body JJ, Borkowski A, Cleeren A, Bijvoet OLM: Treatment of malignancy associated hypercalcemia with intravenous amino hydroxy propylidene diphosphonate. J Clin Oncol 4:1177–1183 1986.
18. Boland PJ, Lane JM, Sundaresan N: Metastatic disease of the spine. Clin Orthop 169:95–102, 1982.
19. Bowers TA, Murray JA: Bone metastases from renal carcinoma: The preoperative use of transcatheter arterial occlusion. J Bone Joint Surg 64(A):749–754, 1982.
20. Breslow L, Cumberland WG: Progress and objectives in cancer control. JAMA 259:1690–1694, 1988.
21. Bridwell KH, Jenny AB, Saul T, et al: Posterior segmental spinal instrumentation (PSSI) with posterolateral decompression and debulking for metastatic thoracic and lumbar spine disease: Limitations of the technique. Spine 13:1383–1394, 1988.
22. Bruckman JE, Bloomer WD: Management of spinal cord compression. Semin Oncol 5:135–140, 1978.
23. Carabell SC: Spinal cord compression. In DeVita VT, Hellman S, Rosenberg SA (eds): Cancer: Principles and Practice of Oncology. 2nd Ed. Philadelphia, JB Lippincott, 1985, pp 1860–1865.
24. Carr BI, Goodkin R: Breast cancer with osseous metastasis and herniated lumbar disc. A cautionary tale. Cancer 56:1701–1703, 1985.
25. Carstens SA, Resnick D: Diffuse sclerotic skeletal metastases as an initial feature of gastric carcinoma. Arch Intern Med 140:1666–1668, 1980.
26. Chien LT, Kalwinsky DK, Peterson G, et al: Metastatic epidural tumors in children. Med Pediatr Oncol 10:455–462, 1982.
27. Citrin DL, Bessent RG, Greig WR: A comparison of the sensitivity and accuracy of the Tc-99 phosphate bone scan and skeletal radiograph in the diagnosis of bone metastases. Clin Radiol 28:107–117, 1977.
28. Clark CR, Keggi KJ, Panjabi MM: Methyl methacrylate stabilization of the cervical spine. J Bone Joint Surg 66(A):40–46, 1984.
29. Constans JP, de Divitiis E, Donzelli R, et al: Spinal metastases with neurological manifestations. J Neurosurg 59:111–118, 1983.
30. Corcoran RJ, Thrail JH, Kyle RW, et al: Solitary abnormalities in bone scans of patients with extra-osseous malignancies. Radiology 121:663–667, 1976.
31. Costigan DA, Winkelman MD: Intramedullary spinal cord metastasis. J Neurosurg 62:227–233, 1985.
32. Cotrel Y, Dubousset J, Guillaumat M: New universal instrumentation in spinal surgery. Clin Orthop Rel Res 227:10–23, 1988.
33. Cramer SF, Fried L, Carter KJ: The cellular basis of metastatic bone disease in patients with lung cancer. Cancer 48:2649–2660, 1981.
34. Cusick JF, Larson SJ, Walsh PR, Steiner RE: Distraction stabilization in the treatment of metastatic carcinoma. J Neurosurg 59:861–866, 1983.
35. Cybulski GR, Von Roenn KA, D'Angelo CM, DeWald RL: Luque rod stabilization for metastatic disease of the spine. Surg Neurol 28:277–283, 1987.
36. Delattre JV, Arbit E, Rosenblum MK, et al: High dose versus low dose dexamethasone in experimental epidural spinal cord compression. Neurosurgery 22:1005–1007, 1988.
37. Denis F: Spinal instability as defined by the three column spine concept in acute spinal trauma. Clin Orthop Rel Res 189:65–76, 1984.

38. DeWald RL, Bridwell KL, Prodromas C, Rodts MF: Reconstructive surgery as palliation for metastatic malignancies of the spine. Spine 10:21–26, 1985.

39. Dick W: Internal Fixation of Thoracic and Lumbar Spine Fractures. Toronto, Hans Huber, 1989.

40. Dorfman LJ, Donaldson SS, Gupta PR, Bosley TM: Electrophysiologic evidence of subclinical injury to the posterior columns of the spinal cord after therapeutic radiation. Cancer 50:2815–2819, 1982.

41. Doubilet PM, Seltzer SE, Hessel SJ: Computed tomography in the diagnosis and management of paravertebral masses. Comput Radiol 8:101–106, 1984.

42. Dunn RC, Kelly WA, Whons RNW, Howe JF: Spinal epidural neoplasia. A 15 year review of the results of surgical therapy. J Neurosurg 52:47–51, 1980.

43. Dunn HK: Anterior stabilization of thoraco-lumbar injuries Clin Orthop 189:116–124, 1984.

44. Elomaa I, Blomqvist G, Grohn P: Long term controlled trial with diphosphonate in patients with osteolytic bone metastases. Lancet 1:146–149, 1983.

45. Falcone AE, Nappi JF: Chemotherapy and wound healing. Surg Clin North Am 64:779–794, 1984.

46. Feldman AR, Kessler L, Myers MH, Naughton MD: The prevalence of cancer: Estimates based on the Connecticut Tumor Registry. N Engl J Med 315:1394–1397, 1986.

47. Fer MF, Greco FA, Oldham RK: Poorly Differentiated Neoplasms and Tumors of Unknown Origin. Orlando, Grune & Stratton, 1987.

48. Fidler MW: Pathological fractures of the cervical spine. Palliative surgical treatment. J Bone Joint Surg 67(B):352–357, 1985.

49. Findlay GFG: Adverse effects of the management of malignant spinal cord compression. J Neurol Neurosurg Psych 47:761–768, 1984.

50. Fink IJ, Garra BS, Zabell A: Computed tomography with metrizamide myelography to define the extent of spinal canal block due to tumor. J Comput Assist Tomogr 8:1072–1075, 1984.

51. Fisher MS: Lumbar spine metastasis in cervical carcinoma: A characteristic pattern. Radiology 134:631–634, 1980.

52. Flatley JJ, Anderson MH, Anast GT: Spinal instability due to metastatic disease; treatment by segmental spinal stabilization. J Bone Joint Surg 66(A):47–52, 1984.

53. Foley KM: The treatment of cancer pain. N Engl J Med 31:84–95, 1985.

54. Fontana M, Pompili A, Cattani F, Mastrostefano R: Metastatic spinal cord compression. Follow-up study. J Neurosurg Sci 24:141–146, 1980.

55. Forbes G, Nichols DA, Jack CR, et al: Complications of spinal cord arteriography: Prospective assessment of risk for diagnostic procedures. Radiology 169:479–484, 1988.

56. Fornasier VL, Horne JG: Metastases to the vertebral column. Cancer 36:590–594, 1975.

57. Friedlander GE: Bone grafts—the basic science rationale for clinical applications. J Bone Joint Surg 69(A):786–790, 1987.

58. Fyfe I, Henry APJ, Mulholland RC: Closed vertebral biopsy. J Bone Joint Surg 65(B):140–143, 1983.

59. Galasko CSB, Bennett A: Relationship of bone destruction in skeletal metastases to osteoclast activation and prostaglandins. Nature 263:508–510, 1976.

60. Galasko CSB: Skeletal Metastases. London, Butterworth, 1986.

61. Galasko CSB: The significance of occult skeletal metastases, detected by skeletal scintigraphy, in patients with otherwise apparent "early" mammary carcinoma. Br J Surg 67:694–696, 1975.

62. Gilbert RW, Kim JH, Posner JB: Epidural spinal cord compression from metastatic tumor; diagnosis and treatment. Ann Neurol 3:40–51, 1978.

63. Godersky JC, Smoker WRK, Knutzon R: Use of magnetic resonance imaging in the evaluation of metastatic spinal disease. Neurosurgery 21:676–680, 1987.

64. Goldberg LD, Ditchek NT: Thyroid carcinoma with spinal cord compression. JAMA 245:953–954, 1981.

65. Goodkin R, Carr BI, Perrin RG: Herniated lumbar disc in patients with malignancy. J Clin Oncol 5:667–671, 1987.

66. Goodwin-Austen RB, Howell DA, Worthing B: Observations on radiation myelopathy. Brain 98:557–568, 1975.

67. Graus F, Krol G, Foley K: Early diagnosis of spinal epidural metastasis: Correlation with clinical and radiologic findings (abstr). Proc Am Soc Clin Oncol 4:269, 1985.

68. Greenberg HS, Kim JH, Posner JB: Epidural spinal cord compression from metastatic tumor: Results with a new treatment protocol. Ann Neurol 8:361–366, 1980.

69. Gurr KR, McAfee PC, Shih CM: Biomechanical analysis of posterior instrumentation systems after decompressive laminectomy. An unstable calf–spine model. J Bone Joint Surg 70(A):680–691, 1988.

70. Hagenau C, Grosh W, Currie M, Wiley RG: Comparison of magnetic resonance imaging and myelography in cancer patients. J Clin Oncol 5:1663–1669, 1987.

71. Hansebout RR, Blomquist GA Jr: Acrylic spinal fusion: A 20-year clinical series and technical note. J Neurosurg 53:606–612, 1980.

72. Harbin WP: Metastatic disease and the nonspecific bone scan: Value of spinal computed tomography. Radiology 145:105–107, 1982.

73. Harper GR, Rodichuk LD, Prevosti L, et al: Early diagnosis of spinal metastases leads to improved treatment outcome (abstr). Proc Am Soc Clin Oncol 1:6, 1982.

74. Harrington KD: Anterior cord decompression and spinal stabilization for patients with metastatic lesions of the spine. J Neurosurg 61:107–117, 1984.

75. Harrington KD: Metastatic disease of the spine. J Bone Joint Surg 68A:1110–1115, 1986.

76. Harrison KM, Muss HB, Ball MR, et al: Spinal cord compression in breast cancer. Cancer 55:2839–2844, 1985.

77. Heller M, McBroom RJ, MacNab T, Perrin R: Treatment of metastatic disease of the spine with postero-lateral decompression and Luque instrumentation. Neuroorthopedics 2:70–74, 1986.

78. Hollis PH, Malis LI, Zapulla RA: Neurological deterioration after lumbar puncture below complete spinal subarachnoid block. J Neurosurg 64:253–256, 1986.

79. Ikeda H, Ushio Y, Hayakawa T: Edema and circulatory disturbances in the spinal cord compressed by epidural neoplasm in rabbits. J Neurosurg 52:203–209, 1980.

80. Jacobs RR, Dakness LE, Gertzbein SD, et al: A locking hook spinal rod: Current status of development. Paraplegia 21:197–200, 1983.

81. Jaeckle KA, Young DF, Foley KM: The natural history of lumbosacral plexopathy in cancer. Neurology 35:8–15, 1985.

82. Johnson JR, Leatherman KD, Holt RT: Anterior decompression of the spinal cord for neurological deficit. Spine 8:396–405, 1983.

83. Kaneda A, Yamamura I, Kamikozuru M, Nakai O: Paraplegia as a consequence of corticosteroid therapy. J Bone Joint Surg 66(A):783–785, 1984.

84. Kaneda K, Abumi K, Fujuja M: Burst fractures with neurological deficits of the thoraco-lumbar spine: Results of anterior decompression and stabilization with anterior instrumentation. Spine 9:788–795, 1984.

85. Kapp DS, LiVolsi VA, Kohorn EI: Cauda equina compression secondary to metastatic carcinoma of the uterine corpus: Preservation of neurologic function and long term survival following surgical decompression and radiation. Gynecol Oncol 20:209–218, 1985.

86. Kato A, Ushio Y, Hayakawa T, et al: Circulatory disturbance of the spinal cord with epidural neoplasm in rats. J Neurosurg 63:260–265, 1985.

87. Kawabata M, Sugiyama M, Suzuki T, Kumano K: The role of metal and bone cement fixation in the management of malignant lesions of the vertebral column. Int Orthop 4:177–181, 1980.

88. Kelly WM, Badami P, Dillon W: Epidural block: Myelographic evaluation with a single puncture technique using metrizamide. Radiology 151:417–419, 1984.

89. Kerber CW, Bank WO: Polyvinyl alcohol (Ivalon): Prepackaged emboli for therapeutic embolization. AJR 139:1193–1196, 1978.

90. Kobayashi S, Hara H, Okudera H, et al: Usefulness of ceramic implants in neurosurgery. Neurosurgery 21:751–755, 1987.

91. Kori S, Foley KM, Posner JB: Brachial plexus lesions in patients with cancer. Neurology 31:45–50, 1981.

92. Kostuik JP, Errico TJ, Gleason TF, Errico CC: Spinal stabilization of vertebral column tumors. Spine 13:250–256, 1988.

93. Krol G, Heier L, Becker R, et al: MRI and myelography in the evaluation of epidural extension of primary and metastatic tumors. In Volk J (ed): Neuroradiology. Amsterdam, Elsevier, 1985, pp 91–99.

94. Kuhlman JE, Fishman EK, Leichner PK, et al: Skeletal metastases from hepatoma: Frequency, distribution, and radiographic features. Radiology 160:175–180, 1986.

95. Lee YY, Glass JP, Wallace S: Myelography in cancer patients: Modified technique. AJR 145:791–795, 1985.

96. Leeson MC, Makley JT, Carter JR: Metastatic skeletal disease in the pediatric population. J Pediatr Orthop 5:261–267, 1985.

97. Lesoin F, Kabbaj K, Debout J, et al: The use of Harrington rods in metastatic tumor with spinal cord compression. Acta Neurochir 65:175–181, 1982.

98. Levy WJ, Latchaw JP, Hardy RW, Hahn JF: Encouraging surgical results in walking patients with epidural metastases. Neurosurgery 11:229–233, 1982.

99. Liskow A, Chang CH, DeSantis P, et al: Epidural cord compression in association with genitourinary neoplasms. Cancer 58:949–954, 1986.

100. Lowenthal DA, Scher HI, Mauskop A, et al: Prospective evaluation of 35 patients with prostatic cancer with suspected epidural metastasis (abstr). Proc Am Soc Clin Oncol 5:108, 1986.

101. Luce EA: The irradiated wound. Surg Clin North Am 64:821–829, 1984.

102. Macedo N, Sundaresan N, Galicich JH: Decompressive laminectomy for metastatic cancer: what are the current indications? Proc Am Soc Clin Oncol 4:278, 1985.

103. Martenson JA, Evans RL, Lie MR, et al: Treatment outcome and complications in patients treated for malignant cord compression. J Neurooncol 3:77–84, 1985.

104. Martin NA, Gutin PH, Newman AB, Pickett JB: Neurogenic claudication due to narrowing of the lumbar canal by extradural metastatic tumor. Neurosurgery 9:436–439, 1981.

105. McAfee PC, Bohlman HH, Ducker T, Eismont FJ: Failure of stabilization of the spine with methacrylate: A retrospective analysis of 24 cases. J Bone Joint Surg 68(A):1145–1157, 1986.

106. McAfee PC, Bohlman HH: Complications following Harrington instrumentation for fractures of the thoraco-lumbar spine. J Bone Joint Surg 67(A):672–676, 1985.

107. McNeil BJ: Value of bone scanning in neoplastic disease. Semin Nucl Med 4:277, 1984.

108. Miles J, Banks AJ, Dervin E, Noori Z: Stabilization of the spine affected by malignancy. J Neurol Neurosurg Psych 47:897–904, 1984.

109. Miller F, Whitehill R: Carcinoma of the breast metastatic to the skeleton. Clin Orthop 184:121–127, 1984.

110. Mundy GR, Ibbotson KJ, K'DSouza SM: The hypercalcemia of cancer: Clinical implications and pathogenic mechanisms. N Engl J Med 310:1718–1727, 1984.

111. Mundy GR, Wilkinson R, Heath DA: Comparative study of available medical therapy for hypercalcemia of malignancy. Am J Med 74:421–432, 1983.

112. Murphy KC, Feld R, Evans WK, et al: Intramedullary spinal cord metastases from small cell carcinoma of the lung. J Clin Oncol 1:99–106, 1983.

113. Murray PK: Functional outcome and survival in spinal cord injury secondary to neoplasia. Cancer 55:197–201, 1985.

114. Nather A, Bose K: The results of decompression of cord or cauda equina from metastatic extradural tumor. Clin Orthop 169:103–108, 1982.

115. Nemoto R, Kanoh S, Koiso K, Harada M: Tumor-bone interaction by transplantable human tumors in nude mice. Cancer 62:1310–1316, 1988.

116. Obbens EAMT, Kim JH, Thaler H, et al: Metronidazole as a radiation enhancer in the treatment of metastatic epidural spinal cord compression. J Neurooncology 2:99–104, 1984.

117. Onimus M, Schraub S, Bertin D, et al: Surgical treatment of vertebral metastasis. Spine 11:883–891, 1986.

118. O'Neil J, Gardner V, Armstrong G: Treatment of tumors of the thoracic and lumbar spinal column. Clin Orthop Rel Res 227:103–112, 1988.

119. Overby MC, Rothman AS: Anterolateral decompression for metastatic epidural spinal cord tumors. J Neurosurg 62:344–348, 1985.

120. O'Carroll MP, Witcombe JB: Primary disorders of bone with "spinal block." Clin Radiol 30:299–306, 1979.

121. O'Rourke T, George CB, Redmond J III, et al: Computed tomography following metrizamide myelography in the early diagnosis of metastatic disease of the spine. J Clin Oncol 4:578–583, 1986.

122. Pratt YZ, Peters RE, Chuang VP, et al: Palliation of pelvic recurrence of colorectal intra-arterial 5-fluouracil and mitomycin. Cancer 56:2175–2180, 1985.

123. Perrin RG, McBroom RJ: Spinal fixation after anterior decompression for symptomatic spinal metastasis. Neurosurgery 22:324–327, 1988.

124. Perrin RG, Livingston KE, Aarabi B: Intradural extramedullary spinal metastasis. A report of 10 cases. J Neurosurg 56:835–837, 1982.

125. Perrin RG, McBroom RJ: Anterior versus posterior decompression for symptomatic spinal metastasis. Can J Neurol Sci 14:75–80, 1987.

126. Perrin RG, Livingston KE: Neurosurgical treatment of pathological fracture-dislocation of the spine. J Neurosurg 52:330–334, 1980.

127. Pilipshen SJ, Heilweil M, Quan SHQ, et al: Patterns of pelvic recurrence following definitive resections of rectal cancer. Cancer 53:1354–1362, 1984.

128. Pittaluga S, Soffer D, Siegal T, Siegal T: Massive hemorrhagic necrosis of the spinal cord in metastatic cord compression. Clin Neuropathol 2:114–117, 1983.

129. Portnoy RK, Lipton RB, Foley KM: Back pain in the cancer patient: An algorithm for evaluation and management. Neurology 37:134–138, 1987.

130. Posner JB, Howieson J, Cvitkovic E: "Disappearing" spinal cord compression: Oncolytic effects of glucocorticoids (and other chemotherapy agents) on epidural metastases. Ann Neurol 2:409–413, 1977.

131. Punt J, Pritchard J, Pincott JR, Till K: Neuroblastoma: A review of 21 cases presenting with spinal cord compression. Cancer 45:3095–3101, 1980.

132. Ralston SH, Gardner MD, Dryburgh FJ, et al: Comparison of aminohydroxy propylidene diphosphonate, mithramycin and corticosteroids, and calcitonin in treatment of cancer associated hypercalcemia. Lancet 2:907–910, 1985.

133. Redmond J, Spring DB, Munderloh SH, et al: Spinal computed tomography in the evaluation of metastatic disease. Cancer 54:253–258, 1984.

134. Rice DP, Hodgson TA, Kopstein AN: The economic costs of illness: A replication and update. Health Care Fin Rev 7:61–80, 1985.

135. Ries LG, Pollack ES, Young JL Jr: Cancer patient survival: Surveillance, Epidemiology and End Results Program 1973–1979. J Natl Cancer Inst 70:693–707, 1983.

136. Rodichok LD, Harper GR, Ruckdeschel JC: Early diagnosis of spinal epidural metastases. Am J Med 70:1181–1188, 1981.

137. Rodichok LD, Ruckdeschel JC, Harper GR, et al: Early detection and treatment of spinal epidural metastases: The role of myelography. Ann Neurol 20:696–702, 1986.

138. Rodriguez M, DiNapoli RP: Spinal cord compression with special reference to metastatic epidural tumors. Mayo Clin Proc 55:442–448, 1980.

139. Roof BS, Gordan GS, Halden A: Skeletal effects of cancer and their management. In Holland JF, Frei E III (eds): Cancer Medicine. 2nd Ed. Philadelphia, Lea & Febiger, 1982, pp 1264–1273.

140. Rosenberg SA: Surgical Treatment of Metastatic Cancer. Philadelphia, JB Lippincott, 1987.

141. Roy-Camille R: Osteosynthese dorso-lumbar d'une metastase vertebrale. Nouv Presse Med 1:2463–2466, 1972.

142. Sarpel S, Sarpel G, Yu E, et al: Early diagnosis of spinal—epidural metastasis by magnetic resonance imaging. Cancer 59:1112–1116, 1987.

143. Schaberg J, Gainor BJ: A profile of metastatic carcinoma of the spine. Spine 10:19–20, 1985.

144. Scharr MM: Diagnosis of spinal cord and cauda equina metastases. Prog Exp Tumor Res 29:93–104, 1985.

145. Scheid V, Buzdar AU, Smith TL, Hortobagyi GN: Clinical course of breast cancer patients with osseous metastasis treated with combination chemotherapy. Cancer 58:2589–2593, 1986.

146. Schiller JH, Rasmussen P, Benson AB, et al: Maintenance etidronate in the prevention of malignancy induced hypercalcemia. Arch Intern Med 147:963–966, 1987.

147. Shaw M, Rose J, Paterson A: Metastatic extradural malignancies of the spine. Acta Neurochir 52:113–120, 1980.

148. Sherman RM, Waddell JP: Laminectomy for metastatic epidural spinal cord tumors. Posterior stabilization, radiotherapy, and preoperative assessment. Clin Orthop 207:55–63, 1986.

149. Sherry MM, Greco FA, Johnson DH, Hainsworth JD: Breast cancer with skeletal metastases at initial diagnosis. Cancer 58:178–182, 1986.

150. Shibasaki K, Harper CG, Bedbrook GM, Kakulas BA: Vertebral metastases and spinal cord compression. Paraplegia 21:47–61, 1983.

151. Siegal T, Siegal T, Shapira Y, et al: Indomethacin and dexamethasone treatment in experimental neoplastic cord compression: Parts 1 and 2. Neurosurgery 22:328–339, 1988.

152. Siegal T, Siegal T, Robin G, Fuks Z: Anterior decompression of the spine for metastatic epidural cord compression: Is it a promising avenue of therapy? Ann Neurol 11:28–34, 1982.

153. Siegal T, Siegal T: Surgical decompression of anterior and posterior malignant epidural tumors compressing the spinal cord: A prospective study. Neurosurgery 17:424–432, 1985.

154. Siegal T, Tikva P, Siegal T: Vertebral body resection for epidural compression by malignant tumors. A Series of 47 consecutive cases. J Bone Joint Surg 67A:375–382, 1985.

155. Slatkin NE, Posner FB: Management of spinal epidural metastases. Clin Neurosurg 30:698–716, 1983.

156. Solini A, Paschero B, Orsini G, Guercio N: The surgical treatment of metastatic tumors of the lumbar spine. Ital J Orthop Traumatol 11:427–442, 1985.

157. Solini A, Paschero B: Surgical management of spinal cord lesions due to metastases. J Neurosurg Sci 28:201–212, 1984.

158. Stark RJ, Henson RA, Evans SJW: Spinal metastases: A retrospective survey from a general hospital. Brain 105:189–213, 1982.

159. Steffee AD, Biscup RS, Sitkowski DJ: Segmental spine plates with pedicle screw fixation—A new internal fixation device for disorders of the lumbar and thoracolumbar spine. Clin Orthop Rel Res 203:45–53, 1986.

160. Suit H: The problem of primary tumor control. Cancer 61:2148–2152, 1988.

161. Sundaresan N, Bains MS, McCormack P: Surgical treatment of spinal cord compression in lung cancer. Neurosurgery 16:350–356, 1985.

162. Sundaresan N, DiGiacinto GV, Hughes JEO: Surgical treatment of spinal metastases. Clin Neurosurg 33:503–522, 1986.

163. Sundaresan N, DiGiacinto GV: Antitumor and anti-nociceptive approaches to cancer pain. Med Clin North Am 71:329–348, 1987.

164. Sundaresan N, Galicich JH, Bains MS, et al: Vertebral body resection in the treatment of cancer involving the spine. Cancer 53:1393–1396, 1984.

165. Sundaresan N, Galicich JH, Lane JM, et al: Treatment of neoplastic epidural cord compression by vertebral body resection and stabilization. J Neurosurg 63:676–684, 1985.

166. Sundaresan N, Galicich JH, Lane JM: Harrington rod stabilization for pathological fractures of the spine. J Neurosurg 60:282–286, 1984.

167. Sundaresan N, Galicich JH, Lane JM: Treatment of odontoid fracture in cancer patients. J Neurosurg 52:187–191, 1981.

168. Sundaresan N, Galicich JH: Treatment of spinal metastases by vertebral body resection. Cancer Invest 2:383–397, 1984.

169. Sundaresan N, Hilaris BH, Martini N: The combined neurosurgical-thoracic management of superior sulcus tumors. J Clin Oncol 5:1739–1745, 1987.

170. Sundaresan N, Krol G, Hughes JEO: Treatment of malignant tumors of the spine. In Youmans J (ed): Neurological Surgery. 3rd ed. Philadelphia, WB Saunders, 1990.

171. Sundaresan N, Scher H, Yagoda A, et al: Surgical treatment of spinal metastases in kidney cancer. J Clin Oncol 4:1851–1856, 1986.

172. Sundaresan N, DiGiacinto GV, Hughes JEO: Surgical approaches to primary and metastatic tumors of the spine. In Schmidek HH, Sweet WH (eds): Operative Neurosurgical Techniques: Indications, Methods, Results. Vol 2. Orlando, Grune & Stratton, 1988, pp 1525–1537.

173. Sundaresan N, Galicich JH, Lane JM, Scher H: Stabilization of the spine involved by cancer. In Dunsker SB, Schmidek HH, Frymoyer J, Kahn III (eds): The Unstable Spine. Orlando, Grune & Stratton, 1986, pp 249–274.

174. Sundaresan N, DiGiacinto GV, Hughes JEO: Treatment of neoplastic cord compression: Results of a prospective study (abstr). AANS 1988.

175. Sundaresan N, DiGiacinto GV, Hughes JEO, Krol G: Spondylectomy for malignant tumors of the spine. J Clin Oncol (in press).

176. Sypert GW: Stabilization procedures for thoracic and lumbar fractures. Clin Neurosurg 34:340–377, 1988.

177. Sze G, Krol G, Zimmerman RD, Deck MDF: Malignant extradural tumors: MR imaging with GD-DTPA. Radiology 167:217–223, 1984.

178. Sze G, Abramson A, Krol G: Gadolinum DTPA in the evaluation of intradural extramedullary spinal disease. AJNR 9:153–163, 1988.

179. Tang SG, Byfield JE, Sharp TR: Prognostic factors in the management of metastatic epidural cord compression. J Neurooncol 1:21–28, 1981.

180. Thiebaud D, Jaeger PH, Jacquet AF, Burkhardt P: Dose response in the treatment of malignancy by a single infusion of biphosphonate AHPrBP. Am J Clin Oncol 6:762–768, 1988.

181. Tomita T, Galicich JH, Sundaresan N: Radiation therapy for spinal epidural metastases with complete block. Acta Radiol Oncol 22:135–143, 1983.

182. Tong D, Gillick L, Hendrickson FR: The palliation of symptomatic osseous metastases: Final results of the study by the Radiation Therapy Oncology Group. Cancer 50:893–899, 1982.

183. Trippel SB: Antibiotic impregnated cement in total joint arthroplasty. J Bone Joint Surg 68(A):1292–1302, 1986.

184. Ushio Y, Posner R, Kim JH, et al: Treatment of experimental cord compression caused by extradural neoplasms. J Neurosurg 47:380–390, 1977.

185. Vick NA: Letter to the editor. J Neurooncol 5:125–128, 1987.

186. Wang GJ, Lewish GD, Reger SI, et al: Comparative strengths of various anterior cement fixations of the cervical spine. Spine 7:717–721, 1983.

187. Warrell RP Jr, Alcock NW, Bockman RS: Gallium nitrate inhibits accelerated bone turnover in patients with bone metastases. J Clin Oncol 5:292–298, 1987.

188. Watkins RG: Surgical Approaches to the Spine. Berlin, Springer Verlag, 1983.

189. Weissman DE, Gilbert M, Wang H, Grossman SA: The use of computed tomography of the spine to identify patients at high risk for epidural metastases. J Clin Oncol 3:1541–1544, 1985.

190. Wenger DR, Carollo JJ, Wilkerson JA Jr, et al: Laboratory

testing of SSI versus traditional Harrington instrumentation for scoliosis treatment. Spine 7:265–269, 1982.

191. Weissman DE, Dufer D, Vogel V, Abeloff MD: Corticosteroid toxicity in neurooncology patients. J Neurooncol 5:125–128, 1987.

192. Weissman DE: Glucocorticoid treatment for brain metastases and epidural cord compression: A review. J Clin Oncol 6:543–551, 1988.

193. White AA III, Panjabi MM: The basic kinematics of the human spine: A review of past and current knowledge. Spine 3:12–30, 1978.

194. Young RF, Post EM, King GA: Treatment of spinal epidural metastases. Randomized prospective comparison of laminectomy and radiotherapy. J Neurosurg 53:741–748, 1980.

195. Zito G, Kadis GN: Multiple vertebral hemangiomas resembling metastases with spinal cord compression. Arch Neurol 37:247–248, 1980.

SURGICAL TREATMENT FOR SPINAL METASTASES:

The Posterolateral Approach

R. G. PERRIN AND R. J. McBROOM

The management of spinal metastases remains a matter of considerable debate. The purpose of this chapter is to examine surgical treatment by the posterolateral approach.

CLASSIFICATION

Spinal secondaries are conveniently classified according to anatomic location.[4, 15, 18, 35, 41] The vast majority occur extradurally. Intradural extramedullary metastases are uncommon, whereas intramedullary spinal metastases are rarely encountered (Table 30–1).

INCIDENCE

Skeletal metastases occur in the majority of patients with systemic cancer, and the spine is most commonly involved. It is estimated that between 5 and 9 per cent of cancer patients will develop spinal cord and nerve root compromise due to spinal metastases.[4, 7, 14, 20, 21]

Symptomatic spinal metastases most frequently originate from carcinoma of the breast, prostate, and lung—consistent with the prevalence of these respective primaries and the recognized propensity for carcinoma of the breast and prostate to metastasize to bone.[3, 4, 7, 17, 22, 28] Some 10 per cent of patients with symptomatic spinal metastases present with no known culpable primary.[7, 17, 28]

The thoracic spine is the most common site for symptomatic spinal metastases, with the segments about T4 and T11 most often affected.[4, 12, 15, 17, 28, 46–48] Intradural extramedullary metastases most frequently occur about the thoracolumbar junction, where they are found entangled among the cauda equina nerve roots.[35]

CLINICAL FEATURES

Symptomatic spinal metastases produce a characteristic clinical syndrome.[28, 34, 35, 46] Local back or neck pain is the earliest and most prominent feature in some 90 per cent of patients. A radicular pain syndrome is frequently present. If the pain is described as severe, burning, and dysesthetic in character, then intradural extramedullary metastases should be suspected. Palpating the spine at a level involved with extradural metastasis usually elicits local tenderness. If the local back and neck pain is aggravated by movement about the involved segment and is relieved by immobilization, then the probability of underlying mechanical instability must be considered.[34] Localized back or neck pain of symptomatic spinal metastases is often initially dismissed as back strain, arthritis, or neurosis, and correct diagnosis may be delayed until more blatant manifestations of spinal cord or nerve root compromise are apparent.[4, 28] It is axiomatic that a cancer patient who develops back or neck pain harbors spinal metastasis until proven otherwise. Pain is followed by weakness, sensory loss, and sphincter dysfunction. Weakness may develop months after the onset of pain, and the rate at which motor dysfunction develops is variable. However, once present, weakness will progress relentlessly to complete and

TABLE 30–1. RELATIVE FREQUENCY OF SPINAL METASTASES ACCORDING TO ANATOMIC CLASSIFICATION

Author	Patients	ED	ID/EM	IM
Rogers and Heard (1958)[41]	17	94%	6% (one case)	—
Barron et al. (1959)[4]	125	98%	—	1.6%
Edelson et al. (1972)[18]	175	97%	—	3.4%
Perrin et al. (1981)[35]	200	94%	5%	0.5%

ED = extradural, ID/EM = intradural/extramedullary; IM = intramedullary.

305

irreversible paraplegia unless timely treatment is undertaken.

IMAGING STUDIES

Plain x-rays of the spine provide a useful screening test for symptomatic spinal metastases.[4, 38, 43, 45] Osteoblastic metastases may occur, particularly with carcinoma of the breast or prostate; however, the majority of plain film findings show lytic bony destruction. Common plain film findings include pedicle erosion (or sclerosis), paravertebral soft tissue shadow, vertebral collapse, and frank pathologic fracture dislocation.

Pedicle erosion is the earliest and most frequent abnormality seen on plain films[25, 28] (Fig. 30–1). An anteroposterior radiograph of the thoracolumbar spine can be likened to a "totem of owls" (Fig. 30–2). Pedicle erosion due to spinal metastases produces a "winking owl" sign.[33] The site of pedicle erosion is often associated with paravertebral soft tissue shadow[4, 25, 42] (Fig. 30–3). Bony destruction may be sufficiently extensive to result in vertebral collapse causing wedge compression (Fig. 30–4). More advanced vertebral destruction can result in pathologic fracture dislocation[34] (Fig. 30–5).

Lumbar myelography will demonstrate a complete block in the majority of patients with symptomatic spinal metastases who are candidates for neurosurgical decompression[26, 28, 43] (Fig. 30–6). A cisternal myelogram is also indicated to accurately define the location and extent of compressing lesions when the

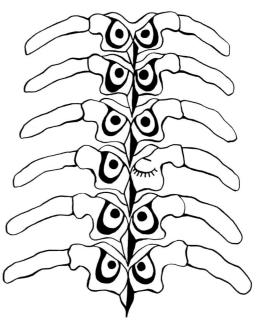

FIGURE 30–2. Anteroposterior radiograph of the thoracolumbar spine resembles a totem of owls. The site of pedicle erosion produces a "winking owl" (and if the erosion occurs bilaterally—a "blinking owl").

anatomic level of a complete lumbar myelographic block does not correspond to the clinical localization, or when multiple levels of involvement are suspected (Fig. 30–7).

Computed tomography (CT) scan may prove useful to demonstrate the disposition of spinal metastases in horizontal cross-section (Fig. 30–8).

Magnetic resonance imaging (MRI) has become the investigation of choice; it is able to display multiple levels of local contiguous as well as remote involvement through sagittal planes extending the length of the spine (Fig. 30–9). The epidural tumor geometry demonstrated by MRI helps to determine the approach for decompression which will be required. The degree of vertebral destruction displayed by MRI helps to anticipate the extent and technique of spinal stabilization which may be necessary.

MANAGEMENT

The treatment of patients with symptomatic spinal metastases is undertaken to relieve pain and to preserve or restore neurologic function. The goal is generally palliation. Nevertheless, relief from pain and preservation or restoration of neurologic function contribute immeasurably to the quality of remaining life.

There has been considerable debate concerning the relative merits of therapeutic irradiation,[7, 17, 19, 20, 22] surgery,[1, 5, 8, 30, 34, 44, 47, 49–51] or a combination of these modalities[10, 11, 28, 29, 47, 48] for the treatment of spinal metastases. Therapeutic irradiation is the initial treatment of choice in the majority of patients and has proven especially effective for lymphoreticular metastases.[6, 17, 20, 22, 31, 45]

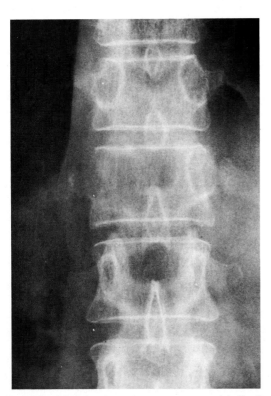

FIGURE 30–1. Pedicle erosion—the most common plain film finding in patients with symptomatic spinal metastases.

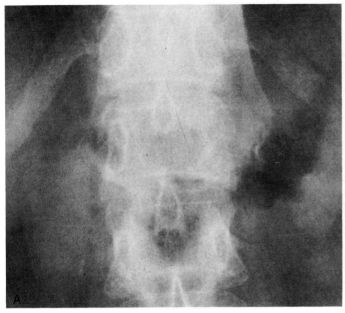

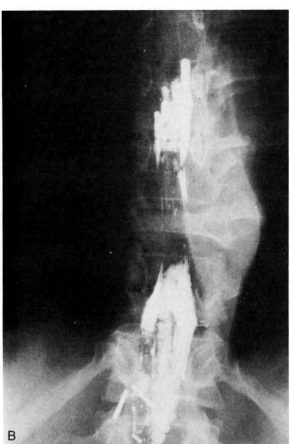

FIGURE 30–3. Paraspinal soft tissues shadow associated (A) with a "winking owl" sign and (B) with a pathologic fracture.

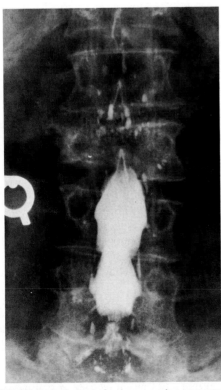

FIGURE 30–4. Pathologic fracture—wedge compression.

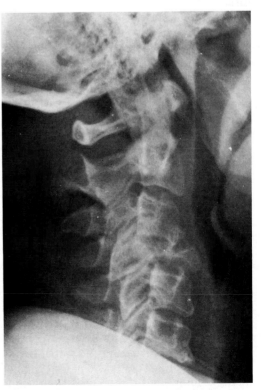

FIGURE 30–5. Pathologic fracture—dislocation of C4.

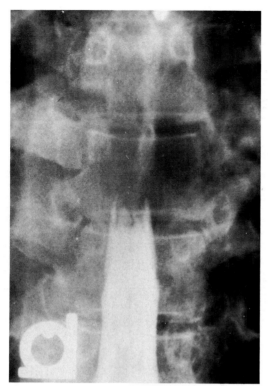

FIGURE 30—6. Complete block on myelography. (Note the "winking owl.")

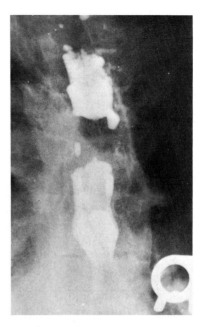

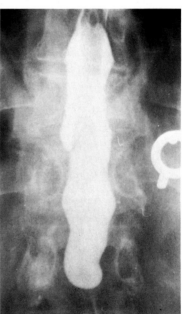

FIGURE 30—7. Composite lumbar and cisternal myelography showing complete blocks bracketing the involved segment.

The indications for surgical intervention include the following (Table 30–2).

Radiation Failure. Surgical intervention is indicated when relapse occurs following therapeutic irradiation. In our experience, the majority of patients with symptomatic spinal metastases who come to surgical decompression have already received the maximum tolerable therapeutic irradiation, and following this spinal cord or nerve roots compromise has occurred due to persistent or recurrent tumor. In addition, patients with spinal metastases judged to be resistant to therapeutic irradiation may be candidates for surgical decompression.

Diagnosis Unknown. Neurosurgical decompression may be diagnostic as well as therapeutic when symptomatic spinal metastases occur without a known primary. Furthermore, surgery is indicated when pathology other than metastatic tumor is suspected (i.e., disc, abscess, hematoma) in a cancer patient.[23]

Pathologic Fracture Dislocation. Compression of spinal cord and nerve roots in patients with pathologic fracture dislocation is usually due to a combination of distortion caused by spinal malalignment and compression produced by extradural tumor.[34] Surgical intervention is then necessary to reduce the dislocation, to achieve decompression of the spinal cord, and to secure stabilization of the spinal column.

Rapidly Evolving or Far-Advanced Paraplegia. Neurosurgical decompression is indicated in patients with rapidly evolving or far-advanced neurologic dysfunction. Therapeutic irradiation may aggravate partial paraplegia.[13, 39] Complete and irreversible def-

icit may then occur before the potential benefits of therapeutic irradiation and/or chemotherapy are realized.

There is general consensus that prompt recognition is essential for treatment to be most effective.[2, 4, 9, 22, 24, 31, 37, 48]

TABLE 30–2. INDICATIONS FOR SURGICAL INTERVENTION IN PATIENTS WITH SYMPTOMATIC SPINAL METASTASES

Radiation failure
Diagnosis unknown
Pathologic fracture dislocation
Rapidly evolving/far-advanced paraplegia

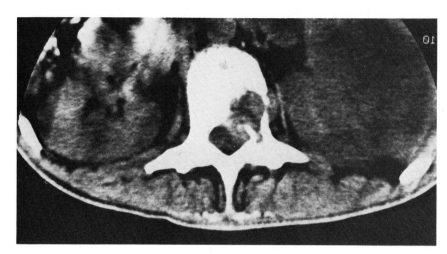

FIGURE 30–8. CT scan of lumbar spine showing anterolateral tumor.

Surgical Strategies

Surgical strategies for spinal metastases must provide for both decompression of the spinal cord and nerve roots as well as stabilization of the spinal column.[36] Decompression of the spinal cord and nerve roots may be accomplished from the front or from behind. Each approach has its place, and neither method is always applicable.[36] The most appropriate surgical approach to a particular patient depends on a number of factors, which may be considered under the following heading.

The Decompression

Symptomatic extradural spinal metastases most commonly arise laterally along the spinal canal, as would be expected given the observed frequency of pedicle erosion ("winking owl" sign), the most common plain film finding. The compressing lesion may be anterolateral—but lateral nonetheless (Figs. 30–8 and 30–10). It is uncommon for symptomatic extradural spinal metastases to be located focally and exclusively anterior or (even less common) posterior along the spinal canal. Occasionally, epidural metastases may extend circumferentially about the dural sac. Moreover, the compressing lesion may consist almost exclusively of epidural tumor lying within the spinal canal and with little or no bone destruction.

The posterolateral approach allows extensive and effective tumor resection around the circumference of the dural sac and the nerve roots, and bilaterally. The posterolateral approach is applicable along the

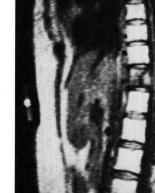

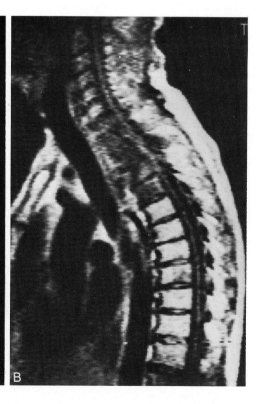

FIGURE 30–9. MRI sagittal spine image showing (*A*) single lower thoracic level involvement and (*B*) multiple contiguous cervicothoracic levels of involvement.

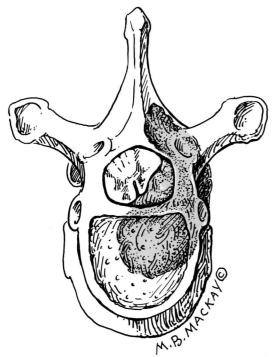

FIGURE 30–10. Diagram depicting typical location of lateral (and anterolateral) extradural metastases.

length of the spinal column and is readily extended longitudinally for additional segments, as is often required.[27, 28, 36]

The anterior approach permits excellent exposure for the majority of the cervical segments with visualization of root sleeves bilaterally. The anterior approach through the chest or abdomen, however, allows access anterolaterally on one side only. The root sleeves on the side opposite the direct approach through the chest or abdomen are difficult to visualize and, consequently, are vulnerable to injury (nerve root damage and cerebrospinal fluid [CSF] fistula) when circumferential decompression is attempted from an anterolateral exposure.[36, 37]

The anterior approach poses significant technical problems at the cephalad and caudad extremes of the spinal column.

Intradural spinal metastases should be approached posteriorly through a simple laminectomy.[35]

The Stabilization

Spinal stabilization is of critical concern in the management of patients with symptomatic spinal metastases. Spinal stability is essential to relieve pain and to prevent recurrent (mechanical) spinal cord and nerve root compromise. Consequently, the ability to achieve secure spinal stability must influence the surgical approach.

Adequate decompression of the spinal cord and nerve roots from behind involves extensive posterolateral resection, which must frequently be applied bilaterally.[28] Consequent spinal instability necessitates fixation of the spinal column, which can be accomplished by segmental instrumentation with sublaminar wires and rods or with pedicular screws and plates.

Posterior decompression procedures performed through an irradiated field, which are followed by spinal stabilization, have been associated with a high incidence of wound dehiscence (with or without infection).[27] Consequently, in the absence of other considerations, an anterior approach would appear to be preferable.

Spinal stabilization is obligatory following anterior decompression procedures that involve vertebral corporectomy.[44] Anterior stabilization poses enormous technical problems at the cephalad and caudad extremes of the spinal column. Furthermore, anterior stabilization is less effective if more than two spinal segments must be spanned.[36, 37]

Whether undertaken from in front or from behind, spinal stabilization techniques are dependent on bony integrity sufficient to accept the fixation devices at levels adjacent to the decompression site.

The Patient

Patients with symptomatic spinal metastases who are in the advanced stages of their disease may be too debilitated to withstand an anterior (transthoracic or transabdominal) procedure. Surgical decompression from behind is less involved and may be better tolerated.

Posterolateral Decompression

Critics of posterior decompression procedures for spinal extradural metastases point out, and correctly so, that simple laminectomy is inadequate. They maintain that the compressing tumor is largely anteriorly or anterolaterally situated and conclude, incorrectly so, that anteriorly disposed spinal metastasis must be removed from in front.

Adequate decompression from behind involves a wide laminectomy exposure extending from a half segment below through a half segment above the compressed cord segment. During the stripping of paraspinal muscles from the spines and laminae, care must be taken to avoid inadvertently plunging through the vertebral laminar layer, which may be deficient owing to tumor destruction. The extradural compressing tissue should be carefully elevated from the dura using, for example, an angled cup curette (Fig. 30–11). The wide resection should be extended posterolaterally about the circumference of the dural sac and anteriorly to beyond the level of the emergence of nerve root sleeves. This procedure generally involves removal of the tumor-destroyed lateral elements and pedicles, which provides access into the vertebral body. The nerve root sleeves are carefully stripped of encasing tumor. Encased nerve roots in the thoracic region may be intentionally crushed if radicular pain attributable to such nerve roots is a prominent feature of the presenting clinical syndrome. Excavation of the tumor-involved vertebral body is accomplished with the aid of an angled cup

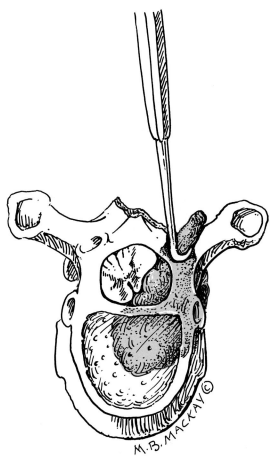

FIGURE 30–11. Elevation of tumor-destroying lamina with up-angled cup curette.

curette and pituitary forceps. A reverse angled cup curette is useful to displace anteriorly disposed tumor mass from the dural sac (Fig. 30–12).

The posterolateral exposure may be undertaken bilaterally with resultant radical and circumferential decompression of the spinal cord and nerve roots (Figs. 30–13 and 30–14).

The posterolateral approach is based on standard laminectomy techniques, affords excellent exposure, permits thorough and circumferential decompression of the dural sac and nerve roots, is applicable along the length of the spinal column, and is readily extended for additional segments (as is often required). The posterior approach avoids a more complicated transthoracic or transabdominal procedure.

Stabilization Following Posterolateral Decompression

The majority of patients who have had an adequate posterolateral decompression of the spinal cord and nerve roots for symptomatic spinal metastases will require stabilization of the spinal column. The combination of vetebral body destruction by tumor and bony resection during surgical decompression will usually result in spinal instability.

The three-column concept used for determining spinal stability in cases of spinal trauma[16] may also

be applied for patients with spinal metastases. Tumor destruction of the anterior and middle columns will eventually lead to failure of the vertebral body under axial load.

The consequent spinal instability may lead to progressive vertebral collapse and frank pathologic fracture dislocation, with mechanical compression of the spinal cord and nerve roots. Posterolateral decompression, by necessity, results in violation of the posterior column and converts a two-column disruption into a three-column disruption. Consequently, rather than improving a patient's pain syndrome, spinal decompression may indeed aggravate discomfort due to mechanical instability.

In the rare circumstance that the symptomatic extradural metastasis is purely posterior to the dural sac, or the tumor is exclusively epidural without bony involvement—that is, the anterior and middle spinal columns remain intact—surgical decompression from behind may be possible without spinal stabilization.

The aim of posterior instrumentation is to provide immediate spinal stability, which will remain intact for the duration of the patient's survival. It is essential to secure multiple levels of fixation to the spine and at a minimum of two levels above and two levels below the decompression site. Spinal fixation may be achieved using sublaminar wires attached to Luque or Harrington rods (Fig. 30–15) or with methyl methacrylate struts. Pedicle screws and plates provide

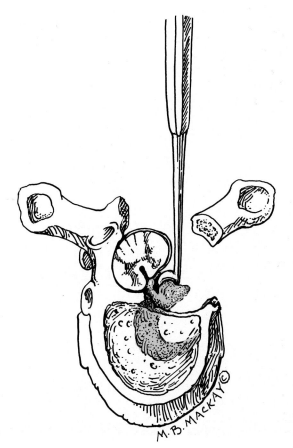

FIGURE 30–12. Displacement of lateral and anterolateral tumor with down-angled cup curette.

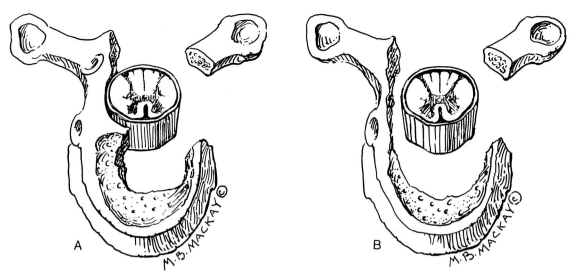

FIGURE 30–13. *A,* Posterolateral decompression of the dural sac and contents. *B,* Bilateral approach results in circumferential decompression.

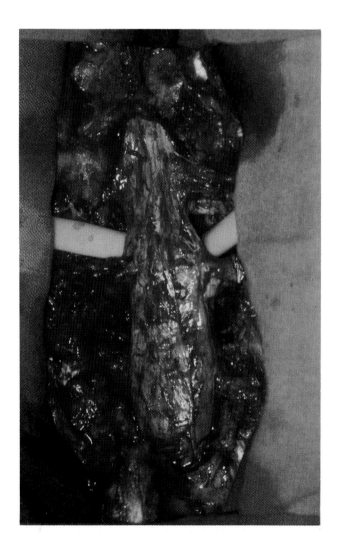

FIGURE 30–14. Operative photograph showing circumferential decompression of the dural sac and nerve roots. Note the surgical clip on the midthoracic root, which was crushed for pain relief.

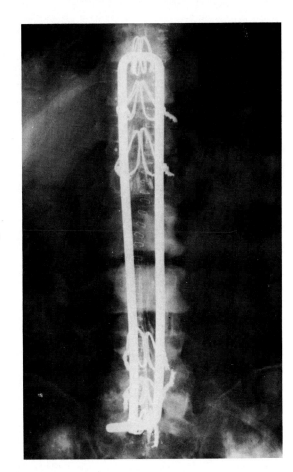

FIGURE 30–15. Luque rod (rectangle) with sublaminar fixation at three levels above and three levels below the posterolateral lumbar decompression site.

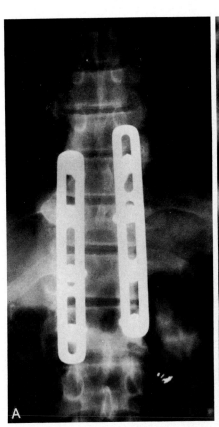

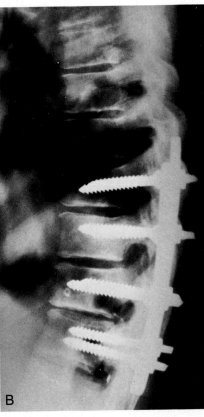

FIGURE 30–16. Anteroposterior (*A*) and lateral (*B*) views showing Steffe plates with pedicular screws for stabilization at the thoracolumbar junction.

an alternative in the lower thoracolumbar area (Fig. 30–16).

Autogenous bone should be used if it is anticipated that the patient may enjoy a prolonged survival. Bone grafts are slow to incorporate in a milieu characterized by osteopenia, residual local tumor, and perioperative therapeutic irradiation. Segmental instrumentation is most appropriate for the majority of cancer patients.

We have encountered few late failures of fixation.[27] The routine use of spinal instrumentation following posterolateral decompression contributes considerably to the patient's postoperative pain relief. Furthermore, spinal deformity and instability are corrected so that recurrent cord compression at the same level is prevented.

CONCLUSION

Our experience with the treatment of symptomatic spinal metastases at the Wellesley Hospital, Toronto, includes some 400 patients. The posterolateral approach has provided beneficial pain relief in 80 per cent of cases. Two thirds of patients have been ambulatory following surgical treatment, compared with 35 per cent who were walking preoperatively. Four per cent of patients were worse after surgery. Forty-three per cent of patients have achieved a satisfactory result,[9] that is, they have been walking and have been continent six months following surgery.

Optimal treatment for patients with symptomatic spinal metastases involves appropriate patient selection, strategic procedural planning, and effective surgical execution.

REFERENCES

1. Alexander E, Davis CH, Field CH: Metastatic lesions of the vertebral column causing cord compression. Neurology 6:103–107, 1956.
2. Andersen EB: Karcinom metastaser i Columna Vertebralis. Ugeskr Laeger 137:2251–2256, 1975.
3. Auld AW, Buerman A: Metastatic spinal epidural tumors. Arch Neurol 15:100–108, 1966.
4. Barron KD, Hirano A, Araki S, Terry RD: Experience with metastatic neoplasms involving the spinal cord. Neurology 9:91–106, 1959.
5. Benson WJ, Scarffe JH, Todd IDH, et al: Spinal cord compression in myeloma. Br Med J 1:1541–1544, 1979.
6. Bhagwati SN, McKissock W: Spinal cord compression in Hodgkin's disease. Br J Surg 48:672–676, 1961.
7. Black P: Spinal metastasis: Current status and recommended guidelines for management. Neurosurgery 5:726–745, 1979.
8. Bogoch ER, English E, Perrin RG, Tator CH: Successful surgical decompression of spinal extradural metastases of liposarcoma. Spine 8:228–235, 1983.
9. Botterell EH, Fitzgerald GN: Spinal cord compression produced by extradural malignant tumors. Can Med Assoc J 80:791–796, 1959.
10. Brady LW, et al: The treatment of metastatic disease of the nervous system by radiation therapy. In Seydel HG (ed):

11. Brice J, McKissock W: Surgical treatment of malignant extradural spinal tumors. Br Med J 1:1341–1344, 1965.
12. Bruckman JE, Bloomer WD: Management of spinal cord compression. Semin Oncol 5:135–140, 1978.
13. Cairns H, Fulton JF: Experimental observations on the effect of radon on the spinal cord. Lancet 2:16, 1930.
14. Clarke E: Spinal cord involvement in multiple myelomatosis. Brain 79:332–348, 1986.
15. Chade HD: Metastatic tumors of the spine and spinal cord. In Vinken PJ, Bruyn GW (eds): Handbook of Clinical Neurology. Vol 20. Amsterdam, North-Holland Publishing Co., 1976, pp 415–433.
16. Denis F: Spinal instability as defined by the three-column spine concept in acute spinal trauma. Clin Orthop 189:75–86, 1986.
17. Dunn RC Jr, Kelly WA, Wohns RN, Howe JF: Spinal epidural neoplasia: A 15-year review of the results of surgical therapy. J Neurosurg 52:47–51, 1980.
18. Edelson RN, Deck MDF, Posner JB: Intramedullary spinal cord metastases: Clinical and radiographic findings in nine cases. Neurology 22:1222–1231, 1972.
19. Eisen HM, Bosworth JL, Ghossein NA: The rationale for whole-spine irradiation in metastatic breast cancer. Radiology 108:417–418, 1973.
20. Friedman M, Kim TH, Panahon AM: Spinal cord compression in malignant lymphoma: Treatment and results. Cancer 37:1485–1491, 1976.
21. Galasko CSB: Skeletal metastases and mammary cancer. Ann R Coll Surg Engl 50:3–28, 1972.
22. Gilbert RW, Kim JH, Posner JB: Epidural spinal cord compression from metastatic tumor: Diagnosis and treatment. Ann Neurol 3:40–51, 1978.
23. Goodkin R, Carr BI, Perrin RG: Herniated lumbar disc disease in patients with malignancy. J Clin Oncol 5:667–671, 1987.
24. Greenberg HS, Kim JH, Posner JB: Epidural spinal cord compression from metastatic tumor: Results with a new treatment protocol. Ann Neurol 8:361–366, 1980.
25. Hall AJ, Mackay NNS: The results of laminectomy for compression of the cord or cauda equina by extradural malignant tumor. J Bone Joint Surg (Br) 55:497–505, 1973.
26. Hatam A, Hindmarsh T, Greitz T: Myelography in metastatic lesions. Acta Radiol (Diagn) 16:321–330, 1975.
27. Heller M, McBroom RJ, Macuds T, Perrin RG: Treatment of metastatic disease of the spine with posterolateral decompression and Luque instrumentation. Neuro-Orthopaedics 2:70–74, 1986.
28. Livingston KE, Perrin RG: Neurosurgical management of spinal metastases. J Neurosurg 49:839–843, 1978.
29. Marshall LF, Langfitt TW: Combined therapy for metastatic extradural tumors of the spine. Cancer 40:2067–2070, 1977.
30. Merrin C, Avellanosa A, West C, et al: The value of palliative spinal surgery in metastatic urogenital tumors. J Urol 115:712–713, 1976.
31. Mullan J, Evans JP: Neoplastic disease of the spinal extradural space. Arch Surg 74:900–907, 1957.
32. Murphy KC, Feld R, Evans WK, et al: Intramedullary spinal cord metastases from small cell carcinoma of the lung. J Clin Oncol 1:99–106, 1983.
33. Perrin RG: Beware the winking owl (cover illustration). J Neurosurg 48(6), 1978.
34. Perrin RG, Livingston KE: Neurosurgical treatment of pathological fracture dislocation of the spine. J Neurosurg 52:330–334, 1980.
35. Perrin RG, Livingston KE, Aarabi B: Intradural extramedullary spinal metastasis. J Neurosurg 56:835–837, 1982.
36. Perrin RG, McBroom RJ: Anterior versus posterior decompression for symptomatic spinal metastasis. Canad J Neurol Sci 14:75–80, 1987.
37. Perrin RG, McBroom RJ: Spinal fixation after anterior decompression for symptomatic spinal metastasis. Neurosurgery 22:324–327, 1988.
38. Rodichok LD, Harper GR, Ruckdeschel JC, et al: Early diag-

nosis of spinal epidural metastases. Am J Med 70:1181–1188, 1981.

39. Rogers L: Malignant spinal tumors and the epidural space. Br J Surg 45:416–422, 1958.

40. Rogers L: The surgery of spinal tumors. Lancet 1:187–190, 1935.

41. Rogers L, Heard G: Intrathecal spinal metastases (rare tumors). Br J Surg 45:317–320, 1958.

42. Rome RM, Nelson JH: Compression of the spinal cord or cauda equina complicating gynaecological malignancy. Gynaecol Oncol 5:273–290, 1977.

43. Sellwood RB: The radiological approach to metastatic cancer of the brain and spine. Br J Radiol 45:647–651, 1972.

44. Sundareson N, Galicich J, Bains M, et al: Vertebral body resection in the treatment of cancer involving the spine. Cancer 53:1393–1396, 1984.

45. Van Woerkom-Eijkenboom WMH, Braakman R: Paraplegia due to spinal epidural neoplasia. Paraplegia 19:100–106, 1987.

46. Vieth RG, Odom GL: Extradural spinal metastases and their neurosurgical treatment. J Neurosurg 23:501–508, 1965.

47. White WA, Patterson RH Jr, Bergland RM: Role of surgery in the treatment of spinal cord compression by metastatic neoplasm. Cancer 27:558–561, 1971.

48. Wild WO, Porter RW: Metastatic epidural tumor of the spine. Arch Surg 87:825–830, 1963.

49. Wilson CB, Fewer D: Role of neurosurgery in the management of patients with carcinoma of the breast. Cancer 28:1681–1685, 1971.

50. Wright RL: Malignant tumors in the spinal extradural space. Ann Surg 157:227–231, 1963.

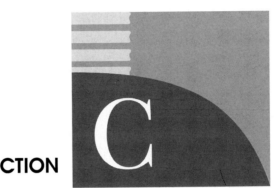

SECTION C

SURGICAL CONSIDERATIONS AND APPROACHES

THE TRANSORAL-TRANSCLIVAL APPROACH TO THE UPPER CERVICAL SPINE

31

VOLKER K. H. SONNTAG, MARK N. HADLEY,
and ROBERT F. SPETZLER

INTRODUCTION

The transoral-transclival surgical approach is the most direct operative approach to pathology ventral to the brain stem and superior cervical spine. This approach can be effectively employed in the treatment of a myriad of extradural cervicomedullary lesions.[1, 2, 4, 6–8, 10, 12, 15, 16, 18, 20–22, 24] The most common applications of the procedure have been for resection of the odontoid process, for basilar invagination especially in rheumatoid disease, or for congenital deformities. Extradural tumor masses can be resected by this approach provided they are not too extensive or broad-based. Although intradural pathology can also be treated via the transoral-transclival approach, there is a high potential morbidity and mortality from cerebrospinal fluid (CSF) fistula, meningitis, and abscess formation.[3, 6, 10, 24]

We will review the indications for the transoral surgical procedure, describe our operative techniques, and highlight our surgical experience. We find that incorporating specific methods of retraction, intraoperative monitoring, and postoperative care make this an effective procedure with minimal patient morbidity and mortality.

INDICATIONS

The transoral operative procedure can be employed in the treatment of pathology ventral to the brain stem and superior cervical spine from the level of the midclivus to the third cervical vertebra. Focal lesions that cause compression of the medulla or upper cervical spinal cord (e.g., a dislocated odontoid) can be removed with ease via this approach. Tumor masses can also be resected using the transoral surgical procedure, provided they do not extend beyond the lateral limits of the operative exposure; apart from nonneoplastic entities, a wide variety of tumors including osteomas, chordomas, sarcomas, schwannomas, epidermoids, and metastatic neoplasms have been resected using this approach.[4, 8, 10, 13, 14, 16, 20, 22, 23]

The precise location of the craniocervical pathology and the mechanism(s) of brain stem or spinal cord compression are the influencing factors when planning a specific surgical approach.[10, 16, 22, 23] A number of patients, particularly those with basilar invagination, will require a combination of surgical procedures to remove offending ventral pathology and to provide posterior fusion and stabilization. We base the decision regarding the surgical approach on a battery of preoperative radiographic studies, including plain roentgenograms (including dynamic flexion and extension view), computed tomography (CT), water-soluble contrast myelography with CT (Fig. 31–1), and magnetic resonance imaging (MRI) (Fig. 31–2). In addition, we have evaluated several patients with complex skull base deformities with three-dimensional CT to help better delineate the precise nature of their bony anatomy.[9]

SURGICAL TECHNIQUE

The patient is intubated with a flexible oral endotracheal tube and is placed in the supine position on the operating room table. The patient's head is secured in a Mayfield fixation device with the head and neck slightly extended, unless the patient was placed in a halo vest prior to surgery (Fig. 31–3). The surgeon sits above the patient's head. A self-retaining McGarver three-ring retractor is inserted, allowing the lips and gums to be spread apart and the tongue and the endotracheal tube to be displaced caudally. Two small red rubber catheters are inserted through the nostrils into the oropharynx and are sutured to the uvula with a 2.0 silk suture. The uvula and soft palate are retracted into the nasopharynx by placing traction on the two rubber catheters and by tying them to the McGarver retraction apparatus (Figs.

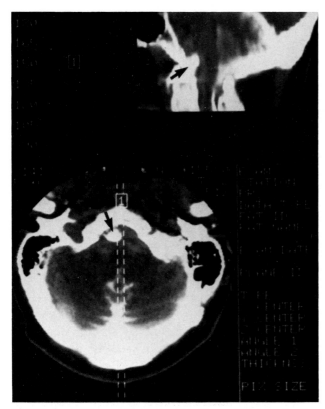

FIGURE 31–1. CT scan with metrizamide. The sagittal reconstruction documents cervicomedullary compression by the displaced odontoid.

31–4 and 31–5). This combination of retraction affords a wide operative exposure of the posterior pharyngeal wall and obviates the need for tracheostomy.[2, 10, 14, 19–21]

The patient's mouth and oropharynx are prepared with iodine solution, the patient is draped, and the operating microscope with a 300-mm lens is brought

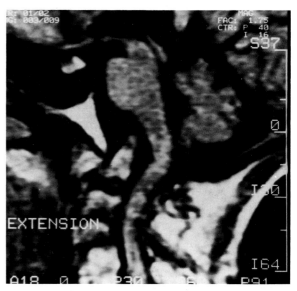

FIGURE 31–2. MRI scan, extension view. Note marked basilar invagination in patient with rheumatoid arthritis.

into position. The tubercle of the atlas can be palpated through the posterior pharyngeal wall and is used as a landmark. A lateral radiograph is used to confirm localization in difficult cases (Fig. 31–6).

A longitudinal midline incision is made in the posterior pharyngeal tissues using the Shaw hemostatic scalpel (Oximetrix Inc., Mountain View, CA), which allows a bloodless opening (Fig. 31–7). For odontoid pathology, the incision is made directly over the tubercle and is extended approximately 2.5 cm inferiorly. For pathology at the lower clivus a more cephalad incision is required, extending upward through the posterior pharyngeal wall of the nasopharynx. The muscles and soft tissues of the posterior pharynx are incised along the midline down to

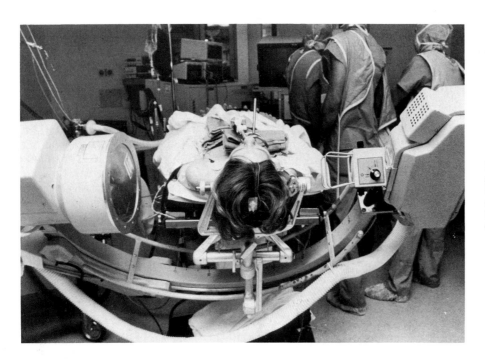

FIGURE 31–3. Patient positioned in supine position. The Mayfield head holder maintains position of slight extension. In this case the C-arm is in position for intraoperative fluoroscopy.

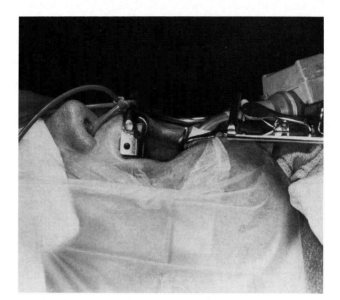

FIGURE 31—4. Lateral view of McGarver 3-ring retractor and use of red rubber catheters through the nostrils.

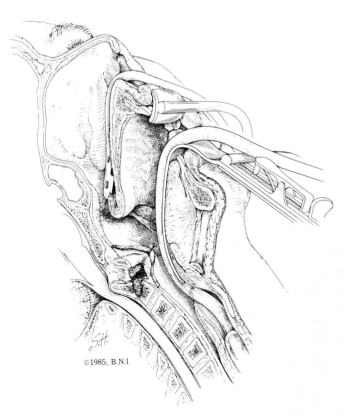

©1985, B.N.I.

FIGURE 31—5. Artist's drawing of retraction system and approach to odontoid pathology.

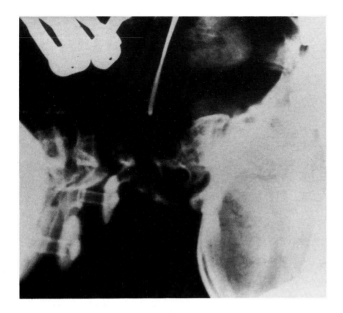

FIGURE 31–6. Intraoperative radiography confirms probe position directly over body of C2.

the periosteum overlying the atlas and axis. A fine periosteal elevator is used to dissect these tissues laterally off of the anterior surface of the vertebrae, and traction sutures or a large eyelid retractor are used to retract them laterally. The C1-C2 and C2-C3 interspaces are identified utilizing an intraoperative radiograph.

A Midas Rex high speed drill (Midas Rex, Ft. Worth, TX) with a small cutting burr is used to perform the bone dissection, either superiorly through the tubercle of the atlas and the inferior clivus or inferiorly at the bodies of C2 or C3 (Fig. 31–8). The depth of bone dissection can be assessed in several ways: (1) by direct inspection and dissection down to the posterior longitudinal ligament, (2) by intraoperative radiography or fluoroscopy, or (3) by placing contrast material into the resection cavity and obtaining lateral (and occasionally anteroposterior) cervical radiographs. The latter technique allows the

most accurate estimates of the depth and width of bone removal. A fine diamond-tipped burr is used to resect the remaining cortical bone layer to expose the posterior longitudinal ligament (dura) at the clivus level. Occasionally the tip of the odontoid can be grasped with a rongeur, elevated away from the brain stem and spinal cord, and dissected free from its ligamentous attachments with straight and angled microcurettes (Fig. 31–9).

When performing this procedure for odontoid resection (Figs. 31–10 through 31–13), we open the posterior longitudinal ligament if it is thick and calcified or if it does not bulge into the resection cavity following odontoid removal. In patients with basilar invagination from rheumatoid arthritis, there may be nonosseous reactive granulation tissue around the odontoid process which may contribute to ventral cervicomedullary compression.[3, 20, 22] This rheumatoid pannus must be excised. The dura mater

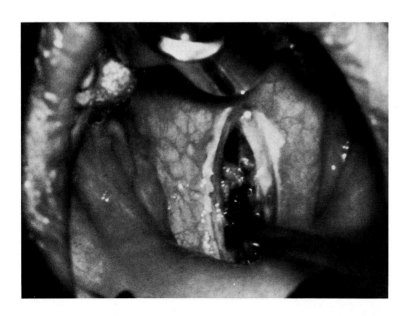

FIGURE 31–7. Intraoperative photograph of the initial midline incision. The surgeon works from above the patient's head. The endotracheal tube is depressed caudally by the McGarver retractor (superior in this photo).

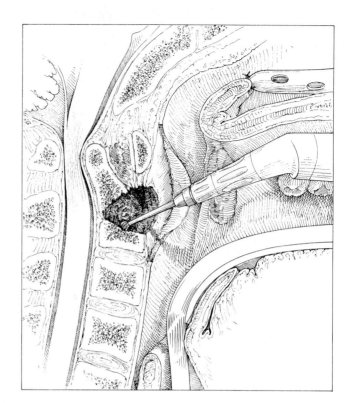

FIGURE 31–8. A high speed drill is used for bony dissection.

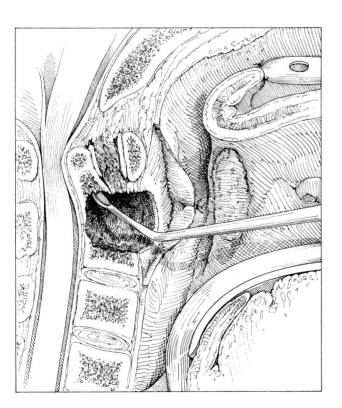

FIGURE 31–9. Artist's representation of use of microcurette to assist with bone removal.

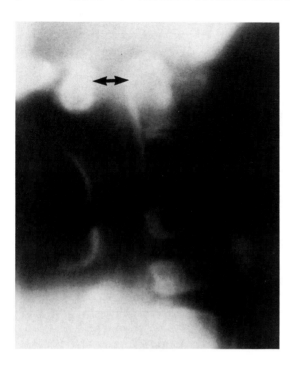

FIGURE 31–10. Tomogram of patient with congenital basilar impression and marked narrowing of cervical canal (*arrows*).

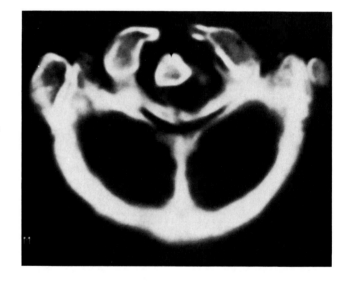

FIGURE 31–11. Metrizamide CT study demonstrates marked cervicomedullary compression by the odontoid process.

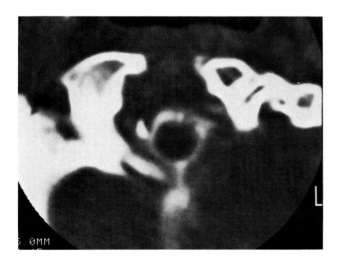

FIGURE 31–12. Postoperative metrizamide CT study documents odontoid resection and decompression of cervicomedullary structures.

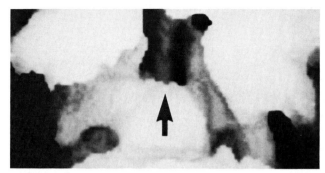

FIGURE 31–13. Three-dimensional CT scan depicts region of odontoid resection (*arrow*).

then assumes a more normal position, a change that can be documented radiographically when contrast material is placed into the resection cavity.

For tumor removal between C3 and the clivus, this approach allows an extensive anterior exposure for excision or biopsy (Figs. 31–14 through 31–19). Utilizing microneurosurgical techniques, we have resected six extradural tumors (two metastatic neoplasms and four chordomas) without operative morbidity or mortality. The transoral-transclival approach affords a generous exposure to ventral intradural pathology as well, and we have used this approach to excise an epidermoid at the pontomedullary junction. The dura mater in these cases is incised in the midline and is retracted laterally. We avoid cauterization of the dural leaves to avoid shrinkage of the dura and to facilitate its reapproximation. Following the intradural procedure, the dura is reapproximated with a continuous 6.0 nylon suture. Autologous fascia lata is then placed over the dural closure and is secured in place with tacking sutures.

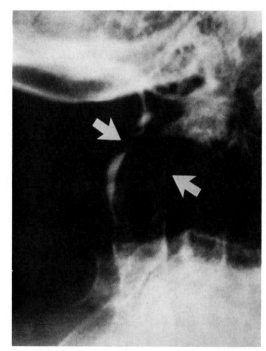

FIGURE 31–15. Myelogram confirms marked compression at C1-C2.

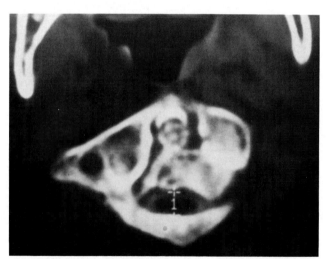

FIGURE 31–16

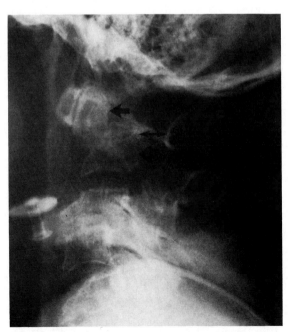

FIGURE 31–14. Lateral radiograph in elderly female with metastatic neoplastic bone destruction, subluxation, and cervical cord compression.

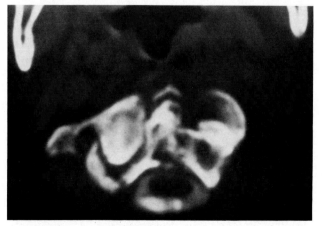

FIGURE 31–17

FIGURES 31–16 and 31–17. Preoperative metrizamide CT study documents neoplastic extradural compression of high cervical cord.

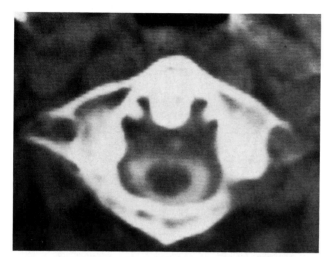

FIGURE 31–18

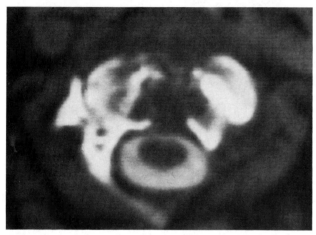

FIGURE 31–19

FIGURES 31–18 and 31–19. Postoperative metrizamide CT scans reveal decompression of cervical cord after transoral procedure to debulk epidural metastatic neoplasm.

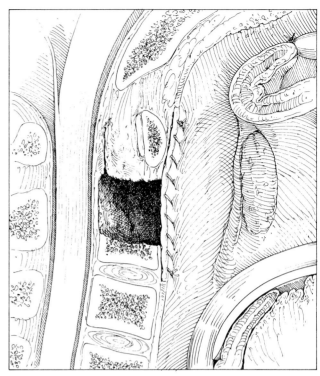

FIGURE 31–20. Artist's representation of completed transoral procedure and watertight closure of posterior pharyngeal tissues.

Prior to closure, the entire wound is irrigated with antibiotic solution, and a multilayer closure of the posterior pharyngeal tissues is performed. The deep muscular layers are approximated with interrupted absorbable sutures, the superficial muscular layers are approximated with a continuous absorbable suture, and finally the posterior pharyngeal muscosa is approximated with a continuous absorbable suture (Fig. 31–20). The posterior pharyngeal wall of the nasopharynx is very thin and fragile, making a good closure at the superior extent of the incision difficult.[10, 11] A lumbar drain is inserted intraoperatively in those cases in which the dura mater has been violated. CSF hypotension is maintained with continuous drainage for 3 to 4 days postoperatively to facilitate a watertight wound closure and to avoid a CSF fistula.

Somatosensory cortical evoked responses and brain stem auditory evoked potentials are recorded throughout the operation. Computerized display screens are utilized intraoperatively to observe minute-to-minute recordings. A hard copy of the improvement in evoked responses can be generated for comparison to preoperative studies.

RESULTS

Over a 10-year period (1977 to 1987), 29 transoral-transclival procedures have been performed by the authors (Table 31–1). Of these, the majority were performed for benign cervicomedullary compression, whereas seven procedures were directed at the treatment of ventral tumors of the clivus or superior cervical spine (C1-C3). Two of the 29 procedures were for treatment of intradural pathology: an arteriovenous malformation (AVM) and an epidermoid tumor at the inferior clivus–C1 level.

One patient with extradural pathology had significant postoperative complications (Table 31–2). This patient, a 64-year-old male with basilar invagination

TABLE 31–1. OUTLINE OF PATHOLOGY AT THE CRANIOVERTEBRAL JUNCTION TREATED VIA TRANSORAL APPROACH

Odontoid pathology	21	
Congenital		7
Rheumatoid arthritis		11
Traumatic C1–C2 sublux		3
Other pathology	8	
Extradural met. neoplasm		2
Extradural tumor		4
Intradural tumor		1
AVM with pseudoaneurysm		1
Total	29	

TABLE 31–2. OUTCOME OF 29 PATIENTS TREATED SURGICALLY VIA THE TRANSORAL APPROACH

FOLLOW-UP TRANSORAL APPROACH	MORBIDITY	MORTALITY
Odontoid pathology		
Congenital	0	0
Rheumatoid	1 vertical sublux with brain stem stroke	1 Severe pneumonitis (9 weeks)
Traumatic C2–C3 sublux	0	0
Other pathology		
Extradural met. neoplasm	0	1 Pulmonary embolus (7 weeks)
Extradural tumor	0	0
Intradural tumor	0	1 Brain infarction (6 months)
AVM with pseudoaneurysm	1 Meningitis	1 Rupture of basilar mycotic aneurysm (8 weeks)

Median follow-up = 24 months.

from rheumatoid arthritis, had two unrelated complications. The superior aspect of this pharyngeal incision dehisced, requiring reexploration and closure. No infection was noted. Two weeks postoperatively the patient returned to the hospital with signs of an acute neurologic deterioration. Radiographic studies revealed what appeared to be vertical occipitoatlantal subluxation, with vertebral artery occlusion and a brain stem stroke. The patient was improving neurologically on the rehabilitation ward but expired from pneumonia 9 weeks after his initial operation. The only other death in this group of patients occurred secondary to a massive pulmonary embolus 6 weeks following a second procedure (posterior decompression, wiring, and fusion) to stabilize the spine.

Both patients with intradural pathology died, one 8 weeks and the other 6 months postoperatively. The first patient was a young male who bled from a C2-C3 level AVM. We repaired a large associated pseudoaneurysm via the transoral-transdural approach. He developed purulent meningitis without evidence of wound dehiscence and died 8 weeks postoperatively of a new mycotic basilar artery aneurysm that ruptured. The second patient (pontomedullary junction epidermoid) improved dramatically after tumor excision and brain stem decompression. Four months postoperatively she developed meningitis of unknown etiology. She did not develop a CSF leak or evidence of wound dehiscence and recovered with antibiotic therapy. Two months later (6 months following the initial surgery), she presented with significant brain stem dysfunction. CT scan revealed tumor recurrence with brain stem and cerebellar compression. A posterior fossa craniotomy was performed to debulk the tumor and relieve compression. She died one week later of massive brain stem infarction. At autopsy the dural closure was intact. There was no postmortem evidence of infection.

The surviving 25 patients have all shown improvement or stabilization of their preoperative neurologic

deficits (median follow-up, 24 months). All four patients with clival chordomas received postoperative radiation therapy. One has required a second surgical procedure (a combination temporal-suboccipital approach) for tumor recurrence (30 months postoperatively). The other three patients are being followed at regular intervals.

DISCUSSION

The choice of a surgical approach to the craniovertebral junction must be made individually. Selection of the proper approach or combination of procedures is a prerequisite for the most beneficial result. In most cases the location of the pathology and the mechanism of brain stem or spinal cord compression are the influencing factors.[1, 2, 10, 15, 20, 23] Ventral craniovertebral junction pathology should be approached anteriorly; dorsal pathology is best treated from a posterior approach. If instability exists following decompression, then a stabilization procedure should follow. A number of patients, particularly those with craniovertebral junction congenital anomalies or degenerative disease, will require a combination of surgical approaches.[10, 15, 23] A detailed neuroradiologic work-up, including dynamic studies, positive contrast myelography with CT, and MRI, will assist in the management of these patients. In the past, significant morbidity and mortality were reported after the transoral-transclival approach; these factors have limited its general acceptance and application. Refinements in microneurosurgical techniques combined with effective retraction, intraoperative neurophysiologic monitoring, and intraoperative radiography all result in a safe and efficacious surgical procedure.[3, 10, 14, 19–21]

We routinely used a flexible oral endotracheal tube secured caudally by the McGarver three-ring retractor. This combination, with the use of the red rubber catheters to retract the uvula and soft palate superiorly, provides a wide exposure of the posterior pharyngeal wall and obviates the need to perform a tracheostomy or to split the mandible, tongue, and palate. The endotracheal tube is left in place for at least 24 hours postoperatively to avoid potential respiratory compromise from glottic swelling. Patients are monitored in the intensive care unit for 24 hours after extubation, and a tracheostomy tray is maintained at the bedside following removal of the endotracheal tube as a precautionary measure should respiratory compromise occur. No airway complications were encountered in our series.

Somatosensory cortical and brain stem auditory potential recordings are sensitive intraoperative neurophysiologic monitoring techniques when performing neurosurgical procedures of high risk.[3, 10, 14, 17, 21] Our experience has demonstrated their predictive value in instances of potential spinal cord or brain stem injury and their correlation between observed intraoperative responses and clinical outcome.

The use of intraoperative radiography (both anteroposterior and lateral planes) is an important surgical adjunct.[10, 14, 19–21] The depth and width of bone dissection and decompression can be accurately assessed, particularly in combination with contrast material that is placed into the resection cavity. Intraoperative fluoroscopy can document the adequacy of spinal cord decompression by the degree of dural elevation following odontoid resection or tumor excision.

The integrity of the dura still remains an obstacle and a challenge for successful outcome.[3, 10, 11, 14, 24] In the 27 procedures we performed for extradural pathology, there was only one complication and no operative mortality (although two patients eventually died). In all cases, the dura mater remained intact. Both patients on whom we performed transoral procedures for intradural pathology died: one 8 weeks, the other 6 months following surgery. Both patients developed meningitis; one, 4 months after surgery, was treated uneventfully. Neither patient had evidence of wound dehiscence. The dura mater was approximated with a primary closure in the young male patient, while a fascia lata patch was secured with both suture and glue in the woman with the brain stem epidermoid. She was treated for 7 days following surgery with head elevation and CSF lumbar drainage.

While our experience is limited, we believe the transoral approach is a viable alternative in the treatment of intradural pathology at the lower clivus or anterior superior cervical spine. Best results can be obtained by using the surgical adjuncts and monitoring techniques outlined above, with close attention to sterile microneurosurgical techniques. Meticulous closure of the dura mater and posterior pharyngeal wall with postoperative CSF decompression will result in proper wound healing. We believe further experience with intradural lesions and dural closure techniques (laser welding or thrombin-fibrin glue)[11] will refine the transoral approach for intradural pathology, reducing the operative morbidity and mortality for these procedures to that seen in patients with extradural lesions.

REFERENCES

1. Apuzzo MLJ, Weiss MH, Heiden JS: Transoral exposure of the atlantoaxial region. Neurosurgery 3(2):201, 1978.
2. Blazier CJ, Hadley MN, Spetzler RF: The transoral surgical approach to craniovertebral pathology. J Neurosci Nurs 18(2):57, 1986.
3. Crockard HA: The transoral approach to the base of the brain and upper cervical cord. Ann R Coll Surg Engl 67:321, 1985.
4. Crockard HA, Bradford RLK: Transoral transclival removal of a schwannoma anterior to the craniocervical junction: Case report. J Neurosurg 62:293, 1985.
5. Croft TJ, Brodkey JS, Nulsen FE: Reversible spinal cord trauma: A model for electrical monitoring of spinal cord function. J Neurosurg 36:402, 1972.
6. Drake CG: Management of aneurysms of posterior circulation. In Youmans JR (ed): Neurological Surgery. Vol 2. Philadelphia, WB Saunders Co., 1973, pp 787–806.
7. Drake CG: Treatment of aneurysms of the posterior cranial fossa. Prog Neurol Surg 9:122, 1978.
8. Fang DL, Leong JCY, Fang HSY: Tuberculosis of the upper cervical spine. J Bone Joint Surg 65B:47, 1983.
9. Hadley MN, Sonntag VKH, Amos MR, et al: Three-dimensional computed tomography in the diagnosis of vertebral column pathological conditions. Neurosurgery 21:186–192, 1987.
10. Hadley MN, Spetzler RF: The transoral surgical approach to the craniocervical junction. In Samii M (ed): Surgery in and Around the Brain Stem and Third Ventricle. Heidelberg, Springer, 1986, pp 467–475.
11. Hadley MN, Martin NA, Spetzler RF, et al: Comparative transoral dural closure techniques: A canine model. Neurosurgery 22:392, 1988.
12. Hashi K, Hakuba A, Ikuno H, et al: A midline vertebral artery aneurysm operated via transclival approach. Neurol Surg 42:183, 1976.
13. Kanavel AB: Bullet located between the atlas and the base of the skull: Technic of removal through the mouth. Surg Clin 1:361, 1917.
14. Masferrer R, Hadley MN, Bloomfield S, et al: Transoral microsurgical resection of the odontoid process. BNI Quarterly 1(3):34, 1985.
15. Menezes AH, VanGilder JC, Graf CJ, McDonnell DE: Craniocervical abnormalities: A comprehensive surgical approach. J Neurosurg 53:444, 1980.
16. Mullan S, Naunton R, Hekmat-Panah J, Vailati G: The use of an anterior approach to ventrally placed tumors in the foramen magnum and vertebral column. J Neurosurg 24:563, 1966.
17. Owen MP, Brown RH, Spetzler RF, et al: Excision of intramedullary arteriovenous malformation using intraoperative spinal cord monitoring. Surg Neurol 12:271, 1979.
18. Pasztor E, Vajda J, Piffko R, Horvath M: Transoral surgery for basilar impression. Surg Neurol 14:473, 1980.
19. Selman WR, Spetzler RF, Brown R: The use of intraoperative fluoroscopy and spinal cord monitoring for transoral microsurgical odontoid resection. Clin Orthop 154:51, 1981.
20. Spetzler RF: Transoral approach to the upper cervical spine. In Evarts CM (ed): Surgery of the Musculoskeletal System. New York, Churchill Livingstone, 1983, pp 4:19–4:24.
21. Spetzler RF, Selman WR, Nash CL, Brown RH: Transoral microsurgical odontoid resection and spinal cord monitoring. Spine 4(6):506, 1979.
22. Stevens JM, Kendall BE, Crockard HA: The spinal cord in rheumatoid arthritis with clinical myelopathy: A computed myelographic study. J Neurol Neurosurg Psych 49:140, 1986.
23. VanGilder JC, Menezes AH: Craniovertebral abnormalities and their treatment. In Schmidek HH, Sweet WH (eds): Operative Neurosurgical Techniques. New York, Grune and Stratton, 1982, pp 1221–1235.
24. Yamaura A, Makino H, Isobe K, et al: Repair of cerebrospinal fluid fistula following transoral transclival approach to a basilar aneurysm. J Neurosurg 50:834, 1979.

TRANSMANDIBULAR APPROACHES TO THE UPPER CERVICAL SPINE

JATIN P. SHAH and ASHOK R. SHAHA

INTRODUCTION

Surgical exposures of the anterior cervical spine are often necessary for the treatment of a variety of benign and malignant conditions. Several operative approaches to this region are described in the literature; these include the transoral, transcervical, transclival, transseptal, transsphenoidal, transantral, and infratemporal approaches.[1-5, 8, 10, 11] However, the exposures obtained are limited, especially for tumors of the upper cervical spine. Our experience in the management of tumors of the oropharynx suggest that wide exposures are obtained via mandibulotomy. Mandibulotomy approaches can be used for anterior exposures of both the upper cervical spine and clivus. The mandibulotomy is usually performed in the midline with a median glossotomy or in a paramedian position with a paralingual extension through the floor of the mouth.

INDICATIONS

Various tumors involving the high cervical spine or the rostrum of the sphenoid and clivus are approachable through a mandibulotomy approach. These include chordoma, chondroma, chondrosarcoma, osteoma, osteogenic sarcoma, craniopharyngioma, dermoid, meningioma, and so forth. Certain benign conditions may also require exposures of the high cervical spine, including invagination of the odontoid process or spondylosis. Infectious processes such as a retropharyngeal abscess are also encountered in this location, including tuberculous involvement of the cervical spine; surgery may be indicated for diagnosis as well as for decompression. Our most common indication for this procedure is excision of tumors, of which the most commonly encountered is chordoma. Chordomas are tumors that are thought to arise in residual or vestigial remnants of the notochord, and approximately 35 per cent of these tumors arise in the sphenooccipital region.

The two surgical approaches to be described in this chapter are (1) median labiomandibular glossotomy, and (2) median mandibulotomy with paralingual extension (mandibular swing approach).[9]

PREOPERATIVE EVALUATION

Radiographic studies of the spine and skull base are indicated to accurately delineate the extent of disease involvement. Lateral and anteroposterior views of the cervical spine should be initially performed (Fig. 32–1). Following these, computed tomography (CT) scan or magnetic resonance imaging (MRI), followed by a myelogram, may be indicated. On occasion, angiography may be necessary to delineate the vascular anatomy of the tumor and the disposition of the carotid and vertebral arteries and intracranial circulation. For patients undergoing mandibulotomy, preoperative dental evaluation is essential. Impressions of the lower dentition are obtained, and a lower alveolar splint is fabricated preoperatively, since it may be necessary to use the splint either intraoperatively or postoperatively to stabilize the two segments of the mandible. Routine preoperative studies such as a chest x-ray, electrocardiogram, and blood chemistry are all essential. Preoperative and perioperative antibiotics are administered routinely since the operation is considered a clean but contaminated procedure.

The operation is performed under general anesthesia. A tracheostomy is performed initially either under local anesthesia or after induction of general anesthesia. Following this, general anesthesia is continued through the tracheostomy tube. Tracheostomy is important because the airway is out of the surgical field during the course of the operation. In the postoperative period, patients are likely to experience difficulty with breathing and coughing due to swelling in the oropharynx. Tracheostomy not only provides a safe airway during the operation but also ensures its maintenance in the postoperative period.

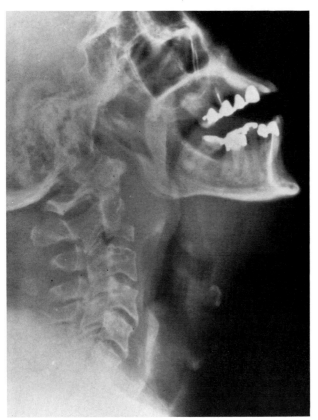

FIGURE 32–1. Lateral x-ray of the cervical spine showing a chordoma arising from C1 and C2 presenting as a retropharyngeal mass.

It also allows access to the tracheobronchial tree for clearance of pulmonary secretions.

MEDIAN LABIOMANDIBULAR GLOSSOTOMY

In 1839 Roux described the approach of splitting the lower lip and mandible directly in the midline for access to tumors of the anterior portion of the tongue. In 1929 Trotter reported a procedure called "median anterior translingual pharyngotomy," in which he extended Roux's midline section of the lower lip and mandible by splitting the tongue sagittally through its median raphe for exposure of the base of the tongue and midportion of the pharynx. The term "median labiomandibular glossotomy" was coined by Hayes Martin in 1961.[6] The principle of this procedure is to split the lower lip, mandible, and tongue in the midline to approach the oropharynx and the upper cervical vertebral column.

Under general anesthesia maintained via the tracheostomy tube, the head and neck area is prepared with antiseptic solution and isolated with sterile drapes (Fig. 32–2). The skin incision begins on the midline of the lower lip by splitting the vermilion border. It continues caudally, dividing the chin and the skin of the submental region up to the hyoid bone. The skin incision is deepened through the subcutaneous tissues of the chin and submental re-

gion until the anterior cortex of the symphysis of the mandible is reached in the upper part of the incision, with the anterior bellies of the digastric muscle being exposed in the lower part. The lower lip is also divided in the midline, but the labial mucosa is not divided all the way up to the gingivolabial sulcus. The incision terminates within approximately 5 mm of the sulcus. At this point, lateral incisions are made in the gingivolabial sulcus on either side, leaving a short cuff of approximately 5 mm of gingival mucosa attached to the gum. These incisions are made to a length of approximately 1.5 cm on both sides of the midline. This is essential since this short cuff of mucosa is required at the time of closure. All soft tissues of the chin are divided up to the bone, and short cheek flaps are elevated on both sides of the midline exposing the central 3 cm of the anterior cortex of the symphysis of the mandible. Care should be exercised to avoid injury to the mental nerve as it exits out of the mental foramen on each side. Injury to it will result in anesthesia of the skin of the chin and should be avoided. Elevation of the short cheek flaps should therefore remain medial to the mental foramen.

If a high speed power saw with an ultrafine blade is available, the mandible can be divided in the midline between the two lower central incisor teeth. If such fine instrumentation is not available, it is advisable to extract one lower central incisor tooth and to perform the mandibulotomy through the socket to avoid loss of both central incisors (Fig. 32–3). Using electrocautery, the mucosa of the attached gingiva and the soft tissues anterior to the mandible

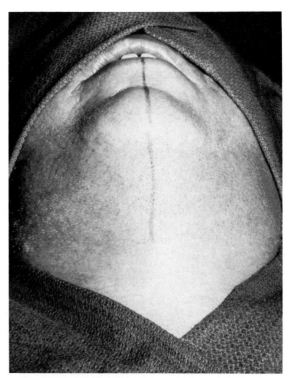

FIGURE 32–2. Lower lip splitting vertical midline incision for median labiomandibular glossotomy.

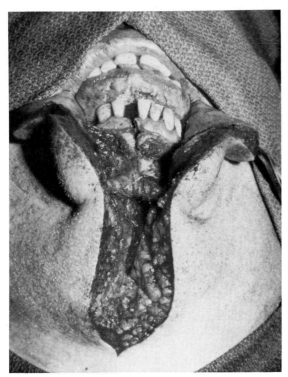

FIGURE 32–3. Exposure of the symphysis for midline mandibulotomy.

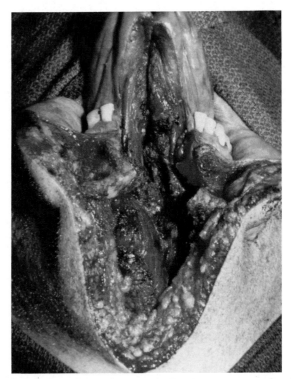

FIGURE 32–4. Median labiomandibular glossotomy completed.

are scored to outline the site of mandibulotomy. The optimal way to divide the mandible is in a zig-zag fashion (shown in Fig. 32–3). The division of the mandible should be carried out sharply with the power saw. Care should be exercised during division of bone to avoid comminuted fractures at the mandibulotomy site. If such a fracture results, all bone fragments should be preserved and reinserted at the time of reapproximation of the mandible. The two sides of the mandible are now retracted apart with a bone hook, putting traction on the soft tissues and the mucosa of the floor of the mouth. Using electrocautery, the mucosa in the midline of the floor of the mouth is incised, while carefully avoiding injury to the Wharton's ducts on either side. As the mucosa is incised, traction on the two mandibular segments puts stretch on the musculature of the floor of the mouth, which is progressively divided in the midline.

The incision in the floor of the mouth is extended through the undersurface of the tongue in the midline up to its tip. The tongue is then divided in the midline. Division of the tongue through the median raphae is relatively bloodless. The incision on the dorsum of the tongue is now carried from its tip all the way back to the glossoepiglottic fold in the posterior third of the tongue (Fig. 32–4). As the tongue is divided, the two halves of the floor of the mouth, tongue, and mandible on each side are retracted laterally, providing progressively increasing exposure of the oropharynx and posterior pharyngeal wall. It must be borne in mind that in order to obtain the widest exposure, the entire tongue needs to be divided through its full thickness from the mucosa of

its dorsum to the hyoid bone. As shown in Figure 32–5, the two halves of the lower part of the oral cavity are retracted laterally with a self-retaining retractor, providing a wide exposure of the posterior pharyngeal wall. In the center of the field inferiorly, the epiglottis can be seen. In the upper part of the center of the field, the stretched soft palate with upturned uvula is seen.

The patient shown in the illustration has a chordoma of the upper cervical spine that was previously biopsied through the mouth. A vertical midline in-

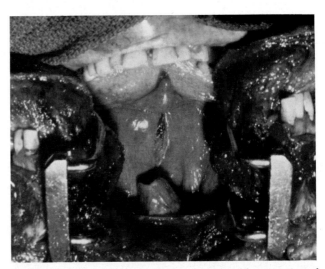

FIGURE 32–5. Posterior pharyngeal wall exposed by retraction of the two halves of the lower part of the oral cavity. Note the uvula at the upper end and the epiglottis at the lower end of the exposed field. A vertical incision is made in the mucosa of the posterior pharyngeal wall.

cision is next made in the posterior pharyngeal wall (Fig. 32–5). The mucosal incision is carried through the musculature of the posterior pharyngeal wall to expose the prevertebral fascia. Dissection now begins in the prevertebral plane superiorly and inferiorly by extending the incision in the posterior pharyngeal wall as necessary. If further cephalad extension is necessary, it is essential to split the soft palate up to the junction of the hard palate (Fig. 32–6). Following division of the soft palate, the mucosal incision of the posterior pharyngeal wall can be carried all the way up to the vault of the nasopharynx. A tumor of the upper cervical vertebral bodies can then be excised under direct vision with ample exposure. The chordoma of the upper cervical spine in this patient was resected using this approach. The surgical defect following excision of the tumor is shown in Figure 32–6.

Following tumor removal, the mucosa of the posterior pharyngeal wall is approximated in the midline with interrupted chromic catgut sutures without a drain. The soft palate is likewise closed in two layers approximating the mucosa of the posterior as well as the anterior surfaces of the soft palate and the intervening musculature. Reapproximation of the tongue is done in three layers using interrupted #00 chromic catgut sutures to accurately align the two halves of the tongue back in the midline. Two layers of muscular sutures and a third layer of mucosal sutures are carried all the way from the glossoepiglottic fold posteriorly up to the tip of the tongue anteriorly, and then on the undersurface of the tongue in the anterior oral cavity. The mucosa of the floor of the mouth is likewise reapproximated. The two halves of the mandible are then held together and retained in position. A two-pronged miniplate is then used to provide internal fixation for the two halves (Fig. 32–7). This mini-plate is appropriately positioned and the screws are tightened. The previously fabricated lower alveolar splint is next applied

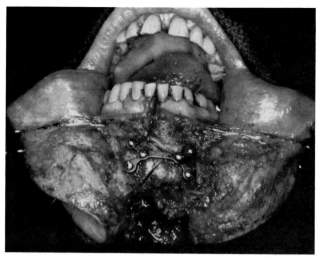

FIGURE 32–7. Realignment of the mandibular segments and internal fixation with miniplate and screws.

by the dentist. The splint is wired to the lower dentition providing additional external support to the mandibulotomy. The remaining incision of the lower lip and skin is closed with a drain in the submental region in the midline.

Postoperative Management

Intensive oral hygiene, early ambulation, and good tracheostomy care are essential for a smooth postoperative recovery. Power sprays with saline or hydrogen peroxide are essential to provide mechanical cleaning of the oral cavity and the suture line. Patients are fed through a nasogastric feeding tube initially. Once the patient is able to swallow his own saliva, oral feedings are started with liquids initially, gradually progressing to a semisolid and regular diet. The tracheostomy tube is retained as long as the patient needs pulmonary support for clearance of secretions. Once the patient is able to restore his normal airway and is able to cough through the mouth, the tracheostomy tube may be removed.

Complications

Massive edema of the tongue is seen occasionally following median glossotomy. Occasionally an intramuscular hematoma produces tremendous painful swelling of the tongue. Small hematomas of modest dimensions can be managed conservatively and will absorb spontaneously. However, massive hematomas require drainage and resuture of the tongue. Sepsis of the mandibulotomy site is occasionally seen, which may lead to a granulating wound in the oral cavity for several weeks. In most instances, the mandibulotomy site heals spontaneously in spite of the fact that it is a compound fracture of the mandible. With intensive and aggressive oral irrigations and cleaning, the mandibulotomy site will usually heal by secondary

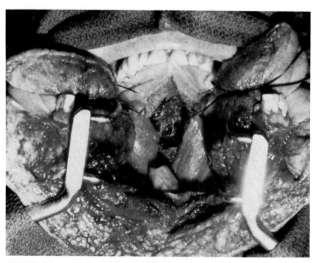

FIGURE 32–6. Soft palate divided in the midline to gain additional exposure, demonstrating the surgical defect following excision of the tumor.

intention even in the event of sepsis in this area. Only rarely does one need to remove the miniplate used for reapproximation of the mandible. Delayed union of the mandible is uncommon. Mandibular stability is usually assumed in approximately 8 weeks, at which time the lower alveolar splint may be removed. If motion is detected at the site of mandibulotomy at this time, the alveolar splint may be reapplied for an additional length of time until bony union is documented. Even if there is no motion detected at the site of mandibulotomy in 8 weeks, calcification at the site of mandibulotomy is not seen on radiographs for up to one year.

MANDIBULAR SWING APPROACH

The mandibulotomy approach with paralingual extension (mandibular swing approach) gives excellent lateral and midline exposure to the nasopharynx, clivus, parapharyngeal space, infratemporal fossa, as well as cervical spine.[7] The initial steps of the operation are essentially the same as described previously. Mandibulotomy is performed in a paramedian position in a zigzag fashion. If a miniplate is not available for fixation of the mandibulotomy, stainless steel wire sutures are used for fixation of the mandible. The zigzag cut in the mandible is made in such a fashion to avoid roots of adjacent teeth (Fig. 32–8). Following mandibulotomy, the intraoral component of the operation differs from median labiomandibular glossotomy.

The two halves of the mandible are retracted laterally, and an incision is made in the mucosa of the lingual gingiva at the site of the mandibulotomy. This mucosal incision is extended laterally through the floor of the mouth all the way up to the anterior pillar of the soft palate. The mucosal incision in the floor of the mouth is made at a distance of approximately 6 to 8 mm from the lingual gingiva in order to permit a cuff of mucosa to remain attached to the lower alveolus. This is essential for reapproximation of the floor of the mouth at the time of the closure. The mucosal incision in the floor of the mouth permits a lateral swing of the mandible exposing the underlying sublingual gland and the mylohyoid muscle. The sublingual gland and the mylohyoid muscle are divided with electrocautery, leaving a stump of the muscle on the medial aspect of the mandible. Division of the mylohyoid muscle permits further lateral swing of the mandible. As the mandible is swung laterally, the lingual nerve straddles the surgical field as it exits from the region of the ascending ramus of the mandible to the lateral aspect of the

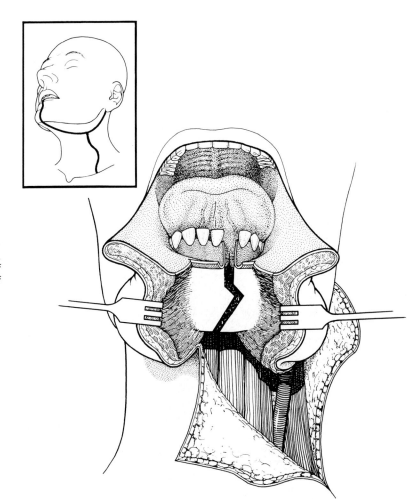

FIGURE 32–8. Skin incision and exposure for median mandibulotomy with paralingual extension. Insert shows a curvaceous vertical component of the incision for completion of a neck dissection if indicated.

tongue. To gain further exposure posteriorly, the lingual nerve should be divided. Similarly, the styloglossus muscle is also divided. An index finger is now introduced in the vallecula, and under direct vision the muscular attachment between the base of the tongue and lateral pharyngeal wall is divided up to the hyoid bone. This provides direct access to the oropharynx (Fig. 32–9).

Further steps of the operative procedure depend on the surgical exposure needed. If the primary problem involves the vertebral column or the parapharyngeal space, division of the muscular attachment between the base of the tongue and pharynx is not necessary. In such instances, the mucosal incision is extended to the soft palate and is carried cephalad up to the maxillary tubercle. A plane can then be developed lateral to the pharyngeal wall through the parapharyngeal space. The lateral wall of the pharynx is dissected by a combination of blunt and sharp dissection, and the pharynx is pushed medially to expose the vertebral column. The posterior pharyngeal wall is likewise dissected in the prevertebral plane; the entire oropharynx is pushed medially and the mandible is swung laterally, providing direct exposure of the cervical vertebral column in its upper part up to the clivus. If further exposure of the skull base is required, the pterygoid muscles are transected from the pterygoid plates, permitting lateral rotation of the mandible on that side. Likewise the styloid group of muscles, that is, the stylohyoid, styloglossus, and stylopharyngeus, may be transected. Further exposure superiorly to the nasopharynx and the infratemporal fossa may require transection of the eustachian tube and the palatine muscles. It is, however, vitally important that the internal carotid artery be identified in the neck and traced cephalad until

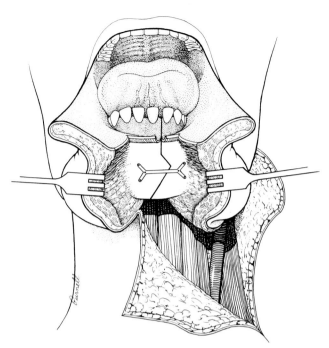

FIGURE 32–10. Closure of the paralingual incision completed with realignment of the mandibular segments using a miniplate.

its entry through the base of the skull. By early identification, the internal carotid artery is protected and retracted laterally, keeping the plane of dissection medial to the vessel. Such extensive dissections provide generous exposures of the upper cervical spine and clivus.

Repair of the surgical incision is relatively simple. After appropriate closure of the pharyngeal wall is performed with interrupted chromic catgut sutures, the mandibulotomy site is reapproximated (Fig. 32–10). The laterally swung mandible is brought back to the midline. The mylohyoid muscle is approximated with interrupted chromic catgut sutures. The mucosa of the floor of the mouth is reapproximated to the cuff of mucosa on the attached lingual gingiva with interrupted chromic catgut sutures. The soft palate is likewise reapproximated if it has been previously divided. Reapproximation of the mandible is done either with a miniplate or with stainless steel wires that are twist-tied. A lower alveolar dental splint is applied for additional support to the repaired mandibulotomy site. The remaining incision in the labial mucosa and the gingivolabial sulcus as well as the lower lip and skin are closed in the usual fashion.

Postoperative care includes, as in the previous case, intensive oral irrigations and cleaning with power sprays using saline and hydrogen peroxide as well as frequent oral suctioning. Tracheostomy care for clearance of pulmonary secretions is essential. Nasogastric tube feedings are begun as early as 24 hours following surgery. Once the patient is able to swallow saliva, clear liquids are started by mouth, and oral intake is gradually advanced to soft and regular diet. The tracheostomy tube is removed when it is no longer necessary for clearance of pulmonary secretions or for maintenance of airway.

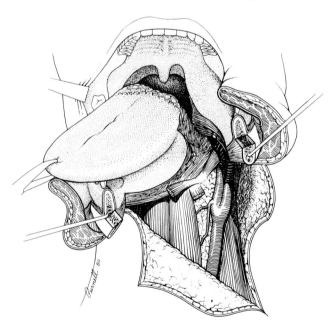

FIGURE 32–9. "Mandibular swing" completed with retraction of the left half of the mandible. Further exposure of the posterior pharyngeal wall and cervical spine is obtained by dividing the musculature of the base of the tongue and extending the mucosal incision in the floor of the mouth to the soft palate.

In our view, the midline mandibulotomy, either with median glossotomy or with paralingual extension, clearly offers obvious cosmetic advantages of retention of the facial contour and the function of the lower alveolus while providing at the same time a generous exposure to the upper cervical vertebrae, base of the skull and clivus.

REFERENCES

1. Biller HF, Sugar JMA, Krespi YP: A new technique for wide field exposure of the base of the skull. Arch Otolaryngol 107:698–702, 1981.
2. Fang HS, Ong FB: Direct anterior approach to the upper cervical spine. J Bone Joint Surg 44A:1588–1604, 1962.
3. Krespi YP, Grady HE: Surgery of the clivus and anterior cervical spine. Arch Otolaryngol Head-Neck Surg 14:73–78, 1988.
4. Krespi YP, Levine TM, Oppenheimer R: Skull base chordomas. Otolaryngol Clin North Am 19:479–504, 1986.
5. Krespi YP, Sisson GA: Transmandibular exposure of the skull base. Am J Surg 148:534–538, 1984.
6. Martin H, Tollefsen R, Gerold FP: Median labiomandibular glossotomy. Am J Surg 102:755–759, 1961.
7. Shah JP, Shemen L, Strong EW: Surgical therapy of oral cavity tumors. *In* Thawley SE, Panje WR (eds): Comprehensive Management of Head and Neck Tumors. Philadelphia, W.B. Saunders, 1986.
8. Southwick WO, Robinson RA: Surgical approaches to the vertebral bodies in the cervical and lumbar regions. J Bone Joint Surg 39A:631–644, 1957.
9. Spiro RH, Gerold F, Strong EW: Mandibular swing approach for oral and oropharyngeal tumors. Head Neck Surg 2:371–378, 1981.
10. Stevenson GC, Stoney RJ, Perlans RK, Adams JE: A transclival approach to the ventral surface of the brain stem for removal of a clivus chordoma. J Neurosurg 24:544–551, 1966.
11. Wood BG, Sadar ES, Levine HL, et al: Surgical problems of the base of the skull. Arch Otolaryngol 106:1–5, 1980.

33

TRANSUNCODISCAL APPROACH TO CERVICAL SPINE TUMORS

AKIRA HAKUBA

INTRODUCTION

In the management of spinal tumors having both an intraspinal and an extraspinal component when the paravertebral mass is small, removal of the extraspinal tumor may be accomplished by unroofing the intervertebral foramen (facetectomy) following removal of the intraspinal component through a standard laminectomy. When the paravertebral mass is large, however, a two-stage operation is often employed: the first to remove the intraspinal portion of the tumor, the second to remove the extraspinal part of the neoplasm. Laminectomy has been employed to surgically manage even ventrally located extraaxial spinal tumors such as meningiomas. With the anterior approach to the spine, often considerable portions of several contiguous vertebral bodies have been removed to expose the tumor. This may often be unnecessary, for example, in cervical neurinomas and meningiomas extending beyond the spinal canal through an enlarged intervertebral foramen. These neoplasms can be removed through an anterolateral approach that involves a transuncodiscal (TUD) exposure[2, 3] using an operative microscope. The procedure involves removal of the uncinate process and posterolateral corners of the vertebral bodies (anterior foraminotomy) by means of a transdiscal (medial) approach. This approach contrasts with the lateral approach to the cervical spine devised by Verbiest.[5] Through the space formed by removal of the tumor from the enlarged intervertebral foramen and by removal of the posterior transverse ridges of the vertebral bodies, an additional limited lateral vertebrectomy can be performed. By maximally widening the intervertebral space (up to 12 to 14 mm) with a specially designed vertebral spreader (Fig. 33–1), a lateral approach to the anterior spinal canal may safely be undertaken. With only minimal retraction of the vertebral artery, we have been able to fully expose tumors located in the anterolateral quadrant of the spinal canal.

We have accomplished total removal of these benign tumors in a one-stage procedure, with excellent results in six patients. We have entitled our exposure the transuncodiscal approach to the spine.

SUMMARY OF CASES

Clinical Material

Our series comprises six intraspinal-extraspinal dumbbell-shaped tumors involving the cervical spine (three in men, three in women). Four of the tumors were neurinomas (one of these was associated with von Recklinghausen's disease [Case 5]), one was a solitary neurofibroma (Case 6), and one was a meningioma. Two of the neurinomas occurred at the C2-C3 level, whereas the remainder were located in the lower cervical spine. The most extensive intradural tumor (Case 1) involved three levels of the cervical

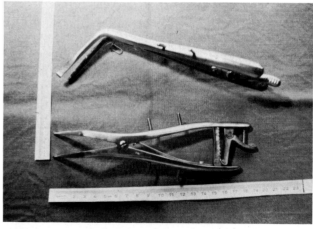

FIGURE 33–1. A vertebral spreader produced by Marui Ika Co., Tokyo, Japan.

Portions of this chapter appeared originally in Hakuba A, Komiyama M, Tsujimoto T, et al: Transuncodiscal approach to dumbbell tumors of the cervical spinal canal. J Neurosurg 61:1100–1106, 1984, and are reprinted with permission.

TABLE 33–1. SUMMARY OF CLINICAL DATA IN SIX PATIENTS WITH DUMBBELL TUMORS OF THE CERVICAL SPINAL CANAL

CASE NO.	AGE (YRS) SEX	PATHOLOGY	PREOPERATIVE NEUROLOGIC FINDINGS	OPERATIVE FINDINGS	FOLLOW-UP	OPERATIVE RESULTS
1	60, M	Meningioma	Complete paralysis of left upper and both lower limbs	Large 1 × 1 × 6 cm intradural extramedullary tumor between C6 and T1 vertebral bodies extending largely (6 × 8 cm) into left paravertebral area through an enlarged left intervertebral foramen at C7–T1	5 yrs	Paralysis of left hand, slight weakness of both lower limbs; able to walk without cane
2	55, M	Neurinoma	Weakness of right hand, hypalgesia below C3	1 × 1 × 1 cm intradural mass between C2 and C3 vertebral bodies, 3 × 3 × 3 cm epidural-intraforaminal mass at left C2–C3	2.5 yrs	No neurologic deficit
3	43, M	Neurinoma	Weakness of right upper and left lower extremities, hypalgesia of right leg	Cystic tumor; 2 × 2 × 2 cm intraforaminal-epidural mass at right C6–C7, 2 × 1 × 1 cm intradural mass between C6 and C7 vertebral bodies	1.5 yrs	Mild hypalgesia in right C7 dermatome
4	55, F	Neurinoma	Weakness and hypalgesia of right upper extremity	5 × 5 × 5 cm extraspinal mass, 3 × 3 × 3 cm intraforaminal mass at right C2–C3, 0.5 × 0.5 cm intradural mass	1.3 yrs	Slight paresis of right 11th nerve
5	25, F	Neurinoma (von Recklinghausen's disease)	Weakness of right upper extremity, hypalgesia of right C5 and C6 dermatomes	4 × 4 × 5 cm extraspinal mass, 3 × 3 × 3 cm intraforaminal epidural mass at right C5–C6	1 yr	Slight weakness of right deltoid muscle
6	40, F	Neurofibroma (solitary)	Slight weakness of right upper extremity, hypalgesia of right C6 dermatome	1 × 2 × 1 cm extraspinal mass, 1 × 1 × 1 cm epidural-intraforaminal mass at right C5–C6, 1 × 1 × 1 cm intradural mass between C5 and C6 vertebral bodies	3 wks	Moderate weakness of right deltoid and biceps muscles, moderate hypalgesia in right C6 dermatome

spine. Table 33–1 summarizes the clinical data of these six patients.

Operative Technique

Exposure of the Anterolateral Cervical Spine Between C2 and C3. With the patient under general endotracheal anesthesia and in the supine position, the neck is rotated to the opposite side and is maximally extended at the craniovertebral junction. A transverse skin incision is made a fingerbreadth (1–2 cm) below the inferior margin of the mandible from about two fingerbreadths (2–3 cm) off the midline to the tip of the mastoid process, sparing the marginal mandibular branch of the seventh nerve. A second incision parallels the anterior margin of the sternocleidomastoid muscle inferiorly from the first incision to the midcervical region (Fig. 33–2A). The sternocleidomastoid muscle is divided near its insertion at the mastoid process. The external and internal carotid arteries and the internal jugular vein are retracted medially, and the mandible is retracted

upward, thereby exposing the prevertebral space. The accessory nerve may have to be sacrificed to gain access to the dumbbell-shaped tumor at this level (Fig. 33–3).

Exposure of the Anterolateral Aspect of the Mid and Lower Cervical Spine. This exposure is identical to that used by Smith and Robinson[4] and Cloward.[1] When the extraspinal portion of the tumor is very large (Case 1, Fig. 33–4), a skin incision is made along the posterior margin of the sternocleidomastoid muscle, starting at the midcervical region and running down to the clavicle, and is then turned forward to run along the upper margin of the clavicle (Fig. 33–2B). The lower end of the sternocleidomastoid muscle is detached from its separate heads of origin at both the clavicle and sternum. The common carotid artery, internal jugular vein, and vagus nerve are retracted medially to provide full exposure of the anterolateral lower cervical spine and of the extraspinal portion of the tumor. The anterior scalene muscle is transversely divided at the level of the tumor while avoiding injury to the phrenic nerve. Following exposure of the tumor, intracapsular de-

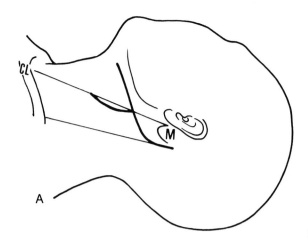

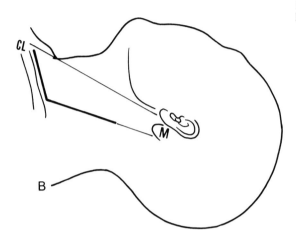

FIGURE 33–2. Skin incision for the transuncodiscal approach. *A*, For exposure of the prevertebral space between C2 and C3. *B*, For exposure of the prevertebral space of the lower cervical spine in the case of a very large paravertebral tumor. CL = clavicle; M = mastoid process.

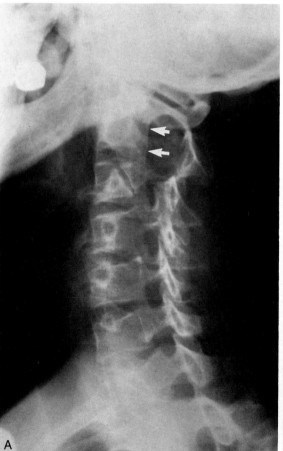

FIGURE 33–3. Case 2. *A*, Left oblique x-ray film of the cervical spine showing a large intervertebral foramen between C2 and C3 on the left side with marked erosion of the pedicles of the left C2 and C3 vertebral bodies (*arrows*). *B*, Metrizamide computed tomography (CT) scans showing a dumbbell-shaped tumor at the left C2-C3 level with marked enlargement of the intervertebral foramen and complete obstruction of the subarachnoid space at C2.

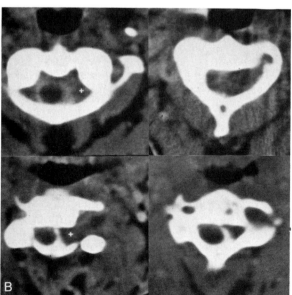

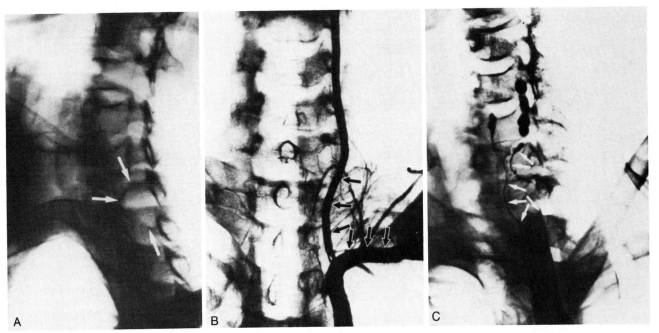

FIGURE 33–4. Case 1. *A*, Left oblique x-ray film of the cervical spine showing a large intervertebral foramen between C7 and T1 on the left with marked erosion of the pedicles on the left C7 and T1 vertebral bodies (*arrows*). *B*, Left retrograde brachial arteriogram showing medial displacement of the proximal portion of the left vertebral artery and downward displacement of the left subclavian artery (*arrows*), with marked stretching of the left thyrocervical trunk and its tributaries. *C*, Ascending myelogram showing an almost complete block at the T1 level with a lobulated tumor shadow between C6 and T1 (*arrows*).

compression is carried out. The common carotid artery and internal jugular vein are then retracted laterally and the trachea and esophagus are retracted medially to expose the prevertebral space and the extraspinal tumor mass. The tumor is excised to the external orifice of the intervertebral foramen.

Exposure of Intraspinal Cervical Tumors. The longus colli and longus capitis muscles are transversely divided at the level of the tumor, and the stumps of these muscles are separated from the vertebral bodies and transverse processes. The bone arches of the foramen transversarium above and below the tumor are removed with an air drill exposing the vertebral artery and vertebral veins (Fig. 33–5A). Under 16-power magnification, an anterior discectomy is performed at the level of the tumor. An intervertebral disc space spreader is inserted into the emptied disc space and is opened to expose the medial surface of the uncinate process by operating through the emptied disc space. An ipsilateral uncectomy and removal of the posterolateral corners of the upper and lower vertebral bodies (anterior foraminotomy) are performed (Fig. 33–5B and C). The posterior longitudinal ligament is exposed as the remaining disc tissue, including the annulus fibrosus, is removed.

The intraforaminal portion of the tumor is removed in piecemeal fashion. The anteromedial portion of the vertebral artery is generally adherent to the tumor and provides it with multiple arterial branches, which must be coagulated with a bipolar coagulator and divided. To obtain a better exposure of the intraspinal segment of tumor, the intraverte-bral foramen is enlarged by removal of the upper and lower posterior and posterolateral portions of the vertebral bodies with an air drill. The next encountered structure, the posterior longitudinal ligament, is divided and removed, exposing the epidural venous plexus. This plexus is usually well developed on the dorsolateral surface of the intraforaminal and epidural tumor, and it is separated from the tumor capsule and coagulated. Bleeding from the venous plexus can usually be controlled either by insertion of Biobond-soaked Oxcel or, alternatively, by insertion of fibrinogen and thrombin-soaked Gelfoam. The vertebral artery is gently retracted back and forth during removal of the intraforaminal and epidural portions of the tumor dorsal to the vertebral artery. Internal decompression of the tumor is performed with the ultrasonic aspirator. Following this, the tumor capsule is removed with microsurgical scissors and forceps. The portion of the tumor extending into the subdural space through the dural neck is exposed by opening the anterolateral part of the dural canal in a longitudinal fashion, thereby exposing the tumor situated ventral and lateral to the spinal cord (Fig. 33–5D). For larger tumors additional exposure is obtained by removal of the lateral portion of the vertebral body (slightly wider than 5 mm) and resection of the pedicles. By these measures one exposes the superior and inferior poles of the tumor and provides room for its manipulation. In Case 1, the largest tumor in the spinal canal in this series, the upper pole of the tumor extended two vertebrae above the enlarged intervertebral foramen (see Fig. 33–4), necessitating the

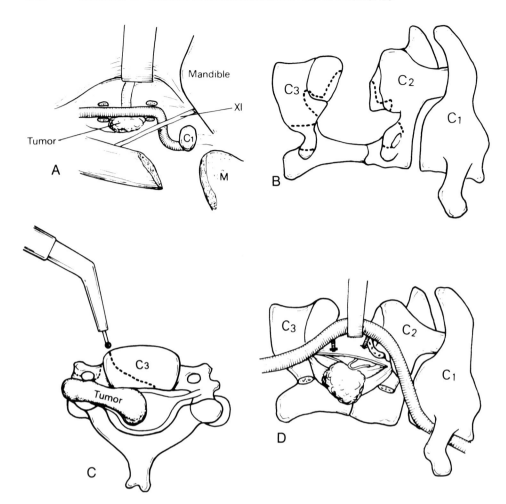

FIGURE 33–5. Case 2. *A,* The sternocleidomastoid muscle is divided at its insertion. The longus colli and longus capitis muscles are transversely divided at the level of the tumor, and their stumps are separated from the vertebral bodies and transverse processes. The bone arches of the foramen transversarium above and below the tumor are removed by an air drill, and the vertebral vein and the vertebral artery are exposed. XI = 11th cranial nerve; M = mastoid process; C1 = left transverse process of the first cervical spine. *B,* Broken lines indicate the limits of the uncectomy, the opening of the foramen transversarium, and the removal of the posterolateral corners and transverse ridges of the C3 vertebral body. *C,* A schematic view of the transuncodiscal approach. Broken lines indicate the limits of the ipsilateral uncotomy, the removal of the posterolateral corner and transverse ridge, and the unroofing of the foramen transversarium of the C3 vertebra. *D,* The left vertebral artery is retracted forward. The intervertebral foramen is enlarged by maximal widening of the intervertebral space and removal of the intraforaminal tumor. Through this space the dural canal is opened, and a small intradural tumor is delivered epidurally.

transuncodiscal approach at the disc space one level above the intraforaminal tumor, and also a lateral vertebrectomy and resection of the pedicles of the two vertebrae (Fig. 33–6*A*). Excellent exposure is obtained through the spaces formed by the uncectomy and anterior foraminotomy, removal of the posterior transverse ridges, lateral vertebrectomy of the two vertebrae, and removal of the intraforaminal tumor. Further exposure is obtained by widening the intervertebral space with the vertebral spreader inserted into the emptied disc space, which is maximally distracted.

The posterior longitudinal ligament is divided along the posterior margins of the exposed vertebrae and is removed. The anterolateral wall of the dural canal is opened in longitudinal fashion, the tumor ventral and lateral to the spinal cord is exposed (Fig. 33–6*B*) and removed (Fig. 33–6*C*), after which the remaining extraspinal tumor is removed. Following completion of this part of the operation, the dura is closed with watertight continuous sutures of 5-0 monofilament nylon and either with a fascia lata graft if a large dural defect is present or with a piece of the muscle if the dural defect is small. The defect of the bone and the intervertebral space are filled with T-shaped iliac bone graft (Fig. 33–7). The accessory nerve, which is often divided in the case of dumbbell-shaped tumors at C2-C3, is reanastomosed

with 9-0 interrupted monofilament nylon sutures, and the divided sternocleidomastoid muscle is reapproximated by interrupted sutures.

Postoperative Management

Cervical traction is maintained with Gardner-Wells tongs applied preoperatively and 4 kg of weight, which is decreased to 1 kg and continued postoperatively. Within two weeks after the operation a halo vest is applied and the patient is allowed to ambulate. The halo vest is removed in about 4 months depending on the serial radiographic studies.

Postoperative Results

The first case for which we employed this approach was a 60-year-old male with a 1 × 1 × 6 cm intraextradural meningioma between C6 and T1 (Case 1), who preoperatively had paralysis of the left hand and paraplegia. Function of his lower limbs gradually improved after surgery. Five years postoperatively the monoplegia of the upper extremity remained unchanged; he had a mild sphincter disturbance and mild weakness of both legs with moderate spastic gait, so that he was able to walk without a cane. One of the two patients with a neurinoma at the C2-C3 level (Case 2) had to have the 11th nerve

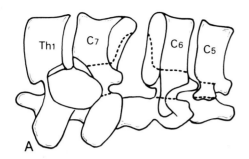

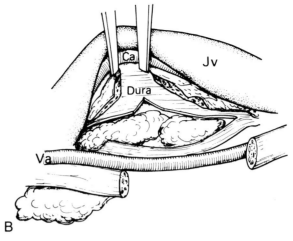

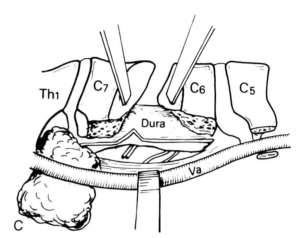

FIGURE 33–6. Case 1. *A*, An anterolateral schematic view of the lower cervical spine including the first thoracic spine. The intervertebral space between the C6 and C7 vertebral bodies is maximally opened. Broken lines indicate the limits for the uncoforaminotomy, the lateral vertebrectomy, the unroofing of the foramen transversarium, and the removal of the pedicles and posterior transverse ridges. *B*, A lateral vertebrectomy slightly wider than 5 mm and a resection of the pedicles as well as of the posterior transverse ridges of the C6 and C7 vertebral bodies are accomplished. The posterior longitudinal ligament is resected and the dura is exposed. The common carotid artery (Ca), the internal jugular vein (Jv), and the vagus nerve are retracted medially, and the vertebral artery (Va) is slightly retracted laterally and backward. The anterolateral dura between the C5-C6 disc space and the T1 vertebral body is opened in longitudinal fashion, and the tumor ventrolateral to the spinal cord is exposed. *C*, Total removal of the intradural tumor is accomplished.

sectioned and reanastomosed. Preoperatively the patient had a weak right hand and truncal hypalgesia below C3. This patient showed excellent neurologic improvement including function of the 11th nerve, and at a follow-up examination 2½ years later had no neurologic deficit. The other one (Case 4) showed only a very mild 11th nerve palsy at the time of the latest follow-up 1 year and 4 months postoperatively. Another patient (Case 3) showed only mild hypalgesia at the right C7 dermatome 1½ years after the operation. The patient with von Recklinghausen's disease

(Case 5) showed very mild residual weakness of the right upper limb 1 year postoperatively. These four patients with neurinomas had returned to their original jobs within 6 months after their operations. The remaining patient (Case 6) with a solitary neurofibroma at the C5-C6 level with complete involvement of the right sixth cervical nerve root had moderate weakness of the right deltoid and biceps muscles with moderate hypalgesia in the right C6 dermatome 3 weeks after the operation. Routine postoperative vertebral angiograms in all of these patients demonstrated this vessel to be patent. Postoperative cervical spine x-ray films demonstrated bony fusion in all of the cases except Case 6, who had the operation performed only 3 weeks before this writing (Figs. 33–8 and 33–9).

The advantages of the transuncodiscal approach include a one-stage operation to remove tumors located in the ventrolateral portion of the spinal canal without retraction of the spinal cord, combined with minimal removal of vertebral bodies by widely opening the intervertebral disc space after disc excision. The operation carries with it the possibility of injury to the vertebral artery and the phrenic, vagus, accessory, and hypoglossal nerves during removal of the dumbbell-shaped tumors. Dangers can be minimized with detailed preoperative studies, including vertebral arteriography, computed tomography, and cer-

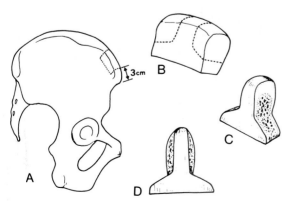

FIGURE 33–7. Diagrams showing preparation of the T-shaped iliac bone graft.

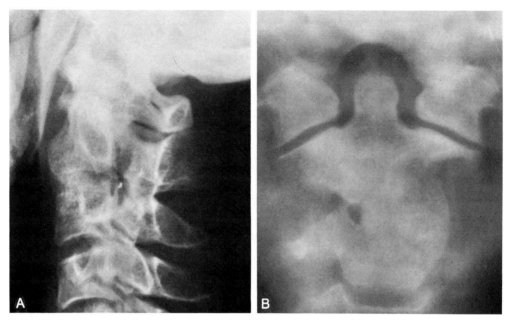

FIGURE 33—8. Case 2. *A*, Lateral cervical spine x-ray film showing good alignment of the cervical spine and complete fusion between C2 and C3. *B*, An anteroposterior tomogram of C2 and C3 showing complete fusion.

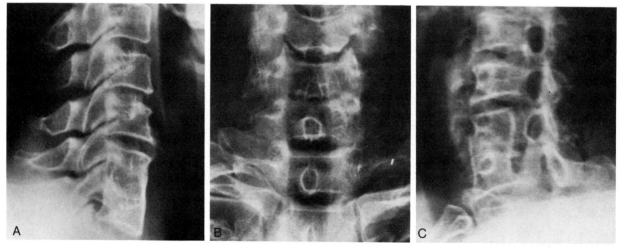

FIGURE 33—9. Case 1. Lateral (*left*) anteroposterior (*center*), and left oblique (*right*) views showing complete fusion between C6 and C7 and good alignment of the cervical spine.

vical myelography and by the application of standard microsurgical techniques. This procedure does require division of the accessory nerve for exposure of dumbbell-shaped tumors located at the high cervical level.

REFERENCES

1. Cloward RB: The anterior approach for removal of ruptured cervical disks. J Neurosurg 15:602–617, 1958.
2. Hakuba A: Transuncodiscal approach. A combined anterior and lateral approach to cervical discs. J Neurosurg 45:284–291, 1976.
3. Hakuba A, Komiyama M, Tsujimoto T, et al: Transuncodiscal approach to dumbbell tumors of the cervical spinal canal. J Neurosurg 61:1100–1106, 1984.
4. Robinson RA, Smith GW: Anterolateral cervical disc removal and interbody fusion for cervical disc syndrome (abstr). Bull Johns Hopkins Hosp 96:223–224, 1955.
5. Verbiest H: A lateral approach to the cervical spine: Technique and indications. J Neurosurg 28:191–203, 1968.

34

ANTERIOR APPROACHES TO THE CERVICAL SPINE

NARAYAN SUNDARESAN and VED P. SACHDEV

INTRODUCTION

Anterior or anterolateral approaches to achieve decompression of tumors as well as to provide access for stabilization are frequently required for tumors involving the cervical spine. The cervical spine can be approached with minimal disruption of normal cervical musculature, and the anterior approach is therefore familiar to most spine surgeons; but a thorough understanding of the complex neurovascular anatomy is required if neural or vascular damage is to be avoided.

The earliest attempts to resect tumors in the cervical spine began in the early 1930s: Crowe and Johnson excised a large tumor of the first, second, and third vertebrae through a transoral approach. This transoral approach was popularized by Fang and colleagues for the drainage of tuberculous infections[4] but has been reported in the past to be associated with a high rate of infection. This can be minimized with microneurosurgical techniques, as well as with perioperative antibiotics. For more extensive anterior approaches to the C1-C3 region, a midline osteotomy of the mandible and median glossotomy is required for a direct anterior approach,[5] or else the temporomandibular joint may have to be dislocated for anterolateral approaches.

In the early 1950s, Lahey and Warren described an extraoral anterior retropharyngeal approach for the repair of an esophageal diverticulum, using the avascular plane between the carotid sheath and the esophagus.[6] At the same time, Robinson, Smith, and coworkers performed anterior cervical discectomy and fusion in a patient with cervical spondylosis and provided a detailed description of the fascial planes of the anterior cervical approach.[10, 11] Similarly, neurosurgeons are familiar with the standard Cloward exposure that is used for disc excisions and anterior fusion.[2] The cervical spine can be divided into three segments by virtue of the limitation imposed by the mandible and hyoid bone in the upper two segments (C1-C2) and by the sternum and clavicle, which hamper access to lower segments (C7-T1). In this chapter, three major approaches will be considered: (1) *high retropharyngeal* approaches for tumors involving the third cervical spine and above; (2) standard *transcervical* exposures for tumors involving C4 through C7; and (3) extended *lateral* and *anterolateral* approaches to the cervical spine. The approach to the C7-T1 junction is considered separately in the next chapter.

As with all segments of the spine, the major indication for anterior approaches to this region is the radiologic demonstration of tumor involvement of the anterior segments; the cervical spine is highly mobile and therefore loss of stability is frequent. In patients with fracture dislocations of the spine, the initial attempt must be to realign the vertebrae by skeletal traction prior to definitive surgery; while halo-traction represents the optimal method of providing external stabilization, it may not always be practical to put all patients in such a device because of the extensive radiologic evaluation required. We therefore suggest the use of the Philadelphia brace with thoracic extension or some other cervicothoracic orthosis.

In all patients, careful evaluation of tumor extent is required by computed tomography (CT) scanning, magnetic resonance imaging (MRI), and angiography. Unlike other levels, the presence of the vertebral artery requires that preoperative visualization of the vascular structures be performed if CT scans show involvement of the foramen transversarium. In view of the relatively small mass that comprises the cervical vertebrae, combined anterior and posterior approaches should be considered when both elements are involved. Single anterior or posterior approaches alone are useful only for palliative decompression or biopsy purposes.

SURGICAL ANATOMY

The anterior triangle of the neck is bounded *medially* by the midline, *laterally* by the anterior part of the sternomastoid muscle, and *superiorly* by the lower border of the mandible and the posterior belly of the digastric muscle. It is subdivided into three auxiliary triangles—the *submandibular, carotid,* and *muscular* triangles—by the anterior and posterior bellies of the digastric muscle and by the superior belly of the omohyoid muscle (Fig. 34–1*A*). Of the various superficial landmarks, the tip of the transverse process of the atlas can be felt between the angle of the jaw and the mastoid process. In the middle, the hyoid bone, the thyroid cartilage, and the cricoid cartilage can be palpated. The hyoid bone lies at the level of the third cervical vertebra, the thyroid cartilage is at the level of the 4th and 5th vertebrae, and the cricoid cartilage is at the level of the 6th cervical vertebra (Fig. 34–1*B*). The platysma muscle extends from the face above as a subcutaneous sheet of muscles to the second rib. Below the platysma muscle lies the investing layer of deep cervical fascia and the right and left anterior jugular veins, which begin in the submental region and pierce this fascia 2 cm above the manubrium to enter the suprasternal space. There are also three superficial nerves in the anterior triangle: (1) the great auricular nerve, (2) the transverse colli nerve or the anterior cutaneous nerve of the neck, and (3) the cervical branch of the facial nerve.

In the median plane, a number of vascular structures run in front of the trachea, which may have to be ligated. These include communications between the anterior jugular vein, the left brachiocephalic vein which passes in the suprasternal notch, the inferior thyroid vein descending to the brachiocephalic veins, and the occasional thyroid ima artery ascending from the brachiocephalic trunk to the thyroid gland. The isthmus of the thyroid gland generally covers the 2nd, 3rd, and 4th tracheal rings. Lateral to these lie the four paired muscles that depress the larynx and hyoid bone and are referred to as the strap muscles. The sternohyoid and omohyoid muscles attach side-by-side to the hyoid body. The superior belly of the omohyoid leaves the sternohyoid below the level of the cricoid cartilage, passes deep through the sternomastoid, and is attached to the upper part of the scapula. The thyrohyoid extends upward to the greater horn and body of the hyoid from the thyroid cartilage, and the sternothyroid extends down to the posterior surface of the manubrium. These strap muscles are supplied by the ventral rami of the cervical nerves 1, 2, and 3 via the hypoglossal nerve and the ansa cervicalis.

The pharynx descends on the front of the spine

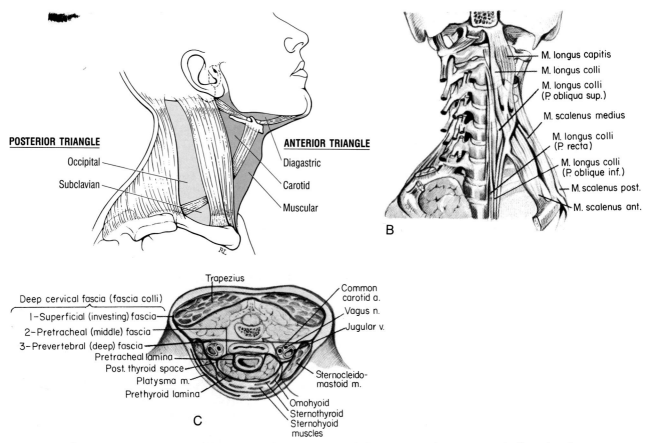

FIGURE 34–1. *A,* Line drawing showing triangles of the neck. For most anterior exposures to the spine, the sternomastoid muscle is retracted laterally. The avascular plane between the trachea and esophagus medially and the carotid sheath laterally is developed. For more extended lateral exposures, the sternomastoid can be detached at its upper or lower end and cut. *B,* Cross-section at the C5 level of the spine indicating the fascial planes and the avascular surgical approach to the anterior spine. *C,* Relationship of the anterior cervical musculature to the cervical spine. (*B* and *C* from Schmidek HH, Smith DA: Anterior cervical disk excision in cervical spondylosis. *In* Schmidek HH, Sweet WH (eds): Operative Neurosurgical Techniques: Indications, Methods, and Results. 2nd ed. Orlando, Grune & Stratton, 1987, pp 1332–1333.)

from the base of the skull to the level of the 6th cervical vertebra, where it becomes continuous with the esophagus. At this level, the larynx becomes continuous with the trachea. Lateral to this level lies the carotid sheath. The common and internal carotid arteries, internal jugular vein, and the vagus nerve descend from the cranial cavity to the thorax and traverse within this condensed sheath of tissue. The arterial stem is medial, the vein is lateral, and the vagus nerve lies posteriorly between the angle of the artery and the vein. Outside the sheath, in front of the rudimentary transverse processes lie the sympathetic trunks. In front of the artery, but outside the sheath, lies the superior root of the ansa cervicalis. At the level of the thyroid cartilage, the common carotid artery ends by dividing into two internal branches of equal size: the internal and external carotid arteries. The internal carotid artery is posterolateral, and the external carotid artery lies anteromedially, and both pass each to the posterior belly of the digastric muscle. The external carotid artery ends in the parotid gland, where it divides into its two terminal branches, and the internal carotid artery passes deep to the parotid gland and the styloid process to the base of the skull. The common and internal carotid artery gives off no branches in the neck, and thus the external carotid artery is the sole supply to the cervical viscera. Three important branches—the superior thyroid, lingual, and fascial—arise from its anterior aspect close to the digastric muscle.

The vagus nerve leaves the skull through the middle compartment of the jugular foramen and descends through the neck within the carotid sheath as far down as the sternoclavicular joint. There it crosses behind the brachiocephalic vein to enter the superior mediastinum. In the superior mediastinum, its course differs on each side. On the right side, it crosses the subclavian artery and descends to the back of the root of the lung, lying first on the side of the brachiocephalic trunk and then on the trachea. On the left side, the vagus nerve continues along the carotid artery to the aortic arch and crosses the left side of the arch to reach the back of the root of the lung. The major branches of importance in the neck include nerve supply to the striated muscles of the pharynx (except stylopharyngeus), soft palate (except tensor palati), and larynx. The pharyngeal branch pierces the superior constrictor and supplies all the muscles of the pharynx and soft palate except the stylopharyngeus, tensor palati, and inferior constrictor. The superior laryngeal nerve passes medial to the internal and external carotid arteries and divides into an internal and external branch. The internal branch pierces the thyrohyoid membrane and is the sensory nerve to the larynx above the level of the vocal cord. The external branch, after supplying the inferior constrictor, ends in the cricothyroid muscle, which is the tensor muscle of the vocal cord. The recurrent laryngeal nerves are important because they may be injured during exposures of the neck. The right nerve arises from the vagus, where it

crosses in front of the subclavian artery, recurs below the subclavian, and ascends upward in the angle between the trachea and esophagus. The left nerve arises where the vagus crosses the aortic arch. It then recurs around the ligamentum arteriosum and ascends in the angle between the trachea and esophagus but has a more constant course on the left side. Both recurrent laryngeal nerves give off cardiac, esophageal, and tracheal branches as well as branches to the inferior constrictor. They supply all muscles of the larynx except the cricothyroid and are sensory to the larynx below the vocal cords.

VERTEBRAL ARTERY ANATOMY

The vertebral artery is divided into two surgical segments in the cervical region: the *pretransverse segment* is that part of the artery between its origin and its entry into the transverse foramina. The *transverse segment* (V2) extends from the point of entry in the foramina to the C2-C3 intertransverse space (Fig. 34–2). The artery itself is approximately 4.5 mm in diameter, and in 40 per cent of the patients the left vertebral artery is dominant. In 35 per cent the right vertebral artery is dominant, and in 23 per cent both arteries are approximately equal. Anatomic variations include direct origins from the aorta (in 3.9 per cent) or from the common carotid artery. Occasionally, there may be a trifurcation of the tracheocephalic trunk or a bifid origin of one vertebral artery.

The C1 segment lies in a triangle above the pleural apex and the vertebral veins and is bounded inferiorly by the subclavian artery, laterally by the longus colli and anterior scalene muscles, and medially by the spine. In the intertransverse segment, the artery passes through the anteromedial part of the transverse foramen in contact with the anterior root of the transverse process, which is about 2.6 mm thick. Each artery is accompanied by a venous plexus, and thus hemostasis may be difficult if these are torn. As

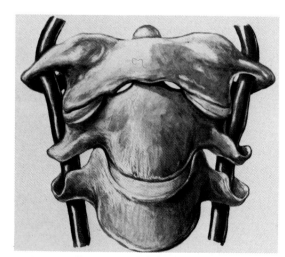

FIGURE 34–2. Relationship of the vertebral artery to the uncovertebral joint. (Reproduced with permission from Watkins RG: Surgical Approaches to the Spine. New York, Springer-Verlag, 1983, p 10.)

the arteries course through the cervical region, they give off branches to the pre- and lateral vertebral muscles, while other spinal arteries enter to supply the radiculomedullary structures.

THE HIGH RETROPHARYNGEAL APPROACH

The operation is performed under general anesthesia in the supine position. If the neck is unstable, skeletal traction using the halo head ring with approximately 5 to 10 lbs of traction is used. While the patient is still awake, both flexion and extension of the neck are tested to determine the extent of safe neck manipulation. It is important to determine the maximum allowable position of neck extension; the patient should be positioned under the maximum possible extension to facilitate exposure. Although intubation while the patient is awake has been proposed, we generally use careful oral intubation under anesthesia in the majority. Fiberoptic nasotracheal intubation may sometimes be necessary for patients with highly unstable spines or marked limitation of neck movement. Monitoring lines for central venous pressure, arterial pressures, and Foley catheter are then inserted. Occasionally, the C-arm of the image intensifier may be positioned if multiple radiographic visualizations are necessary.

The skin incision should be as high as possible (approximately 1 to 2 cm below the mandible) (Fig. 34–3). The side of exposure is usually chosen to allow maximal tumor visualization and resection. To minimize bleeding, we infiltrate the skin with 0.5 per cent zylocaine solution with 1:200,000 epinephrine solution. To extend the skin exposure, a vertical line extending inferiorly is performed either in the midline or in the middle of the transverse incision to form a T. The submandibular incision is carried through the platysma muscle with cautery, and the superficial fascia and skin are mobilized in the form of flaps in the subplatysmal plane down to the investing layer of superficial fascia. These flaps are then everted and sewn to the skin towels.

The marginal mandibular branch of the facial nerve should be identified and preserved. The retromandibular veins drain to the common facial vein, and these can be ligated. By ligating the retromandibular vein and keeping the dissection deep to the vein, the superficial branches of the facial nerve are protected.

The anterior border of the sternomastoid muscle is mobilized by transecting the superficial layer of deep cervical fascia. To enhance exposure, the sternomastoid may also be cut transversely with cautery or stripped from its origin at the mastoid tip. This maneuver allows localization of the carotid sheath by palpation of the arterial pulse. The submandibular salivary gland is resected, and its duct is carefully isolated and sutured to prevent a salivary fistula. All lymph nodes in this vicinity are also resected. The posterior belly of the digastric muscle and the stylo-

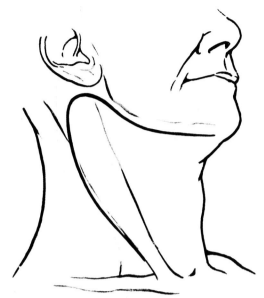

FIGURE 34–3. Skin incision for extended cervical exposures which allows detachment or sectioning of the sternomastoid. (Reproduced with permission from Watkins RG: Surgical Approaches to the Spine. New York, Springer-Verlag, 1983, p 51.)

hyoid are identified, and the digastric tendon is divided intact for later repair (Fig. 34–4A). It is important to avoid retraction of the origin of the stylohyoid muscle, since this may cause injury to the facial nerve as it exists from the skull. Dividing the digastric and stylohyoid muscles allows mobilization of the hyoid bone and the pharynx medially. At this point, the hypoglossal nerve should be identified and mobilized from the base of the skull to the anterior border of the hypoglossal muscle. It is carefully retracted superiorly for the remainder of the procedure. The dissection should proceed to the retropharyngeal space between the contents of the carotid sheath laterally and the pharynx medially (Fig. 34–4B). Superior exposure is facilitated by ligating the branches of the carotid artery and internal jugular vein. By beginning inferiorly and progressing superiorly, several vascular pedicles including the superior thyroid bundle, lingual artery and vein, ascending pharyngeal artery and vein, and facial artery and vein are ligated. This will allow the carotid sheath to be mobilized laterally. The superior laryngeal nerve is carefully identified and mobilized from its origin near the nodose ganglion to its entrance in the larynx.

The prevertebral fascia is then transected longitudinally to expose the longus colli muscles, which are attached to the anterior aspect of the cervical vertebrae (Fig. 34–4C). The midline between the two muscles is carefully noted, as orientation may be lost as the longus colli muscles are detached from the anterior surface of the first vertebra. The anterior atlantooccipital membrane is not disturbed, but the anterior longitudinal ligament is removed.

Tumor resection and decompression are initiated by removal of discs above and below the level of involvement, together with gradual removal of the

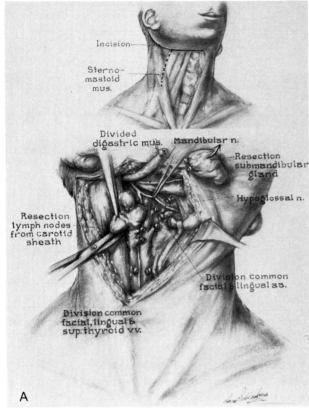

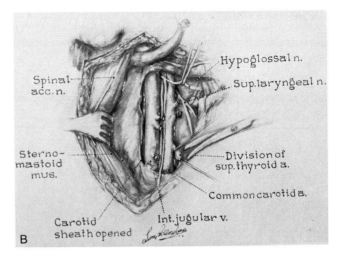

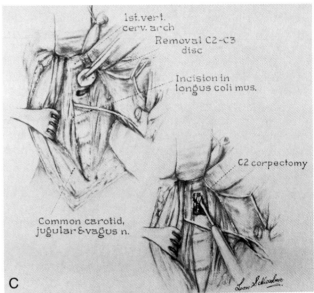

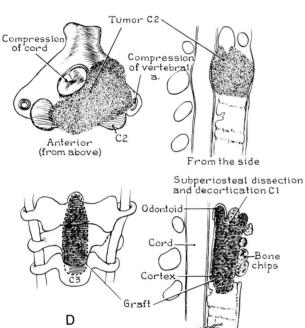

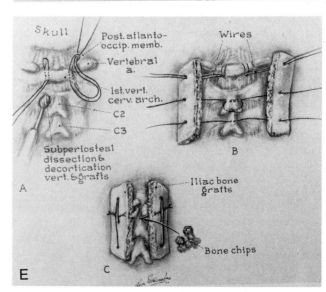

FIGURE 34–4. *See legend on opposite page*

involved bodies piecemeal with curettes and rongeurs. Visualization of the uncovertebral joints between the vertebrae will help the surgeon to confirm the orientation of the midline, and discectomy should proceed to allow complete visualization of the posterior longitudinal ligament. Since blood loss may be profuse during the procedure, it should be minimized by the use of Gelfoam, Avitene, bone wax, or bipolar cautery. Once tumor resection is complete, anterior fusion may be accomplished by either a bone strut or a methyl methacrylate construct. If the hypopharynx has been inadvertently entered, a nasogastric tube should be inserted while the hole is repaired under direct vision in two layers with absorbable sutures. The nasogastric tube should be left in place for 7 to 10 days postoperatively to prevent esophageal or pharyngeal leak with fistula formation. Patients are kept under traction and monitored when they are awake to confirm the absence of a fresh neurologic deficit after operation. The nasal intubation is sometimes maintained for 24 to 48 hours postoperatively. If the neck is still considered unstable, the halo head ring is attached to a vest to allow mobilization. If the spine is unstable, additional posterior cervical fusion may be required. This posterior stabilization may be performed in a one-stage combined procedure, or several days later. In those patients requiring a second posterior fusion, we have delayed operation to the second week (Figs. 34–4D and E and 35–5).

McAfee and colleagues have recently reported their experience with this approach and have described a series of 17 patients, of whom 10 had various tumors involving the spine.[8] In 13 patients, an additional iliac or fibular strut graft was used to provide stabilization. In contrast to the results of infections reported by transoral approaches, there were no infections or iatrogenic neurologic deficits of the spine. The benefits of this approach include both the avoidance of tracheostomy, which is frequently required in the midline mandibulotomy approach, as well as the ability to use a strut graft.

When the operative procedure proceeds expeditiously, this extrapharyngeal approach will allow simultaneous posterior stabilization and arthrodesis to be performed at the same sitting.

STANDARD ANTERIOR APPROACH (C3-C7)
(Figs. 34–6 through 34–10).

For the Cloward or Smith-Robinson approaches, the operation is performed in the supine position under general endotracheal anesthesia. In patients with fracture dislocations, skeletal traction is used intraoperatively. Again, it is important to test the range of flexion and extension in the awake patient prior to induction of anesthesia. The head is turned slightly away from the operative side, and folded sheets are placed underneath the shoulders for extension of the head. A sandbag should be placed underneath the hip if a bone graft is contemplated.

Some surgeons may prefer to identify the level of the skin incision with an intraoperative radiograph prior to making the skin incision. Two operative fields are generally prepared: the cervical region for the tumor resection, and the iliac region for the bone graft. The anesthesiologist should be positioned at the head of the table; ideally, the C-arm of the image intensifier should also be available if instrumentation is contemplated.

For standard cervical lesions, a left-sided approach is generally recommended because of the anatomic differences in the course of the left and right recurrent laryngeal nerves. However, many neurosurgeons may prefer to approach the cervical spine from the right side (Figs. 34–6 and 34–7A and B). The side that allows maximal tumor removal should be chosen in all cases. Either a horizontal incision or an oblique incision along the anterior sternomastoid can be used. We prefer to infiltrate the skin incision with epinephrine to minimize bleeding. The skin and subcutaneous tissues are incised with a knife to expose the platysma muscle, and thereafter most of the

---

FIGURE 34–4. *A,* The high extrapharyngeal exposure to the upper cervical vertebrae. Key features include a high submandibular incision, resection of the submandibular gland, and division of the digastric tendon. The inferior limb of the T is not used unless exposure to the midcervical spine is desired. *B,* After dividing the superficial layer of deep fascia, the carotid sheath is mobilized laterally. This requires division of the superior thyroid pedicle, as well as branches of the internal jugular vein that course medially. The hypoglossal nerve should be identified and preserved; the superior laryngeal nerve is inferior to the hypoglossal nerve and needs to be mobilized and retracted medially. Small branches of the ansa cervicalis (hypoglossus) lie on the carotid sheath and supply the strap muscles. *C,* After the vertebral bodies are exposed, the longus colli muscles are stripped from the front of the spine by cautery and periosteal elevators. The disc between C2 and C3 is identified and removed. Intraoperative radiographs should be taken to confirm the correct level. The body of C2 is then removed with curved curettes and pituitary rongeurs. Occasionally a high speed drill may be required. *D,* Line drawing illustrating involvement of the second cervical vertebra by various tumors; in most patients, both anterior and posterior elements are generally involved, and the vertebral artery is frequently embedded in the tumor. Vertebral angiography with occlusion of the artery should be considered in selected cases. Following tumor resection, stability must be maintained by a strut graft harvested from the ilium, which should be carefully wedged below the anterior arch of the atlas. Postoperatively, patients should be kept immobilized in a halo device. *E,* In most patients, additional posterior fusion with wiring and bone graft from the first to the third cervical vertebrae may be required. Occasionally, the posterior fusion may be performed prior to anterior resection of the tumor. We prefer to supplement bone grafts with Luque instrumentation. (*A* through *E* reproduced with permission from McAfee PC, et al: Anterior retropharyngeal approach to the upper part of the cervical spine. J Bone Joint Surg 69A:1371–1383, 1987.)

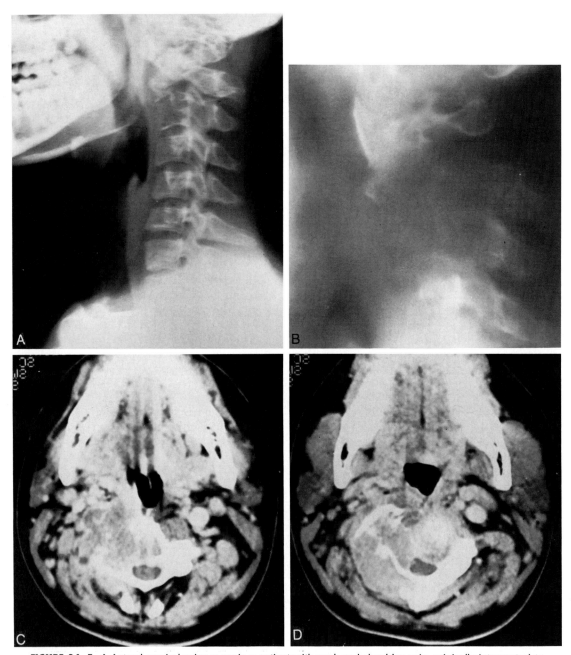

FIGURE 34–5. *A,* Lateral cervical spine x-ray in a patient with neck and shoulder pain, originally interpreted to be normal. *B,* Lateral tomogram in the same patient showing destruction of the C2 and C3 vertebrae secondary to tumor. *C* and *D,* CT scans through the upper cervical spines showing destruction of both anterior and posterior elements by tumor, which encases the left vertebral artery. Biopsy revealed chordoma.

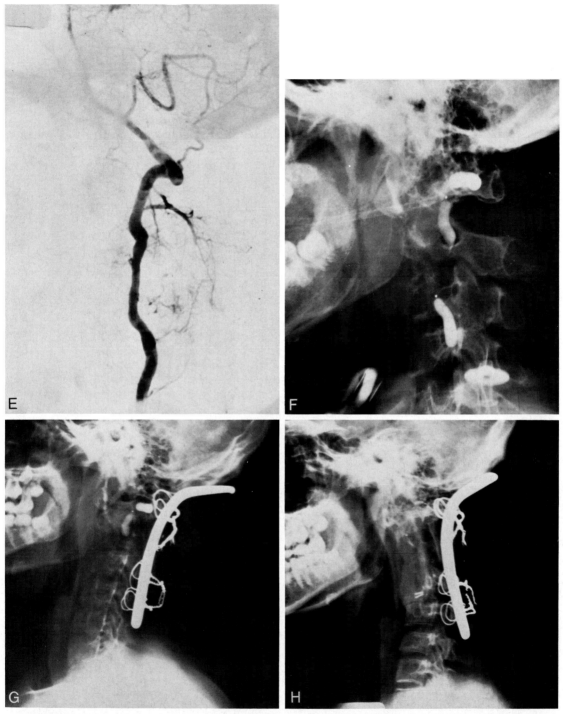

FIGURE 34–5 *Continued.* Left vertebral angiogram (*E*) showing tumor neovascularity typical of chordoma; to facilitate complete tumor resection, the involved segment was occluded with balloon catheters (*F*). *G,* Complete resection of the tumor was carried out in two stages: initially, a posterior decompression and resection of the tumor was performed, and stabilization was achieved with bone grafts and Luque rectangles. At a second stage, the tumor was resected through an anterior retropharyngeal approach. *H,* Postoperative lateral x-ray after removal of tumor and bone graft in position.

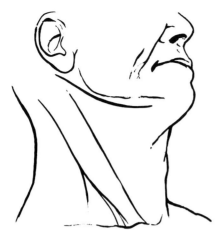

FIGURE 34–6. The high submandibular incision (at or above the hyoid bone) is also used for tumors involving the C3 vertebra. (From Watkins RG: Surgical Approaches to the Spine. New York, Springer-Verlag, 1983, p 13.)

dissection is carried out with fine-tipped electrocautery. The platysma is transsected either in the same plane of the skin incision or parallel to its muscle fibers. Skin flaps should be raised both superiorly and inferiorly to maximize craniocaudal exposure. Hemostasis is achieved by electrocoagulation. Once the skin flaps have been developed, they are held open either with Gelpi retractors or by suturing them to the skin.

The next step is to develop an avascular plane through the investing layer of superficial fascia just anterior to the sternomastoid muscle. This is achieved by grasping the anterior sternomastoid sheath with forceps and dissecting along its anterior border with sharp dissecting scissors. The sternomastoid is retracted laterally, and the trachea and esophagus are retracted medially with small Richardson or Cloward retractors. This maneuver stretches the pretracheal (middle cervical) fascia surrounding the subhyoid

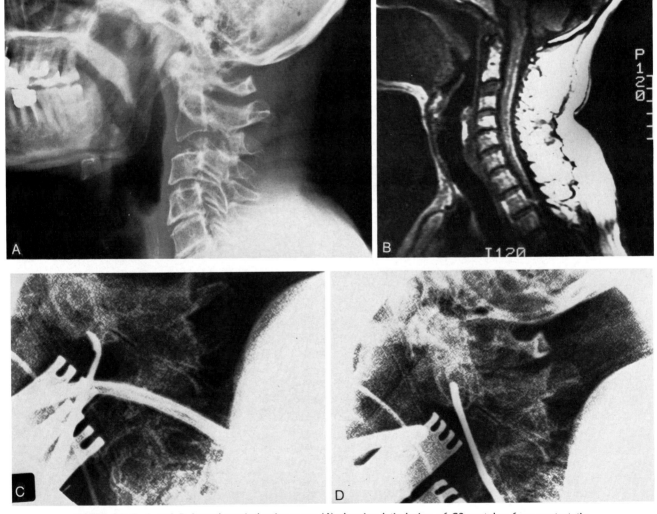

FIGURE 34–7. *A* and *B,* Lateral cervical spine x-ray (*A*) showing lytic lesion of C3 vertebra from metastatic sarcoma. Note that both anterior and posterior elements are involved; MRI (*B*) shows involvement of a single vertebral body and compression of the thecal sac, obviating need for myelography. *C,* Intraoperative x-ray using a C-arm showing accurate identification of the correct vertebral level; the curved curette is showing the inferior rim of the axis and identifies a small remnant of the body of C3 which has to be removed. *D,* Following tumor resection, a heavy Steinmann pin is placed between C2 and C4, and an intraoperative x-ray is taken to confirm accurate positioning of the pin.

muscles. The pretracheal fascia is then opened, and the superior belly of the omohyoid muscle is seen to cross the operative field obliquely. The superior belly of the omohyoid is isolated with a curved hemostat and transected with cautery. A combination of blunt and sharp dissection in the areolar tissue within the avascular plane allows the surgeon to reach the anterior aspect of the spine, which is covered by the longus colli muscles and fascia.

Structures that require ligation with 00 silk sutures during this dissection include the middle thyroid vein and sometimes the inferior thyroid vein. In the upper cervical region, a large venous trunk (Farabeu's trunk) or one of its branches to the jugular vein may also be encountered. The midline is gradually developed by progressively retracting the carotid sheath and the sternomastoid laterally, and the trachea and esophagus medially. The prevertebral fascia is cauterized in the midline and incised longitudinally, which exposes the anterior longitudinal ligament. At this point, a disc space is identified with a Keith or spinal needle, and an intraoperative radiograph is

taken for confirmation of the proper level (Fig. 34–7C and D). While the x-ray is being developed, the medial aspects of the longus colli muscle are cauterized and stripped laterally with a periosteal elevator. This helps keep the wound relatively bloodless and is vital to the proper placement of the sharp self-retaining Cloward or Caspar retractors. Self-retaining Cloward or Caspar blades are placed beneath the edges of the longus colli muscle, and the retractor is positioned for proper exposure. Failure to position the blades correctly is often responsible for many traction-related complications. After the lateral retractors are positioned, the smaller blunt self-retaining retractors that allow craniocaudal visualization may be positioned. The disc spaces above and below the level of tumor involvement are identified. The disc spaces are then incised with No. 15 blades, and the discs removed with a combination of sharp-angled curettes and rongeurs. Once the disc spaces above and below the site of pathology have been identified, the vertebral body or bodies are removed with Adson or Leksell rongeurs. By this process of

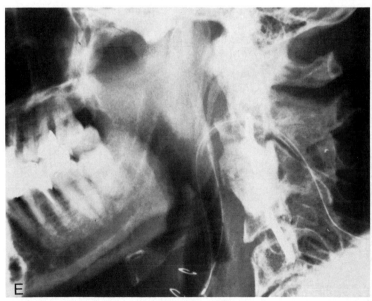

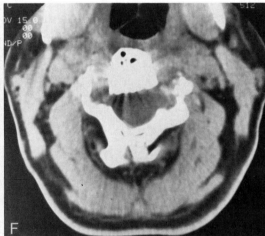

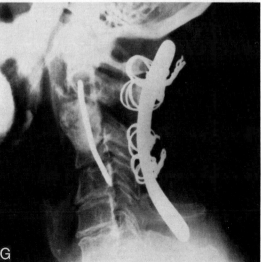

FIGURE 34–7 *Continued. E,* The resected vertebra is then replaced with methyl methacrylate, which is allowed to polymerize in situ. *F,* The extent of resection is further evaluated by a postoperative CT scan; although the vertebral body has been removed, there is persistent tumor in the pedicle and facets which is accessible only through a posterior approach. *G,* During the second stage posterior procedure, the laminae, facets, and pedicles are resected. Stabilization is carried out with bone grafts and contoured Luque ³⁄₁₆-inch rectangles.

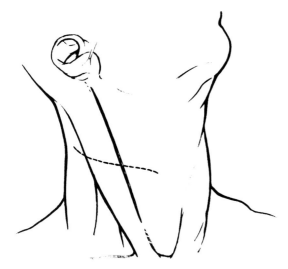

FIGURE 34–8. For cervical lesions C4 through C7, a standard transcervical skin incision is used. By raising skin flaps, it is possible to expose several vertebrae in a superior-inferior direction. (From Watkins RG: Surgical Approaches to the Spine. New York, Springer-Verlag, 1983, p 27.)

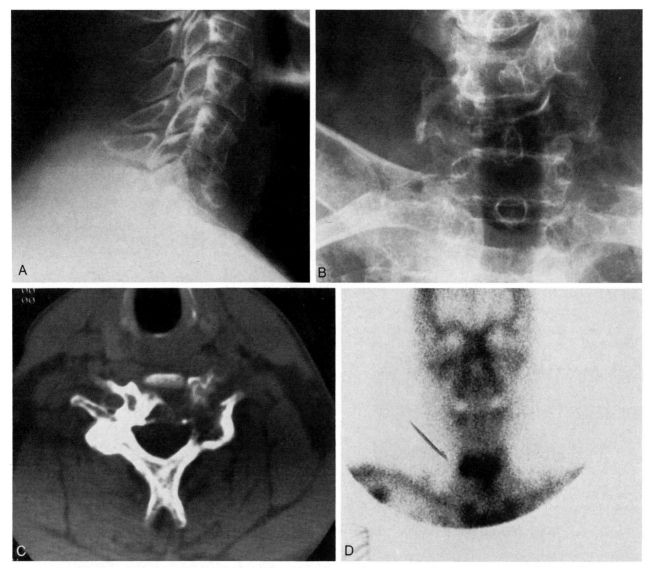

FIGURE 34–9. A through D, Anteroposterior and lateral cervical spine x-rays showing compression fracture of the C6 vertebra from metastatic osteogenic sarcoma. Note that the anteroposterior view shows tumor extension into the facet and pedicle. CT scan (C) confirms involvement of anterior and posterior elements in the patient. For curative resection, both an anterior and posterior approach is necessary. Radionuclide bone scan (D) confirms that this is a solitary focus within bone; with the advent of modern chemotherapy regimens, solitary relapse sites within bone are becoming increasingly common. In patients with solitary relapse sites within the spine, resection is indicated prior to the onset of neurologic deficit.

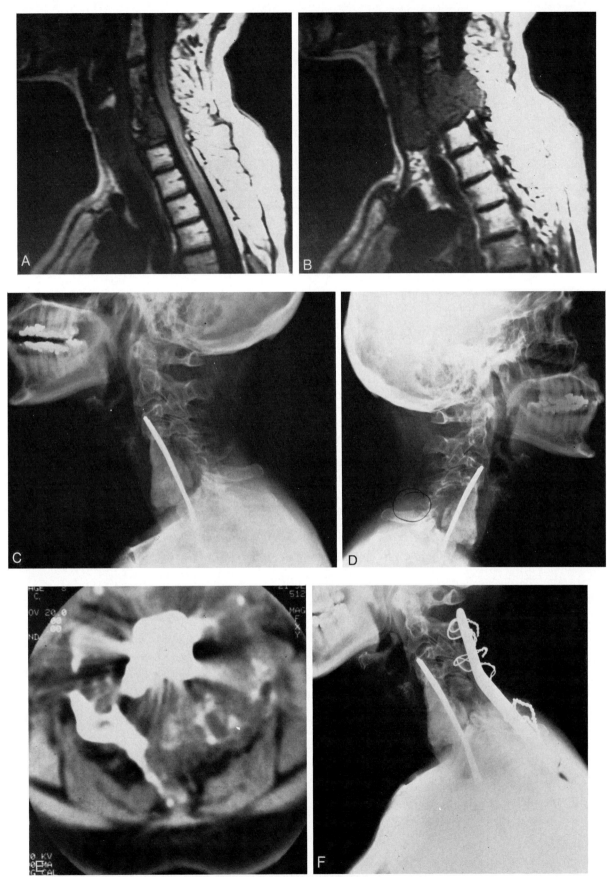

FIGURE 34–10. *A* and *B*, Sagittal MRI scans showing destruction of C4 through C6 vertebrae from breast cancer. Note that the abnormal signal extends to the posterior elements as well, indicating involvement. *C*, At initial Stage I resection, the anterior elements are resected through an anterior approach, and stabilization is carried out with methyl methacrylate and Steinmann pins. Several months later while on hormonal therapy, progressive destruction of the posterior elements is noted on spine x-ray (*D*) and confirmed by CT scan (*E*). A second-stage posterior resection and stabilization were then carried out; patient is currently alive and free of neurologic deficits more than three years following operation. *F*, Lateral cervical spine x-ray in the same patient showing posterior resection and stabilization with Luque rods and bone grafts.

intralesional curettage, the pathologic bodies are gradually removed down to the posterior longitudinal ligament. To maintain proper orientation, the end plates below should be curetted cleanly. The raised edges of the uncovertebral joint will help orientate the surgeon to the lateral margins of the body; beyond the joints lie the vertebral arteries and their associated plexuses. Laterally, dissection should extend to free the nerve roots. Generally, a diamond burr or other high speed drill should be used to thin the posterior bony cortex, after which the remaining shelf can be resected with fine 3-mm Kerrison punches. The posterior longitudinal ligament appears as a structure with glistening fibers that are vertically aligned and tenaciously adherent to the dura. It is important to remove this structure completely, since tumor remnants are often present underneath it. Tumor dissection is continued down to the dura and is aided using magnification with 3.5- to 4.5-powered loupes. The final stages of the operative procedure requires sharp dissection with micro instruments to free the dura from adherent tumor. If a bone fusion is decided upon, a piece of bone graft with three cortical edges is taken from the ilium. It is important to measure the graft bed accurately, so that a graft approximately 2 to 3 mm longer than the bed is harvested. This graft is then countersunk with bone tamps while traction is applied. For immediate stabilization, we prefer to use our technique of Steinmann pin fixation: the pins should clearly straddle at least one vertebra above and below the resected segment, and their position checked intraoperatively by x-ray to avoid misdirection (Fig. 34–7D). A piece of Gelfoam is placed in the wound, and methyl methacrylate is poured in and allowed to solidify. If the Steinmann pins are difficult to position, an alternate technique may be to use anterior distraction rods, such as Knodt rods, or anterior cervical plates, which allow screws to be placed above and below the resected vertebra. The wound is then irrigated and a drain placed through the anterior aspect of the wound through a separate incision. The muscles are approximated, and the platysma muscle and skin are closed with fine sutures. The drain is removed in 24 to 48 hours.

The postoperative management is generally straightforward, and a Philadelphia brace or cervicothoracic orthosis is used for immobilization if a bone graft is used. If several vertebrae have been resected or if there is marked instability, the halo should be used to prevent dislodgement of the graft.

Although this procedure is relatively simple, a wide variety of complications have been reported. In patients with benign disc disease, complication rates have ranged from 10 to 20 per cent. Retraction-related problems result in laryngeal edema, hoarseness, dysphagia, or the sensation of a lump in the throat. This can be minimized by accurate placement of the Cloward retractor blades underneath the longus colli muscle. A short course of steroid therapy may be helpful for the edema, and a tracheostomy should rarely be necessary.

Bleeding from the epidural space is common especially when the posterior longitudinal ligament is removed; in most cases, such bleeding can be controlled with hemostatic agents such as Avitene. However, occasionally such epidural bleeding may result in compression of the dura. If a neurologically intact person deteriorates in the early hours following operation, epidural bleeding should be suspected and the patient taken immediately back to the operating room for reexploration.

Injury to the carotid artery or sympathetic trunk has been reported with resulting ischemia and Horner's syndrome. Injury to the vertebral artery has also resulted in excessive bleeding and occasionally in a carotid-cavernous fistula. Occasionally, esophageal and tracheal perforation may result from the retractors. If an esophagus perforation occurs, this should be repaired immediately with nonabsorbable sutures.

When grafts are used, various bone graft/donor site problems may occur in approximately 5 per cent of cases. These may result from graft extrusion, nonunion, or infections around the donor site.

If the tumor involves both anterior and posterior elements, the second-stage posterior approach may be performed one to two weeks later (Fig. 34–7G). We prefer to use Luque fixation for posterior stabilization in the cervical spine.

LATERAL APPROACH

In 1968, Verbiest described an anterolateral approach to the cervical spine which was used to decompress lateral spondylotic ridges compressing the vertebral artery.[14] This approach was originally described by Henry for exposure of the vertebral artery within the intraosseous cervical spine[5] (Fig. 34–11). In occasional patients with tumors involving the brachial plexus or laterally placed cervical tumors, this operation is indicated alone or in combination with posterior laminectomy. Patients are positioned in the supine position, with the head in neutral position. We prefer to use a transverse incision, but an oblique incision along the anterior border of the sternomastoid is just as acceptable. After cutting the platysma muscle, two cutaneous nerves will be in view: the great auricular nerve and the transverse cutaneous nerve of the neck. Although Verbiest suggested that the sternomastoid be retracted laterally, we prefer to detach it at its cephalad insertion or to section it with cautery. Using blunt dissection, the carotid sheath is identified and retracted laterally. The trachea and esophagus are then retracted medially with Cloward retractors. This allows identification of the anterior tubercles of the transverse processes, the most prominent of which is the Chassaignac tubercle of the C6 vertebra. The anterior tubercles give attachment to the prevertebral fascia, the longus colli, longus capitis, and the anterior scalene muscles. The attachments of the longus colli, which runs from the C2-T3 region, are detached from the anterior tubercles and

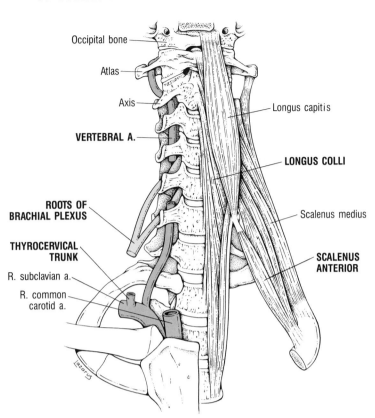

FIGURE 34–11. Line drawing showing pertinent anatomy of the anterolateral approach described by Verbiest.

retracted medially. While retracting the longus colli muscle medially, it is important to avoid injury to the cervical sympathetic chain that runs just in front of the transverse processes behind the carotid sheath. After dissecting all muscular attachments to the anterior tubercle, the anterior roots of the transverse processes as well as the costotransverse lamellae are removed. Bleeding may be encountered from both veins and from pathologic vessels draining into the vertebral plexus. The bone itself is removed by fine rongeurs or a high speed drill. The nerve root lies posterior to the vertebral artery at the level of the foramen transversorium. The joint of Luschka lies at the superior medial portion of the costotransverse lamella; in Verbiest's approach, lateral retraction of the vertebral artery was suggested. Following tumor resection, the wound is approximated in layers after placing a drain.

REFERENCES

1. Bailey RW, Badgley CE: Stabilization of the cervical spine by anterior fusion. J Bone Joint Surg 42A:565–594, 1960.
2. Cloward R: Ruptured Cervical Intervertebral Discs—Codman Signature Series 4. Randolph, MA, Codman & Shurtleff, 1974.
3. DeAndrade JR, MacNab I: Anterior occipito-cervical fusion using an extra-pharyngeal exposure. J Bone Joint Surg 51A:1621–1626, 1969.
4. Fang HSY, Ong GB: Direct anterior approach to the upper cervical spine. J Bone Joint Surg 44A:1588–1604, 1962.
5. Henry AK: Extensile Exposure. Baltimore, Williams & Wilkins, 1959, pp 53–72.
6. Lahey FH, Warren KW: Esophageal diverticula. Surg Gynec Obstet 98:1–28, 1954.
7. Johnson RN, Southwick WO: Surgical approaches to the cervical spine. In Rothman RH, Simeone FA (eds): The Spine. Philadelphia, WB Saunders, 1982, pp 93–147.
8. McAfee PC, Bohlman HH, Riley LH, et al: Anterior retro-pharyngeal approach to the upper part of the cervical spine. J Bone Joint Surg 69A:1371–1383, 1987.
9. Riley LH Jr: Surgical approaches to the anterior structures of the cervical spine. Clin Orthop 91:16–20, 1973.
10. Robinson RA, Smith GW: Antero-lateral cervical disc removal and interbody fusion for cervical disc syndrome (abstr). Bull Johns Hopkins Hosp 98:223–224, 1955.
11. Robinson RA, Riley LH: Techniques of exposure and fusion of the cervical spine. Clin Orthop 109:78–84, 1975.
12. Schmidek HH, Smith DA: Anterior cervical disc excision in cervical spondylosis. In Schmidek HH, Sweet WH (eds): Operative Neurosurgical Techniques—Indications, Methods, Results. Philadelphia, WB Saunders, 1988, pp 1327–1345.
13. Tew JM Jr, Mayfield FH: Complications of surgery of the anterior cervical spine. Clin Neurosurg 23:424, 1976.
14. Verbiest H: Antero-lateral operations for fractures and dislocations in the middle and lower parts of the cervical spine. J Bone Joint Surg 51A:1489–1530, 1969.
15. Watkins RG: Surgical Approaches to the Spine. New York, Springer-Verlag, 1983, pp 1–50.
16. Whitesides TE Jr, Kelly RP: Lateral approach to the upper cervical spine for anterior fusion. South Med J 59:879–883, 1966.

35

SURGICAL APPROACHES TO THE CERVICOTHORACIC JUNCTION

NARAYAN SUNDARESAN and GEORGE V. DiGIACINTO

INTRODUCTION

The choice of surgical approaches to the cervicothoracic junction should be dictated by the location and extent of the pathology, the scope of planned surgery, as well as the need for stabilization. With the advent of computed tomography (CT) scans, it is apparent that the majority of tumors in the cervicothoracic junction predominantly involve the anterior segments of the spine, thus dictating an anterior approach for adequate exposure. Frequently, adjacent vertebral bodies as well as the rib cage may be involved, and the tumor may invade the lower cord of the brachial plexus. In those patients in whom a direct anterior approach is indicated, two physiologic constraints limit direct anterior exposures to the spine: (1) the shape of the thoracic inlet, and (2) the degree of anterior kyphosis resulting from possible pathologic collapse of the vertebra.[4] Since the cervicothoracic junction forms the apex of two physiologic curvatures, anterior stabilization is technically difficult to accomplish and frequently needs to be supplemented by additional posterior stabilization. Primary tumors are infrequently found at this region, and by far the most common tumor encountered is a carcinoma of the lung (superior sulcus tumor) with direct extension to the spine and brachial plexus. The majority of such tumors have extensive anterolateral paraspinous components and also directly invade the perineurium of intercostal nerves. These tumors should not be resected through the direct anterior approach described here, but are more appropriately approached by posterolateral thoracotomy by virtue of the necessity to resect the extensive paraspinal tumor. Most metastases to the cervicothoracic region, however, should be candidates for this procedure; in our experience, tumors in this region arise most often from the breast, kidney, lung, and/or soft parts (sarcomas), in addition to the occasional primary tumor such as osteosarcoma and Ewing's sarcoma.

The initial surgical efforts to approach this region were directed toward the drainage of Pott's abscesses. Both Capener[1] and Menard[5] initially described lateral costotransversectomy approaches that allow biopsy of tumors as well as limited neural decompression, but these approaches do not allow access for stabilization. In 1957, Nanson[6] described an anterior approach for upper dorsal sympathectomy which is rarely used today. Most dorsal sympathectomies are currently performed by the transaxillary approach. The supraclavicular approach may occasionally be used for biopsy of tumors in this region prior to a more definitive procedure. Before the development of magnification techniques and effective illumination, direct anterior approaches to the upper thoracic vertebrae carried considerable morbidity (up to 30 per cent), and Hodgson suggested that this approach be abandoned in favor of posterolateral thoracotomy.[3]

SURGICAL ANATOMY

The thoracic inlet is kidney-shaped with an average anteroposterior diameter of 5 cm and a transverse diameter of 10 cm. It is bounded by the first thoracic vertebra posteriorly, the top of the manubrium anteriorly, and the first ribs on each side (Fig. 35–1A). Its plane slopes forward and downward, but there is considerable variation in the size, shape, and obliquity of the inlet. The sternomastoid muscle arises from the sternum and clavicle by two heads. The sternal head is a rounded fasciculus that is tendinous and arises from the upper part of the anterior surface of the manubrium. The clavicular head is more fleshy

A portion of this chapter appeared originally in Sundaresan N, Shah J, Feghali J: The trans-sternal approach to the upper thoracic vertebra. Am J Surg 198:473–477, 1984, and is reprinted with permission.

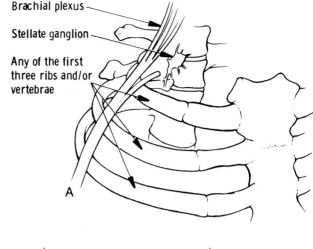

Brachial plexus

Stellate ganglion

Any of the first
three ribs and/or
vertebrae

A

FIGURE 35–1. *A,* Line drawing showing thoracic
inlet and relationship of bony structures to the
stellate ganglion and brachial plexus. *B,* Surgical
anatomy at the base of the neck.

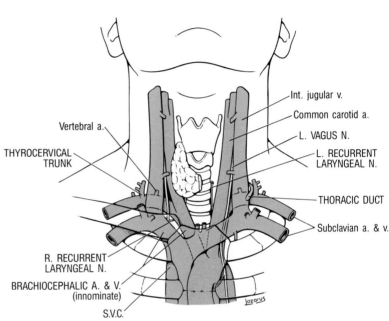

Vertebral a.

THYROCERVICAL
TRUNK

Int. jugular v.

Common carotid a.

L. VAGUS N.

L. RECURRENT
LARYNGEAL N.

THORACIC DUCT

Subclavian a. & v.

R. RECURRENT
LARYNGEAL N.

BRACHIOCEPHALIC A. & V.
(innominate)

S.V.C.

and arises from the superior border and anterior
surface of the medial third of the clavicle. More
posteriorly lie the infrahyoid strap muscles. The
sternohyoid muscle arises from the posterior surface
of the medial end of the clavicle, the posterior sternoclavicular ligament, and the posterior surface of
the manubrium and medial end of the first rib.
Important vascular structures in the superior mediastinum include the innominate, common carotid,
and left subclavian arteries arising from the arch of
the aorta (Fig. 35–1*B*). The innominate artery originates from the convexity of the aortic arch and passes
obliquely upward, backward, and to the right. A
high-riding arch with a more distal origin of the
innominate artery may necessitate considerable retraction if a right-sided approach is used. The recurrent laryngeal nerve arises from the vagus and
courses around the subclavian artery on the right
and around the aortic arch on the left. It traverses
the operative field obliquely at a higher level on the
right and around the aortic arch on the left. On the
left side, it reaches the tracheoesophageal groove

more caudally and is thus less liable to injury with
this exposure. In a recent report of 1000 thyroidec-
tomies, Sanders and colleagues[7] noted that the right
recurrent laryngeal nerve was not "recurrent" in 1
per cent of his study patients and arose at a higher
level in the neck. On the left side, no anatomic
variations were noted. Another important structure
that is potentially vulnerable is the thoracic duct. At
this level, it usually lies to the left of the midline and
empties at the junction of the internal jugular and
subclavian veins posteriorly. Occasionally it may divide into two branches, one emptying on the left side
and the other into the right subclavian vein with the
right lymphatic duct. The right lymphatic duct is
much less prominent and should not be encountered
during this dissection.

The blood supply of the spinal cord in the lower
cervical region is derived from radicular arteries that
take origin from the vertebral, thyrocervical, and
costocervical branches of the subclavian artery. In
the upper thoracic region, radicular vessels originate
from the supreme intercostal arteries. The cervico-

thoracic junction thus represents a watershed zone between these two major arterial zones and is therefore more vulnerable to ischemic injury.

CLINICAL FEATURES AND RADIOLOGIC EVALUATION

The majority of patients with lesions involving the upper thoracic region present with pain in the neck or in the interscapular region. Involvement of the nerve roots (C8 through T2) may produce radiation of pain, with associated numbness and tingling down the arm. A Horner's syndrome may result if the lesion involves the superior sympathetic ganglion, which lies in the paravertebral gutter. With tumor extension superiorly and laterally, there may be signs of involvement of the brachial plexus.

Radiologic studies should include plain roentgenograms, although this region is difficult to evaluate by plain radiography alone. Computed tomography and sagittal tomography are almost invariably required (Figs. 35–2 through 35–5). CT scan is the best modality for revealing soft tissue tumor extension into the paravertebral gutters or the brachial plexus (Fig. 35–2). Myelography is required in all

patients. Frequently, a pronounced anterior defect will be noted from bony subluxation of one vertebra over the other; on occasion, a complete block may be noted (Fig. 35–3). For adequate decompression of the spinal cord, all vertebrae involved in a kyphotic deformity must be resected. Radionuclide bone scans are valuable in detecting concomitant disease in adjacent or distant sites. In patients presenting with a pathologic compression fracture at this region, abdominal examination by a CT scan should be carried out to exclude a primary lesion in the kidney.

SUPRACLAVICULAR APPROACH

For the supraclavicular approach, the patient is positioned supine with the neck hyperextended and rotated slightly away from the side. A transverse incision is made 1 to 2 cm above the clavicle, and the platysma muscle is divided in the plane of the incision (Fig. 35–6). The incision should extend from the midline anteriorly and beyond the sternomastoid posteriorly. Both anterior and external jugular veins should be divided. The external investing fascia, which contains the sternomastoid, is incised with cautery, and the sternomastoid itself is cut from a

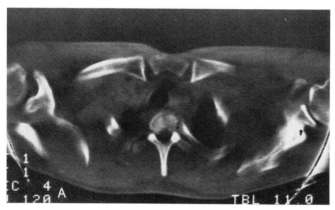

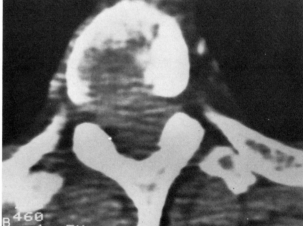

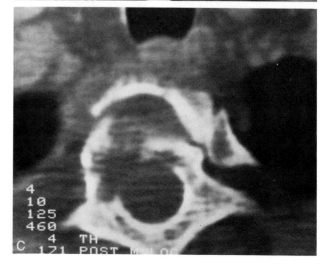

FIGURE 35–2. *A,* CT scan showing tumor involving the second thoracic vertebra (osteosarcoma). *B,* CT scan discloses destructive lesion involving second thoracic vertebra (metastatic breast carcinoma). *C,* CT scan showing subluxation of T1 on T2 vertebra caused by inappropriate laminectomy for tumor involving the anterior elements.

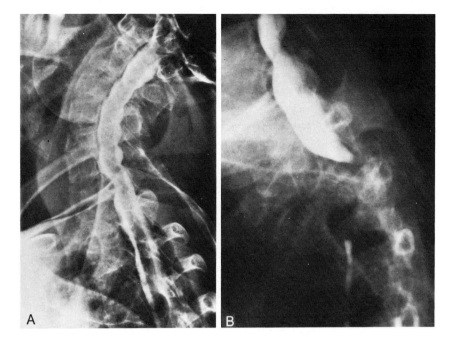

FIGURE 35–3. *A,* Myelogram with patient in swimmer's position shows tumor with epidural compression at the T1-T2 level. *B,* Myelogram through C1-C2 puncture showing complete block resulting from laminectomy, and secondary bony subluxation.

lateral to medial direction while the structures posterior to it are protected with a right-angled clamp or by the finger of the surgeon. The inferior strap muscles (omohyoid and sternohyoid muscles) are then sectioned, which exposes the anterior scalene muscle lateral to the prevertebral fascia (Fig. 35–7). The phrenic nerve lies on the anterior scalene muscle and must be protected from injury. By retracting the phrenic nerve, carotid sheath, and the internal jugular vein medially, the anterior scalene muscle is exposed. This muscle is covered by the Sibson's fascia, which connects the transverse processes of the 7th cervical vertebra to the first rib. This fascia is continuous with the endothoracic fascia on the inner surface of the first rib. The anterior scalene muscle may be divided and the Sibson's fascia freed from the transverse process of the 7th cervical vertebra, which will then allow inferior retraction of the lung. The recurrent laryngeal nerve should be identified within the operative field and retracted medially. A limited exposure of the spine is afforded by opening the prevertebral fascia over the midline of the bodies of the vertebra. Important structures that require protection include the subclavian artery and the thyrocervical trunk; this trunk consists of the vertebral artery, which courses medially to enter the foramen transversarium at the sixth cervical vertebra, the anterior cervical artery, and the transcervical artery, which courses posteriorly into the posterior cervical triangle (Fig. 35–8). In addition, if the approach is from the left, the junction of the internal jugular vein and subclavian veins will contain the thoracic duct. While the supraclavicular approach is useful for biopsy of tumors of the lung apex, it does not provide adequate access for resection of more extensive tumors involving either the paraspinal or midline regions.

MEDIAN STERNOTOMY

In 1957, Cauchoix and Binet[2] described their experience with a direct transsternal approach to the cervicothoracic region. The skin incision consists of two parts: a cervical one along the anterior border of the sternomastoid muscle, and a thoracic extension along the midline of the sternum down to the xyphoid process (Fig. 35–9). The cervical incision is carried out first, and the periosteum is stripped off the sternum. A median sternotomy is then performed. A Finochietto retractor is then placed in the sternotomy wound and gradually opened. The two operative areas are then joined by dividing the inferior strap muscles, that is, the sternohyoid and the sternothyroid. The pleura is carefully dissected on both sides and retracted. The left innominate vein is divided between ligatures, and the upper portion of the aortic arch is exposed. The trachea and esophagus are retracted toward the right side, and the cervicothoracic vertebrae from the 4th cervical to the 3rd dorsal can be visualized. The left recurrent laryngeal nerve, which runs in the tracheoesophageal junction, must be seen and retracted in the exposure. In the original report, Cauchoix and Binet described a 19-year-old patient with a chondroma in whom tumor resection was performed but noted that lateral extension precluded total resection of the tumor. We have used this approach only for extensive tumors that involve both the cervical and thoracic vertebrae, especially if profuse bleeding is expected.

TRANSAXILLARY APPROACH

An alternative approach to the upper thoracic spine and pleural apex is the transaxillary approach

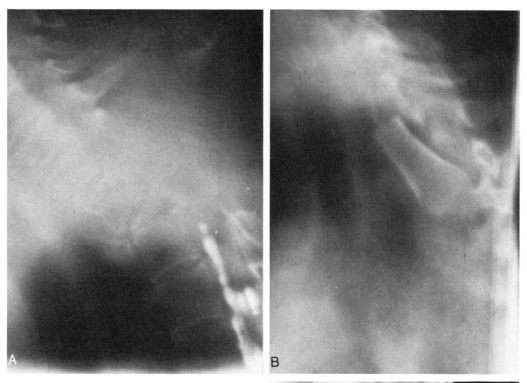

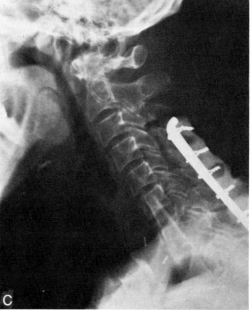

FIGURE 35—4. *A,* Lateral tomogram showing subluxation of T1 on T2 caused by laminectomy; to correct this deformity, tumor resection of the involved vertebrae and anterior fusion through the transsternal approach was necessary. *B,* Lateral tomogram showing resected vertebra and fusion with resected clavicle. *C,* At junctional segments, secondary posterior stabilization with Luque rods may be necessary for adequate fixation in long-term survivors.

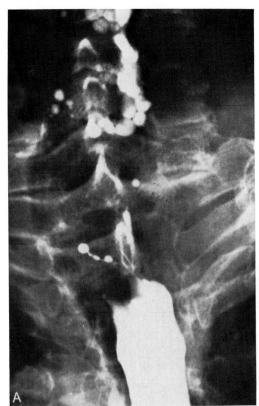

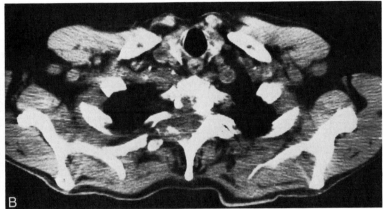

FIGURE 35–5. *A,* Myelogram showing block at the T1-T2 level secondary to carcinoma of the esophagus. *B,* CT scan in same patient showing tumor is predominantly *lateral* to the midline; in such cases, a direct anterior approach is contraindicated.

FIGURE 35–6. Line drawing showing supraclavicular incision.

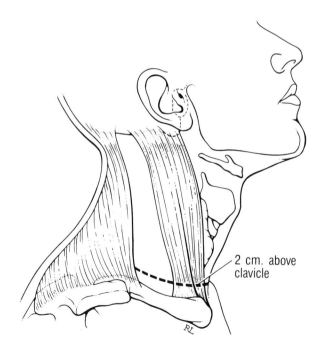

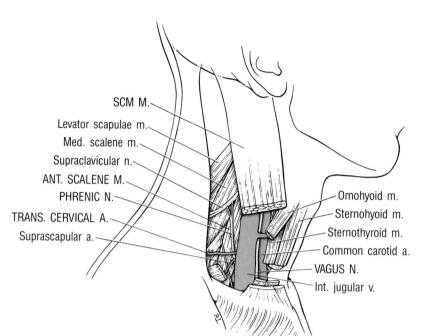

SCM M.
Levator scapulae m.
Med. scalene m.
Supraclavicular n.
ANT. SCALENE M.
PHRENIC N.
TRANS. CERVICAL A.
Suprascapular a.

Omohyoid m.
Sternohyoid m.
Sternothyroid m.
Common carotid a.
VAGUS N.
Int. jugular v.

FIGURE 35–7. Vascular and neural structures seen after section of the sternomastoid and strap muscles.

FIGURE 35–8. Deep vascular and neural structures exposed in the supraclavicular approaches.

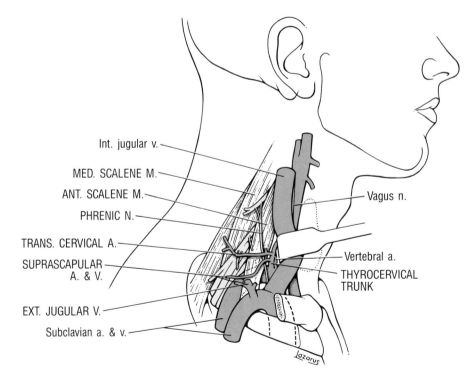

Int. jugular v.
MED. SCALENE M.
ANT. SCALENE M.
PHRENIC N.
TRANS. CERVICAL A.
SUPRASCAPULAR A. & V.
EXT. JUGULAR V.
Subclavian a. & v.

Vagus n.
Vertebral a.
THYROCERVICAL TRUNK

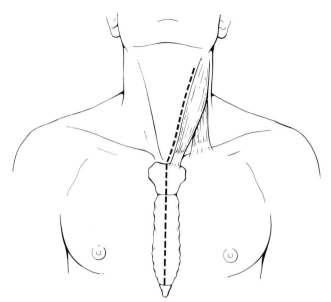

FIGURE 35–9. Incision for combined cervicothoracic exposures via median sternotomy.

used for upper dorsal sympathectomy. A major advantage of this approach is its minimum morbidity, since no major muscles need to be sectioned.

Patients are positioned in the lateral position with the arm abducted and the elbow flexed. The forearm is held in position with padded dressings attached to an ether screen. The skin incision is made from the anterior to the posterior axillary folds, opposite the third intercostal space. The incision is deepened down by cautery to the chest wall, and the axillary fat pad is pushed cephalad. The intercostobrachial nerve exits through the second interspace and should be carefully identified and sectioned. By palpation with fingers, the third rib can be identified. The pleural cavity is entered either through the second or third interspace, and the operation may or may not always require rib resection. In general, it is preferable to enter the third interspace directly without rib resection, and a small Finochietto retractor is positioned and gradually opened. If a rib resection is decided upon, cautery is used to strip the periosteum off the third rib, and the periosteum is dissected free with the Alexander periosteal elevator. The rib is then removed with rib shears or box rongeurs, and the self-retaining lung retractor is placed. The apex of the lung is then deflated and held down by sponge sticks. The sympathetic chain and the first two vertebral bodies are generally visible through the pleura. The parietal pleura is opened over the bodies of T1 through T3 and is dissected medially to expose the anterior surfaces of the vertebral bodies. Once biopsy or resection is completed, the pleural cavity is drained with a chest tube for 48 to 72 hours following surgery. In view of the limited exposure afforded of the upper thoracic inlet, this approach is not advocated for major tumor resection.

TRANSSTERNAL APPROACH TO THE UPPER THORACIC VERTEBRAE

The operation is performed under general endotracheal anesthesia and with the patient placed in the supine position. The neck is extended slightly using a folded sheet under the shoulders and a donut under the head. The range of extension and flexion of the neck should be tested preoperatively with the patient awake. In patients with instability of the spine, a halo traction device is applied and traction maintained intraoperatively. A T-shaped skin incision is used (Fig. 35–10). The horizontal limb is made 1 cm above the clavicle and extends to the lateral margin of the sternocleidomastoid muscle on either side. The vertical limb is extended down to the body of the sternum. Subplatysmal flaps are elevated and retained by sutures (Fig. 35–11). Several veins (the anterior jugular veins and the jugular venous arch) and the medial supraclavicular nerve may cross the site and need to be sectioned. The sternal and clavicular heads of the sternocleidomastoid muscle are detached from their bony origins by cautery and are retracted superiorly and laterally. The strap muscles (sternohyoid and sternothyroid muscles) on the ipsilateral side are sectioned just above the clavicle and sternal notch. They are cut and retracted superiorly and medially (Fig. 35–12). The fatty and areolar tissues in the suprasternal space are cleared. The sternal origin of the pectoralis major muscle is stripped laterally off the body of the sternum, and at the same time the medial half of the clavicle is stripped subperiosteally of all muscle insertions. The medial third of the clavicle is sectioned using a Gigli wire saw. This segment of clavicle is then disarticulated from the manubrium. A power drill is used to thin the edges of a rectangular piece of manubrium, which is then cut with heavy scissors (Fig. 35–13).

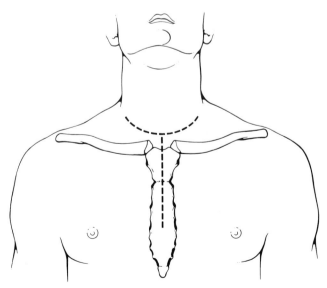

FIGURE 35–10. The position of the skin incision is represented by the broken lines.

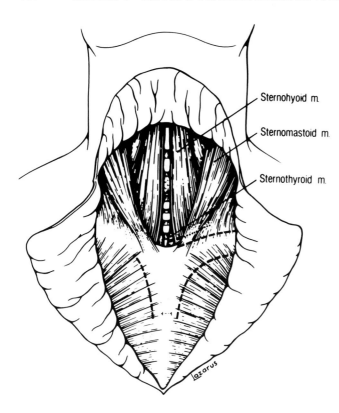

Sternohyoid m.

Sternomastoid m.

Sternothyroid m.

FIGURE 35–11. With skin flaps elevated, the pectoralis major, sternomastoid, and strap muscles are exposed. Broken lines indicate the level at which these muscles are transected before retraction.

The underlying periosteum is preserved to protect the mediastinal structures, which are separated by gentle blunt dissection. The periosteum is then removed to expose the vascular structures beneath. Then the inferior thyroid vein is doubly ligated and sectioned, but we have rarely needed to ligate the innominate vein. The thymus and surrounding fat should be dissected free and resected if present. In the lower neck, the avascular plane between the carotid sheath laterally and the trachea and esopha-gus medially is identified and developed down to the prevertebral fascia (Fig. 35–14). An attempt should be made to identify the recurrent laryngeal nerve, which lies in the tracheoesophageal groove in this location. The plane between the esophagus and the prevertebral fascia is developed, and the trachea and esophagus, including the recurrent laryngeal nerve, are mobilized for better exposure. Self-retaining retractors are placed, preferably under the longus colli muscle if it is well developed.

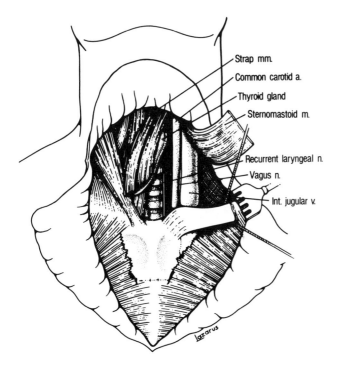

Strap mm.

Common carotid a.

Thyroid gland

Sternomastoid m.

Recurrent laryngeal n.

Vagus n.

Int. jugular v.

FIGURE 35–12. Retraction of the muscles exposes the carotid sheath, the tracheoesophageal complex, the manubrium sterni, and the clavicle. (Note Gigli's wire saw in position.)

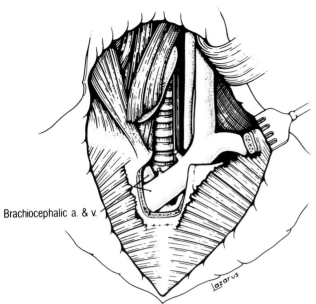

FIGURE 35–13. Exposures after bone resection. All tributaries to the brachiocephalic artery (innominate) and vein must be doubly ligated, but the vein itself is usually retracted downward.

Using periosteal elevators, ligaments and periosteum overlying the vertebral bodies are stripped laterally as far as possible (Fig. 35–15). The disc spaces above and below the involved vertebral segments are identified. Excellent lighting and the use of magnifying loupes or the operating microscope are prerequisites for this stage of the procedure.

Sharp-angled curettes and rongeurs are used for piecemeal removal of the diseased vertebra. On occasion, especially in the presence of marked sclerosis, a high speed drill may be necessary. Since bone and tumor tissue may be compressing the dura, it is vital to curette upward to prevent undue pressure on the spinal cord (Fig. 35–16, *left*). All involved bone is removed down to the posterior longitudinal ligament. If epidural tumor is present, this is also removed with pituitary rongeurs and curettes. Decompression should extend laterally to free involved nerve roots that may be compressed by bone fragments.

Meticulous hemostasis is obtained using the bipolar cautery under constant irrigation with saline solution. A sheet of Gelfoam is then used to protect the dura. The clavicle is dissected free from associated ligamentous and cartilaginous tissues. It is used as a strut graft and should be impacted in place while the neck is gently stretched by the anesthesiologist (Fig. 35–16, *right*). Additional cancellous bone from the sternum is also laid along the strut and is packed as tightly as possible to augment the fusion. As an alternative, immediate stability can be achieved by the use of Steinmann's pins and methyl methacrylate that is allowed to polymerize in situ. Suction drains are placed, and the wound is closed in layers. An appropriate orthotic device is used for postoperative immobilization.

DISCUSSION

Our experience with this procedure suggests that it is well tolerated and associated with minimal mor-

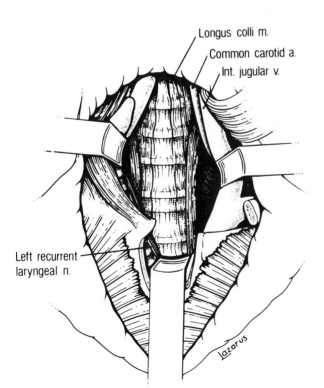

FIGURE 35–14. The prevertebral plane is exposed; the carotid sheath is retracted laterally; and the trachea, esophagus, and left recurrent laryngeal nerve are retracted medially across the midline.

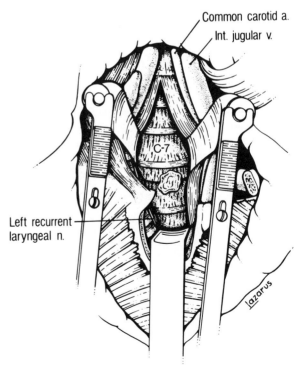

FIGURE 35–15. Self-retaining retractors are placed under the prevertebral muscles. Note collapse of the T1 vertebra secondary to tumor involvement.

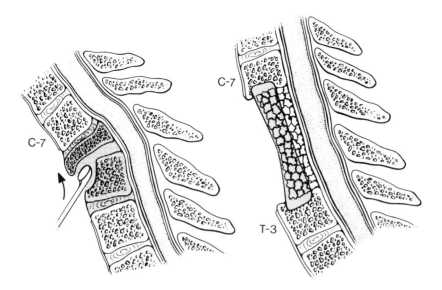

FIGURE 35–16. Note resection of involved bone and tumor with curettes, which should be directed away from the dura (*left*). Following tumor resection, the clavicle is used as a strut graft, and bone chips are packed around it (*right*).

bidity. In a small series of 10 patients, complete pain relief was seen in all patients, and improvement in motor deficit was noted in all those who presented with radiculopathy or myelopathy.[11] This direct approach is indicated for the surgical management of all lesions affecting the upper two thoracic vertebrae. A complete median sternotomy as originally proposed by Cauchoix and Binet is not necessary, but we believe resection of the clavicle adds to the exposure and allows vascular control. This is important for vascular neoplasms involving the spine, since arterial feeders originate from the subclavian or innominate arteries.[8] Involvement of the posterior elements (laminae and pedicles) in addition to the vertebral body is a contraindication to this approach, as is the presence of a large anterolateral soft tissue mass. For such patients, we prefer a posterolateral thoracotomy and resection of the first three ribs, which allows tumor resection as well as combined anterior and posterior fusion.

Postoperatively, the neck has to be kept immobilized with a Philadelphia collar to allow the bone graft to fuse. Bone fusion may take 2 to 3 months, and tomograms are obtained at periodic intervals to check for alignment and callus formation. Despite the use of radiation, successful bone fusion occurred in all our patients. After more extensive resections, if stability is in doubt, more rigid immobilization with a halo vest may be required. In addition, because of the mobility of the cervical vertebrae, additional posterior fusion with bone graft or Luque instrumentation may be required in patients whose life expectancies exceed a year.

Although the upper thoracic region is thought to be a rare site for neoplasms, involvement of the first three vertebrae accounted for 15 per cent of patients with neoplasms of the spine in our series.[9, 10] Although this procedure may be seemingly complex, palliation of pain as well as maintenance of ambulation represent important goals of therapy in patients with neoplasms involving this region.

REFERENCES

1. Capener N: The evolution of lateral rhacotomy. J Bone Joint Surg 36(A):173–179, 1954.
2. Cauchoix J, Binet J: Anterior surgical approaches to the spine. Ann R Coll Surg Engl 27:237–243, 1957.
3. Hodgson AR, Stock FE, Fang HSY, Ong GB: Anterior spinal fusion: The operative approach and pathologic findings in 412 patients with Pott's disease of the spine. Br J Surg 48:172–178, 1960.
4. Johnson RM, Southwick WO: Surgical approaches to the spine. *In* Rothman RH, Simeone FA (eds): The Spine. 2nd ed. Philadelphia, WB Saunders, 1982, pp 67–187.
5. Menard V: Causes de la paraplegie dans le maladie de Pott. Rev Orthop 547–564, 1894.
6. Nanson EM: The anterior approach to upper dorsal sympathectomy. Surg Gynecol Obstet 104:118–120, 1957.
7. Sanders G, Uyeda RY, Karlan MS: Nonrecurrent inferior laryngeal nerves and their association with a recurrent branch. Am J Surg 146:501–503, 1983.
8. Standefer M, Hardy RW, Marks K, Cosgrove DM: Chondromyxoid fibroma of the cervical spine: A case report and a description of an operative approach to the lower anterior cervical spine. Neurosurgery 11:288–292, 1982.
9. Sundaresan N, Galicich JH, Bains MS: Vertebral body resection in the treatment of cancer involving the spine. Cancer 53:1393–1396, 1984.
10. Sundaresan N, Galicich JH, Land JM, et al: The treatment of neoplastic epidural cord compression by vertebral body resection and stabilisation. J Neurosurg 63:676–684, 1985.
11. Sundaresan N, Shah J, Feghali J: The trans-sternal approach to the upper thoracic vertebra. Am J Surg 198:473–477, 1984.

ANTERIOR APPROACHES TO THE THORACIC AND THORACOLUMBAR JUNCTION

NARAYAN SUNDARESAN, JAMES E. O. HUGHES,
and HENRY H. SCHMIDEK

INTRODUCTION

As at other levels of the spine, the choice of surgical approach to the thoracic spine should be tailored to the site of pathology. The transthoracic approach, which provided extensive access to the anterior spine, was used originally for the treatment of tuberculous (Potts) disease. With the development of anesthetic techniques and postoperative ventilatory support, this approach is increasingly used in the management of patients with neoplasms involving the spine.[14–16] In addition, the use of broad-spectrum antibiotics used prophylactically, as well as careful preoperative management, has greatly diminished the incidence of postoperative complications, including pneumonia. This is particularly important in minimizing surgical morbidity in elderly patients and others with impaired host defenses.

Although there have been successful reports of thoracotomy in the early literature, Hodgson reported the first extensive description of the exposures gained by thoracotomy to debride tuberculous abscesses of the spine.[10] He noted that thoracotomy allowed complete resection of all devitalized bone and necrotic tissue associated with this disease, and provided access for anterior fusion with bone grafts to be performed after debridement. He noted that these operations were difficult to perform through the more limited exposure afforded by posterolateral costotransversectomy. Hodgson's mortality and complication rate (2.9 per cent in a large series of over 400 cases) provided the impetus for others to use this approach in other pathologic conditions, particularly neoplasms. In addition to the treatment of tumors, transthoracic anterior spinal surgery is indicated to correct kyphotic and kyphoscoliotic deformities of the spine.[20] It is generally accepted that kyphosis that measures more than 40 degrees tends to be progressive, results in neurologic deficit, and

requires correction by anterior decompression and stabilization through the chest. All kyphotic deformities have a high rate of success when fusion is performed from in front, since posterior fusion across a kyphosis stresses the bone graft, which tends to attenuate over time. In patients with loss of the posterior elements, as in meningomyelocele, anterior spine fusion is combined with instrumentation. In addition, the transthoracic approach is indicated for midline thoracic disc protrusions as well as for traumatic spinal injuries with protruding disc and bone fragments in the canal.[4, 11]

A limited alternative to the open thoracotomy approach is costotransversectomy. This operation involves resection of the transverse process and approximately 5 cm of adjacent rib. This exposure can be used at any level of the thoracic spine and is technically easier for the neurosurgeon. In the management of tumors, its use should be limited to biopsy and for palliative decompression of metastatic disease in patients with advanced cancer. This operation may require instrumentation with posterior stabilization, since the exposure does not provide adequate access for anterior stabilization.

Although all segments of the thoracic spine may be exposed by transthoracic surgery, exposures of different segments may be categorized into three groups.

1. The upper three thoracic vertebrae can be exposed by a direct anterior approach, which may or may not require median sternotomy, depending on the level. However, when a large paraspinal component is present, posterolateral thoracotomy with resection of the 3rd rib provides the needed access.

2. The 4th to the 9th vertebrae are the easiest to expose through a posterolateral thoracotomy.

3. The thoracolumbar region of the spine from the 10th thoracic to the 1st lumbar vertebrae form a separate segment hidden by the rising dome of the

diaphragm and can be exposed by a variety of techniques.[3, 18]

Although most surgical texts recommend a left posterolateral thoracotomy to expose the spine because of ease of mobilizing the aorta, we believe a right-sided approach is preferable in most patients with midline lesions for the upper thoracic segments. In the past, the thoracic veins, which were often incorporated by necrotic tumor or inflammation, were considered difficult to retract because of their fragility and hemorrhage that was sometimes difficult to control. However, we have found that they are easily controlled with bipolar cautery or hemostatic clips. We preferentially use a left-sided approach for the thoracolumbar region, because the liver is more difficult to retract when compared with the spleen. With these generalizations, however, the operative approach is chosen to allow maximal tumor resection. Detailed radiologic evaluation using computed tomography (CT) and magnetic resonance imaging (MRI) scans are used to determine the optimal side of approach. If these studies are not available, the side that shows the greater collapse or destruction on the plain anteroposterior x-ray should be chosen.

In general, thoracic exposures can be performed with or without rib resection. In view of the natural thoracic kyphosis and the caudal angulation of the posterior portion of the ribs posterior to the angle, it is much easier for most surgeons to work from above downward in the thoracic spine. Therefore, an interspace at least two levels above the level of vertebral body involvement should be entered, and the rib below it resected. It is not always necessary to remove the entire rib, since adequate access is available by removing the posterior 5 to 10 cm only. For the thoracolumbar segments, a transthoracic exposure requires removal of a rib at least *two* levels above the site of involvement. The diaphragm is then detached from its costal insertion to the lower ribs. A concern regarding surgery of the thoracic spine is the arterial supply of the spinal cord. In *elective* surgical cases at the thoracolumbar junction, spinal angiography may be indicated to determine the exact configuration of the arterial supply to the spinal cord. Spinal angiography is also routinely used in the management of highly vascular tumors to minimize intraoperative blood loss during surgery.

In semielective and urgent cases precise evaluation of lung function, including preoperative pulmonary function tests and blood gas estimations, should be carried out. Almost all complications and deaths following transthoracic surgery with lung resection are cardiorespiratory in nature, and a basic understanding of pulmonary and cardiac risk factors should be a prerequisite for spine surgeons. While careful patient selection can be used to achieve low morbidity and mortality rates, this does not always equate with better care because borderline and high-risk patients may often be deprived of the benefits of operation.[12]

In patients with apparently normal cardiorespiratory systems, it is important to understand that advancing age is associated with decreased overall physiologic functions, with rapidly decreasing cardiovascular performance noted after the age of 70. Thus risk of surgery in patients 90 years and above is about twice that in patients 75 to 84, which in turn is twice that of those under 70.[12, 13] We have noted a steep rise in mortality following pulmonary resection and transthoracic surgery in patients over 70 years, which should be taken into account in considering therapeutic options.

It is also not infrequent that cancer (especially of the lung) is associated with chronic pulmonary disease. This is particularly true in smokers, who are more likely to have increased respiratory secretions, a decreased ability to clear them, and impaired pulmonary function. A complete history and physical examination with regard to smoking history, productive cough, and the ability to clear secretions, as well as evaluation by a pulmonary physician, may be helpful in minimizing postoperative complications.

Following thoracotomy under general anesthesia, virtually all patients develop postoperative decrease in functional residual capacity related to the spontaneous collapse of alveoli, atelectasis secondary to decreased clearance of secretions, and alteration of the normal pattern of ventilation with decreased or absent sigh breaths, as well as a mismatch of ventilation perfusion.[2, 8, 9] Postoperative studies show that the vital capacity (VC), forced expiratory volume in one second (FEV1), and functional residual capacity (FRC) decrease to approximately one third of preoperative values on days 1 through 5 after operation, and rise to 70 per cent of preoperative values on day 7. Several studies have shown that preexisting pulmonary disease increases mortality rate following lung surgery tenfold but has a lesser effect in those over 65. In many studies, postoperative morbidity and mortality correlate well with preoperative abnormal lung function.[2, 6, 8, 9, 17, 19]

Simple spirometric tests can be used to identify patients at increased risk of complications. The three tests that provide the best information in predicting postoperative difficulties include forced vital capacity (FVC), maximum breathing capacity (MBC), and the FEV1. Patients posing lower respiratory risks are those with FVC greater than 70 per cent of that predicted, FEV1 greater than 70 per cent of that predicted, and MBC greater than 60 per cent of that predicted. However, no single test should be used as a contraindication for operation. Careful preoperative preparation as well as perioperative care are essential to reduce the risk of pulmonary complications. Smoking should clearly be discontinued, preferably for weeks if possible. Reversible factors in patients with chronic obstructive pulmonary disease (COPD) such as bronchial edema or increased bronchial tone should be identified, and preoperative therapy with bronchodilators may be helpful. Patients with chronic bronchitis should be treated with nebulizers, chest physical therapy, and postural drainage. Those with infections should receive proper antibiotic coverage.

In addition to pulmonary risk factors, the risk of

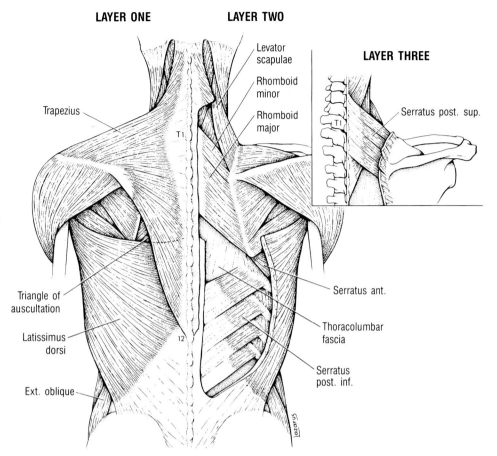

LAYER ONE

LAYER TWO

Levator scapulae

Rhomboid minor

Rhomboid major

Trapezius

LAYER THREE

Serratus post. sup.

T1

Serratus ant.

Thoracolumbar fascia

Serratus post. inf.

Triangle of auscultation

Latissimus dorsi

Ext. oblique

FIGURE 36–1. Line diagram illustrating various muscle layers of the posterior thoracic cage.

operation is clearly increased in patients with pre-operative cardiovascular disease, who are five times more likely to suffer postoperative mortality and twice as likely to develop major complications. The presence of an "old" myocardial infarction (more than 6 months) is associated with a postoperative infarction rate ranging from 0.13 to 5 per cent. The presence of cardiac arrhythmias also increases peri-operative risk because it correlates with other more severe heart disease. In addition, the presence of heart failure has been noted to be one of the most important predictors of outcome after noncardiac operations.[7] Preoperative heart failure should be controlled with diuretics, inotropic drugs, and after-load reduction agents; in patients with arrhythmias, temporary pacing should be considered.

In addition to the above factors, several others are particularly important in the cancer patient: a combination of poor nutrition and debilitation clearly affects wound healing and morbidity. Hypoalbuminemia has been associated with increased pulmonary and steroid-related complications. The use of intensive chemotherapy in conjunction with steroids clearly adds to the risk of infection, since host defense mechanisms may be impaired. Thus steroid therapy for greater than 8 weeks clearly increases morbidity from both sepsis and pulmonary emboli. Drugs such as doxorubicin may affect cardiac performance and require tests of ventricular function prior to operation. In addition, conditions of the bony cage, such

as kyphoscoliosis, as well as radiation fibrosis may increase morbidity by their restrictive effects on lung function.

SURGICAL ANATOMY

In the standard posterolateral thoracotomy, several muscles of the posterior thorax must be divided to enter the rib cage (Fig. 36–1). The *trapezius* muscle extends from the spinous processes and attaches to the spine of the scapula all the way from the cervical region to the T12 level. Its fibers run obliquely and laterally to the scapular spine. Underneath the trapezius lie the *rhomboids*, which arise from the spinous processes to the 6th cervical and upper five thoracic vertebrae. In the lower thorax, the *latissimus dorsi* muscle arises beneath the trapezius from the lower six thoracic vertebrae and extends as a broad sheet across the back to the axilla. The *serratus posterior inferior* arises as muscular bundles from the lower four ribs, while the *serratus posterior superior* arises from the upper three ribs medially.

In addition to the muscles, a series of ligaments join the ribs, transverse processes, and vertebral bodies (Fig. 36–2). The costotransverse ligaments run from the transverse process of one vertebra to the rib. They are divided into the superior, posterior, and inferior costotransverse ligaments. In addition, the capsular ligament secures the neck of the rib to

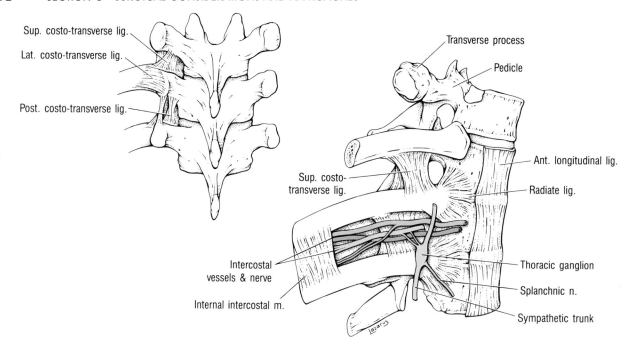

FIGURE 36–2. Line diagrams illustrating attachment of the various costotransverse ligaments from the head of the rib to the transverse process and the vertebral body.

the front of the transverse process. More laterally, the lateral costotransverse ligament extends from the tip of the transverse process to the posterior tubercle of the same rib. Finally, the costovertebral radial ligament binds the head of the rib to its respective vertebral body and articulation. The *head of the rib* articulates generally with the corresponding body, as well as with the disc *above* it. The pedicle lies directly in front of the base of the transverse process and *directly underneath the head and neck of the rib* (Fig. 36–3). In addition, the pertinent vascular anatomy within the thoracic cage is shown in Figures 36–4 and 36–5. On the left, the aortic arch reaches the level of the fourth thoracic vertebra and is closely applied to the anterior aspects of the vertebral bodies on the left of the midline. Above the level of the arch, the esoph-

agus, thoracic duct, and subclavian artery are in close proximity to the vertebral body. In the lower thorax, the aorta lies to the left of the midline, and the azygos vein and the thoracic duct lie to the right of the midline immediately anterior to the vertebral bodies. Both the aorta and the azygos system are held to the vertebral bodies by intercostal vessels that are draped between the disc spaces and join the intercostal nerve lateral to the sympathetic trunk.

OPERATIVE TECHNIQUE

For formal posterolateral thoracotomy approaches, patients should be positioned in the lateral decubitus position and tilted forward about 15 degrees. We prefer to use the Olympic Vac-Pac unit to maintain this position. Axillary rolls are placed beneath the lower axilla, and a pillow is placed between the legs (Fig. 36–6). Generally, the lower leg is kept extended at the knee, and the upper leg is flexed. Patients are further secured by wide (2-inch diameter) tapes attached to the iliac crest; however, the iliac crest must be made available for a possible bone graft. The upper arm may be draped by protecting it with pads attached to an overhanging ether screen or by allowing it to rest on folded sheets. In all patients, arterial blood gas monitoring, central venous lines, and a Foley catheter are inserted. In elderly patients and others with impaired cardiac function, a Swan-Ganz catheter may be placed.

For exposures requiring lung retraction, a double-lumen endotracheal tube is inserted so that the exposed lung can be selectively deflated. The skin is prepared with Betadine and soap solution, the skin incision is marked, and the skin towels are held in

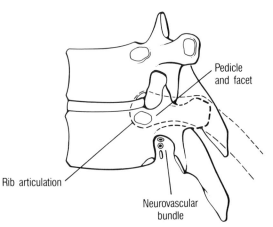

FIGURE 36–3. Line diagram illustrating relationship of the head of the rib to the pedicle. Note that the head of the rib articulates with the disc space and with the upper portion of the vertebral body.

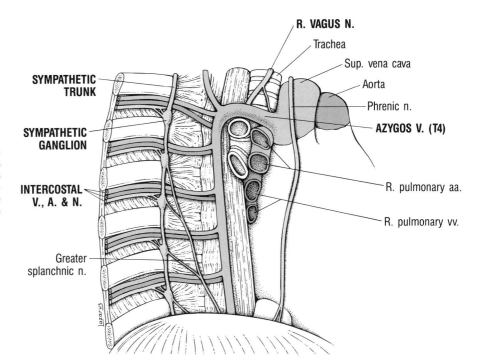

FIGURE 36—4. Vascular structures visualized when the right thorax is opened. Note that the azygos vein is at the level of the fourth thoracic vertebra. The right vagus nerve lies in the tracheoesophageal groove, and the phrenic nerve runs more anteriorly.

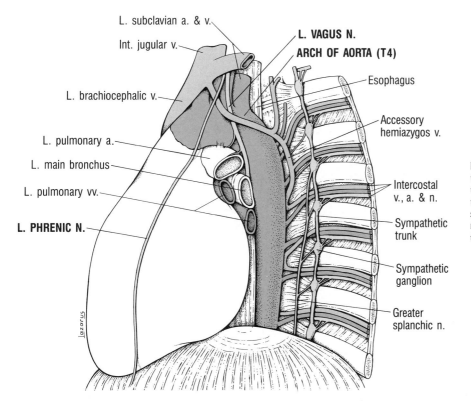

FIGURE 36—5. Anatomy visualized through the left thoracic cage. Note that the arch of the aorta lies at the fourth thoracic level, and that segmental vessels have to be ligated before the anterior portion of the fourth thoracic vertebra can be visualized.

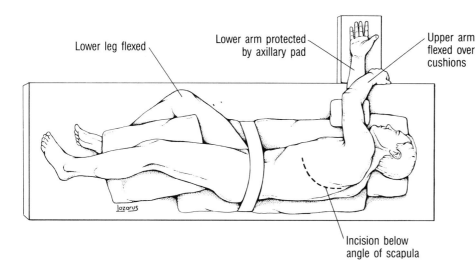

Lower leg flexed

Lower arm protected by axillary pad

Upper arm flexed over cushions

lazarus

FIGURE 36–6. Patient positioning in the lateral position for standard posterolateral thoracotomy.

Incision below angle of scapula

place with staples. The skin incision begins close to the spine of the scapula, passes along the lateral border of the paraspinous muscles 2 or 3 cm below the inferior angle of the scapula, and then swings anteriorly beyond the anterior axillary line. For the upper spine, the incision should also be below the angle of the scapula, which has to be retracted upward after mobilizing the scapula.

After the skin incision is made, we prefer to use electrocautery to cut down to the chest wall. With scissors and fingers, the triangle of auscultation is dissected, which allows mobilization of the latissimus muscle. Both the latissimus dorsi muscle and the serratus anterior muscle are mobilized by blunt dissection with a finger underneath the muscles and are transected with cautery along the line of the incision (Fig. 36–7). Larger bleeding vessels require clamping with hemostats and electrocoagulation. Posteriorly, the dissection should proceed to divide the trapezius and rhomboids. Anteriorly, depending upon the level of access to the chest, the pectoralis major is retracted

or split. In general, preserving major muscles by retraction rather than transection will ensure a smoother postoperative course. By retracting the scapula and the lateral margin of the trapezius, the appropriate rib level is determined. This is done by counting from the top, and generally the second is the uppermost rib that can be palpated from this approach. The first rib is generally inside the second rib, and when palpating from the outer aspect it may not always be identified. The periosteum of the rib to be resected is cut with electrocautery, and bleeding is sealed with coagulation. A Cushing or Alexander periosteal elevator is used to strip the periosteum from the external surfaces of the ribs (Fig. 36–8). Once this is done, curettes or the Doyen periosteal elevator is used to strip the remaining superior and inferior surfaces of the ribs of their periosteum, while preserving the adjacent neurovascular bundle.

To gain exposure of the ribs posteriorly, a longitudinal incision is made along the anterior border of the paraspinal muscles, which will allow them to be

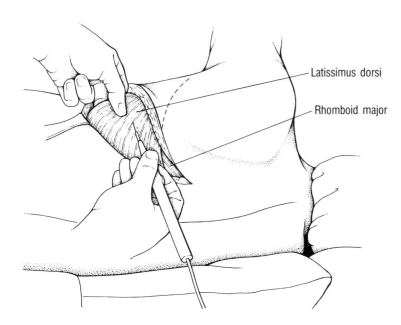

Latissimus dorsi

Rhomboid major

FIGURE 36–7. Once the triangle of auscultation is opened, the latissimus dorsi muscle is cut with electrocautery along the line of the incision.

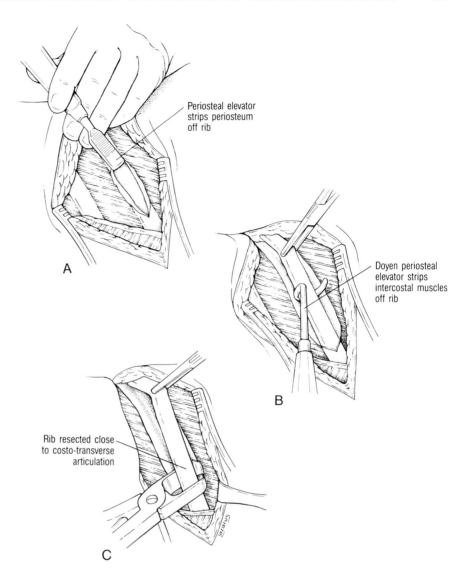

FIGURE 36–8. *A,* Stripping of periosteum from the rib using the Alexander periosteal elevator. *B,* The undersurface of the rib is dissected free with a Doyen elevator while the neurovascular bundle is preserved. *C,* After mobilizing the rib anteriorly, the posterior portion is resected close to the costotransverse articulation.

retracted posteriorly past the rib angle. The rib is then cut with rib shears as far posteriorly as possible near its angle. For patients with metastatic disease, we sometimes remove only the posterior 5 to 10 cm of rib (Fig. 36–9) to facilitate closure of the thoracotomy. The neurovascular bundle is identified with right-angled clamps and is ligated with 00 or 000 silk ties; the intercostal nerve is cut to prevent its stretching, which may be responsible for severe postoperative pain. The intercostal space is then held open by a retractor, and the thorax is entered through the periosteal bed. Alternatively, one could enter the intercostal space (which is easier), but closure is slightly more difficult.

During the entry into the chest, the lung is protected underneath with a sponge stick, and the rest of the pleura is opened with either cautery or scissors. The self-retaining Finochietto retractor is now placed in the open pleural cavity and is gradually opened. In addition, the self-retaining Hurson retractor is attached to maintain retraction of the lung.

The vertebral bodies can now be seen and are usually covered by the pleura. Often, the tumor can

be seen protruding through the anterior longitudinal ligament and pleura. If the tumor is intraosseous, the intervertebral discs protrude prominently, while the involved vertebral bodies between them are concave. It is important to leave the head of the rib intact during the initial dissection because it protects the pedicle and helps avoid neural injury.

It is important to *establish the correct level if tumor is not evident* by counting from within the thoracic inlet, and we routinely obtain radiographic confirmation to establish the vertebral level in the operating room after the spine has been exposed. The parietal pleura is picked up with long DeBakey forceps and the pleura carefully reflected over the vertebral bodies (Fig. 36–10). Depending on the extent of tumor pathology, we prefer to identify intact discs above and below the site of involvement. The disc itself is more prominent, softer, and avascular. The neurovascular bundle generally crosses the middle portion of the body. Once the pleura is reflected, intercostal vessels that course over the vertebral bodies should be carefully identified and ligated with 000 silk sutures as well as with clips. At this point, additional

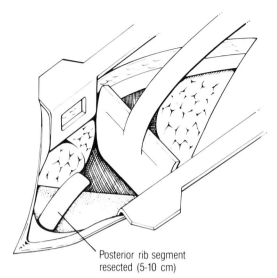

FIGURE 36–9. Thoracotomy exposure with retractor in place. For limited exposures, only the posterior 5 to 10 cm of rib needs to be removed.

Posterior rib segment
resected (5-10 cm)

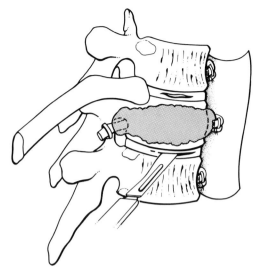

FIGURE 36–11. Line diagram illustrating technique of isolating tumor by cutting into disc spaces above and below the level of involvement.

posterior exposure may be gained by piecemeal removal of the posterior end of the rib, but it is important not to remove the rib entirely, since it forms a useful landmark that identifies the pedicle.

The paraspinal soft tissue mass is then carefully isolated, and the whole area is packed off with moist pads. After removal of all soft tissues attached to the spine, the disc space is incised either with a long-handled scalpel or with a small straight osteotome (Fig. 36–11). Curve-angled curettes, #0 or #1, are

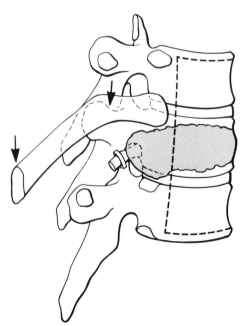

FIGURE 36–10. Dotted lines indicate the pleura to be reflected to expose tumor. Notice that the arrows indicate that the posterior segment of rib should be preserved until the end of procedure to protect the pedicle, which may have been destroyed by tumor. Shaded area indicates tumor.

introduced into the disc spaces, and the initial procedure begins by isolating the involved segments that are to be resected. Following partial curettage, straight and curved osteotomes are used to remove the anterior portion of the vertebral bodies. The remaining vertebral bodies are then removed with curettes, rongeurs, and occasionally the high speed air drill. The dissection should proceed so that the dura is not exposed until the entire bony segment has been thinned out. Dissection then proceeds with removal of the discs and the vertebral bodies down to the posterior longitudinal ligament. Lastly, the head of the rib is removed, allowing identification of the pedicle. The pedicle is also removed. During this process, brisk bleeding may be encountered, and intermittently the procedure may need to be stopped to allow the patient's condition to be stabilized. For tumor resection to be complete, magnification is used and the posterior longitudinal ligament is removed to enable tumor removal until the dural surface is free of tumor. When a malignant tumor is present, we prefer to remove enough of the vertebral body so that, at a subsequent operation, a complete spondylectomy can be performed by removal of the remaining spine. Additional posterior extension of tumor may be removed by combining the anterior resection with a hemilaminectomy (Fig. 36–12).

Following tumor resection hemostasis is secured with a bipolar current. If frozen sections have revealed a malignant tumor, stabilization of the resected vertebral bodies is then performed by using Steinmann pins and methyl methacrylate that is allowed to polymerize in situ. We insert two Steinmann pins by holding them with specially designed holders and allowing these pins to straddle intact vertebral bodies above and below the level of involvement (Fig. 36–13). Careful positioning of the Steinmann pins is required to prevent inadvertent penetration of the opposite pleural cavity or vascular injury. In the

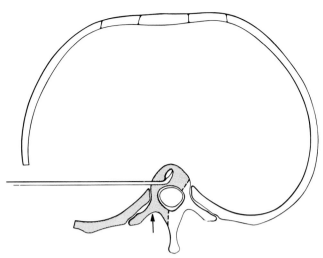

FIGURE 36–12. Diagram shows extent of resection possible from a one-sided thoracotomy approach. Note that the posterior extensions can be removed by performing a hemilaminectomy on the side of the approach.

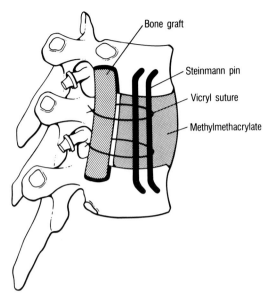

FIGURE 36–14. Technique of stabilization with methyl methacrylate replacement. Occasionally, the bone graft from the resected rib may be used laterally as a fusion mass. It is then held in place with heavy vicryl sutures anchored to the Steinmann pins.

cervical region, pin positioning is checked with an intraoperative x-ray. After this has been done, the dura is covered with Gelfoam, and liquid methyl methacrylate is injected into the cavity with a 50-cc syringe. During the heat of polymerization, saline irrigation is used to dissipate heat. It is important to keep blood from forming a loculated collection within the epidural space. Thus, packing of the epidural space is not advocated, and blood should be allowed to drain out into the pleural cavity. In patients with benign spine tumors or in those who do not require radiation, an iliac crest graft may be harvested, and this can be keyed in between the vertebral bodies. Alternatively, the rib that was harvested can be used as a lateral fusion mass next to the acrylic (Fig. 36–14).

When the thoracotomy is closed, two chest tubes are inserted. A posterior tube is directed superiorly to collect air, and an anterior tube is positioned inferiorly over the diaphragm to evacuate blood. A purse-string suture is placed in the skin around each tube, and the ribs are reapproximated with a rib approximator. Between three and six pericostal sutures are placed, using either Vicryl or Dexon sutures. When pericostal sutures are placed, care should be taken to prevent the intercostal nerve's being crushed by the sutures. The muscular layers (serratus anterior, trapezius, latissimus dorsi, and rhomboids) are then carefully approximated. The subcutaneous tissues and skin are closed, and the chest tubes are attached to waterseal constant suction.

Thoracolumbar Region

For surgical approaches to the thoracolumbar junction, a variety of transthoracic, extrapleural, and extraperitoneal approaches are available.[18] It has been stated that large exposures require opening both the thoracic and the abdominal cavities, which may increase the morbidity of operation. For many spinal procedures, it is possible to expose the thoracolumbar vertebrae (T11-L1) by resection of the 10th or 11th ribs; by staying largely extrapleural, morbidity can be minimized. To understand the various exposures in this region, a knowledge of the anatomy of the diaphragm is required (Fig. 36–15). For thoracolumbar exposures, the peripheral (costal) portion of the diaphragm has to be divided to allow exposure of the anterior spine. This peripheral detachment of the diaphragm is associated with minimal disruption of diaphragmatic function.

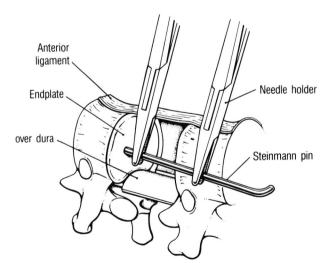

FIGURE 36–13. Technique of inserting Steinmann pins into vertebral bodies above and below the resected site. The Steinmann pins are held in place with special needle holders and should be carefully placed to avoid vascular injury.

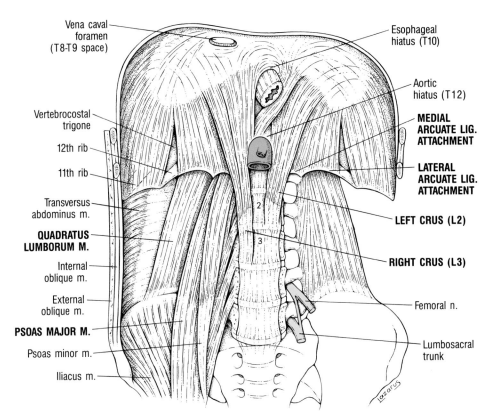

Vena caval foramen (T8-T9 space)

Esophageal hiatus (T10)

Aortic hiatus (T12)

MEDIAL ARCUATE LIG. ATTACHMENT

Vertebrocostal trigone

12th rib

11th rib

LATERAL ARCUATE LIG. ATTACHMENT

Transversus abdominus m.

QUADRATUS LUMBORUM M.

LEFT CRUS (L2)

Internal oblique m.

RIGHT CRUS (L3)

External oblique m.

PSOAS MAJOR M.

Femoral n.

Psoas minor m.

Lumbosacral trunk

Iliacus m.

FIGURE 36–15. Anatomic attachments of the diaphragm. Detachment of the costal origin and stripping the crura from the front of the vertebral bodies are required to expose the thoracolumbar segments.

The diaphragm is a dome-shaped muscle that is muscular in its periphery and is tendinous centrally. Anteriorly and laterally, it originates from the cartilaginous ends of the lower six ribs and xyphoid cartilage. Posteriorly, it originates from the upper lumbar vertebra through the crura, the arcuate ligaments, and the 12th ribs. The *medial arcuate ligament* arises from the crura and crosses over the psoas muscle to insert on the transverse process of the first lumbar vertebra. The *lateral arcuate ligament* arises from the transverse process of the first lumbar vertebra and extends over the quadratus lumborum muscles to the tips of the 12th ribs. The *right crus* extends down the right side of the bodies of L1, L2, and L3; the *left crus* attaches to the bodies of L1 and L2 on the left side. These crura extend cephalad to the T11-T12 area in the midline and form the aortic hiatus. In addition to the aorta, the aortic hiatus gives passage to the azygos vein and the thoracic duct. The esophagus and the vena cava enter by separate foramina in the anterior wall of the diaphragm. The esophageal hiatus is at the level of the 10th thoracic vertebra and also transmits the vagus nerve. In addition to these, there are small apertures for the splenic nerves and the hemiazygos vein. The sympathetic trunk is usually found under the medial arcuate ligaments. Both the inferior and superior surfaces of the diaphragm are covered by the endothoracic fascia of the chest and abdomen. The pleural cavity extends over the majority of the 11th rib and the medial portion of the 12th rib.

The skin incision is generally made in the plane of the 10th rib. The incision is then deepened down through the thoracic muscles, and the latissimus dorsi and serratus anterior muscles are transected. The incision is carried over the periosteum of the 10th rib, and the rib is resected as previously described. The endothoracic fascia and pleura are carefully stripped from the inner surface of the rib to minimize the actual pleural opening. The opening is gradually spread with a Finochietto retractor. Using a sponge stick, the diaphragm is kept under tension, and a circumferential incision is made in the medial portion of the diaphragm adjacent to the costal margin. By using cautery, it is possible to detach the diaphragm from its costal insertion with minimal blood loss. This allows exposure of the upper retroperitoneal space, which is gradually developed by blunt dissection. The spleen, kidney, and stomach are retracted medially and downward, using a broad malleable retractor. The entire anterior surface of the thoracolumbar junction, the vertebral bodies, and the aorta can then be visualized. The aorta is carefully mobilized by both sharp and blunt dissection, and the corresponding segmental vessels are carefully ligated with hemostatic clips and divided. The sympathetic trunks extend over the anterolateral aspects of the bodies just next to the psoas muscle and should be spared if possible. The crus of the diaphragm is stripped from the anterior longitudinal ligament using a Cobb periosteal elevator. The arcuate ligament is divided at its insertion to the lumbar transverse process and 12th rib. Using the Cobb periosteal elevator, the anterior longitudinal ligament and the anterior surface of the bodies are now carefully stripped of all soft tissues and are exposed for tumor resection.

Following tumor resection and stabilization, the cut edges of the diaphragm are resutured. A single chest tube or two tubes are placed and the wound is closed in layers.

POSTOPERATIVE MANAGEMENT

In the postoperative period, most patients are monitored in the recovery room for at least 24 hours following surgery. We prefer to keep patients intubated for at least 12 hours after surgery to minimize atelectasis. Prior to extubation, physical examination of the chest should reveal good breath sounds. A chest film taken after admission to the recovery room should confirm the absence of pleural space abnormalities as well as collapse of the lung. Important complications of thoracotomy include atelectasis, pneumonia, and airway obstruction. Congestive heart failure and pulmonary edema may occur if fluid replacement is excessive, especially in elderly patients, and if venous pressures are not closely monitored. Careful monitoring of fluid requirements and appropriate pulmonary care is important to minimize the possibility of adult respiratory syndrome.

Most tumor resections of the spine may be accompanied by considerable bleeding, and chest tube output should be closely monitored. To minimize pulmonary complications, we allow patients to be ambulated or to sit up in bed by the next day. Chest tubes are removed when the 24-hour drainage is less than 100 cc, generally by the fourth postoperative day. During this period, patients are treated with broad-spectrum antibiotics while steroid therapy is carefully tapered. The persistence of pleural drainage for more than a week should arouse the suspicion of cerebrospinal fluid (CSF) fistula from nerve roots transected during operation. Although we allow patients to be out of bed by the second day, pulmonary embolism represents a major threat in cancer patients and in those with weakness in the lower extremities. For this reason, we recommend the use of subcutaneous heparin, 5000 units every 12 hours in the perioperative period. There should be no hesitation in considering anticoagulation with systemic heparin if deep vein thrombosis is present.

For comfort, a prefabricated clam shell jacket is used, and intensive physical therapy is begun as soon as possible. If radiation or chemotherapy is required, such treatment can be started after a week. Most patients are ready for discharge from hospital within two weeks if no complications are encountered.

REFERENCES

1. Bernard GR, Bradley RB: Adult respiratory distress syndrome: Diagnosis and management. Heart and Lung 15:250–255, 1986.
2. Boysen PG, Block AJ, Moulder PV: Relationship between preoperative pulmonary function tests and complications after thoracotomy. Surg Gynecol Obstet 151:813–815, 1981.
3. Burrington JD, Brown C, Wayne ER, Odom J: Anterior approach to the thoraco-lumbar spine—technical considerations. Arch Surg 111:456–463, 1976.
4. Cook WA: Trans-thoracic vertebral surgery. Ann Thorac Surg 12:54–68, 1971.
5. Crawford FA, Kratz JM: Thoracic incisions. *In* Sabiston DC Jr, Spencer FC (eds): Surgery of the Chest. 4th Ed. Philadelphia, WB Saunders, 1983, pp 143–145.
6. Gass GD, Olsen GN: Preoperative pulmonary function testing to predict postoperative morbidity and mortality. Chest 89:127–135, 1986.
7. Goldman L: Cardiac risk and complications of non-cardiac surgery. Ann Intern Med 98:504–513, 1983.
8. Gracey DR. Divertie MB, Didier EP: Preoperative pulmonary preparation of patients with chronic obstructive pulmonary disease: A prospective study. Chest 76:123–129, 1979.
9. Harman E, Lillington G: Pulmonary risk factors in surgery. Med Clin North Am 63:1289–1297, 1979.
10. Hodgson AR, Stock FE, Fang HSY, Ong GB: Anterior spinal fusion: The operative approach and pathologic findings in 412 patients with Potts disease of the spine. Br J Surg 48:172–178, 1960.
11. Johnson RM, Southwick WD: Surgical approaches to the spine. *In* Rothman RH, Simeone FA (eds): The Spine. 2nd Ed. Philadelphia, WB Saunders, 1982, pp 147–171.
12. Roth JA: Preoperative assessment of patients undergoing lung resection for cancer. *In* Roth JA, Ruckdeschel JC, Weisenburger TH (eds): Thoracic Oncology. Philadelphia, WB Saunders, 1989, pp 156–175.
13. Seymour G: Medical assessment of the elderly surgical patient. Rockville, MD, Aspen Publishers, 1986.
14. Sundaresan N, DiGiacinto GV, Hughes JEO: Surgical treatment of spinal metastases. Clin Neurosurg 33:503–522, 1986.
15. Sundaresan N, DiGiacinto GV, Hughes JEO: Surgical approaches to primary and metastatic tumors of the spine. *In* Schmidek HH, Sweet WH (eds): Operative Neurosurgical Techniques: Indications, Methods, Results. Vol 2. Orlando, Grune & Stratton, 1988, pp 1525–1537.
16. Sundaresan N, Galicich JH, Lane JM, Scher H: Stabilization of the spine involved by cancer. *In* Dunsker SB, Schmidek HH, Frymoyer J, Kahn III (eds): The Unstable Spine. Orlando, Grune & Stratton, 1986, pp 249–274.
17. Tisi GM: Preoperative evaluation of pulmonary function. Am Rev Respir Dis 119:293–310, 1979.
18. Watkins RG: Surgical Approaches to the Spine. New York, Springer-Verlag, 1983.
19. Wenly JA, DeMeester TR, Kirchner PT: Clinical value of quantitative ventilation-perfusion lung scans in the surgical management of bronchogenic carcinoma. J Thorac Cardiovasc Surg 80:533–543, 1980.
20. Winter RB, Moe JH, Wang JF: Congenital kyphosis, its natural history and treatment as observed in a study of 130 patients. J Bone Joint Surg 55(A):223–256, 1973.

SURGICAL INTERVENTION FOR NEOPLASTIC INVOLVEMENT OF THE LUMBAR SPINE

TZONY SIEGAL and TALI SIEGAL

INTRODUCTION

Neoplastic involvement of the lumbar spine may be divided into two major surgical categories: (1) Conus and/or cauda equina compression by an epidural tumor, illustrated by a high-degree myelographic block. The clinical manifestations include pain and neurologic impairment of variable severity. (2) Vertebral involvement leading to spinal instability with or without some epidural extension. The main clinical manifestation is pain with or without signs of nerve root compression.

Indications for surgical intervention differ according to the surgical category. In the presence of cauda equina compression, surgical intervention is aimed primarily at obtaining prompt decompression of the neural elements and at the same time maintaining spinal stability. For cauda equina compression, surgery is recommended[4, 11] when

1. The nature of the compressing tumor is in doubt and rapid decompression is advisable;

2. Radiotherapy cannot be used due to previous irradiation;

3. The compressing tumor is known to be radioresistant;

4. Neurologic deterioration occurs during radiotherapy;

5. A pathologic fracture produces bone retropulsion and compression of the neural structures.

Progressive neoplastic involvement of the vertebral elements will cause painful segmental instability or frank fracture-dislocation with potential neurologic worsening. Here, the role of surgery is

1. To reinstate spinal stability;

2. To alleviate pain by tumor debulking, nerve root decompression, restoration of vertebral height, and abolishment of the painful segmental instability;

3. To prevent the oncoming neurologic dysfunction secondary to progressive spinal instability.

When debulking of a retroperitoneal paraspinal tumor is considered,[10] contiguous vertebral and epidural involvement will require spinal decompression and, if indicated, adequate stabilization. Unlike the previous category, surgical intervention in these patients is on an elective rather than an emergency basis.

PREOPERATIVE EVALUATION

Preoperative studies are essential for selection of the appropriate surgical approach and stabilization technique (Table 37–1). The location of the main tumor mass dictates the surgical approach, whether anterior or posterior. The tumor position and extent of bone involvement are determined by the information obtained from spinal x-rays, computed tomography (CT), and myelography (Table 37–1). Magnetic resonance imaging (MRI) studies are most useful because spinal structure visualization is superb and diagnosis can be made immediately without morbidity or inconvenience to the patient. The selection of an anterior, posterior, combined, or staged surgical approach should be determined by the main site of instability as well as by the location of the tumor inside and outside the spinal canal.

Laminectomy is indicated when the bulk of tumor is in a posterior or posterolateral location. It may also be required as a second-stage procedure if considerable residue of the encircling tumor is left beyond the equator of the dura at the end of an anterior decompression. Although in most instances the preoperative evaluation will correctly assess the potential postoperative spinal instability, the decision to add posterior stabilizing instumentation is taken at the conclusion of the decompressive procedure.

Anterior decompression of the lumbar spine is indicated when: (1) the bulk of the compressing tumor is situated in an anterior or anterolateral

TABLE 37–1. PREOPERATIVE ASSESSMENT OF TUMOR LOCATION AND EXTENT OF PATHOLOGY IN NEOPLASTIC INVOLVEMENT OF THE LUMBAR SPINE

Bone involvement (spinal radiography + CT) or MRI:
- Vertebral body and pedicles, posterior elements, or a combination of both
- Number of vertebrae involved
- Percentage of bone mass loss of the vertebral cut surface

Myelography (+ CT) or MRI:
- Block related or unrelated to the bone lesion
- Number of segments involved
- Position of the epidural mass: anterior, posterior, and/or encircling

Spinal stability (spinal radiography + CT) or MRI:
- Involvement of two or more adjacent vertebrae
- Involvement of both anterior and posterior elements at the same level
- Loss of more than 50 per cent of the vertebral width
- Any combination of the above will increase instability

Retroperitoneal paravertebral mass (CT) and MRI:
- Location
- Extent
- Involvement of adjacent structures (kidneys, ureters, large vessels)
- Involvement of posterior abdominal wall

CT = Computed tomography; MRI = magnetic resonance imaging.

position in the spinal canal; (2) the epidural compression is caused by retropulsion of bone into the canal as a result of a pathologic fracture of the vertebral body; (3) the painful spinal instability is a result of destruction of one or more vertebral bodies (not necessarily associated with compression); and (4)

there is need for debulking of a contiguous paravertebral mass in an anterior or anterolateral position to the spinal column.

THE ANTERIOR APPROACH TO THE LUMBAR SPINE (L2-L5)

The intubated patient is placed in a right or left lateral decubitus position according to the tumor location as assessed by the preoperative studies. The acute bend of the table (Fig. 37–1) is placed under the lumbar area. Thus, a stretch is put on the lateral abdominal wall, which faces the surgeon, and after incision the wound stays widely open with minimal need for retraction. The incision is started at the lateral border of the paraspinous muscle mass at the level of the second lumbar vertebra and is carried in an oblique fashion laterally, ventrally, and distally to the lateral border of the rectus abdominis muscle. These paraspinous muscles should not be incised, as bleeding is usually profuse. Cutting through them does not improve the surgical exposure, and, when intact, they contribute to spinal stability. The incision is deepened by cautery to the peritoneum. By digital blunt dissection, the peritoneum is detached from the undersurface of the diaphragm. Attention is then directed centrally to the iliopsoas muscle: the peritoneum is peeled off the muscle medially until the lumbar spine is visualized. This is carried out staying close to the iliopsoas muscle, and no intentional

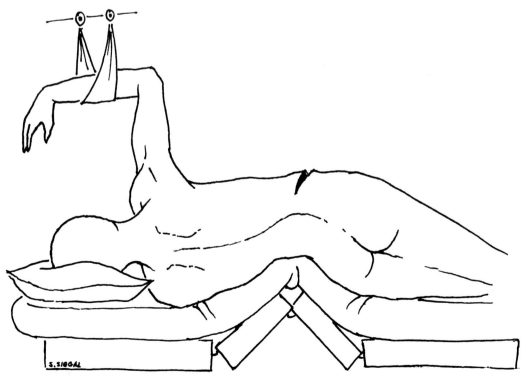

S. SIEGAL

FIGURE 37–1. Patient positioning for the lumbar vertebral replacement. The acute bend of the table, over which the patient is placed in the lateral decubitus position, puts a stretch on the lateral abdominal wall, deepening the incision with minimal retraction. This is an important detail as it improves exposure and facilitates the surgery.

dissection is done to reveal the ureter or kidney. When the peritoneum has been entirely detached from the diaphragm, the posterior abdominal wall, the iliopsoas muscle, and the spine, the abdominal contents will fall forward, opening the way for surgery on the vertebral bodies.

The iliopsoas muscles cover the lateral and anterolateral aspects of the lumbar spine; between them is the anterior longitudinal ligament, which runs as a white strong strip in the midline, segmentally elevated by the bulge of the intervertebral discs. For intraoperative location of the diseased vertebra, the surgeon inspects the iliopsoas muscle for a swelling that indicates an underlying or infiltrating paravertebral tumor. In addition, discoloration or bulging of the anterior longitudinal ligament, presence of frank anterior penetrating tumor, or an abnormally short interdiscal distance are all good localizing signs of the area to be decompressed. If the tumor is contained within the vertebra and its level is difficult to identify, it is wise to take an anteroposterior intraoperative x-ray of the lumbar spine, with a heavy intravenous needle hammered lightly into the lateral aspect of the vertebra. To retract the iliopsoas muscle and expose the lumbar spine, a round-ended retractor is placed under the medial border of the muscle and is kept in close contact to the vertebral bodies and pulled laterally to the intervertebral foramina. Normally, the vertebral body's circumference is significantly smaller than that of the intervertebral disc, causing it to appear as a depression between the bordering discs. The segmental arteries and veins usually cross the narrow midportion of the vertebral body. Most tumors will present a swelling with a red or blue tint (or black in the case of melanoma) localized to one or two vertebral bodies. The swelling may be soft or rubbery and must be palpated for pulsations. A pulsating tumor usually has substantial vascular feeders that must be looked for and ligated. The longitudinal structures usually encountered are sympathetic nerves that may be cut or preserved at the discretion of the surgeon.

Bleeding is minimized by ligation of the vascular bundles as they cross the waists of the vertebral bodies. The vertebral waist, covered by areolar tissue, is searched to find the segmental bundle, which may sometimes show through. The tip of a curved long hemostat is brought down on the bone close to one disc. It is made to sweep toward the other disc with its tip closed tight to the bone surface. As it emerges near the other disc, the vascular bundle will be elevated on the hemostat's jaws. Opening the instrument will stretch the vessels across the jaws and so will allow clipping or ligating on both sides of the instrument. No effort is made to separate the segmental artery from the vein, as both are contained in the same ligature. The two ligatures are placed as far away from each other as possible. The vascular bundle is then cut at mid-distance. The procedure is repeated at each level of interest. With the segmental vessels ligated, a thorough subperiosteal dissection is carried out anteriorly across the midline of the vertebral bodies, displacing the aorta or vena cava and protecting it with a malleable retractor inserted between it and the spine. The anterior longitudinal ligament is spared, if possible. In other cases, the vessel is embedded within the tumor capsule. Every effort is made to localize and ligate these vessels, although a torn segmental artery can be controlled. The dissection is continued laterally, elevating all soft tissues off the vertebral bodies and discs to the anterior margin of the intervertebral foramina. Dissection is not carried onto the pedicles unless there is need for lateral decompression as well.

Starting the excision of the tumor is the event that all participants, especially the anesthesiology team, must be made aware of, in view of the possibility of serious bleeding. In the case of a vertebra soft with tumor, after an initial incision with a No. 15 blade, large curettes are appropriate for expedient removal of large lumps of tissue. It also provides the pathologist with a better, noncrushed specimen for examination. In case of a hard vertebral shell, chisels may be used. The vertebral body is removed all the way back to the posterior longitudinal ligament. If there is evidence of tumor in the spinal canal, the ligament, if still present, has to be removed to visualize the dura and to decompress it. Pulsations of the dura, if present, signify opening of the myelographic block. Reaching the epidural space safely can also be achieved by following the segmental nerve exit at the intervertebral foramen, where it is decompressed. Once in the epidural space, a curved No. 2 curette is used in this fashion: it is introduced in the space, with the active edge hugging the posterior wall of the vertebral body. By slowly rotating the curette, the rounded blunt end will gently peel off the soft tissue adhering to the bone. When the surgeon is confident of the dissection, a short controlled pull will dislodge the bone segment forward. Care is taken not to pull on the segmental nerve.

The segmental roots may be encased in tumor tissue. There is also a possibility of direct penetration of the nerve root by the tumor, which may lead to intractable pain. Neurolysis must be attempted to lessen pain and maintain motor function of the lower extremities.

When the main bulk of the tumor has been removed, the anatomy is assessed. Bleeding may interfere with the inspection, so it is wise to palpate posteriorly to correctly locate the decompressed dura. Passing a thin rubber tubing above and below the decompressed area is an innocuous method of assessing the patency of the epidural space. When necessary, more vertebral segments are decompressed in the same fashion.

Bleeding during anterior decompression of the spine is usually 1500 ml or less, but in some cases (carcinoma of the thyroid, hypernephroma, multiple myeloma) it may be horrendous. The bleeding may originate from overlooked major vascular feeders of the tumor, from pathologic vessels within the tumor that when severed will not contract, from the spongy vertebral bone, or from the epidural venous plexus.

We have not experienced accidental tears of big vessels. Expeditious removal of the tumor is recommended because after a major debulking the bleeding is likely to lessen, more so in cases of complete excision. When bleeding continues, we usually apply Gelfoam or Surgicel on a gauze to the bleeding area and wait for the anesthesiology team to catch up with the fluid replacement. With bleeding under good or even partial control, decompression is completed and vertebral body replacement is considered. We have repeatedly observed that the replacement exerts a local hemostatic effect.

The vertebral body replacement is a spine-stabilizing procedure. Adequate decompression of the spinal cord, correction of deformity, and stabilization of the spinal column are inherent to the technique and, if obtained, will maximize spinal cord function. We have reported on our experience with vertebral body replacement using components of the Harrington instrumentation system, namely threaded rods, nuts, and hooks.[11] In our hands it has proven efficient and durable, with the additional advantage of not having to enlarge the surgical armamentarium.

THE VERTEBRAL BODY REPLACEMENT TECHNIQUE

A heavy threaded Harrington rod is cut about 1½ inches longer than the distance to be spanned by the vertebral replacement construct. On one end of the rod, a sharp sacral Moe hook is fastened in place by two nuts, one on each side (Fig. 37–5). Another nut is added, followed by the second hook facing the other way. Clamps are applied to both hooks to allow insertion of the assembly into the spinal gap in a coronal plane. The assembly is positioned at the widest vertebral diameter with the blades of the hooks reaching across the midline of the intact vertebral bodies, above and below. The hooks are then distracted to have their blades sink into the vertebral bodies. After the initial manual distraction, a large lamina spreader is positioned between and in direct contact with the hooks rather than with the clamps. Opening the spreader will gently drive the hook blades into the vertebral bodies. Backing up the mobile hook on the rod in the advanced position is accomplished by moving the nut on the thread. The gentle distraction is done in stages, ascertaining that the distraction forces are correctly directed and do not dislodge the assembly. Special care is taken to avoid impingement on the spinal canal. The spreader and hook clamps are removed when optimal height of the replacement has been obtained and the kyphosis has been corrected. A manual testing of the stability of the inserted assembly is carried out by pulling lightly on the rod. A thorough rinsing with warm saline is followed by gauze packing of the decompressed area.

A longstanding kyphosis will resist correction due to ligamentous or bony tethers. To overcome this, the anterior longitudinal ligament is sectioned and the residual vertebral shell on the opposite side of the decompression may have to be removed as well. Radiopaque methyl methacrylate (bone cement) is used to reconstruct the excised vertebral bodies. It is digitally inserted into the gap while still soft and is applied around and over the metal instrumentation (see Fig. 37–2). The cement is pushed into the spongy bone interstices of the proximal and distal vertebrae to improve the purchase on the bony elements and then the rest of the cavity is filled up. The cement must cover the sharp edges of the rod and hooks to avoid direct contact with the pulsating big vessels. Special care is taken not to exert any pressure on the dura mater. While hardening, the cement is kept at a distance from the dura by a Freer elevator, and so a cleft is formed leading from the epidural space into the retroperitoneum, allowing free drainage of postoperative bleeding. Excess of bone cement is removed. When the methyl methacrylate has set the area is rinsed again, and one large bore thoracic drain is inserted in the midaxillary line, preferably distal to the incision. The operating table is straightened and the wound is closed in layers. The skin is meticulously approximated and sutured without tension. The drain is connected to a suction system.

The surgical approach and vertebral replacement technique described above are suited to the lumbar spine (L2-L5). A few points deserve special notice:

(1) Regardless of the number of vertebrae to be replaced, the steps of anterior instrumentation of the spine (vertebral body replacement) are essentially the same. (2) The lumbar spine column at its lower segments is in close contact with the bifurcations of the aorta and vena cava, and the lateral aspects of L5 are in close relation to the iliac arteries and veins. Therefore, careful manipulation and retraction are indicated, and the vertebral replacement construct should not be in the way of the pulsating large vessels. We have not encountered any vascular complications, such as tears of the vena cava or iliac veins, nor late occurrence of iatrogenic aneurysms.

Postoperative Management

Turning in bed is not restricted. In case of paraplegia, turning is done every three hours and is noted on the bed chart. Regular hospital beds are used because turning frames are uncomfortable. Intravenous antibiotics are continued for 48 hours postoperatively. When the drainage for 24 hours is less than 50 ml, the drain is removed. The wound is covered again and left undisturbed until the 20th postoperative day. Sutures are then removed. If wound dehiscence is probable or edge necrosis begins to show, stitch removal is delayed. The patient is seated on the first or second postoperative day, and ambulation is considered the day after drain removal. There is no need for corsets, plaster jackets, or any other external fixation devices. Evaluation of stability at the site of the vertebral body replacement is by spine x-rays taken with the patient standing and supine. Assessment of patency at the site of the preoperative myelographic block is done by watching on fluoroscopy the movement of the Pantopaque remaining in the subarachnoid space.

Complications

Surgical mortality rate following vertebral body resection in cancer patients falls within the same range as after laminectomy, with an average rate of 8 per cent.[8, 12, 14]

Neurologic deterioration is a rare complication in vertebral body resection and occurs in only 2 to 4 per cent of patients.[8, 12, 14] The incidence of nonneurologic complications following vertebral body resection is similar to the reported rate following laminectomy. Dislodgement of the vertebral replacement construct can cause severe pain and neurologic deterioration due to spinal instability and subluxation. This occurred in 5 per cent of our patients prior to June, 1982, due to faulty anchorage of the construction to adjacent vertebrae.[11] Since the introduction of our improved technique, no dislodgement has occurred in 80 patients who underwent vertebral body replacement procedures. However, the operation and instrumentation techniques require considerable expertise. The anterior approach to the spine may subject the patient to a variety of potentially serious complications, such as severe bleeding, damage to the adjacent vital organs, infection, and poor healing of irradiated tissues. Therefore, we believe that these procedures should be undertaken by a surgeon familiar with the anterior surgical approach to the spine and with the technique of spinal instrumentation and its different options. Neurologic examination is carried out at 3-month intervals and stability is reassessed. Recurrence of instability is heralded by local or radicular pain that is elicited by motion or physical activity. Recurrence of pain in a persistent or radicular pattern may indicate nerve root compression and/or infiltration by tumor. Recurrence of neurologic symptoms suggests either severe instability or regrowth of the epidural tumor. In these situations, reassessment and repeat myelography are indicated. If a high-degree myelographic block is present or instability is evident, decompression and additional stabilizing instrumentation are considered.

POSTERIOR DECOMPRESSION AND INSTRUMENTATION

The intubated patient is placed face down on a spinal frame. This will prevent an increase in intraabdominal pressure and will lessen epidural bleeding during surgery. If a frame is not available, the patient is placed on rolls so that the weight-bearing areas are lateral on the chest and pelvis, leaving the abdomen and lower chest free for breathing movement. The head is positioned on a horseshoe headrest which allows free access to connections of the anesthesia apparatus. After prepping, when covering the back, a wide operative field is allotted for large skin flaps and possible incision lengthening. Skin incisions through radiation portals must be avoided at all costs. Some of these surgical wounds may dehisce and some will never heal, being further complicated by chronic discharge. Therefore the area of intended decompression is reached through an incision placed laterally in healthy tissue, circumventing the irradiated area, and a generous skin flap is created to be elevated and retracted. The extent of the lateral placement of the incision is dictated by the width of the radiation portal, which can usually be perceived by discoloration of the skin or, in inveterate cases, by the loss of subcutaneous fat. The incision is usually placed 8 to 10 cm lateral and parallel to the midline, long enough to allow exposure of four to five spinal segments above and below the planned area of decompression if spinal instrumentation is anticipated (Fig. 37–2). The incision is carried down to the fascia, and the flap is elevated medially to reach the spinous processes and 5 cm beyond them. Traction on the flap is by sutures in the subcutaneous tissue, with hemostats on their ends.

The fibrous caps of the spinous processes are split in midline by diathermy, and subperiosteal dissection of the paravertebral soft tissues is carried out. Tissues even mildly resistant to dissection are released by cautery. Possible undetected involvement with tumor of the posterior arch elements dictates caution: a bone fragment may be pushed or turned into the dura during elevation of the paravertebral muscles. In most cases, a posterior arch involvement will point to the level in need of decompression. However, it is not unusual to detect tumor deposits at other levels, which may have been designated for anchorage of the stabilizing instrumentation. This necessitates the dissection of additional segments to ensure firm placement of rods and wires.

Identification of the spinal levels by an intraoperative x-ray is mandatory, as it determines the site at which laminectomy is carried out and avoids unnecessary removal of posterior elements. The x-ray must include either the thoracolumbar or the lumbosacral junction, the one closest to the area of the intended decompression. In that area, a towel clip is attached to the base of a spinous process close to its superior margin. If so placed, the location of the tongs of the towel clip corresponds on the posteroanterior view of the x-ray with the midportion of the vertebral body at the same level. When the x-ray has been obtained, the spinous process is nicked for future reference and the towel clip is removed. Counting is done in reference to this vertebra. Laminectomy is carried out starting one level distal to the lower border of the myelographic block. Decompression is continued cephalad, carefully removing the posterior elements and refraining from insinuation of instruments between the lamina and the underlying compressing tumor, especially in the presence of neurologic deficit. Only after both proximal and distal

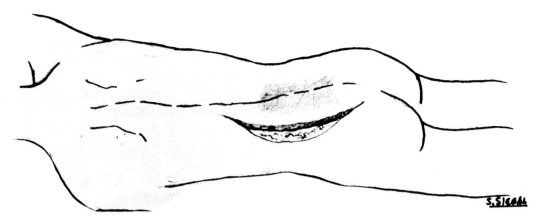

FIGURE 37–2. The surgical incision for posterior decompression in previously irradiated patients. The incision is placed 8 to 10 cm lateral and parallel to the midline, long enough to allow adequate exposure. Radiation portals (*shadowed area*) must be spared incisions at all costs.

tumor borders have been exposed is the tumor's removal considered. Neurologic deterioration as a direct result of laminectomy in cancer patients is not uncommon,[1, 4–7, 12] so that every effort must be made to minimize possible iatrogenic insult. Magnification loupes or operative microscopy may be indicated in some cases.

The neoplasm is most conveniently approached from its distal margin. In the area adjacent to the tumor, the epidural fat is split in midline with a Freer elevator to reach the normal dura underneath. The split is advanced until the tumor margin is encountered. A dissection plane is sought, gently elevating the tumor edge from the dura. Some tumors present no problem at removal because they are flexible or friable or easily detachable. Other tumors are of firm consistency; elevating one end may turn the other to impinge on the dura. Removal is piecemeal with sharp instruments. Tumors that adhere tenaciously to the dura (e.g., osteoblastoma, lung carcinoma) deserve special notice. They also are excised piecemeal, but in these cases one must accept neoplastic residue on the dural surface. Caution must be exercised not to violate the dura during tumor scraping. The malignant remnants are treated by radiation, if practical.

In many cases the tumor encircles the dura. The tumor sleeve is cut open either by sharp incision or by bipolar diathermy; it is elevated off the dura and then incised in midline from its undersurface up. This is continued until a grasp can be purchased on the cut margin of the tumor, which then can be gently peeled off laterally. The segmental nerves are looked for, and, if possible, the tumor is peeled off them too. In the lateral compartment, the overlying tumor is removed by sharp instruments, preferably sharp curettes of appropriate size. These cut the tumor against the local bone elements and so allow its evacuation without pulling on the dura or the tumor itself. The dura mater is usually an effective barrier to tumor penetration. The segmental nerves are protected by the dural sleeve up to their point of exit at the intervertebral foramen. Distally, however,

tumor invasion of the nerves may and does occur. This is one of the causes of intractable pain often encountered in these unfortunate patients. Gentle peeling of the tumor off the nerves is attempted to preserve motor function.

Intraoperative bleeding may be very significant. It is controlled by application of either Gelfoam or Surgicel with gentle pressure onto the bleeding surface. Vascular feeders of the tumor mass are difficult to control from the posterior aspect of the spine. The walls of tumor vessels may be devoid of contractile components and thus lack the ability to contract. The continuous gentle pressure is to encourage coagulation. Removal of excess local bleeding is by suction only. Rubbing an oozing tumor surface by gauzes removes already formed plugs of coagulum.

When tumor removal is completed or is optimal for the specific case, the bare dura and roots are routinely covered with free fat grafts harvested from the available subcutaneous tissues at the incision site. The fat graft is fixed with a few sutures to soft tissues to prevent displacement.

Evaluation of residual spine stability is done at this stage. The spine is considered unstable if tumor excision has necessitated removal of apophyseal joints bilaterally at the same and/or adjacent level(s) or if a pathologic fracture is present (Table 37–1). Even if in doubt as to whether decompression has led to an unstable situation, it is best to go ahead with spine stabilization. A stable spine will maximize neurologic function and save the patient the severe intractable pains of instability. We usually use the double Harrington rod distraction system supplemented by segmental sublaminar wiring. This system satisfies two main requirements for reestablishing spinal stability: distraction and fixation. The gradual distraction obtained by Harrington instrumentation will cause optimal tension in the spinal and paraspinal soft tissues (ligaments, joint capsules, muscles), taking out the slack that accompanies vertebral compression. It may also correct local deformity (kyphosis), restore lost vertebral height, and lessen compression at the level of the intervertebral foramina. When coupled with

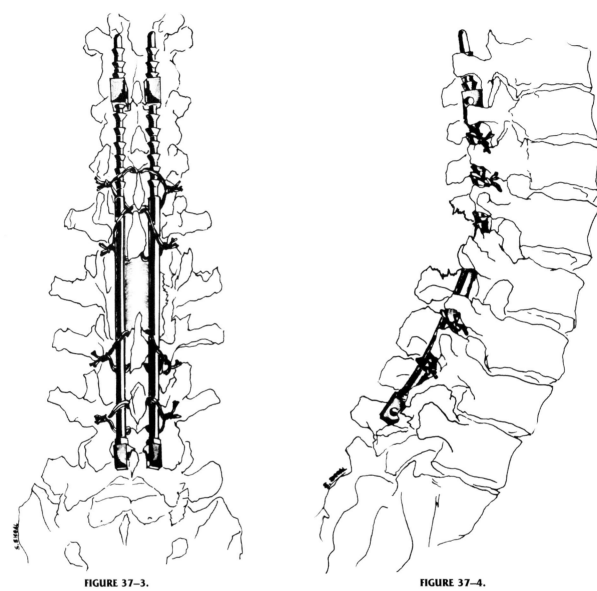

FIGURE 37–3.   **FIGURE 37–4.**

FIGURE 37–3 and 37–4. Posterior intrumentation of the lumbar spine with Harrington distraction rods and segmental wiring. The Harrington distraction instrumentation, coupled with segmental sublaminar wiring, results in instant spinal stability. (1) The upper hooks are placed in the apophyseal joints. (2) The lower hooks are placed on the laminae of a vertebra, two levels distal to the laminectomy. In case of a decompressive laminectomy extending to levels caudal to L3, distal laminar hooks will be replaced by the longer sacral alar hooks, which are then placed on both alae of the sacrum. (3) Following incision of the ligamenta flava above and below the laminae, double 18-gauge stainless steel wire is passed under the laminae, two levels above and two levels below the decompression area. To restrict dangerous wandering, the wires are bent on the laminae. (4) The Harrington rods are then chosen of a total length, longer by 3 to 4 cm than the distance between the upper and lower hooks. (5) The rods are given a bend to accommodate the lumbar lordosis. The ratchet end is never bent to avoid rod breakage (Fig. 37–4). (6) The ratchet end of the rods is inserted in the upper rods and then pulled back to be firmly seated at the collar end, on the lower hooks. (7) The Harrington spreader is placed on the ratchet under the upper hook to incrementally advance the distraction hook along the ratchet portion of the rod. The optimal distraction depends on the surgeon's skill and experience. (8) The segmental wires are tightened on the rods. (9) The exposed dura is covered by a free fat graft.

sublaminar wiring, which will fix the spine segmentally to the parallel rods, it results in a firm and solid internal fixation with instant spinal stability (Fig. 37–3). No external appliances (braces, jackets, and so forth) are required. The technique entails placement of two upper Harrington hooks (No. 1251, Zimmer, Warsaw, IN) in the apophyseal joints, under the inferior facets of the third or fourth vertebra above the laminectomy. Either two lower laminar hooks (Zimmer No. 1256) are placed on the laminae of a vertebra, two levels caudal to the distal end of the laminectomy, or two sacral hooks are placed on the sacral alae. Double 18-gauge wire is passed under the intact laminae on each side, above and below the laminectomy site.

Passing the sublaminar wires bilaterally requires incision of the flaval ligaments above and below the laminae. If spinous processes are in the way, their overhang is osteotomized. The stainless steel wires, 18 gauge and 30 centimeters in length, are bent in their middle in a hairpin fashion. This straight double wire is now given a gentle bend to allow surfacing of the hairpin end after its passage underneath the lamina. It is usually introduced under the caudal edge of the lamina to surface cephalad. As it is pulled out, the wire ends are crossed on the lamina to restrict wandering of the wire, which may be pushed against the dura during further instrumentation endeavors. At this point, the distance between the upper and lower hooks is measured. Two Harrington rods, longer by 3 centimeters than the measured distance, are bent to accommodate or restore lumbar lordosis and are then positioned in the hooks (Fig. 37–4). The upper hooks are moved up on the ratchets until optimal tension is reached for both rods. Next the segmental wires are tightened on the rods. The use of the twofold wire is aimed to resist breakage but also to distribute on a larger surface the pressure on the laminae and so possibly avoid a cutout. The tightening is done by crossing the wire ends forcefully across the rod. In the tightened position, fixation is obtained by twisting the wire ends around each other. Excess twisting may cause wire breakage, therefore no more than three full circle twists are allowed. The wire ends are cut and the "braids" are bent toward the rod shaft to avoid future discomfort.

Bone Grafts

Prior to wound closure one must consider the advisability of bone grafting to achieve bony arthrodesis. This is a matter of debate. Orthopedic surgeons have traditionally regarded bone grafting as an integral part of spine fusion with internal fixation. Experience has shown that single or even double Harrington rodding may end in rod breakage, especially in young and active people, if solid bony arthrodesis of the spine has not been obtained. However, the great majority of patients with primary or metastatic spinal deposits are not young, and with the advent of segmental instrumentation rod break-

age is a rare occurrence. In many cases, activity is restricted by some neurologic deficit, by pain, or by less-than-optimal medical status. It is therefore reasonable to assume that in these conditions the internal fixation alone will provide durable spinal stability.

When considering addition of bone grafts, the time factor must also be taken into account. If bone autografts are employed, the time required for spinal arthrodesis to occur is about 6 months, and to mature 6 more months. When one resorts to bank bone (allografts), the required time is longer, especially if postoperative radiation is scheduled. The median survival of patients with spinal cord compression due to metastatic spread is 12 to 18 months.[2, 3, 9, 12, 15] Therefore, our main indication for adding iliac cancellous bone grafts is a benign or slow-growing tumor in children and young adults (osteoblastoma, giant cell tumor, aneurysmal bone cysts, and the like).

There are three additional arguments against bone grafting: (1) it requires a separate incision with an increase in operating time and morbidity in patients with active disease; (2) the iliac bone graft may be microscopically involved with tumor; and (3) the bone graft incorporation may be inhibited by postoperative radiation.

When a decision has been reached to employ bone grafts, either autologous or bank bone, decortication is limited to the transverse and spinous processes, since access to the lamina is obstructed by the presence of rods and segmental wiring. An ample quantity of grafts is applied to the decorticated areas in continuity. If internal fixation obtained by instrumentation is adequate, there is no need for external appliances.

Closure of Surgical Wound

Postoperative bleeding from residual tumor or tumor bed may account in some cases for the neurologic deterioration observed after surgery. Therefore we routinely cover the dura and segmental nerves with a free fat graft and then place a large-bore noncollapsible drain by the side of one of the Harrington rods near the decompression area. Care is taken that the rod separates the fat graft from the drain, because with suction the free fat graft may dislodge, obstruct the drain, halt the evacuation of the hematoma, and leave the dura bare. Further care is taken to position the drain so that it does not get caught in the wire ends on removal. The drain exit is lateral (posterior axillary line) and certainly not through irradiated tissue.

Meticulous technique is employed in closing the wound. The paravertebral muscles are tightly closed over the rods. The skin flap is brought down by sutures in sequential rows to cause adherence of the flap to its bed and eliminate potential spaces. These sutures will also release tension on the flap edges, having the skin on both sides of the incision lean toward each other to a touch. No skin overriding is acceptable. Sutures are used only for the alignment

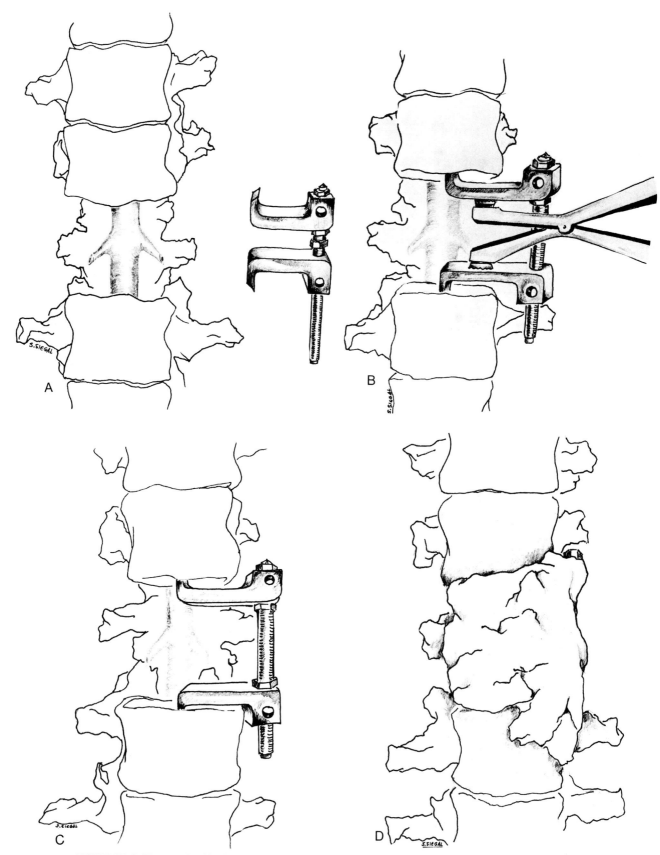

FIGURE 37–5. The vertebral body replacement technique. *A,* Two sharp sacral Moe hooks on a heavy threaded rod cut to measure. One hook is fastened in place by two nuts; the other is mobile. *B,* Positioning of the assembly is by clamps (not shown) at the widest vertebral diameter in the coronal plane. Gradual distraction by a lamina spreader will gently drive the sharp hooks into the vertebral bodies. *C,* The third nut is advanced on the thread to back up the mobile hook in the final distracted position. *D,* Final shape of vertebral body replacement: the methylmethacrylate covers the metal components and spans the space between them.

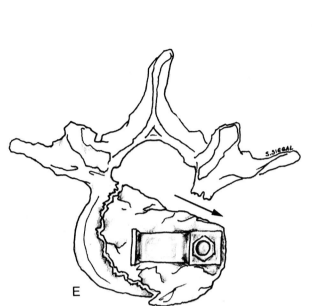

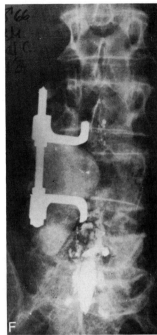

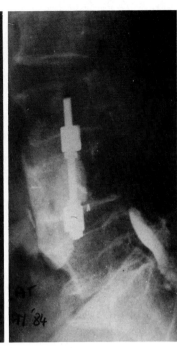

FIGURE 37–5 *Continued. E,* While hardening, the cement is kept away from the dura, and so a cleft is formed leading from the epidural space into the retroperitoneum. This will allow free drainage of postoperative bleeding *(arrow). F,* The anteroposterior and lateral x-rays of a vertebral body replacement at L4. Note coronal positioning of the instrumentation and its coverage by methyl methacrylate to avoid direct contact with the pulsating large vessels.

of the skin flap and need not be tight. Since sutures are routinely left in place for at least 20 days, a tight suture will submerge, knot and all, under the skin.

Postoperative Management

The patient is kept flat on his back for at least 10 hours following surgery. Heels and sacrum are protected from weight-bearing contact with the mattress. Turning frames are not used, even for paraplegics, as all patients find them very uncomfortable. Regular beds are used, and following the first 12 postoperative hours, free turning in bed is allowed. Perioperative antibiotics are discontinued on the third postoperative day unless otherwise indicated, and the drain is removed. The patient is seated on the second postoperative day and is walked on the fourth, if able to do so. Radiotherapy, when indicated, can be administered during the fourth postoperative week, provided healing of the surgical wound is per primum. Prior to discharge, x-rays of the spine are obtained, with the patient both standing and supine, to evaluate stability. A fluoroscopic remyelogram is also routinely obtained. Since some Pantopaque is usually left in the subarachnoid space at the time of the preoperative myelogram, there is no need for repeated lumbar punctures for periodic assessments of the patency at the site of the previous myelographic block.

Complications

Complications related to posterior decompression and instrumentation include neurologic worsening, bleeding, hook cutout, skin breakdown, infection, and rod breakage. The risk of neurologic deterioration as a direct result of laminectomy is of major concern, but exact figures related to the lumbar area are lacking. The overall rate of worsening is about 12 per cent in cancer patients.[4, 5]

Bleeding from the cut surface of residual tumor may continue for a few days. Patent large bore drainage is essential to prevent collection of epidural hematoma. Spine instrumentation in the elderly differs from that in the young due to aging of bone, ligaments, joints, and discs. Osteoporosis may weaken the apophyseal joint components, and ligamentous elasticity may be reduced, causing the lumbar spine to be more rigid and brittle. In this situation tightening the upper hooks on the ratchets may end in late hook cutout. This complication and that of rod breakage can be markedly diminished by the routine use of segmental wiring.

Skin breakdown occurs almost regularly when incisions cross irradiated areas and may be complicated by chronic discharge. Sometimes, granulation tissue may fill the gap over a course of several months.

In our earlier cases, when bone cement (methyl methacrylate) was used to better the purchase of the instrumentation on the posterior spinal elements, we commonly encountered a sterile serous accumulation at the cement site. The routine use of segmental sublaminar wiring vastly improved spine stabilization, obviated the need for use of cement, and eliminated the sterile serous accumulations related to it.

CONCLUSION

The problem of neoplastic involvement of the spine is of a magnitude that cannot be ignored. The spinal surgeon in command of modern surgical techniques is called upon to contribute skills in spine reconstruction to alleviate the suffering of these unfortunate patients and to improve the quality of their lives. It is a new frontier open for innovation.

REFERENCES

1. Barcena A, Lobato RD, Rivas JJ, et al: Spinal metastatic disease: Analysis of factors determining functional prognosis and the choice of treatment. Neurosurgery 15:820–827, 1984.
2. Benson H, Scarffe J, Todd ID, et al: Spinal cord compression in myeloma. Br Med J 1:1541–1544, 1979.
3. Bernat JL, Greenberg ER, Barrett J: Suspected epidural compression of the spinal cord and cauda equina by metastatic carcinoma. Cancer 51:1953–1957, 1983.
4. Black P: Spinal metastases: Current status and recommended guidelines for management. Neurosurgery 5:726–746, 1979.
5. Findlay GFG: Adverse effects of the management of malignant spinal cord compression. J Neurol Neurosurg Psych 47:761–768, 1984.
6. Gilbert RW, Kim JH, Posner JB: Epidural spinal cord compression from metastatic tumor: Diagnosis and treatment. Ann Neurol 3:40–51, 1978.
7. Hall AJ, Mackay NNS: The results of laminectomy for compression of the cord and cauda equina by extradural malignant tumor. J Bone Joint Surg (Br) 55:497–505, 1973.
8. Harrington KD: Anterior cord decompression and spinal stabilization for patients with metastatic lesions of the spine. J Neurosurg 61:107–117, 1984.
9. Martenson JA, Evans RG Jr, Lie MR, et al: Treatment outcome and complications in patients treated for malignant epidural spinal cord compression. J Neurooncol 3:77–84, 1985.
10. Shafir M, Holland JF, Cohen B, Aufses AH Jr: Radical retroperitoneal tumor surgery with resection of the psoas major muscle. Cancer 56:929–933, 1985.
11. Siegal TZ, Siegal T: Vertebral body resection for epidural compression by malignant tumors. Results of forty-seven consecutive operative procedures. J Bone Joint Surg 67A:375–382, 1985.
12. Siegal TZ, Siegal T: Surgical decompression of anterior and posterior malignant epidural tumors copressing the spinal cord: A prospective study. Neurosurgery 17:424–432, 1985.
13. Siegal TZ, Siegal T: The management of malignant epidural tumors compressing the spinal cord. In Schmidek HH, Sweet WB (eds): Operative Neurosurgical Techniques: Indications, Methods, and Results. Orlando, Grune & Stratton, 1988, pp 1539–1562.
14. Sundaresan N, Galicich JH, Bains MS, et al: Vertebral body resection in the treatment of cancer involving the spine. Cancer 53:1393–1396, 1984.
15. Vieth R, Olson G: Extradural spinal metastases and their neurosurgical management. J Neurosurg 23:501–508, 1965.

38

SURGICAL CONSIDERATIONS IN PELVIC TUMORS WITH INTRASPINAL EXTENSION

KALMON D. POST and PAUL C. McCORMICK

INTRODUCTION

Tumors involving the sacrum and related neural, pelvic, and retroperitoneal structures constitute a heterogeneous group of neoplasms. Although uncommon in occurrence, sacral and presacral tumors can present at any age and encompass a wide range of histopathology. The intrasacral space is unique in its capacity for regional expansion, resulting in a delayed clinical presentation as the slowly growing mass fills the sacrum. It then can advance cephalad in the spinal canal, exit through the sacral foramina, or erode through the walls of bone by either invasion or pressure.

The surgical approach to these lesions is complex and frequently multidisciplinary, requiring the involvement of neurosurgeons, orthopedists, and abdominal surgeons. Accurate preoperative assessment and detailed knowledge of both surgical and functional anatomy are necessary in the management of these lesions.

Symptoms and signs such as root pain, neurologic deficits, urinary and bowel complaints, and bone changes may not discriminate between benign and malignant tumors. Urinary and bowel complaints, if neurogenic in nature, suggest malignancy, whereas bone destruction is seen only with malignant tumors.[12, 47]

SURGICAL ANATOMY

Sacrum

The sacrum is a triangular bone formed by the fusion of five sacral vertebrae (Fig. 38–1). Superiorly, the base of the sacrum articulates with the 5th lumbar vertebra through the intervertebral disc and two facet joints; inferiorly, the narrow sacral apex is connected to the coccyx via a rudimentary intervertebral disc.

The sacrum attaches laterally to the iliac bones. The pelvic surface of the sacrum forms the posterior bony wall of the lesser pelvis. Below the sacral promontory, the ventrally projecting portion of the S1 vertebral body, the sacrum is ventrally concave in both the horizontal and vertical planes.[34] This concavity, which is more pronounced in women, serves to increase the volume of the pelvis.

The pelvic surface of the sacrum presents four sets of foramina, the ventral sacral foramina, which transmit the primary ventral rami of the first four sacral nerves. Transverse ridges of bone extending between each set of ventral sacral foramina represent the points of fusion between the sacral bodies. The bars of bone separating ipsilateral foramina are medial extensions of the costal processes which are fused to the vertebral bodies. Lateral to the first three sacral foramina are the sacral ala. They are formed by the fusion of the costal and transverse processes of the first three sacral vertebrae. The lateral surfaces of the sacral ala articulate with both ilia through the sacroiliac joints.[34]

The posterior surface of the sacrum is convex dorsally and presents a series of vertically oriented bony crests. The middle sacral crest represents the fusion of the upper three or four spinous processes of the sacral vertebrae. Inferiorly, the middle sacral crest is interrupted by the sacral hiatus, which results from the failure of fusion of the fifth and, occasionally, the fourth sacral vertebral laminae.

Just lateral to the sacral hiatus, the inferiorly projecting sacral cornua represent the partially formed inferior articular facets of the fifth sacral vertebra. It is through the sacral hiatus that anesthesiologists administer caudal anesthesia. On either side of the middle sacral crest are the intermediate crests formed from fused laminae and articular facets. The lateral sacral crests represent the union of the transverse processes of the upper three sacral vertebrae. Between the intermediate crests and the lateral sacral

391

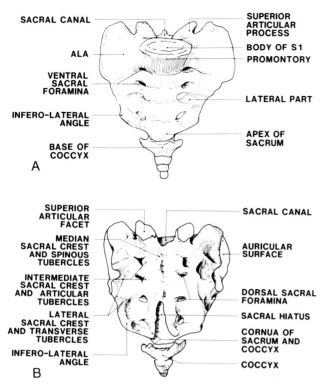

FIGURE 38–1. Pelvic (A) and dorsal (B) surfaces of the sacrum and coccyx. (Reprinted with permission from Levine E, Batnitzky S: Computed tomography of sacral and perisacral lesions. CRC Crit Rev Diag Imaging 21:307–373, 1984. Copyright CRC Press, Inc., Boca Raton, FL.)

crests are four sets of foramina, the dorsal sacral foramina, through which pass the primary dorsal rami of the first four sacral nerves. The fifth sacral nerve exits the spinal canal between the fifth sacral vertebra and the coccyx.[34]

The complex embryologic development of the sacrum results in the frequent occurrence of anomalies of this bony structure. There is about a 5 per cent incidence of sacralization of the fifth lumbar vertebra.[34] However, in only about 20 per cent of sacralized lumbar vertebrae is the fusion so complete that just four lumbar vertebrae are present. Conversely, there is a 6 per cent incidence of either partial or complete lumbarization of the first sacral vertebra, resulting in six lumbar vertebrae.[34] About 4.5 per cent of the general population possess a simple spina bifida occulta.[24, 27, 83] The bifida usually involves only S1 but may include the entire sacral spine. Whereas most anomalies of the sacrum are clinically insignificant, their presence should be kept in mind when planning a surgical approach to the sacrum.

The sacrum forms the lowest portion of the bony spinal canal. Transverse section of the sacrum at the S1 level demonstrates the canal to be triangular; in lower sections the canal becomes progressively smaller and assumes an elliptical shape.[45] The upper half of the sacral spinal canal contains the caudal dural sac, the subarachnoid space filled with cerebrospinal fluid (CSF), and the vertically oriented cauda equina and filum terminale.

Below the termination of the dural sac, at the level of the lower part of the S2 vertebra, the spinal canal encloses a variable amount of epidural fat and blood vessels, as well as the lower sacral roots and the filum terminale, and continues caudally to insert into the periosteum of the coccyx.

Laterally, the sacral canal is continuous with four sets of intervertebral foramina. These foramina contain the dorsal root ganglia of the first four sacral nerve roots. In the lateral portion of the foramina, both dorsal and ventral sacral roots join to form the sacral spinal nerves. The dorsal and ventral sacral foramina are continuous with the intervertebral foramina. While the dorsal sacral foramina pass mainly posterolaterally, the course of the ventral sacral foramina is inferior and slightly lateral. This results in the primary ventral rami taking a nearly vertical course as they pass from the sacral canal into the presacral space.[71]

The blood supply to the sacrum is primarily from the medial and lateral sacral arteries.[34] The medial sacral artery is a branch of the aorta and descends along the midline on the surface of the lumbar and sacral vertebrae into the pelvis. The lateral sacral arteries are branches of the posterior division of the internal iliac arteries. Typically, two lateral sacral arteries descend bilaterally on the ventral surface of the sacrum. They send branches into each of the ventral sacral foramina to supply the sacrum and the dural sheaths of the sacral nerve roots.

There are numerous anastomoses between the medial and lateral sacral arteries. Occasionally, a foraminal branch of these vessels will ascend along the roots of the cauda equina and participate in the blood supply to the cauda equina and the conus medullaris. Most tumors arising from the sacrum or presacral space, as well as some intraspinal neoplasms, derive at least part of their blood supply from the medial and lateral sacral arteries. Depending on the tumor type, angiography may demonstrate enlargement, displacement, or encasement of these vessels.

The stability of the sacrum comes mostly from the articulation between the lateral sacral ala of the first three sacral vertebrae and the iliac bones. This sacroiliac articulation consists of a synovial joint and a strong interosseous sacroiliac ligament which lies just posterior to the joint cavity. The articular surfaces of the sacrum cause the sacrum to wedge firmly between the ilia.[34] This articular configuration, plus the presence of the interosseous ligament, tends to pull both iliac bones closer together in response to a vertical load.

The ventral and dorsal sacroiliac ligaments, which lie on the ventral and dorsal surfaces of the sacroiliac joint, function to reinforce the stability of the joint.[34] Degenerative changes in the sacroiliac joint, resulting in the fusion of the articular surfaces of the joint cavity, are especially common in men over 50 years of age.[34] Two large ligaments, the sacrotuberous and sacrospinous ligaments, prevent rotation of the lower sacrum in the vertical plane when weight is applied to the upper surface of the sacrum.[34]

It is not clear how much of the sacroiliac joint can

be removed without jeopardizing stability. Stener and colleagues[31, 71] presented both clinical and experimental evidence suggesting that the sacroiliac joint may be removed up to the level of the S1 foramen without sacrificing stability. Most of their subjects, however, were males over the age of 50 in whom the sacroiliac joints may have been ankylosed.

Presacral Space

The presacral space is a crescent-shaped, potential space located between the posterior wall of the rectum and the anterior surface of the sacrum and coccyx. According to lateral views during barium enema, the space is usually under 1 cm in length. Measurements above 2 cm are considered abnormal and warrant a search for pathology in the presacral space.[13]

The presacral space is lined with two fascial layers. The anterior lining is the fascia proprius of the rectum, and the posterior sheath is the fascia pelvis parietalis, or Waldeyer's fascia, covering the anterior surface of the sacrum.[13, 37] The presacral space is limited superiorly by the peritoneal reflection at about the S2 level and inferiorly by the anococcygeal ligament and the levator ani muscles, which also form the floor of the lesser pelvis. The lateral border of the presacral space is defined in a rostral-caudal direction by the ureters and internal iliac arteries, and the piriformis and coccygeus muscles, respectively.

The contents of the presacral space include loose areolar tissue, lymph nodes, medial and lateral sacral arteries, sacral sympathetic chain, and branches of both the inferior hypogastric plexus and sacral plexus, including the nervi erigentes.[37]

Bowel/Bladder Innervation

Micturition is largely a reflex function.[53] The afferent and efferent arcs are carried by the sacral parasympathetic plexus, the nervi erigentes. Sensory fibers in the bladder wall respond primarily to increased intravesicular pressure. Their central processes project cranially in the spinal cord to provide the conscious sensation of bladder fullness. Collaterals of these sensory processes synapse on the preganglionic parasympathetic cell bodies at the S2-S4 cord level to participate in the micturition reflex. Fibers from the preganglionic cells synapse on the postganglionic cell bodies located in the bladder wall. Muscarinic ACH receptors on the smooth muscle of the bladder wall, the detrusor, are innervated by the short postganglionic fibers (Fig. 38–2).

Increased intravesicular pressure above a critical level activates the micturition reflex. Supraspinal control of the micturition reflex is exerted through a loosely organized group of cells located in the dorsolateral pons. Through a direct projection of the frontal lobes, this collection of cells brings the micturition reflex under voluntary control.[61]

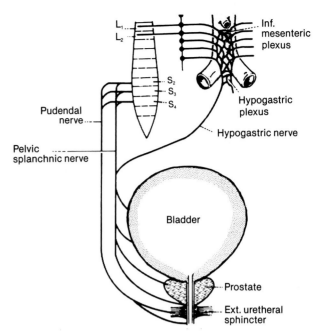

FIGURE 38–2. Diagrammatic representation of somatic, sympathetic, and parasympathetic innervation of the urinary bladder. (From Gray SG, Singhabhandhu B, Smith RA: Sacrococcygeal chordoma: Report of a case and review of the literature. Surgery 78:573–582, 1975; with permission.)

Sympathetic innervation of the bladder arises from preganglionic cells in the intermediolateral cell columns at the T12-L2 cord level. Their fibers project into the pelvis via the hypogastric plexus, where they synapse on postganglionic cell bodies. Sympathetic receptors in the bladder are both alpha and beta adrenergic. Alpha receptors, located on the smooth muscle of the internal sphincter at the bladder neck, produce contraction of the internal sphincter in response to sympathetic stimulation. Beta receptors are found on the smooth muscle of the bladder, predominantly in the region of the trigone. Activation of the beta receptors produces smooth muscle relaxation resulting in increased bladder compliance.[53] Thus sympathetic innervation of the bladder aids in maintaining continence.

Somatic efferents from the anterior horn cells at the S2-S4 cord level travel via the pudendal nerve to innervate the skeletal muscle of the external sphincter located between the pelvic diaphragm. The external sphincter surrounds the urethra as it pierces the pelvic floor. Voluntary contraction of the external sphincter maintains urinary continence during periods of increased abdominal pressure (e.g., coughing or straining). Contraction of the external sphincter can also temporarily delay micturition during active detrusor contraction.

The clinical effects of lower motor neuron dysfunction depend on the number and level of sacral nerve root section of compression. Bilateral loss of sacral nerve roots below the S1 level during high sacrectomy produces urinary retention with overflow incontinence.[53] The initially hypotonic bladder will eventually hypertrophy, leading to small bladder volumes as a result of increased bladder outlet resistance from unopposed sympathetic innervation.

The risk of recurrent urinary tract infections and reflux resulting in hydronephrosis is high in these patients. Early institution of intermittent self-catheterization is mandatory, and in some patients augmentation cystoplasty may be necessary to increase bladder volume. Unilateral loss of S2-S5, although producing perineal anesthesia on the affected side, generally does not result in significant bladder dysfunction.[30, 52] It has been our experience that bilateral function of the S2 nerve roots, as well as unilateral function of S3, is required for adequate bladder performance.

Innervation of the lower bowel and rectum is predominantly parasympathetic. Somatic fibers carried by the pudendal nerve innervate the external anal sphincter. Neurogenic disturbances of defecation usually accompany bladder dysfunction. These disturbances generally can be managed successfully with bowel training, maintenance of formed stool, and periodic use of laxatives or enemas when necessary.[29]

EMBRYOLOGY

The finding that congenital tumors and cysts account for the majority of the pathology in the sacrococcygeal region reflects the complexity of the developmental events occurring in the caudal portion of the embryo. Most of these lesions are the direct effect of disordered embryogenesis resulting from persistence of embryonic cell rests, failure of regression, or defective cleavage of germ cell layers.

The transformation of the rounded cell mass, the blastocyst, to a recognizable embryo with a longitudinal axis commences with the appearance of the primitive streak at the caudal end of the embryonic disc. Cells from either side of this longitudinal groove migrate through an opening in the primitive streak, the primitive pit, and extend cranially between ectoderm and endoderm. These cells differentiate into the paraxial mesoderm, which eventually undergoes somite formation, and they are responsible for the development of the vertebral column, skeletal muscles, and the connective tissue of the body wall.[75]

Hensen's node, a heaped-up cell mass located just rostral to the primitive streak, gives rise to cells that migrate cranially between the sheets of paraxial mesoderm. These cells form a cylindrical structure, the notochord, which is presumed to play a role in the induction of both neural tube formation and segmentation of the paraxial mesoderm into somites. The continuity of the notochord is interrupted by the development of the vertebral bodies; by the fourth month of fetal life the notochord remains only in the center portion of the intervertebral disc known as the nucleus pulposis.

Development of the vertebrae at the sacrococcygeal level consists of the formation of several vertebrae, followed by a reduction in number of these vertebrae and fusion of the remaining ones. Autopsy studies have shown coiling and budding of the caudal notochord, presumably resulting from this process of reduction and fusion of the caudal vertebral units.[35] Budding of the notochord has also been described at its rostral end in the region of the clivus, and embryonic rests of notochordal tissue in the adult have been found in both locations. These findings may explain why over 75 per cent of chordomas arise either in the sacrococcygeal region or in the area near the upper portion of the clivus.

The neural tube begins its formation at 18 days and is completed by the 28th day of fetal life.[75] The most caudal portion of the neural tube, the posterior neuropore, is located just rostral to Hensen's node and the primitive streak. The latter two structures coalesce and canalize, thereby forming a second tube of neural ectoderm which becomes attached to the caudal portion of the neural tube during the period of canalization of the tail bud (28 to 40 days).[44] By the ninth week of fetal life, the primitive spinal cord occupies the entire length of the spinal canal. From this period until birth most of the caudal neural tube formed by the tail bud undergoes regression and is present in the adult as the filum terminale.[72]

Following fusion of the neural tube, the surface ectoderm, which was initially attached to the lateral margins of the neural plaque, separates from the plaque and fuses in the midline to cover the dorsal aspect of the neural tube. A failure of this cleavage may result in the inclusion of surface ectoderm with subsequent tumor formation.

Abnormal formation of the gut may also be responsible for developmental tumors in the sacrococcygeal region. Initially the gut develops from the endodermal vesicle and is divided into the foregut and the hindgut. Early in embryogenesis, before closure of the neural tube, a communication known as the neurenteric canal exists between the caudal portion of the neural tube and the hindgut. This communication is transitory in nature, being present for about two days. Persistence of this connection may result in cyst formation or, as postulated by some authors, may be responsible for teratomatous neoplasms.

The most caudal portion of the hindgut, the postanal gut, is present in the 3.5- to 8.0-mm stage when the embryo possesses a true tail.[25] It is located caudal to the proctodeum, which is the future site of the rectum and anus. The postanal gut eventually fills with epithelial debris and is obliterated, but persistence of this structure is the presumed pathogenesis of postanal gut cysts (Fig. 38–3).

INCIDENCE AND CLASSIFICATION

Tumors of the sacrum and presacral space are decidedly rare. In three large hospital series, tumors in this region accounted for a combined incidence of 1 per 46,000 admissions.[63, 81] The first recorded presacral tumor was reported by Middeldorpf in

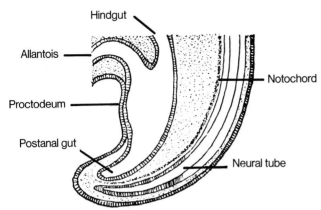

FIGURE 38–3. Diagrammatic illustration of caudal embryo at 4-mm stage. (From Campbell WL, Wolfe M: Retrorectal cysts of developmental origin. Am J Roentgenol 117:307–313, 1973; © by American Roentgen Ray Society.)

TABLE 38–1. DIFFERENTIAL DIAGNOSIS OF SACRAL AND PRESACRAL TUMORS IN 328 PATIENTS

CLASSIFICATION	NUMBER OF CASES	PERCENTAGE
Congenital	188	57.3
Developmental cysts	79	
Dermoid cyst		
Enteric cyst		
Postanal gut cyst		
Anterior sacral meningocele		
Tumors	109	
Teratoma	35	
Chordoma	74	
Inflammatory	31	9.5
Neurogenic	29	8.8
Ependymoma	13	
Neurofibroma	7	
Neurofibrosarcoma	2	
Schwannoma	4	
Ganglioneuroma	2	
Neuroblastoma	1	
Osseous	29	8.8
Giant cell tumor	12	
Osteogenic sarcoma	8	
Cartilaginous tumor	6	
Osteoma	2	
Ewing's sarcoma	1	
Metastatic Tumors	24	7.3
Miscellaneous	27	8.2
Adrenal rest tumor	1	
Aneurysmal bone cyst	2	
Dermoid	1	
Fibroma	2	
Fibrosarcoma	2	
Hemangioendothelioma	4	
Hemangioma	1	
Hemangiopericytoma	2	
Leiomyoma	2	
Lipoma	2	
Liposarcoma	3	
Lymphangioma	1	
Plasmacytoma	3	
Undifferentiated sarcoma	1	
Total	328	100

1885.[54] The patient was a one-year-old child with a sacrococcygeal teratoma. For a period following this report all tumors involving the sacrum and presacral space were classified as "Middeldorpf tumors." With the subsequent identification of many additional tumor types in this region, the term Middeldorpf tumor has been largely abandoned.

A comprehensive classification was proposed by Lovelady and Dockerty in 1948 when they reported on 127 women with extragenital pelvic tumors.[48] Since then this classification has been expanded and modified, but the general form has been retained. Table 38–1 shows a current classification, as well as the diagnoses of 328 patients collected from several clinical series of sacral and presacral tumors.[9, 21, 47, 51, 77, 80] These tumors may also be classified as tumors of the bony sacrum, lesions arising primarily in the presacral space, and cauda equina tumors and cysts.

PRESENTATION

Benign tumors are often asymptomatic (50 per cent), while the majority of malignant lesions present with symptoms, most frequently pain.[12] Prior history of trauma may lead to the discovery of the previously asymptomatic mass, or it may be appreciated on routine rectal or pelvic examination.

Pain is often sacrococcygeal, buttock/low back, or rectal, with radiation to the legs. It is present in 65 to 90 per cent of patients with malignant lesions, with a mean duration of 6 to 12 months.[12, 47] Bladder and bowel dysfunction are noted in 15 to 20 per cent of malignancies.[12, 47] Median tumor size is 8 to 9.4 cm, and almost all can be palpated on rectal examination.[12, 47] Primary sacral tumors are fixed in position, while others may be movable.

RADIOGRAPHIC EVALUATION

Plain radiographs of the sacrum, including anteroposterior and lateral views, are often difficult to interpret owing to overlying intestinal gas and the curvature of the sacrum. The lateral view often shows poor bony detail because of the large amount of soft tissue that the x-rays must traverse, the thinness of the sacrum, and the dorsal curvature.[45, 76] Characteristics of each tumor type have been reviewed recently.[11, 45, 70, 76] Barium enema and IVP may help, but these still often underestimate the size of the presacral soft tissue mass.

Computed tomography (CT) is very sensitive in detecting intraosseous neoplasms and the presacral soft tissue masses which often are not evident on plain x-rays.[70] The total extent of each lesion is readily determined using CT scan, but this method is diagnostically nonspecific, and differentiation between primary and secondary tumors of the sacrum generally is not possible from the CT appearance alone (Fig. 38–4). In some specific instances, such as teratomas, CT scan is potentially helpful when plain films may be normal. CT scanning with intravenous

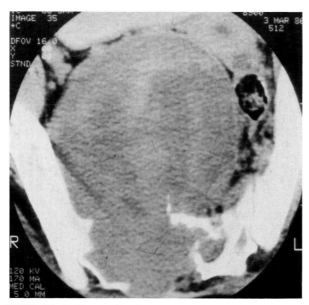

FIGURE 38–4. CT scan showing giant sacral neurofibroma producing expansion of the sacral canal with a huge presacral component almost completely filling the lesser pelvis.

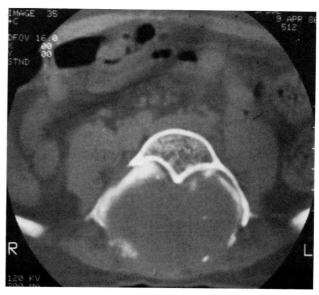

FIGURE 38–6. CT scan of ependymoma, demonstrating expansion of the sacral canal with smooth sclerotic margins of the sacrum surrounding the tumor.

contrast, as well as with oral barium and rectal Renografin, may help delineate the anatomy.[70]

When evaluating patients with primary sacral tumors, CT scan is of limited value in determining the pathology of the lesion. Widening of the sacral canal suggests a neural tumor such as a neurofibroma or ependymoma (Fig. 38–5). The presence of a well-defined sclerotic border implies a benign lesion (Fig. 38–6), whereas an extraosseous soft tissue mass would strongly favor a diagnosis of malignant tumor (Fig. 38–7).[70] As in all patients with sacral lesions, a metrizamide- or iohexol-assisted study will determine the relationship of the thecal sac to the lesion (Fig. 38–8).

CT scan is particularly useful in the postoperative period. After abdominosacral resection, early changes may be suggestive of tumor, although they also may be secondary to surgery.[40] Serial CT scans will be necessary. After radiation treatment, CT scans may show widening of the presacral space, thickening of the perirectal fibrous tissue, and visualization of a fibrotic connection between the sacrum and rectum.[17] Magnetic resonance imaging (MRI) scans are now available and may show a high degree of soft tissue contrast in imaging of musculoskeletal structures.[59, 62] Involvement of gluteal muscles and other soft tissues may elude detection even with contrast-enhanced CT.

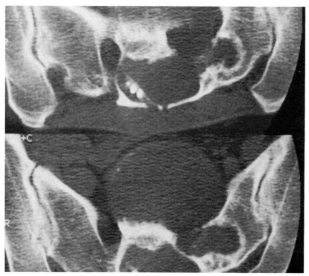

FIGURE 38–5. CT scan showing sacral schwannoma with both sacral and presacral components communicating through an enlarged sacral foramen. Note the widening of the sacral canal.

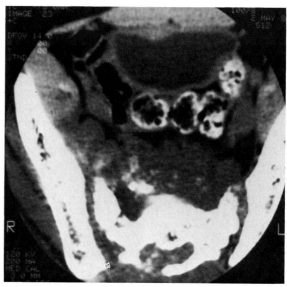

FIGURE 38–7. CT scan of Ewing's sarcoma. Note the mottled irregular erosion of the sacrum indicative of malignant invasion.

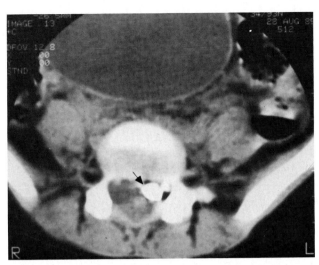

FIGURE 38–8. Metrizamide CT scan showing ventral and lateral displacement of the sacral thecal sac *(arrow)* by extradural neuroblastoma.

SURGICAL APPROACHES

Biopsy is sometimes considered for a radio- or chemosensitive tumor such as neuroblastoma or lymphoma. Thereafter, surgery can be less aggressive. However, transrectal biopsy should not be considered as it may spread disease and necessitate rectal resection.[71]

The transsacral approach has had wide acceptance for many years.[1, 6, 47, 52, 65] It is familiar and offers epidural and intradural exposure with clear demarcation between tumor and neural tissue. There is, however, limited presacral accessibility, and vascular control is not possible except from within the tumor. This approach is ideal for predominantly intraspinal masses with limited or no presacral component. It is, however, inadequate for total excision of most presacral tumors, especially those with high presacral extension. We have used this approach predominantly in staged operations with a transabdominal approach.

CASE 1

A 5½-year-old girl presented with a one-week history of abdominal pain and vomiting. Physical examination revealed a large pelvic mass. Neurologic evaluation, including bowel and bladder function, was within normal limits. A CT scan of the abdomen and pelvis showed a large well-encapsulated mass originating in the pelvis with extension above the pelvic brim into the retroperitoneum. The ventral aspect of the sacrum appeared effaced, but no obvious erosion was identified. Further evaluation was notable for markedly elevated urinary vanillylmandelic acid levels, suggesting the diagnosis of neuroblastoma. A thorough search, including bone scan, liver-spleen scan, and bone marrow biopsy, revealed no evidence of disseminated disease. Celiotomy was performed by the pediatric surgery service, which revealed a large, well-encapsulated tumor in the pelvis and retroperitoneum. Gross total removal of this portion of the tumor was achieved. Near the completion of the resection,

however, an intraspinal extension of the tumor through the S1 foramen was appreciated. No attempt was made to remove the intraspinal portion of the tumor at that time. Postoperatively, the patient did well without complications. Histologic examination of the tumor specimen revealed neuroblastoma.

The patient was transferred to the neurologic service for further evaluation and treatment of the intraspinal tumor. Metrizamide myelography revealed an extradural mass extending up to the level of the L5 vertebra (Fig. 38–9A). A CT scan further delineated the intraspinal mass, which appeared to completely fill the sacral canal (Fig. 38–9B).

The tumor was approached through a lumbosacral laminectomy extending from L5 through S4. A large extradural tumor was encountered on the dorsal aspect of the thecal sac (Fig. 38–9C). Laterally, small extensions of tumor followed the exiting dural sleeves of the L5-S3 roots on both sides (Fig. 38–9D). A gross total removal of all evident tumor was performed, except for a small portion of the tumor which appeared to be invading the right S1 nerve root (Fig. 38–9E).

Postoperatively, the patient did well except for moderate weakness of the right leg, which has improved. She has received chemotherapy and is currently without clinical evidence of recurrence 22 months after the second operation.

Rectal electromyographic continuous monitoring can be used to assess S2 and S3 function during dissection. If S4 and S5 are sacrificed bilaterally and S3 unilaterally, bladder and bowel function will remain normal with only perineal anesthesia. Function will be impaired if S3 is taken bilaterally. This is of less concern if preoperative losses exist. When tumor is predominantly extradural as in Case 1, we have been able to spare the roots with greater frequency. Intradural lesions are often far more difficult.

The transabdominal approach allows mobilization of the rectum anteriorly and the ureters laterally. Control of the internal iliac vessels and the middle sacral vessels is also readily achieved.[47, 58] The access to the presacral space can be quite extensive. This is the preferred approach for large presacral masses with little or no intraspinal extension. It is, however, inadequate for tumors with significant intraspinal components. Tumor/neural differentiation is not easy.

CASE 2

A 39-year-old woman presented with a 6-month history of progressive loss of movement in the left foot, associated with progressive numbness over the buttocks and backs of both legs. She also had recent pain and fullness in the left lower quadrant of the abdomen.

One and one half years previously she had undergone a total hysterectomy and had noticed total loss of vaginal sensation. She also developed increasing low back pain that radiated into both legs.

At age 10, she underwent an extensive lumbar laminectomy for "malignant tumor of the spine," followed by local radiotherapy. She did well, except for weakness and atrophy of the left leg. At age 27 she became

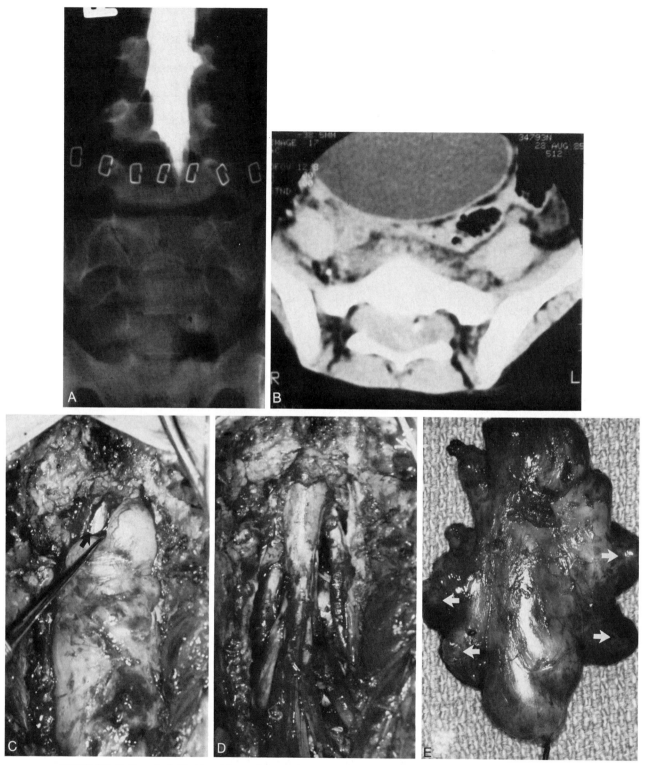

FIGURE 38–9. Case 1. *A*, Metrizamide myelogram demonstrating truncation and displacement of thecal sac by extradural mass. Skin staples from previous celiotomy are also seen. *B*, CT scan of sacrum showing intraspinal mass. *C*, Operative photograph of dorsally placed extradural tumor within the sacral canal. The thecal sac can be seen on the ventral aspect of the tumor *(arrow)*. *D*, Operative photograph of cauda equina following tumor resection. *E*, Photograph of tumor specimen. Note the extensions on either side of the tumor conforming to the foramina of the sacrum *(arrows)*.

pregnant and was delivered by cesarean section because she was "unable to feel labor."

Examination showed atrophy and weakness of the entire left leg. Perineal hypesthesia and hypalgesia were present in the S2-S5 segments. Anal reflexes were absent and rectal tone was markedly reduced.

Myelography demonstrated a large intraspinal mass beginning at L3 and extending caudally into the sacral canal. Sacral expansion and erosion laterally and anteriorly were noted (Fig. 38–10A). A CT scan of the pelvis revealed a large tumor mass extending to the anterior abdominal wall (Fig. 38–10B–D).

Barium enema with air contrast showed no gross filling defects from the cecum to the rectum. The distal sigmoid and rectum were displaced anteriorly. The mucosal pattern was normal. Urodynamic studies showed a severe incomplete lower motor neuron deficit involving the bladder and sphincter. The patient could not elicit voluntary contraction of the bladder, and no voiding was produced during abdominal straining.

A posterior lumbosacral exposure was carried out, demonstrating an enormous tumor filling the entire thecal sac from L3 to the bottom of the sacrum. The consistency was that of a hard rubber ball, and pathology was myxopapillary ependymoma. An aggressive removal was performed, leaving only a small amount of tumor entwined with the right L5 and S1 roots.

Subsequently, a transabdominal approach was performed with removal of the pelvic component of tumor (Fig. 38–10E and F). Excellent exposure of the pelvic tumor was obtained allowing complete removal.

Sparing of pudendal nerves is necessary for S2 and S3 function. In Case 2, however, bladder function was already lost. There is considerable difficulty removing an intraspinal component through this approach and far less safety when dissecting tumor from the nerve roots.

The transperineal approach of Kraske[42] is simple, with minimal morbidity. It can be done in the flexed prone or lithotomy position, with either a vertical or transverse incision. The anococcygeal rephe, gluteal musculature, and sacrospinous/sacrotuberous ligaments are divided, offering access to the retrorectal space. The rectum is mobilized anteriorly, yielding access to small benign tumors and cysts of the low presacral space. While it is possible with this approach to resect tumor and sacrum in continuity, it is difficult to remove large tumors.

The combined abdominosacral approach has many advocates.[1, 12, 47, 58, 71] Some recommend it for all lesions greater than 5 cm in size,[21] especially for presacral benign or malignant teratomas, carcinomas of the rectum, uterus, ovary, bladder, and prostate, and all chordomas. It is appropriate in one stage for radical en bloc resection of localized malignant tumors. It can be staged for benign tumors with intraspinal involvement and a large presacral component. En bloc resections may leave significant neurologic sequelae, especially if the sacral nerve roots are taken bilaterally.

Surgical cures are rare for malignant tumors, however, and aggressive resections for palliation must be tempered by rational expectations of survival and by considerations of surgical morbidity.

DEVELOPMENTAL CYSTS

Common to all developmental cysts occurring in the sacrococcygeal region is an abnormality of embryogenesis responsible for their origin. Each type of cyst is more common in women. Since the majority of patients with developmental cysts are asymptomatic, the lesions are usually discovered on routine gynecologic examination during childbearing years.[8, 39] Because it is usually not possible to distinguish the type of cyst based on the history, clinical findings, or radiographic features, final categorization of the cyst rests on the histologic identification of the epithelial lining and associated structures.

Dermoids are midline cysts that can arise anywhere along the craniospinal axis. About 25 per cent of spinal dermoids are found in the sacrococcygeal region, making them the most common developmental sacrococcygeal cyst.[22] These cysts may be located within the spinal canal or ventral to the sacrum in the presacral space.

Dermoids frequently communicate with the skin via an epithelial-lined dermal sinus tract which predisposes these patients to recurrent infection. The relationship between dermoids and dermal sinus tracts is not constant. While over 50 per cent of patients with dermal sinus tracts harbor dermoid cysts, less than one third of patients with dermoid cysts have demonstrable dermal sinus tracts.[22] Nevertheless, a patient with a history of recurrent low back pain and fever or multiple episodes of meningitis should undergo a thorough search for a midline dermal sinus tract. The association of dermoids and dermal sinus tracts suggests a failure of surface ectoderm cleavage from the developing neural tube as the etiologic cause of dermoid cyst formation.

Dermoids appear grossly as smooth, often lobulated, cysts filled with sebaceous fluid, epithelial debris, and, occasionally, hair. Microscopic examination of the cyst wall reveals a stratified squamous epithelial lining and the presence of dermal appendages, such as sweat glands, hair follicles, and sebaceous glands. The identification of dermal structures is necessary to make the diagnosis of a dermoid cyst, since squamous metaplasia can occur in other types of developmental cysts if subjected to repeated inflammation.[8]

The clinical picture of a patient with a dermoid cyst depends largely on the location of the cyst. Since intraspinal dermoids and presacral dermoids also differ with respect to radiographic features and surgical treatment, they will be discussed separately.

Intraspinal dermoids are occasionally asymptomatic; more commonly, they present before 10 years of age with either cauda equina dysfunction secondary to compression or multiple episodes of meningi-

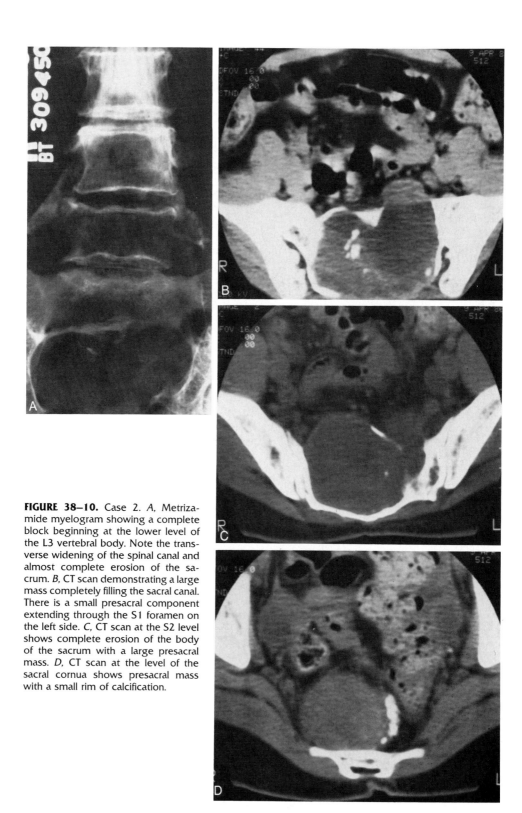

FIGURE 38–10. Case 2. *A,* Metrizamide myelogram showing a complete block beginning at the lower level of the L3 vertebral body. Note the transverse widening of the spinal canal and almost complete erosion of the sacrum. *B,* CT scan demonstrating a large mass completely filling the sacral canal. There is a small presacral component extending through the S1 foramen on the left side. *C,* CT scan at the S2 level shows complete erosion of the body of the sacrum with a large presacral mass. *D,* CT scan at the level of the sacral cornua shows presacral mass with a small rim of calcification.

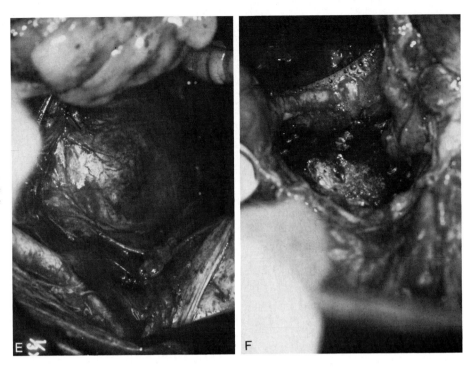

FIGURE 37–10 *Continued. E,* Operative photograph of large well-encapsulated presacral mass. *F,* Operative photograph following resection of the presacral tumor.

tis.[22] In cases in which the dermoid is adherent to the filum terminale, a tethered cord syndrome may be the presenting feature. The identification of a dermal sinus tract suggests the presence of a dermoid cyst; as already noted, however, the absence of a dermal sinus tract does not preclude the existence of a dermoid.

Plain films of the sacrum may be normal, but about two thirds of patients will demonstrate a posterior spina bifida.[22] In addition, if the dermoid is large, plain films may reveal bony erosion of the posterior aspect of the sacral bodies. CT scan has proved to be extremely valuable in identifying intraspinal dermoids. The appearance of a cystic mass with attenuation values often lower than those of water is suggestive of a dermoid cyst. However, intraspinal lipoma, a tumor commonly associated with spina bifida occulta and the tethered cord syndrome, also will demonstrate an attenuation coefficient lower than that of water.

Although CT scan is the imaging procedure of choice for dermoids, myelography is recommended in all patients with intraspinal dermoids for two main reasons. First, because of the ascent of the spinal cord during fetal development, the dermoid cyst may also migrate cranially if attached to neural elements. The location of the dermoid, therefore, may be several vertebral segments higher than the dural sinus opening. In this situation, myelography usually will identify the dermoid, while the CT scan limited to the sacral segments will be negative. The second reason for including myelography in the preoperative evaluation is the association of other types of occult spinal dysraphism that may be located more rostrally in the spinal canal.

The treatment of an intraspinal dermoid is surgical removal. This is accomplished through a posterior laminectomy. If a dermal sinus tract is present, it should be followed to the posterior vertebral elements or ligaments. This will identify the level of the dermoid and define the limits of the laminectomy. The dermoid may be located in the epidural space; more commonly, it is inside the dura, requiring entry into the subarachnoid space. An attempt should be made to remove the dermoid in toto, since spillage of the contents of the cyst may cause a chemical meningitis that can lead to chronic arachnoiditis. If the dermoid is densely adherent to the cauda equina, total removal may not be possible and recurrences may result.

Unlike intraspinal dermoids, dermoids located in the presacral space are usually asymptomatic and are discovered during routine examination. About 40 per cent of patients with presacral dermoids are symptomatic and generally fit into one of three clinical syndromes.[8, 39, 48] They may present with the subacute onset of low back pain and fever secondary to abscess formation or may give a history of recurrent draining sinus with the purulent drainage through a perianal sinus or a fistulous communication with the rectum. Many of these patients have previously undergone multiple surgical procedures for the presumed diagnosis of perirectal abscess. A second group of patients presents with vague complaints of low back pain, pelvic pressure, and constipation. These complaints are often of several years' duration. The third group of patients presents with dystocia.

Examination usually will reveal a smooth cystic mass on the posterior wall of the rectum. Unless the cyst is infected, the mass will be nontender and freely movable. Neurologic function, including bowel and bladder control, is usually normal.

The radiologic evaluation of patients with presacral

dermoids generally consists of plain films of the sacrum, CT scans, and barium enema if there is suspicion of a fistulous communication. Plain films are most often normal, but up to one third of patients will show posterior spina bifida of all or part of the sacral vertebrae. Erosion of the sacrum is uncommon, but if the dermoid is large, bony erosion of the anterior aspect of the sacrum can occur. CT scan will accurately identify the dermoid and its relationship to surrounding structures.

The treatment of patients with presacral dermoids is surgical removal through a perineal approach into the presacral space. Resection of the coccyx and division of the muscles of the pelvic floor as well as the anococcygeal ligament often will be necessary to permit adequate exposure. Even large dermoids located high in the presacral region are indistinguishable from presacral dermoids with respect to clinical and radiographic features. The postanal gut cyst probably takes its origin from persistence of the postanal gut, which has been described previously. Although there is no general agreement on the precise embryologic event responsible for the development of enteric cysts, several theories have been proposed. These explanations include splitting of the entodermal vesicle, persistence of diverticula normally present in the second month of fetal life, and sequestration of gut epithelium.[8]

Identification of the cyst type is determined by microscopic examination. Postanal gut cysts are lined by cuboidal or columnar epithelium and contain mucin-secreting goblet cells. Enteric cysts demonstrate glandular epithelium, as well as one or more layers of smooth muscle in the wall of the cyst. A serosal covering also may be present.[8] The treatment of postanal gut cysts and enteric cysts is through a

low posterior approach into the presacral region, already described for presacral dermoids.

Anterior sacral meningocele is a rare congenital lesion that arises as a result of a unilateral defect in the formation of a variable number of sacral vertebral bodies. The meningocele, lined with dura and arachnoid, herniates into the pelvis through the hemisacral defect (Fig. 38–11A). It is filled with CFS which is in direct communication with the spinal subarachnoid space. Neural elements are occasionally contained within the meningocele, but the majority of patients have a normally formed spinal cord and cauda equina. The frequent association of anterior sacral meningocele with other anomalies, including genitourinary duplications, anorectal malformations, and congenital tumors such as teratomas and dermoids, suggests that the anterior sacral meningocele is part of a generalized dysraphic state involving the caudal portion of the embryo (Fig. 38–11B).[57]

Anterior sacral meningocele is usually diagnosed in women during the second and third decades of life.[57] The female predominance reflects the frequency of gynecologic and obstetric symptoms caused by the meningocele, since the sex incidence is equal when the anterior sacral meningocele is discovered in infancy and childhood. Patients also may present with rectal and urinary complaints secondary to local compression by an enlarging meningocele. In some patients, a history of headache related to coughing or sneezing is elicited.[7] This is presumably caused by raised intrapelvic pressure, which is transmitted through the meningocele to the subarachnoid space, resulting in increased intracranial pressure. There are reports of meningocele rupture into the rectum causing meningitis and death.

The diagnosis of anterior sacral meningocele gen-

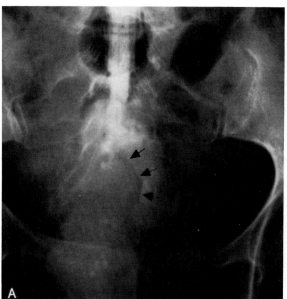
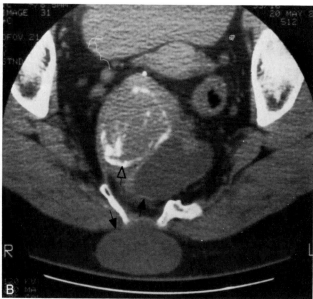

FIGURE 38–11. *A,* Metrizamide myelogram showing ill-defined collection of contrast within a large anterior sacral meningocele in a 48-year-old woman with back pain. Note the classic hemisacral defect known as the scimitar sacrum *(arrows). B,* CT scan shows both dorsal and ventral meningocele sacs *(closed arrows).* Note the calcified mass anterior to the ventral meningocele sac *(open arrow).* This was confirmed at operation to be a benign teratoma.

erally is made by plain films of the sacrum and is confirmed by myelography. Plain films reveal a classic sickle-shaped sacral defect known as a scimitar sacrum (Fig. 38–11*B*). Myelography demonstrates filling of the meningocele with contrast material through the hemisacral defect. CT scan is useful in defining the relationships of the surrounding pelvic structures, as well as in identifying associated anomalies of tumors.

The treatment of anterior sacral meningocele is obliteration of the communication between the spinal subarachnoid space and the meningocele. The surgical approach is through a posterior laminectomy and transdural ligation of the neck of the meningocele. A small dural opening is recommended to inspect the meningocele before ligation is performed. If functional neural tissue is found within the meningocele, plication of the neck of the meningocele should be performed with preservation of the neural elements.[18] Following closure of the neck, the meningocele may be aspirated, but excision is not required since the meningocele does not produce CSF and eventually will collapse.

TERATOMA

Teratoma is the most common primary tumor of the sacrococcygeal region in children.[80] Girls are affected three times as frequently as boys.[2, 16, 49] This tumor usually presents at birth as a large mass protruding from below the coccyx. The cell of origin is not precisely known but generally is believed to be derived from Hensen's node, which is pushed caudally into the region of the coccyx during development of the neural tube.

Teratomas contain elements of all three germ cell layers. The microscopic appearance varies between the "primitive" form, which demonstrates only immature cellular morphology, and the "mature" form, which shows recognizable organ differentiation. The majority of these tumors are cystic, and up to 75 per cent have histologically confirmed calcification.

About 30 per cent of sacrococcygeal teratomas are malignant.[16] Embryonal carcinoma is by far the most common malignancy found in these tumors, but malignant growth can arise from derivatives of all three germ cell layers. About 15 per cent of malignant teratomas have already metastasized to lung, liver, or bone by the time of diagnosis, and all of them exhibit locally invasive growth into pelvic structures.[16] Both of these factors preclude surgical cure. Even when the tumors are contained locally, allowing en bloc resection, the vast majority will recur.

Current treatment of malignant sacrococcygeal teratomas involves aggressive resection, followed by local radiotherapy and combination chemotherapy consisting of vincristine, actinomycin D, and cyclophosphamide. Adriamycin to a total dose of 300 mg/m[2] has been used in some patients. Patients with pulmonary metastases receive, in addition, local radiotherapy to the lung fields.[60] Despite these treatment modalities, the prognosis is extremely poor with very few long-term survivors.

Benign teratomas, on the other hand, have a favorable prognosis. En bloc resection of these tumors, which includes removal of the coccyx, results in a cure in most patients. Failure to remove the coccyx as part of the resection has resulted in a recurrence rate of 31 per cent.[16]

Accurate distinction between benign and malignant teratomas is ultimately determined by microscopic examination. However, clinical information obtained during preoperative evaluation can be helpful in identifying which tumors are malignant. This information often alters treatment strategies. For example, malignant teratomas more frequently arise in the presacral space, whereas most tumors located below the pelvic floor in the region caudal to the coccyx are benign.

The age of the patient at the time of diagnosis is a sensitive predictor of malignancy. In one study,[16] patients with sacrococcygeal teratomas presenting under the age of two months had a 10 per cent incidence of malignancy, while 91 per cent of patients who presented after the age of two months had malignant tumors. Many investigators suggest that the high rate of malignancy in the older age group represents malignant degeneration of a previously benign teratoma. However, in a group of patients presenting with sacrococcygeal teratomas at birth but not operated upon until after four months of age, the malignancy rate was only 30 per cent.[16, 33]

The clinical examination at the time of diagnosis also is helpful in distinguishing benign from malignant teratomas. Most patients with benign teratomas do not present with any functional abnormalities, whereas patients harboring malignant teratomas frequently have bowel/bladder dysfunction as well as evidence of compression of pelvic lymphatics and venous structures.[16]

Sacrococcygeal teratomas can occur in the adult. However, in a review of 60 adult patients with sacrococcygeal teratomas, almost 60 per cent of these patients had either a mass or symptoms referrable to the tumor that could be traced to childhood.[32] In this group of 60 patients, 8 (11 per cent) had histologically proven malignancy.

In the radiologic evaluation of these tumors, CT scan provides accurate preoperative localization and delineation of the extent of the tumor. The majority of benign teratomas are cystic, and about 60 per cent have visible calcification. Despite the often large size of these tumors, there is usually no bone destruction. However, up to 10 per cent will show evidence of sacral anomalies. Intraspinal extension is unusual but can occur in greater than 50 per cent. In cases involving sacral anomalies or suspected intraspinal extension, myelography should be performed.

CHORDOMA

Chordomas are the most frequent primary tumor arising in the sacrococcygeal region in the adult.

Although chordomas have been described in patients ranging from 3 months to 89 years of age, they are essentially a phenomenon of adult life, with over 50 per cent occurring between the ages of 50 and 70 years.[28] After the age of 40, men are affected twice as frequently as women; this male predominance is absent in patients younger than 40 years who have chordomas.[28]

Chordomas are considered congenital in origin because their microscopic appearance of vacuolated, "physaliferous" cells is similar to that seen in the notochordal remnants known to occur in the sacro-coccygeal region. The observation that chordomas arise primarily within the substance of bone, and not outside the sacrum where notochordal cell rests occur, casts doubt on the relationship of these cells to the future development of chordomas. It has been suggested that, in addition to extraosseous notochordal remnants, there may be trapping of notochordal cells during cartilage formation of the sacrococcygeal vertebrae, resulting in intraosseous cell rests capable of neoplastic transformation in adult life.[78]

The most common initial symptom in patients with sacrococcygeal chordomas is pain. The pain is usually localized in the lower back, but a sciatic distribution of pain also may be present in up to 30 per cent of patients.[28] Complaints of constipation usually follow the onset of pain after a variable amount of time. This probably occurs as a result of rectal compression from an increasing presacral mass. Later, these patients inevitably exhibit evidence of sacral plexus involvement with bowel/bladder dysfunction and lower extremity paresis.

The mean duration of symptoms before diagnosis ranges from one to three years. This finding takes on additional significance when one considers the slow rate of chordoma growth and the unresectability of these tumors by the time of diagnosis. Despite the fact that most chordomas can be appreciated by rectal examination, many patients carry the diagnosis of chronic low back pain for months to years before the correct diagnosis is made. Theoretically, this delay in diagnosis reduces the possibility of effecting surgical cure.

The radiologic evaluation of these patients consists primarily of CT scan. Although plain films of the sacrum will identify erosion and enlargement in the anteroposterior diameter of the sacrum in 85 per cent of patients, CT scan is more sensitive and allows for accurate localization of the presacral soft tissue mass.[45, 70] The usual CT scan shows a mixed lytic and sclerotic picture.[45] Between 50 and 60 per cent of chordomas also show calcification on CT scan. Recent MRI evaluation of chordomas demonstrates these tumors to be relatively homogeneous in appearance, with long T1 and T2 relaxation times.[62] The main advantage of MRI over CT scan is better contrast between the tumor and the surrounding soft tissue structures.

Since chordomas may extend intraspinally, a myelogram should be considered in all patients, especially in those with suspected cauda equina involvement.

Electrodiagnostic studies consisting of nerve conduction velocity (NCV) and electromyogram (EMG) are often useful in differentiating plexus from cauda equina dysfunction. Angiography, though not usually necessary in the preoperative evaluation, most often shows an avascular mass with displacement and occasionally encasement of iliac and sacral vessels.[73] Bone scan demonstrates either reduced uptake or normal distribution of the isotope at the midline site.[64] Therefore, a midline sacral tumor that is cold on bone scan is very likely to be a chordoma.

The treatment of sacrococcygeal chordomas is primarily surgical. Radiotherapy has met with only anecdotal success, and chemotherapy has been proven to be of no value. Despite aggressive resection, the overall prognosis is poor, with eventual recurrence and death usually less than six years after the diagnosis of chordoma.[14, 28] It is advisable to resect as much of the sacrum, coccyx, and surrounding structures as possible without producing major disability. The limiting factor, in large part, is the second sacral vertebra, since its removal may lead to loss of sacral stability as well as permanent and severe neurologic damage.

Most patients cannot be cured surgically because their tumors already involve the S2 vertebra by the time of presentation. These patients are best treated by a combination of aggressive surgery followed by radiation in the hope of significant palliation. About 10 to 40 per cent of sacrococcygeal chordomas will metastasize, most frequently to lung, liver, muscle, bone, and skin.[10, 28, 74] A search for metastatic deposits should be undertaken before proceeding with a radical and often debilitating resection.

Recently, there have been reports of more aggressive resections of these tumors.[12, 36, 47, 71] The concern over sacral stability, as well as the proximity of the sacral nerve roots and plexus, has been reevaluated in light of the natural history of these tumors. Stener[71] reported on five patients with chordomas on whom he performed high sacral amputations. In one case, the amputation extended above the S1 foramen. He found no incidence of functional sacral instability and no evidence of tumor recurrence, although the mean follow-up in these patients was only about four years. Bowel, bladder, and sexual function were sacrificed in all patients, although he reported that these deficits were well tolerated. A longer follow-up will be required to better evaluate the efficacy of this radical approach.

INFLAMMATORY LESIONS

The presacral space can be the site of abscess formation resulting from the contiguous spread of inflammatory processes affecting the lower bowel. The cause may be local, as in diverticular or anal crypt infections, or the abscess may occur as a complication of more systemic inflammatory diseases, such as ulcerative colitis or Crohn's disease. Penetrating trauma to the rectum or anus is also recognized as a cause of presacral abscess formation. The spread of infection from the presacral space is confined superiorly by the peritoneal reflection, posteriorly by the sacrum, and inferiorly by the muscular floor of the pelvis. The result is formation of an abscess that may be walled off and act as a mass lesion with compression of the rectum. Alternatively, the abscess may be decompressed periodically through a fistulous communication with the rectum or perianal skin.

Patients presenting with presacral abscess generally complain of low back pain and pressure in the rectum and pelvis. The pain occasionally radiates into the buttocks and legs, but neurologic deficits do not occur. There may be a history of purulent drainage if a fistula is present. Rectal examination will usually reveal a tender mass compressing the posterior wall of the rectum.

Plain films of the sacrum are normal, although there may be evidence of a soft tissue mass in the presacral space. CT scan will identify the abscess in most cases. There may be poor definition of pelvic structures, reflecting an ongoing inflammatory process. Barium enema will demonstrate anterior displacement of the rectum. If a rectal fistula is present, a barium enema may reveal its location.

The treatment of presacral abscess consists of providing adequate drainage. This can be performed through either a transrectal or a perianal approach. Distinguishing a presacral abscess from a secondarily infected developmental cyst is important because drainage alone is inadequate treatment for an infected cyst. In patients with recurrent abscess formation despite multiple drainage procedures, the presence of a developmental cyst should be suspected. In these patients, excision of the cyst is the appropriate treatment.

NEUROGENIC TUMORS

Ependymoma

Ependymomas account for 10 to 15 per cent of spinal cord tumors.[68] The majority occur in the region of the conus medullaris and cauda equina. Spinal ependymomas are more common in men, with the peak incidence occurring during the fourth decade of life.

Spinal cord ependymomas are believed to arise from ependymal cells which line the central canal of the spinal cord. The filum terminale, which represents the vestigium of the caudal neural tube present during early embryologic development, also contains ependymal cells that are believed to be the cell of origin of ependymomas arising at the level of the cauda equina. Ependymomas of the filum terminale are unique in that, unlike their intracranial counterparts, the majority are either papillary or myxopapillary in appearance.[66] The myxopapillary form is only found in ependymomas of the filum terminale. In general, these forms are more benign and, in terms of prognosis, are similar to grades I and II of cellular ependymomas found intracranially.

Tumors arising from the sacral portion of the filum terminale cause expansion of the sacral canal and thinning of its bony margins. These lesions may result in erosion of the anterior sacral cortex and present as soft tissue masses in the presacral area (Fig. 38–10B–D). Rarely, an ependymoma may originate in the presacral soft tissue from heterotopic ependymal tissue.[23]

Pain is the most frequent initial symptom in patients with ependymomas of the filum terminale. The pain either is localized in the lower back or is present in a sciatic distribution.[56] Weakness, sphincter disturbances, or sensory complaints are rarely initial symptoms, although the majority of patients will exhibit some form of a cauda equina syndrome by the time of diagnosis.[20, 56] The duration of symptoms before diagnosis averages between two and three years, which reflects the slow growth rate of these tumors.

Myelography is the most useful preoperative study in patients with ependymomas of the filum terminale. The appearance of an extradural, frequently loculated, filling defect is the characteristic finding. MRI and CT scans are helpful in identifying the caudal extent of the tumor, especially if there is a total block present on myelography.

The treatment of ependymomas of the filum terminale is primarily surgical removal. Intraoperative sensory evoked potentials are frequently useful, since dissection of the tumor from the roots of the cauda equina may be difficult. Improved microsurgical techniques have resulted in complete removal in 50 to 80 per cent of these tumors, according to recent reports.[3, 69] Radiotherapy should be given in cases of known subtotal removal, since it has been shown to lengthen the disease-free interval before recurrence.[79]

Schwannoma and Neurofibroma

Schwannomas and neurofibromas together constitute about 25 per cent of spinal cord tumors.[55] Men and women are affected equally, and the peak incidence occurs during the fourth and fifth decades of life. These tumors are fairly evenly distributed throughout the most frequent site of occurrence. About 20 per cent of spinal schwannomas and neurofibromas arise from the cauda equina.

There is controversy over the cell of origin of schwannomas and neurofibromas. This is reflected in confusion in the literature regarding the distinction between the two tumors. Many authors use the labels schwannoma and neurofibroma interchangeably, while use of synonymous terms such as neuroma, neurinoma, and neurilemmoma have added to the lack of clarity.

Schwannomas are generally believed to arise from Schwann cells, which form the myelin of peripheral nerves, whereas the perineural cell, found in the perineurium of peripheral nerves, is thought to be the originating cell of neurofibromas. Both the Schwann cell and the perineural cell are histologically similar and may, in fact, represent the same cell.[67] However, there are morphologic differences between schwannomas and neurofibromas, demonstrable on both light and electron microscopy, which appear to justify a distinction between the two tumor types. It is understandable that schwannomas and neurofibromas are often grouped together, since it usually is not possible to distinguish between the two based on clinical or radiographic features, and the treatment for both tumors is the same.

When they occur in multiples, schwannomas and neurofibromas are usually associated with von Recklinghausen's neurofibromatosis.[67] Solitary neurofibromas are also frequently an expression of neurofibromatosis, while this is not true for solitary schwannomas. Malignant transformation of these tumors is rare and usually occurs only in patients with neurofibromatosis.

Intraspinal schwannomas and neurofibromas usually arise from a posterior nerve root, and the majority are entirely intradural. About 30 per cent, however, either are totally extradural or are dumbbell-shaped with both intradural and extradural components.[55] It is the extradural component that may extend through the intervertebral foramen into an extraspinal location, where it frequently grows to a large size before diagnosis (Figs. 38–4, 38–5, and 38–12). The most common initial complaint in patients with schwannomas and neurofibromas arising from the sacral portion of the cauda equina is pain.[1, 20] The pain is initially localized in the lower back but frequently evolves to include a radicular component, suggesting the nerve root origin of the tumor. There is often a dysesthetic quality to the pain, and objective sensory deficits in the sacral dermatomes are common. The Achilles deep tendon reflexes may be absent, but motor weakness and bowel/bladder dysfunction are unusual.

The duration of symptoms before diagnosis is variable, usually in the range of several years.[1, 20] This is probably due to the fact that the sacral dural sac is capacious, containing only the filum terminale and the cauda equina. Compression of the spinal cord, which has ended several vertebral segments higher, does not occur. This allows the tumor to grow to a large size before the appearance of objective neurologic complaints. In one series of 13 giant sacral schwannomas,[1] 11 of 13 patients had a rectal mass noted on palpation.

Plain films, CT scans, and myelography are the most useful diagnostic studies in the preoperative evaluation of these patients. Plain films of the sacrum usually reveal expansion of the sacral canal with erosion of the posterior aspect of the sacral bodies. There may be enlargement of a sacral foramen through which the tumor has grown into the presacral space. If there is a large presacral component, an irregular area of bone erosion with smooth sclerotic margins may be seen on the anterior aspect of the sacrum.

CT scans will define both the intraspinal and presacral tumor mass. These tumors usually appear isodense with respect to surrounding soft tissue structures and exhibit variable, but usually homogeneous, enhancement with intravenous contrast agents (Fig. 38–12). Myelographic examination is necessary to define the extent of the intradural portion of the tumor. If the tumor is located below the termination of the dural sac, myelography may be normal. In some cases, cephalad extension of tumor in the epidural space may produce truncation of the lower portion of the dural sac.

CASE 3

A 35-year-old woman presented with a 12-year history of low back pain with radiation down the left leg. Sacral palpation often caused similar radiating pain. A pregnancy was carried successfully 12 years before, but intense back and pelvic pain developed and delivery was by cesarean section. Menses became irregular and painful. During a routine pelvic examination a large pelvic presacral lesion was discovered. Ultrasound and CT scan confirmed the lesion (Fig. 38–12).

Examination showed mild thoracic scoliosis but was otherwise normal except for mild hyperesthesia over the left lateral upper thigh. Myelography showed the dural sac cut off at the L5 level and deviated to the right. An intrasacral mass filled the left side and the entire sacral region. A laminectomy of S1 through S3 was performed with a gross total removal of an intrasacral schwannoma. It exited the canal via a left midsacral foramen into the presacral space. The CSF space was not entered. A transabdominal pelvic approach is planned as a second stage to complete the removal.

The surgical approach to sacral schwannomas and neurofibromas is dependent on the size and location of the presacral component of the tumor, as well as on the degree of intraspinal involvement. Tumors that occupy the presacral space and are entirely extradural, with little or no intraspinal component, should be removed through an anterior transabdominal approach. This approach affords excellent exposure of the presacral space, allowing identification and isolation of the tumor's vascular supply, which usually comes from both medial and lateral sacral

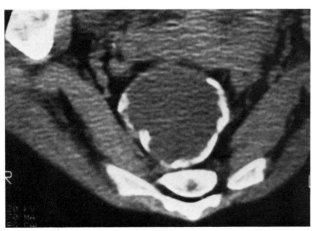

FIGURE 38–12. CT scan showing presacral schwannoma. Note rim of calcification. Same patient as in Figure 38–5.

vessels as well as from the hypogastric plexus. A diffuse venous complex may encompass the mass and drain into the iliac veins.

For intraspinal tumors, both intradural and extradural, the posterior transsacral approach is the procedure of choice. In addition to allowing intradural and extradural access, this approach provides direct visualization of the relationship between sacral nerve roots and the tumor. In cases in which a small presacral extension of the tumor is present, limited access to the space can be obtained by transforaminal resection of the sacrum up to the S2 foramen, removal of the coccyx, and division of the anococcygeal muscles from the coccyx. A large presacral component, especially if located high in the presacral space, generally is not amenable to removal through this approach. Preoperative needle biopsy is not recommended.

Unfortunately, most sacral schwannomas and neurofibromas have both intraspinal involvement and a large presacral component. In these patients, a combination of both approaches, either staged or performed under the same general anesthetic, usually will be necessary to completely remove the tumor. We prefer a staged approach, first removing the intraspinal component through a posterior transsacral approach and following in a few weeks with a transabdominal removal of the remaining tumor. We believe that the risks of CSF leak, meningitis, and sacral nerve root injury are reduced by first removing the intraspinal portion of the tumor. Hemostasis has not been a problem when first approaching the tumor through the transsacral route.

GANGLIONEUROMAS

Ganglioneuromas are slow-growing tumors presumed to arise from mature sympathetic ganglion cells. They probably represent the benign counterpart of malignant neuroblastomas.[26] Ganglioneuromas occur most frequently during adolescence and early adulthood. Like neuroblastomas, the majority of ganglioneuromas occur in the abdomen, where they usually arise from the adrenal gland. A small percentage occur in the pelvis, probably originating in the sacral extension of the sympathetic chain. Because ganglioneuromas are slow-growing tumors, they frequently attain a large size in the pelvis before producing symptoms. They may grow through a sacral foramen into the epidural space and produce signs of sacral nerve root compression. The treatment of these tumors is surgical removal. Since ganglioneuromas are usually benign encapsulated tumors, complete extirpation is generally possible. For dumbbell-shaped tumors with intraspinal extension, this is best achieved through the staged posterior and anterior approach already described.

NEUROBLASTOMA

Neuroblastomas may present during early childhood as presacral masses. About 10 per cent of pelvic neuroblastomas will extend through the sacral foramen into the epidural space, producing dumbbell-shaped tumors.[41] In these patients, signs of bladder/bowel dysfunction and lower extremity weakness may result. Plain films may show enlargment of the sacral foramen, but CT scans and myelography are necessary to define the extent of intraspinal involvement (see Fig. 38–9*A* and *B*).

Treatment of patients with neuroblastoma requires removal of the intraspinal portion of the tumor through a posterior approach, followed by transabdominal resection of the presacral component. The biologic aspects of neuroblastoma as they relate to treatment and prognosis will be fully discussed in Chapter 39 (Case 1).

OSSEOUS TUMORS

Primary bone tumors are generally phenomena of long bones, with less than 10 per cent occurring in the vertebral skeleton.[46] An exception is the benign osteoblastoma, which has a 35 per cent incidence of vertebral involvement.[38] As is the case with bone lesions in other locations, tumors arising from the osseous matrix of the sacrum usually occur during childhood and early adult years. Males and females are affected with about equal frequency, although individual tumor types do show an uneven sex distribution.

Primary bone tumors occurring in older age groups often are associated with Paget's disease. There is a 10 to 15 per cent incidence of malignant bone tumors in patients with extensive and long-standing Paget's disease, but bone tumors also may occur in patients with monostotic involvement. Osteogenic sarcoma is by far the most common tumor complicating Paget's disease, but giant cell tumor and fibrosarcoma also have been reported.[46]

The most common presenting symptom in patients with primary bone tumors of the sacrum is pain. The pain usually is localized in the sacrum and often is worse at night. The duration of symptoms before diagnosis is characteristically short, ranging from several weeks to a few months. In some patients with benign tumors, however, the history may date back as far as a year or longer. In patients harboring malignant tumors, signs of sacral nerve or plexus involvement often will appear shortly after the onset of pain. Osteogenic sarcoma, giant cell tumor, and Ewing's sarcoma frequently extend into the presacral space as a soft tissue mass that can be appreciated on rectal examination.

Plain films and CT scans of the sacrum usually provide adequate preoperative localization of sacral bone tumors. Myelography is reserved for those patients with evidence of intraspinal extension. A chest x-ray should be included in the preoperative work-up, since osteogenic sarcoma and Ewing's sarcoma frequently have metastasized to the lung by the time of diagnosis.[46]

The information obtained during radiographic evaluation is often helpful in predicting the tumor type. Certain features, such as location of the tumor in the sacrum, pattern of bone erosion, and presence of new bone formation within the tumor, may suggest the tumor histology. However, there is enough variability and overlap of these features to usually preclude specific tumor identification based solely on radiographic studies. The role of surgery in the treatment of primary bone tumors is dependent on the histology of the tumor. Osteoid osteoma and osteoblastoma are benign tumors that can be managed successfully with surgery alone. Adequate curettage of these lesions usually results in resolution of pain and a very low incidence of recurrence.[38] Osteogenic sarcoma and Ewing's sarcoma are histologically malignant tumors that exhibit locally invasive growth. Furthermore, the majority of these tumors have already metastasized to the lung by the time of diagnosis.

The surgical management of these tumors consists of careful subtotal resection for decompression and obtaining adequate tissue for diagnosis. Surgery should be followed by chemotherapy and local radiotherapy. Improvement in the long-term survival of these patients over the past 10 years has resulted from advances in chemotherapy, as well as from aggressive surgical resection of metastatic pulmonary deposits.[46]

The treatment of giant cell tumors remains controversial.[15, 19, 43] Despite the fact that this tumor is histologically benign, recurrence rates approaching 60 per cent occur in patients treated with curettage alone.[19, 46] Significant morbidity and mortality result from these recurrences. Local radiotherapy, sometimes to a dose of 10,000 cGy, reduced the recurrence rate, but was complicated by the later development of sarcomatous tumors in about 20 per cent of patients.[46] Improved surgical techniques and the introduction of liquid nitrogen cryotherapy have dramatically improved the prognosis of patients with giant cell tumors. When combined with localized radiotherapy in doses limited to 3500 cGy, recurrence rates of less than 10 per cent are now being reported.[19, 50]

METASTATIC TUMORS

The vertebral skeleton is commonly the site of metastatic disease, ranking behind only the lung and liver in incidence of metastatic involvement.[5] Primary tumors arising in lung, breast, prostate, and kidney, as well as lymphomas, are the most frequently reported neoplasms that metastasize to the spine. Most vertebral bodies, suggesting both hematogenous spread from distant sites and an appropriate metabolic environment within the marrow, are capable of supporting metastatic tumor growth.

In addition to hematogenous metastases originating from distant neoplasms, the sacrum is frequently involved by local spread from tumors arising in pelvic viscera. The sacrum may be invaded by contiguous spread of tumor growth, as in the case of recurrent rectal carcinoma, or it may be involved by localized spread of genitourinary neoplasms via lymphatics or possibly through connection in pelvic venous plexuses first described by Batson.[4]

Unlike the centrally located metastatic deposits resulting from hematogenous spread, secondary involvement of the sacrum by pelvic neoplasms usually seed the cortical surface through external compression. In some cases, the periosteum provides an effective barrier to advancing tumor growth, while in others there is frank invasion of the sacrum by neoplastic cells.

In patients with a known neoplasm, pain in the sacral region should be assumed secondary to metastatic involvement until proven otherwise. The pain is often severe and poorly controlled by analgesics. Plain films and CT scans will usually confirm the diagnosis. The presence of an irregular lytic or blastic lesion, which may be multiple, is the usual appearance on radiographic studies.[45] The metastasis may extend into the presacral space or break through the posterior cortex of the sacrum into the spinal canal.

Metastatic involvement of the sacrum usually signifies advanced disease. In most cases, the appearance of sacral metastases occurs many months to several years after the diagnosis and initial treatment of a known primary neoplasm. The goal of treatment in these patients is palliation. This generally is accomplished by local radiotherapy to the pelvis or, in cases of breast or prostatic metastatic disease, by hormonal manipulation. In rare cases, surgical decompression of neural or pelvic structures may be indicated. Although these modalities are usually effective in ameliorating pain, the overall prognosis is poor, with most patients dying from the disease within two years of the diagnosis of metastatic lesion.

MISCELLANEOUS TUMORS

Most of the tumors in this group arise from mesenchymal derivatives either contained within the nonosteoid-forming matrix of the sacrum or arising from the supporting connective tissue and muscle of the pelvis. There are generally no unifying clinical or radiographic features that serve to separate these tumors from the more commonly encountered neoplasms in this region. An exception is soft tissue sarcomas, which usually appear in patients who have had radiotherapy to the pelvis several years earlier. The treatment and prognosis of tumors in this group vary, depending on the histologic type of the lesion.

REFERENCES

1. Abernathy CD, Onofrio BM, Scheithauer B, et al: Surgical management of giant sacral schwannomas. J Neurosurg 65:286–295, 1986.
2. Altman RP, Randolph JG, Lilly JR: Sacrococcygeal teratoma: American Academy of Pediatric Surgical Section Survey—1973. J Pediatr Surg 9:389–398, 1974.
3. Barone BM, Elvidge AR: Ependymomas: A clinical survey. J Neurosurg 33:428–438, 1970.

4. Batson OV: The function of the vertebral veins and their role in the spread of metastases. Ann Surg 112:132–148, 1940.

5. Boland DJ, Lane JM, Sundaresan N: Metastatic disease of the spine. Clin Orthop 169:95–102, 1982.

6. Brindley GV: Sacral and presacral tumors. Ann Surg 121:721–734, 1945.

7. Brown MH, Powell LD: Anterior sacral meningocoele. J Neurosurg 2:535–538, 1945.

8. Campbell WL, Wolfe M: Retrorectal cysts of developmental origin. Am J Roentgenol 117:307–313, 1973.

9. Castro AF: Presacral tumors. South Med J 54:969–977, 1960.

10. Chambers PW, Schwinn CP: Chordoma: A clinicopathologic study of metastasis. Am J Clin Pathol 72:765–776, 1979.

11. Ciapetta P, Di Lorenzo N, Delfini R: CT evaluation of sacral tumors with neural involvement. J Neurosurg Sci 25:89–94, 1981.

12. Cody HS, Marcove RC, Quan SH: Malignant retrorectal tumors. Dis Colon Rectum 24:501–506, 1981.

13. Crispin AR, Fry IK: The presacral space shown by barium enema. Br J Radiol 36:319–322, 1963.

14. Dahlin DC, McCarty CS: Chordoma: A study of 59 cases. Cancer 5:1170–1178, 1952.

15. Di Lorenzo N, Spallone A, Nolletti A, et al: Giant cell tumors of the spine: A clinical study of six cases, with emphasis on the radiological features, treatment, and follow up. Neurosurgery 6:29–34, 1980.

16. Donnelan WA, Swenson O: Benign and malignant sacrococcygeal teratomas. Surgery 64:834–846, 1968.

17. Doubleday LC, Bernardino ME: CT findings in the perirectal area following radiation therapy. J Comput Assist Tomogr 4:634–638, 1980.

18. Dyck P, Wilson CB: Anterior sacral meningocoele. J Neurosurg 53:548–552, 1980.

19. Eckardt JJ, Grogan TJ: Giant cell tumor of bone. Clin Orthop 204:45–58, 1986.

20. Fearnside MR, Adams CBT: Tumors of the cauda equina. Neurosurg Psych 41:24–31, 1978.

21. Freier DT, Stanley JC: Retrorectal tumors in adults. Surg Gynecol Obstet 132:681–686, 1971.

22. French BN: Midline fusion defects and defects of formation. In Youmans JR (ed): Neurological Surgery. Vol 3. Philadelphia, WB Saunders, 1982, pp 1236–1380.

23. Gerston KF, Suprun H, Cohen H, et al: Presacral myxopapillary ependymoma presenting as an abdominal mass in a child. J Pediatr Surg 20:276–278, 1985.

24. Giles RG: Vertebral anomalies. Radiology 17:1262–1266, 1931.

25. Gius JA, Stout AP: Perianal cysts of vestigial origin. Arch Surg 37:268–287, 1938.

26. Glennen GG, Grimley PM: Tumors of the extra-adrenal paraganglion system. In Tumors of the Peripheral Nervous System. Washington, DC, Armed Forces Institute of Pathology, 1974.

27. Golding FC: Discussion of the significance of congenital abnormalities of the lumbosacral region. Proc R Soc Med 43:636–638, 1950.

28. Gray SG, Singhabhandhu B, Smith RA: Sacrococcygeal chordoma: Report of a case and review of the literature. Surgery 78:573–582, 1975.

29. Gunterberg B, Kewenter J, Petersen I, et al: Anorectal function after major resections of the sacrum with bilateral or unilateral sacrifice of sacral nerves. Br J Surg 63:546–554, 1976.

30. Gunterberg B, Norlen L, Stener B, et al: Neurourologic evaluation after resection of the sacrum. Invest Urol 13:183–188, 1975.

31. Gunterberg B, Romanus B, Stener B: Pelvic strength after major amputation of the sacrum. Acta Orthop Scand 47:635–642, 1976.

32. Head HD, Gerstein JD, Muir RW: Presacral teratoma in the adult. Am Surg 41:240–248, 1975.

33. Hickey RC, Layton JM: Sacrococcygeal teratoma: Emphasis on the biological history and early therapy. Cancer 7:1031–1043, 1954.

34. Hollinshead WH: Textbook of Anatomy. 3rd Ed. Hagerstown, MD, Harper and Row, 1974.

35. Horowitz T: Chordal ectopia and its possible relation to chordoma. Arch Pathol 31:354–362, 1941.

36. Huth JF, Dawson EG, Elber FR: Abdominosacral resection for malignant tumors of the sacrum. Am J Surg 148:157–161, 1984.

37. Jackman RJ, Clark PL: Retrorectal tumors. JAMA 145:956–962, 1951.

38. Jackson RP, Reckiling FW, Mantz FA: Osteoid osteoma and osteoblastoma. Clin Orthop 128:303–313, 1977.

39. Johnson WR: Postrectal neoplasms and cysts. Aust NZ J Surg 50:163–166, 1980.

40. Kelvin FM, Korobkin M, Heaston DK, et al: The pelvis after surgery for rectal carcinoma: Serial CT observations with emphasis on nonneoplastic features. AJR 141:959–964, 1983.

41. King D, Goodman J, Hawk T, et al: Dumbbell neuroblastoma in children. Arch Surg 110:888–891, 1975.

42. Kraske P: Zur exstirpation hochsitzender mastarmkrebse. Arch Klin Chir 33:563–569, 1886.

43. Larsson SE, Lorentzon R, Boquist L: Giant cell tumor of the spine and sacrum causing neurological symptoms. Clin Orthop 111:201–211, 1975.

44. Lemire RJ: Variation in the development of the caudal neural in human embryos. Teratology 2:361–370, 1969.

45. Levine E, Batnitzky S: Computed tomography of sacral and perisacral lesions. CRC Crit Rev Diag Imaging 21:307–373, 1984.

46. Lichtenstein L: Bone Tumors. 4th ed. St. Louis, CV Mosby Co, 1972.

47. Localio SA, Eng K, Ranson JHC: Abdominosacral approach for retrorectal tumors. Ann Surg 191:555–560, 1980.

48. Lovelady SB, Dockerty MB: Extragenital pelvic tumors in women. Am J Obstet Gynecol 58:215–236, 1949.

49. Mahour GH, Wolley MM, Trivedi SN, et al: Teratomas in infancy and childhood: Experience with 81 cases. Surgery 76:309–318, 1974.

50. Marcove RC, Weis LD, Vaghaiwalla MR, et al: Cryosurgery in the treatment of giant cell tumors of bone: A report of 52 consecutive cases. Clin Orthop 134:275–289, 1978.

51. Mayo CW, Baker GS, Smith LR: Presacral tumors: Differential diagnosis and report of case. Proc Staff Meet Mayo Clinic 28:616–622, 1953.

52. McCarty CS, Waugh JM, Mayo CW, et al: The surgical treatment of presacral tumors: A combined problem. Proc Staff Meet Mayo Clinic 27:73–84, 1952.

53. McGuire EJ: The innervation and function of the lower urinary tract. J Neurosurg 65:278–285, 1986.

54. Middeldorpf K: Zur kinntnis der angebornen sacralgeschwulste. Virchows Arch A 101:37–44, 1885.

55. Nittner K: Spinal meningiomas, neurinomas, and neurofibromas and hourglass tumors. In Vinken PJ, Bruyn BW (eds): Handbook of Clinical Neurology. Vol 20. Amsterdam, North Holland Publishing Co, 1976, pp 177–322.

56. Norstrom CW, Kernohan JW, Love JG: One hundred primary caudal tumors. JAMA 178:93–99, 1961.

57. Oren M, Lorber B, Lee SH, et al: Anterior sacral meningocoele. Dis Colon Rectum 20:492–504, 1977.

58. Pack GT: A plea for the synchronous combined abdominoperineal surgical approach for certain pelvic tumors. Surgery 57:613–614, 1965.

59. Pettersson H, Hudson T, Hamlin D, et al: Magnetic resonance imaging of sacrococcygeal tumors. Acta Radiol Diagn 26:161–165, 1985.

60. Raney RB, Chatten J, Littman P, et al: Treatment strategies for infants with malignant sacrococcygeal teratomas. J Pediatr Surg 16:573–577, 1981.

61. Rockswold GL, Chou SN: Urological problems associated with central nervous system disease. In Youmans JR (ed): Neurological Surgery. Vol 2. Philadelphia, WB Saunders, 1982, pp 1031–1050.

62. Rosenthal DI, Scott JA, Mankin HJ, et al: Sacrococcygeal chordoma: Magnetic resonance imaging and computed tomography. AJR 145:143–147, 1985.

63. Ross ST: Sacral and presacral tumors. Am J Surg 76:687–693, 1948.

64. Rossleigh MA, Smith J, Yeh SDH: Scintigraphic features of primary sacral tumors. J Nucl Med 27:627–630, 1986.

65. Rowe RJ, Brock DT: The surgical management of presacral tumors. Am J Surg 92:710–726, 1956.

66. Russell DS, Rubinstein LJ: Pathology of Tumors of the Nervous System. 4th ed. Baltimore, Williams and Wilkins, 1977, pp 213–216.

67. Russell DS, Rubinstein LJ: Pathology of Tumors of the Nervous System. 4th ed. Baltimore, Williams and Wilkins, 1977, pp 372–396.

68. Sloof JL, Kernohan JW, McCarty CS: Primary Intramedullary Tumors of the Spinal Cord and Filum Terminale. Philadelphia, WB Saunders, 1982.

69. Sonneland PRL, Scheithauer BW, Onofrio BM: Myxopapillary ependymoma: A clinicopathologic and immunocytochemical study of 77 cases. Cancer 56:883–893, 1985.

70. Soye I, Levine E, Batnitzky S, et al: Computed tomography of sacral and presacral lesions. Neuroradiology 24:71–76, 1982.

71. Stener B, Gunterberg B: High amputation of the sacrum for extirpation of tumors. Spine 3:351–366, 1978.

72. Streeter GL: Factors involved in the formation of the filum terminale. Am J Anat 25:1–12, 1919.

73. Sundaresan N: Chordomas. Clin Orthop 204:135–142, 1986.

74. Sundaresan N, Galicich JH, Chu FCH, et al: Spinal chordomas. J Neurosurg 50:312–319, 1979.

75. Tuchmann-Duplessis H, Auroux H, Haegal P: Illustrated Human Embryology. Vol 3. New York, Springer-Verlag, 1975.

76. Turner ML, Mulhern CB, Dalinka MK: Lesions of the sacrum: Differential diagnosis and radiological evaluation. JAMA 245:275–277, 1981.

77. Uhlig BE, Johnson RL: Presacral tumors and cysts in adults. Dis Colon Rectum 18:581–596, 1975.

78. Ulich TR, Mirra JM: Ecchorosis physaliphora vertebralis. Clin Orthop 163:282–289, 1982.

79. Wara WM, Sheline: Radiation therapy of tumors of the spinal cord. In Youmans JR (ed): Neurological Surgery. Vol 5. Philadelphia, WB Saunders, 1982, pp 3222–3226.

80. Werner JL, Taybi H: Presacral masses in childhood. Am J Roentgenol 109:403–409, 1970.

81. Whitaker LD, Pemberton JD: Tumors ventral to the sacrum. Ann Surg 107:96–106, 1938.

82. Willis RA: Pathology of Tumors. 4th ed. London, Butterworths, 1967, p 937.

83. Willis TA: An analysis of vertebral anomalies. Am J Surg 6:163–168, 1929.

TECHNIQUE OF HIGH SACRAL AMPUTATION

BERTIL STENER

INTRODUCTION AND ANATOMIC PRINCIPLES

In the past surgical attempts to remove malignant tumors of the sacrum have been unsuccessful at least partly due to the reluctance on the part of the surgeon to sacrifice urogenital and anorectal function. What we have learned since then is that if the surgeon is not prepared to make this sacrifice, the tumor eventually produces this result and, if not completely removed, will eventually threaten the patient's life. The sacral nerves pass in a lateral and anteroinferior direction through canals that end with the anterior sacral foramina. The S1 nerves pass between the first and second sacral vertebrae, the S2 nerves between the second and third sacral vertebrae, and so on (Fig. 39–1). Thus, if a malignant tumor involves the third sacral vertebra, the S2 nerves must be included in the specimen; if the tumor involves the second sacral vertebra, the S1 nerves must be sacrificed in addition to the other lower sacral nerve roots. In both of these cases, this will result in a loss of the parasympathetic, voluntary motor, and sensory pathways to and from the pelvic visceral organs which are mediated through the S2-S4 roots. Sympathetic innervation can be preserved since these nerve fibers are mediated through the superior hypogastric plexus.

Malignant tumors of the sacrum which expand anteriorly will usually respect the preformed fibrous barrier of the periosteum and the presacral fascia, and because of this property this barrier should not be violated by a transrectal biopsy. If such a biopsy has been performed before the patient is referred for definitive surgery, the rectum must be excised along with the surgical specimen, since the tumor may have spread to the retrorectal space as a consequence of the biopsy.

When a primary malignant tumor originates in the body of a sacral vertebra, usually the case with a sacral chordoma, the rudimentary intervertebral disc may serve as a temporary barrier to the tumor's cephalad extension. By growing into the sacral canal the tumor may by-pass this barrier and invade an adjacent vertebra. This invasion may not be radiographically evident. The sacrum should be amputated to cover this possibility in these cases.

Three muscles are attached to the sacrum—the sacrospinalis, gluteus maximus, and piriformis. These muscles need to be transected well beyond the level of palpable tumor since they may be infiltrated by the malignancy.

SURGICAL PROCEDURE AND TECHNIQUE

There are two levels of high sacral amputation: that between the first and second sacral vertebrae passing through the canals of the S1 nerves (Fig. 39–2A, C, and E), and that performed through the first sacral vertebra, above the canals of the S1 nerves (Fig. 39–2B, D, and F). The former level permits the preservation of the S1 nerves; the latter does not.

Two different surgical approaches are required, an anterior approach and a posterior approach. If the rectum is to be preserved, the operation is started anteriorly and finished posteriorly; whereas if the rectum is to be resected en bloc with the specimen, the operation is started anteriorly, continued posteriorly, and finished anteriorly. For the anterior approach the patient is placed in the supine position. The legs are elevated in a lithotomy position, and the anus is sutured closed (temporarily if the rectum can be preserved). For the posterior approach the patient is placed in the prone position onto a Wilson frame in order to avoid compression of the inferior vena cava.

The incision for the anterior approach varies depending on whether the rectum is to be sacrificed. If the rectum can be preserved, a good exposure can be obtained without opening the peritoneal cavity. A large semicircular incision is made through the skin and the subcutaneous layers (Fig. 39–3). The tendon of the rectus abdominis muscle is severed bilaterally 1 cm above its insertion on the pubic bone, and the

This chapter is to a large extent based on a publication by Stener B, Gunterberg B: High amputation of the sacrum for extirpation of tumors. Principles and technique. Spine 3:351–366, 1978, with permission.

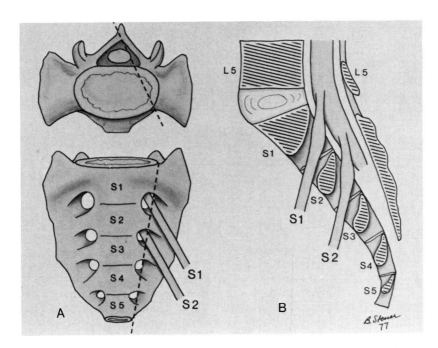

FIGURE 39–1. The course of the S1 and S2 nerves through the sacrum. Interrupted lines in *A* show the plane in which the sacrum has been osteotomized in *B*. The canals of the sacral nerves run obliquely in a lateral and anteroinferior direction. The S1 nerves leave the dural sac behind the lumbosacral disc, the S2 nerves behind the S1–S2 disc. (Reproduced with permission from Stener B, Gunterberg B: High amputation of the sacrum for extirpation of tumors. Principles and technique. Spine 3:351–366, 1978.)

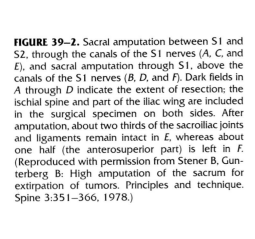

FIGURE 39–2. Sacral amputation between S1 and S2, through the canals of the S1 nerves (*A, C,* and *E*), and sacral amputation through S1, above the canals of the S1 nerves (*B, D,* and *F*). Dark fields in *A* through *D* indicate the extent of resection; the ischial spine and part of the iliac wing are included in the surgical specimen on both sides. After amputation, about two thirds of the sacroiliac joints and ligaments remain intact in *E*, whereas about one half (the anterosuperior part) is left in *F*. (Reproduced with permission from Stener B, Gunterberg B: High amputation of the sacrum for extirpation of tumors. Principles and technique. Spine 3:351–366, 1978.)

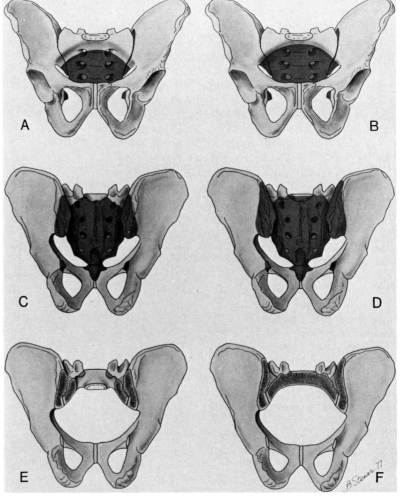

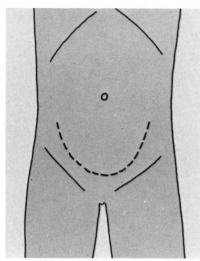

FIGURE 39–3. Representation of incision of skin and subcutaneous layers used for extraperitoneal anterior approach when rectum can be preserved. (Reproduced with permission from Stener B, Gunterberg B: High amputation of the sacrum for extirpation of tumors. Principles and technique. Spine 3:351–366, 1978.)

abdominal muscular wall is cut through on both sides along the lateral border of the aponeurotic sheath of the rectus abdominis. The peritoneum is displaced bilaterally to expose the area where the common iliac artery and vein bifurcate into the external and internal iliac vessels. The dissection is then carried out bilaterally in a medial direction behind the peritoneum, the ureter, and the branches of the superior hypogastric nerve plexus. Finally the right and left dissections meet to provide exposure of the sacral promontory and the superior part of the sacrum.

If the rectum has to be resected en bloc, the peritoneal cavity is opened through an inferior midline incision which may be extended above the umbilicus. After dividing and ligating the superior rectal vessels, the bowel is transected at the rectosigmoid junction, and its open ends are closed by invagination. Bilaterally the middle rectal vessels are divided

and ligated. The peritoneum is cut in the bottom of the rectovesical pouch or rectouterine pouch, and the rectum is released anteriorly as far distally as possible from above. With the patient in the lithotomy position an inverted U-incision is made around the anus (previously sutured closed), and the anal canal and rectum are freed anteriorly and bilaterally from below.

The surgical procedure subsequently is the same regardless of whether the rectum is spared or resected. The internal iliac arteries and veins are divided bilaterally, and the ends are secured by suture-ligatures. The lateral and median sacral arteries and veins are also divided and ligated. If the sacrum is to be amputated through the first sacral vertebra, above the canals of the S1 nerves, it is advisable to divide and ligate the iliolumbar vessels. The periosteum is then stripped from the uppermost sacrum, starting at the promontory and proceeding distally to the level selected for amputation (Figs. 39–4 through 39–7). This entails cutting the sympathetic nerve trunk where it passes the sacral wing level with the ipsilateral sacral foramina. The lumbosacral nerve trunk (L4 and L5), which passes the sacral wing more laterally (Fig. 39–7B), is released so that it can be protected later when the sacral amputation is performed. If the S1 nerves can be preserved, they are exposed where they emerge through the first anterior sacral foramina. With a suitable osteotome or chisel the anterior cortex of the sacrum is cut through transversely at the level of these foramina or, if indicated, above them (Fig. 39–7B).

It is advantageous to carry the osteotomy tract past each sacroiliac joint (see Fig. 39–2A and B) under the lumbosacral nerve trunk. It will then be easier to determine the correct level for the completion of the resection. This osteotomy tract can be palpated from behind during the posterior stage of the operation by a finger inserted under the edge of the ilium in the bottom of the greater sciatic notch (see Fig. 39–2C and D).

If the rectum has been preserved, the anterior

FIGURE 39–4. A, Sacral amputation between S1 and S2. The anteriorly protruding part of the tumor is covered by periosteum and the presacral fascia. To avoid the risk of penetrating this fibrous barrier inadvertently, the periosteum of S1 and the anteroinferior part of this vertebra are included in the specimen. B, After removal of the lumbosacral ligamentum flavum with its bony attachments, the dural sac has been ligated and divided between the S1 and S2 nerves. Dark fields indicate the extent of bone resection. The inferior half of the canal of the S1 nerve is included in the specimen while the nerve itself is preserved.

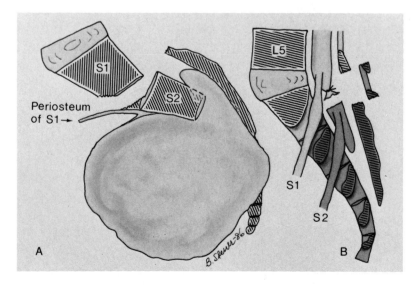

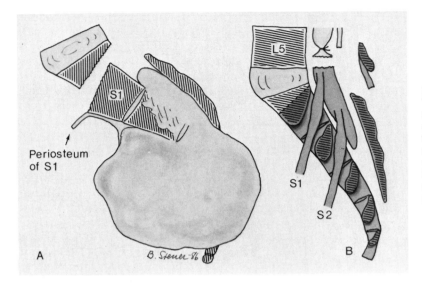

FIGURE 39–5. *A,* Sacral amputation though S1. The periosteum of the vertebra is included in the specimen. *B,* After complete laminectomy of L5 and removal of the lumbosacral ligamentum flavum, the dural sac has been ligated and divided superior to the S1 nerve. Dark fields indicate the extent of bone resection. The whole canal of the S1 nerve is included in the specimen. The first sacral vertebra is transected obliquely, somewhat more being preserved anteriorly than posteriorly.

wound is now permanently closed after insertion of two suction tubes; if the rectum is sacrificed, the anterior wound is closed temporarily. The patient is then turned to the prone position.

With the posterior exposure, it is important to include in the specimen to be resected the skin and subcutaneous layers over the inferior part of the sacrum especially overlying the hiatus of the sacral canal through which the tumor might have penetrated (see Fig. 39–4A). If a previous biopsy has been performed, the entire track of the biopsy should be removed along with an adequate margin of healthy tissue. If the rectum has to be removed along with the tumor, the posterior incision lines join the U-incision previously made around the anus. Superior to the area of skin to be removed, a midline incision is extended cephalad to permit a good exposure of the posterior elements of L5. On each side, after raising a flap of skin and subcutaneous tissue, the gluteus maximus muscle is transected well away from the sacrum, and the underlying piriformis muscle is

severed at its musculotendinous junction. The superior and inferior gluteal vessels are divided and ligated. An attempt is made to preserve the superior gluteal nerve, which innervates the gluteus medius and minimus and the tensor fasciae latae muscles; it runs under the edge of the ilium in the bottom of the greater sciatic notch. The sacrotuberous ligament is transected near the ischial tuberosity, and the underlying sacrospinous ligament and coccygeus muscle are released by chiseling off their common pelvic attachment, the ischial spine, which is included bilaterally in the specimen (see Fig. 39–2A–D). If the rectum can be preserved, the anal region is released by severing the bands that attach it to the coccyx. If the rectum has to be included in the specimen, the levator ani muscle is transected on each side.

At the lumbosacral level, the sacrospinalis muscles are severed transversely, exposing the underlying skeletal parts. If the sacral amputation is intended to be done with the S1 nerves preserved, the dural sac is exposed by removal of the lumbosacral ligamentum

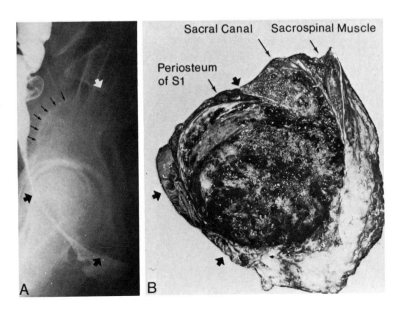

FIGURE 39–6. Sacral amputation between S1 and S2 as in Figures 39–2A, C, and E, and 39–4A and B. A, Lateral preoperative roentgenogram in 56-year-old man with a large chordoma whose superior pole (*thin black arrows*) almost reaches the level of the promontory. *B,* An approximately median sagittal section of the surgical specimen. Anteroinferior part of S1 is indicated by white arrow in *A* and by black arrow in *B*. Rectum is indicated by large black arrows in both figures. The patient has been free from evidence of tumor for 11½ years. (Reproduced with permission from Stener B, Gunterberg B: High amputation of the sacrum for extirpation of tumors. Principles and technique. Spine 3:351–366, 1978.)

FIGURE 39–7. Sacral amputation through S1 as in Figures 39–2B, D, and F, and 39–5A and B. A, Chordoma in 55-year-old man extends cephalad in the sacral canal causing deformation of the dural sac. Interrupted line indicates level of sacral amputation. B, Surgical field after extraperitoneal anterior approach. White arrow indicates track made by chisel in the right sacral wing, above the first sacral foramen (see Fig. 39–2B). Black arrow indicates the right lumbosacral nerve trunk. Round dot indicates periosteum reflected from the right sacral wing. Asterisk indicates the lumbosacral disc. C, Surgical specimen (superior part) divided in the middle sagittal plane. Having destroyed the body of S3, the tumor protrudes anteriorly elevating the periosteum and the presacral fascia (*white arrow*); extending cephalad in the sacral canal, it also affects the body of S2. The disc between S2 and S3 (*black arrow*) serves as a temporary barrier. The patient has been free from evidence of tumor for 6½ years after operation. Despite the loss of the S1 nerve he is able to walk even on tiptoe. (From Stener B: Surgical treatment of giant cell tumors, chondrosarcomas, and chordomas of the spine. *In* Uhtoff H (ed): Current Concepts of Diagnosis and Treatment of Bone and Soft Tissue Tumors. Berlin, Springer-Verlag, 1984, pp 233–242.)

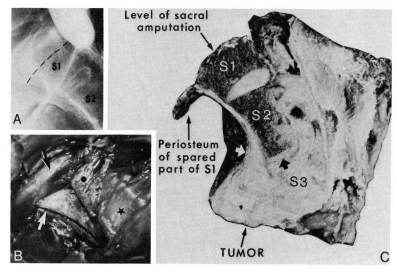

flavum including its bony attachments above and below (see Fig. 39–4B); an inferior partial laminectomy is done on L5; and the roof of the sacral canal is removed as far distally as level with the first posterior sacral foramina (see Fig. 39–2C). If the sacral amputation is intended to be done with the S1 nerves included in the specimen, the dural sac is exposed by a complete laminectomy of L5 and removal of the lumbosacral ligamentum flavum (see Fig. 39–5B). The dural sac is ligated and divided at such a level that the S1 nerves are either preserved or not, depending on the choice of level for the sacral amputation (see Figs. 39–4B and 39–5B).

After the dural sac is ligated and transected, the sacrum itself is resected. When the S1 nerve can be preserved the sacrum is osteotomized between the first and second sacral vertebrae, with the inferior half of the canals of the S1 nerves included in the specimen (Figs. 39–2A, C, and E, and 39–4A and B), and a posteroinferior part of each ilium is also included (Fig. 39–2A and C). The osteotomy is performed posteriorly, guided by a finger that palpates the track previously chiseled through the anterior cortex of the sacrum and ilium through the greater sciatic notch. It can be helpful for the orientation to introduce a dissector through each of the canals of the S1 nerves. Once the transection of bone has been completed, the sacral nerves, exclusive of S1, are cut where they converge to form the sciatic nerve.

If the S1 nerves are to be sacrificed, an osteotomy is performed through the first sacral vertebra at a level that includes the canals of these nerves (Figs. 39–2B, D, and F, and 39–5A and B). Since these canals course obliquely in an anteroinferior direction, the sacrum is transected obliquely, with somewhat more of the first sacral vertebra being preserved anteriorly than posteriorly (Fig. 39–5A and B). Laterally on each side the osteotomy is done so that a large posterior part of the ilium is included in the

specimen (Fig. 39–2B and D). For orientation while performing this osteotomy, it is helpful first to deeply notch the iliac crest at the level of the transverse process of L5. This facilitates palpation from behind of the anterosuperior surface of the sacral wing and the sacroiliac joint, and the osteotomy is done about 1 cm posteroinferior and parallel to this surface. The osteotomy track previously chiseled through the anterior cortex of the sacrum and ilium is also helpful to orient the osteotomy plane. Once the bone has been transected and the sacral nerves severed bilaterally at the level of the greater sciatic foramen, the specimen is removed. After establishing hemostasis, the posterior operation is completed by suturing the skin flaps in the midline, with an opening being left for drainage at the inferior end. A compression bandage is applied. If the midline incision is closed completely (which may be advisable especially if the rectum is preserved), adequate regional drainage can be effected through a separate incision in each gluteal region.

If the rectum has been resected the patient is again turned to the supine position and the previous, temporarily closed, abdominal incision is reopened in order to accomplish a pelvic closure of the peritoneal cavity and to perform a colostomy. The sigmoid colon, previously invaginated at its distal end, is released from its mesentery by cutting near the wall of the bowel. This mesentery, with preserved vascular supply, is used to close the peritoneal defect in the lesser pelvis. The periphery of the mesentery is sutured to the peritoneum that has previously been cut transversely in the bottom of the rectovesical pouch (rectouterine pouch in females). Through a circular opening made in the abdominal wall on the left side, the released sigmoid colon is drawn out extraperitoneally. The midline abdominal wound is closed, and a colostomy is done at the level where the vascular supply of the bowel is judged to be adequate.

PERSONAL EXPERIENCE OF SACRAL AMPUTATIONS

The author has performed four operations according to Figure 39–2A, C, and E (all for chordoma) and three operations according to Figure 39–2B, D, and F (two for chordoma and one for malignant ependymoma). Figure 39–6 illustrates a case of the former type, Figure 39–7 a case of the latter type; these two patients (both with chordoma) have been free from evidence of tumor for 14 years and 9 years, respectively. Of the four other patients with chordoma, one underwent the operation as a secondary procedure (he eventually succumbed to the disease); one was free of tumor when she died from myocardial infarction after 2 years and 4 months (confirmed at autopsy); one has been free from evidence of local recurrence for more than 14 years but has been treated with radiation for a supposedly malignant lesion in the lumbar spine (no biopsy); and one is free from evidence of disease after 6 years despite the fact that tumor tissue was transected unexpectedly during the osteotomy through the first sacral vertebra (she received postoperative radiation because of this). The patient who had a malignant ependymoma died from metastases after 1 year and 3 months.

REFERENCES

1. Stener B: Surgical treatment of giant cell tumors, chondrosarcomas, and chordomas of the spine. *In* Uhtoff H (ed): Current Concepts of Diagnosis and Treatment of Bone and Soft Tissue Tumors. Berlin, Springer-Verlag, 1984, pp 233–242.
2. Stener B: Complete removal of vertebrae for extirpation of tumors. A 20-year experience. Clin Orthop 245:72–82, 1989.
3. Stener B, Gunterberg B: High amputation of the sacrum for extirpation of tumors. Principles and technique. Spine 3:351–366, 1978.

40

SURGICAL APPROACHES TO TUMORS OF THE PELVIS INVOLVING THE AXIAL SKELETON

CONSTANTINE KARAKOUSIS

INTRODUCTION

Tumors in the sacroiliac area often present difficulties in exposure and safe resection, as well as in adequacy of surgical margins. Only recently have surgical techniques been developed to a degree permitting deliberate and accurate dissection similar to other anatomic areas which have a longer history of surgical endeavors.

The presentation of the approaches in this chapter follows a description of various surgical techniques I have found useful for this region; in addition, the indications, according to tumor location, are described.

THE ABDOMINOINGUINAL INCISION

The abdominoinguinal incision is applicable for tumors located in the iliac fossa, around the iliac vessels, or on the wall of the lesser pelvis when there is no osseous involvement, although fixation to the soft tissues may be present (Fig. 40–1). It is also applicable for tumors involving the pubic bone (Fig. 40–2), with or without involvement of the adjacent soft tissue, when there is no need to remove the acetabulum.[5, 7]

In the past, tumors located in the iliac fossa were deemed unresectable through the usual abdominal exposure or were treated with hemipelvectomy, that is, the removal of the entire ipsilateral extremity and hemipelvis. With abdominal or low-flank incisions there is proximal exposure but not distal exposure and control. The abdominoinguinal incision involves a lower midline incision from above or just below the umbilicus to the pubic symphysis. An exploration is first performed (Fig. 40–3) to rule out evidence of metastatic disease; this also allows some dissection between the tumor mass and ureter, rectosigmoid, and bladder. The incision is then extended along the pubic crest to the side of involvement (right or left) up to the middle of the inguinal ligament and then vertically for a few centimeters over the femoral vessels. The rectus sheath and muscle are divided near the crest and the inguinal ligament at the pubic tubercle. The femoral vessels are exposed. In the male the spermatic cord is identified and the floor of the inguinal canal is incised to the internal inguinal ring. At this level the internal spermatic vessels may be divided if they are crossing over the tumor, without endangering the viability of the testis if the latter has not been extricated off the scrotal pouch during the manipulations. The vas deferens is displaced medially. If on palpation from inside, these structures are too close to the tumor, the ipsilateral testis may be removed en bloc with the tumor.

With further dissection under the medial portion of the inguinal ligament, the inferior epigastric vein and artery are serially ligated and divided at their origin (Fig. 40–4), and the lateral third of the inguinal ligament is detached off the iliac fascia. The

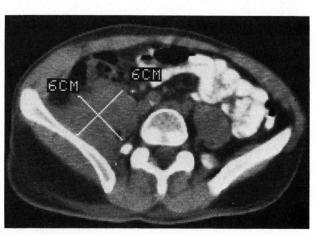

FIGURE 40–1. Soft tissue sarcoma in the right iliac fossa.

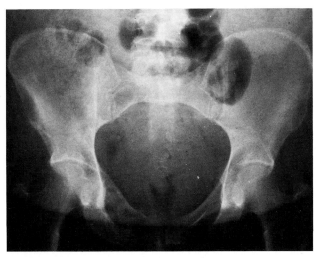

FIGURE 40–2. The posterior pubic ramus is destroyed by a malignant fibrous histiocytoma.

corner of the skin flap, previously belonging to the lower end of the midline incision, is now displaced lateral to the anterosuperior iliac spine. The operative field includes the abdominal cavity, the iliac fossa on the side of involvement, and the femoral triangle in one continuous, uninterrupted view (Fig. 40–5). The iliac vessels are exposed from the aorta to the femoral vessels in one field. Vessel loops may be passed proximally and distally around these vessels, and if there is any question of proximity to the tumor, dissection may be carried out along these vessels starting from the proximal or distal portion. If the tumor involves these vessels, ideally the dissection should first be completed around the tumor, separating it with whatever margin is possible from

other structures. As the last act in the resection, following heparinization, the vessels may be divided proximally and distally and replaced with a standard synthetic graft. This certainly would be necessary for the artery, but the vein can simply be ligated proximally and distally. Although the rate of thrombosis in venous synthetic grafts is high, in our experience a short segment of the iliac vein replaced by a polytetrafluoroethylene graft may remain open. When the vein is ligated or a venous graft clots postoperatively, leg elevation is essential for avoiding excessive edema.

If the tumor involves the inner aspect of the lower abdominal wall and inguinal ligament, after the skin incision is made dissection may be carried out on the surface of the external oblique aponeurosis, or between the external oblique and internal oblique muscles to the extent necessary, as guided by palpation on the abdominal side, to remove the involved portion of the abdominal wall en bloc with the tumor. When a narrow strip of the external oblique aponeurosis along with the inguinal ligament has been removed, it is often possible to close the gap by using a relaxing incision above. When a larger defect has been created, the missing portion of the abdominal wall may be replaced with a synthetic mesh. Care should be exercised in the process of reconstruction so that the mesh is not in direct contact with the femoral vessels, in order to avoid possible later arterial erosion and hemorrhage. This event is more likely to happen if the vessels have been previously radiated. The sartorius muscle or the straight head of the rectus femoris muscle may be moved to cover the vessels. If the skin of the groin is also involved and has to be removed, the resulting defect is covered with a tensor fascia lata myocutaneous flap.[11]

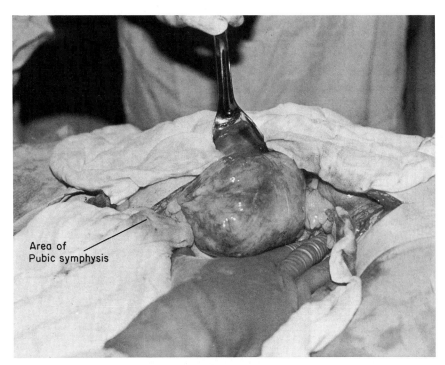

FIGURE 40–3. Through a lower midline incision an exploration is first performed. This tumor has a broad base of attachment to the right iliac fossa. The exposure is inadequate through the abdominal incision.

Area of
Pubic symphysis

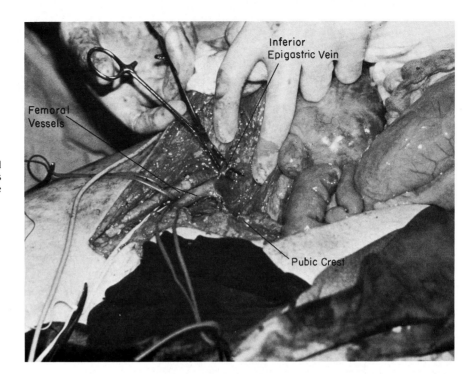

FIGURE 40–4. Dissection, ligation, and division of the inferior epigastric vessels at their origin permit mobilization of the inguinal ligament with the flap.

For a tumor in the iliac fossa, its relation to the femoral nerve should be explored early in the dissection. It is easy to identify the femoral nerve lateral to the artery in a plane posterior to the artery, as this nerve lies behind the continuation of the iliac fascia. When this fascia is incised the nerve is exposed and can be traced proximally as it dips between the iliac and psoas muscles. If a "clean" plane of dissection between the tumor and the femoral nerve is found, the latter is preserved. If the nerve is involved, it should be removed en bloc with the tumor. Follow-

ing sacrifice of the femoral nerve, patients experience inability to extend the knee and initially have to walk with the aid of crutches or a cane. After six months or so, patients usually manage to walk without external support, as shown by our experience with anterior compartment resections of the thigh whenever the femoral nerve is divided at the level of the groin.

Tumors involving the pubic bone can be easily removed by dividing the pubic symphysis medially and laterally, and the anterior and posterior pubic rami just medial to the acetabulum. Adjacent in-

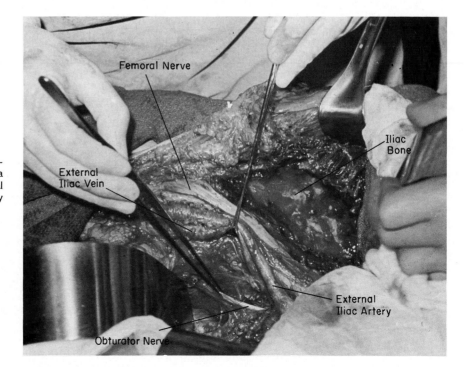

FIGURE 40–5. The operative field following resection of a soft tissue sarcoma within the right iliac muscle. The femoral nerve and iliofemoral vessels are clearly shown.

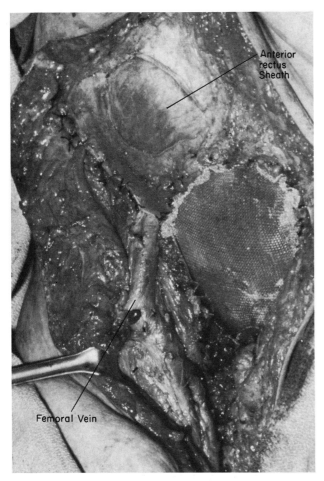

FIGURE 40–6. The right pubic bone has been removed with en bloc resection of the adductor group of muscles. The defect has been replaced with a mesh.

volved soft tissues such as the medial compartment of the thigh may also be resected en bloc. In this procedure, the obturator nerve crossing through the obturator foramen is sacrificed by dividing its trunk as well as the obturator vessels above. Removal of the obturator nerve does not cause any appreciable functional deficit and the gait remains normal. Following resection, the resulting defect may be closed with the use of a mesh sutured anteriorly to the external oblique aponeurosis and rectus sheath, medially to the fascia in front of the pubic symphysis, and posterolaterally to aponeurotic muscle structures (Figs. 40–6 and 40–7). Muscle or omentum should be interposed between the iliac vein and the mesh.

The closure of the abdominoinguinal incision is fairly simple. The inguinal ligament, lateral to the femoral artery, is approximated to the iliac fascia (if the iliopsoas muscle has been removed, to the capsule of the hip joint) and medial to the femoral vein, to Cooper's ligament. The rectus sheath and muscle are reapproximated to the pubic crest.

INTERNAL HEMIPELVECTOMY

This procedure is applicable to primary bone tumors involving the iliac or entire innominate bone,

with no or moderate soft tissue involvement, so that the major nerves to the extremity, that is, the sciatic and femoral nerves, and the iliofemoral vessels, can be preserved.

Although other incisions have also been described, we have found most effective the use of a reverse-Y incision.[6] This incision starting at the posterosuperior iliac spine is carried along the iliac crest to the anterosuperior iliac spine. The medial limb of the incision is then continued along the inguinal ligament to the pubic symphysis. The lateral limb of the incision is extended between the anterosuperior iliac spine and a point behind the greater trochanter (Fig. 40–8). Medial to the iliac crest, the anterolateral abdominal wall muscles are divided and the retroperitoneal space is opened, permitting exploration and assessment of the tumor resection and any soft part involvement.

The inguinal ligament is divided off the anterosuperior iliac spine, and its lateral third is dissected off the iliac fascia. By dividing the inferior epigastric vessels at their origin, it is mobilized sufficiently to be divided at the pubic tubercle. The ipsilateral rectus sheath and muscle are divided off the pubic crest. The iliac and femoral vessels are now exposed in one continuous field and tapes are passed around them. If the psoas muscle is not involved it may be included in the tapes (Fig. 40–9). The pubic symphysis is divided with a Gigli saw, the adductor group of muscles are divided off their origin, and (following division of the sartorius, tensor fascia lata, and rectus femoris muscles near their origin) the neck of the femur is divided or, alternatively, the head of the femur is disarticulated (Fig. 40–10). More laterally the fascia lata and insertion of gluteus maximus to the femur are incised, and the sciatic nerve is exposed and traced proximally. The plane deep to the gluteus maximus, if not involved by the tumor, is developed until the sacroiliac joint is exposed. The sacroiliac joint is divided with an osteotome. If the tumor reaches the joint area, the bone may be divided through the sacral ala. In this case, the lumbosacral

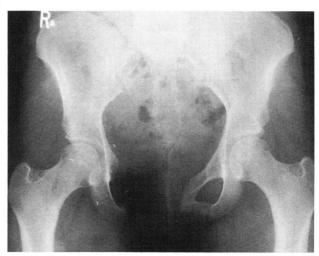

FIGURE 40–7. X-ray appearance following removal of the pubic bone.

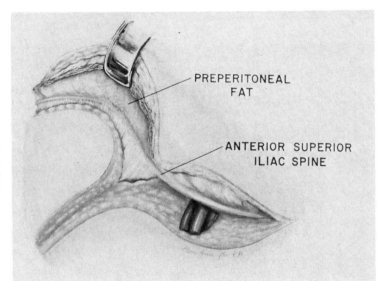

FIGURE 40–8. The reverse-Y incision used for internal hemipelvectomy. The retroperitoneal space has been entered. The inguinal ligament will be detached from the anterior superior iliac spine and, following ligation of the inferior epigastric vessels, from the pubic tubercle.

PREPERITONEAL FAT

ANTERIOR SUPERIOR ILIAC SPINE

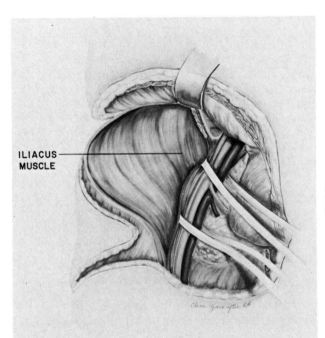

ILIACUS MUSCLE

FIGURE 40–9. Tapes have been passed around the iliofemoral vessels, femoral nerve, and psoas muscle to aid in their retraction and preservation.

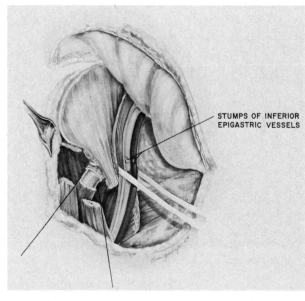

STUMPS OF INFERIOR EPIGASTRIC VESSELS

FIGURE 40–10. The neck of the femur is divided with a Gigli saw. (From Karakousis CP: Internal hemipelvectomy. Surg Gynecol Obstet 158:279–282, 1984. Reprinted by permission of Surgery, Gynecology & Obstetrics.)

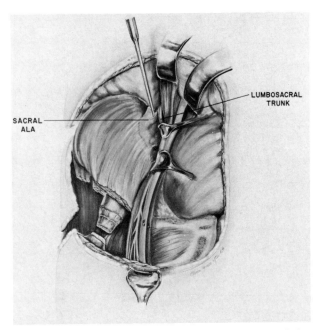

FIGURE 40–11. The lumbosacral trunk coursing on the sacral ala is at risk of being injured with a transection of the bone, if not retracted medially. (From Karakousis CP: Internal hemipelvectomy. Surg Gynecol Obstet 158:279–282, 1984. Reprinted by permission of Surgery, Gynecology & Obstetrics.)

trunk (L4-L5 roots) en route to forming the sciatic nerve should be retracted medially to avoid accidental injury (Fig. 40–11).

The hamstring muscles are divided off the ischial tuberosity posteriorly, the levator ani muscle medially, and finally the sacrotuberous and sacrospinous ligaments. The specimen, that is, the entire hemipelvis with the adjacent iliac and gluteus medius and minimus muscles, can thus be removed (Fig. 40–12). Skeletal traction is often recommended on the op-

erated extremity for about 3 weeks in order to avoid excessive shortening. Crutch walking initially without bearing weight on the operated side is practiced for 3 to 4 months; then partial and gradually full weight-bearing are slowly permitted. Following internal hemipelvectomy, patients have normal movement at ankle and knee joints but no hip movement. They require crutches indefinitely, but remain quite mobile, and are able to walk up and down stairs. The functional and cosmetic results are definitely superior to hemipelvectomy. Since extensive rehabilitation is required, this procedure is most suitable for young patients eager to have limb salvage.

When there is no evidence of soft tissue involvement in the buttock areas, the incision can be simplified by omitting the lateral limb of the reverse-Y (Figs. 40–13 and 40–14). Formal exposure of the sciatic nerve is not required. Following exposure of the iliac crest, the gluteal muscles can be detached off the lateral aspect of the iliac bone using a periosteal elevator until the greater sciatic notch is exposed.

When only the pubic bone is involved it can be removed through the abdominoinguinal incision as shown above. When only a portion of the iliac bone is involved above the acetabulum, a portion of the previously described incision may be used (Figs. 40–15 and 40–16). Preservation of the acetabulum, when feasible, is of course of great functional value, since walking is then nearly normal without any support.

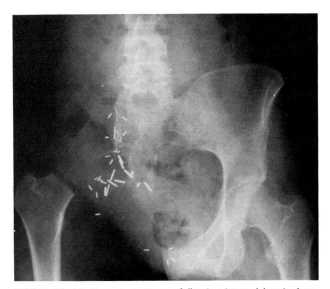

FIGURE 40–12. X-ray appearance following internal hemipelvectomy on the right side.

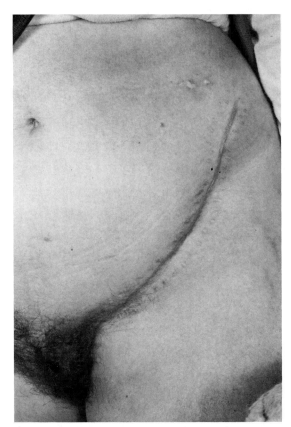

FIGURE 40–13. The incision employed for resection of the pubic bone and a portion of the iliac bone including the acetabulum.

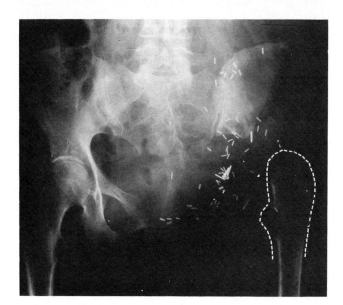

FIGURE 40–14. Postoperative x-ray appearance of the patient in Figure 40–13.

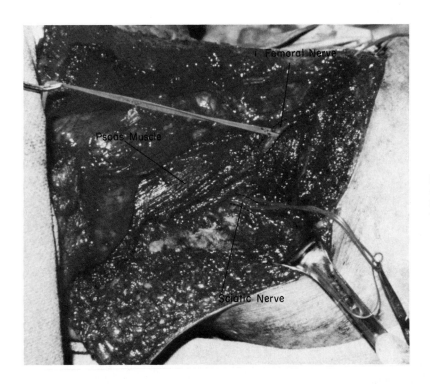

FIGURE 40–15. Operative field following resection of the iliac bone above the acetabulum and the iliac muscle for an osteogenic sarcoma arising from the iliac bone and extending into the iliac muscle.

FIGURE 40–16. The closed incision. It consisted basically of an incision along the iliac crest and inguinal ligament, with a proximal T-extension for extra exposure in that area.

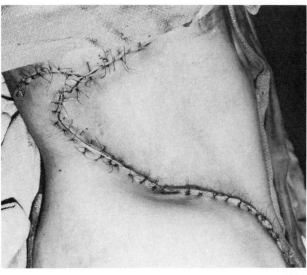

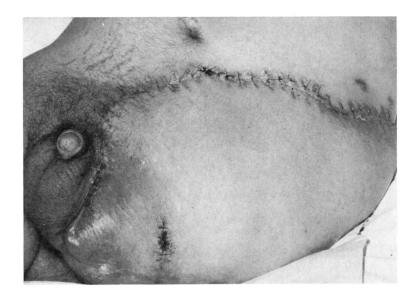

FIGURE 40–17. Even a long posterior flap reaching to the level of the umbilicus or above maintains its viability when the gluteus maximus muscle is left attached to it.

HEMIPELVECTOMY

This surgical procedure implies the removal of the entire lower extremity and a portion of or the entire hemipelvis on the ipsilateral side. It is indicated for tumors extensively involving the soft tissues and bone, so that satisfactory resection with limb salvage cannot be performed.[1, 4]

In patients requiring this procedure, a posterior flap is fashioned; regardless of the level of division of the iliac vessels, the viability of the posterior flap is assured only when the gluteus maximus is left attached to the flap (Fig. 40–17).[4] For extensive tumors located in the buttock, an anterior flap is made. In our experience, a long anteromedial flap from the thigh composed of skin, subcutaneous fat, and the fascia lata muscle, with the iliofemoral vessels attached, provides good, reliable coverage.[4, 8] When the tumor extends on the medial side or when a particularly broad flap may be needed, a flap composed of skin, subcutaneous tissue, and the quadri-

ceps muscle, with the femoral vessels in the middle of the flap, may be preferable.[12]

For tumors located proximally and extending from the iliopsoas muscle to the lumbar spine, the usual hemipelvectomy incision is inadequate. A combination with a lower midline incision in these cases provides the necessary proximal exposure (Fig. 40–18).[4]

For most cases of posterior flap hemipelvectomy, the patient is placed in a supine position with the buttock on the affected side elevated on folded sheets, so that the area of the gluteal fold and below can be prepped and included in the operative field. However, if it is anticipated that a high division of the bone will be required, a lateral or semilateral position is preferable because the bone may be divided proximally at a high level if necessary, that is, along the row of posterior sacral foramina of the affected side.

For an anterior flap hemipelvectomy, a semilateral position is preferable because of the necessity to have adequate exposure both anteriorly and posteriorly.

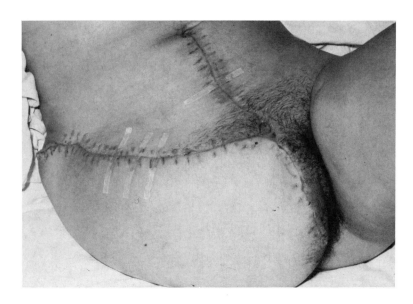

FIGURE 40–18. The combination of a posterior flap hemipelvectomy incision and a lower midline incision provides excellent proximal exposure and heals well.

DISCUSSION

Tumors in the sacroiliac area are often diagnosed at a locally advanced stage because clinical symptoms or evidence of a mass in this area are not appreciable by the patient in early stages. Swelling of the lower extremity may occur as a result of compression by the tumor and thrombosis of the iliac vein, which often is misdiagnosed as thrombophlebitis and is treated as such for several months. Some patients present with neurologic symptoms in the distribution of the femoral, obturator, or sciatic nerves due to compression of these nerves by the tumor. Delay in diagnosis often results from the assumption that these symptoms are secondary to benign musculoskeletal conditions that cause low back pain with or without radiation to the peripheral nerves.

A high index of suspicion is essential in making an early diagnosis. With radiologic techniques such as computed tomography (CT) and magnetic resonance imaging (MRI) scans, small tumor masses can now be detected.

Tumor masses involving the soft tissues of the pelvis with lateral fixation can be removed, often with the abdominoinguinal incision. When the bone is involved unilaterally, resection can be performed with the technique of internal hemipelvectomy. It is only for the occasional, extensive tumor that a hemipelvectomy is required. In most of these, lacking wide surgical margins, adjuvant radiation may be considered. Our experience with chordomas and soft tissue sarcomas[9, 10] suggests that the combination of resection and radiation is highly effective in securing local control. The rate of distant relapse is dependent, of course, on the histologic grade of the tumor. For high grade tumors adjuvant chemotherapy should be considered, although its effectiveness has not been firmly established.

REFERENCES

1. Ariel IM, Shah JP: The conservative hemipelvectomy. Surg Gynecol Obstet 144:406–413, 1977.
2. Gunterberg B, Kewenter J, Petersen I, Stener B: Anorectal function after major resections of the sacrum with bilateral or unilateral sacrifice of sacral nerves. Br J Surg 63:546–554, 1976.
3. Karakousis CP: Sacral resection with preservation of continence. Surg Gynecol Obstet 163:270–273, 1986.
4. Karakousis CP: Atlas of Operations for Soft Tissue Tumors. New York, McGraw-Hill, 1985, pp 335–369.
5. Karakousis CP: The abdominoinguinal incision in limb salvage and resection of pelvic tumors. Cancer 54:2543–2548, 1984.
6. Karakousis CP: Internal hemipelvectomy. Surg Gynecol Obstet 158:279–282, 1984.
7. Karakousis CP: Exposure and reconstruction in the lower portions of the retroperitoneum and abdominal wall. Arch Surg 117:840–844, 1982.
8. Karakousis CP, Vezeridis MP: Variants of hemipelvectomy. Am J Surg 145:273–277, 1983.
9. Karakousis CP, Emrich LJ, Fleminger R, Friedman M: Chordomas: Diagnosis and management. Am Surg 53:497–501, 1981.
10. Karakousis CP, Emrich LJ, Rao U, Krishnamsetty RR: Feasibility of limb salvage and survival in soft tissue sarcomas. Cancer 57:484–491, 1986.
11. Nahai F, Hill HL, Hester TR: Experiences with the tensor fascia lata flap. Plast Reconstr Surg 63:788–799, 1979.
12. Sugarbaker PH, Chretien PA: Hemipelvectomy for buttock tumors utilizing an anterior myocutaneous flap of quadriceps femoris muscle. Ann Surg 197:106–115, 1983.

SURGICAL APPROACHES TO THE SACROILIAC JOINT

JESSOP McDONALD and JOSEPH M. LANE

INTRODUCTION

In recent years, improved diagnostic and staging methods coincident with the advancement of en bloc resection techniques have resulted in operative treatment of many tumors of the posterior pelvis heretofore left untouched or incompletely excised. As a result of these developments, tumors involving the sacroiliac area are now increasingly amenable to surgical therapy. Anatomically, this area lies deep within the confines of the pelvis behind the viscera, making anterior approaches both indirect and complex. Posteriorly, the sacroiliac joint is covered by the overlying medial projection of the iliac tuberosity, necessitating osseous manipulation to gain access. In this chapter, we describe anterior, posterior, and combined anteroposterior approaches to the sacroiliac joint and adjacent musculoskeletal anatomy. In addition, a method of percutaneous aspiration of the joint is reviewed. In Table 41–1, the spectrum of malignant tumors involving this region is presented together with long-term results.

ANTERIOR APPROACH

The patient is placed in the semisupine position supported by a sandbag on an operating table that permits usage of intraoperative radiograph. An anterior incision is made extending from the anterosuperior iliac spine approximately 10 to 12 cm posteriorly, coursing 1 to 5 cm above and parallel to the

iliac crest (Fig. 41–1). The incision is deepened through the subcutaneous fat to expose the underlying aponeurosis of the external oblique muscle. The inferior margin of the incision is then elevated to expose the superior aspect of the crest of the ilium, from which the aponeurotic attachments of the internal and external oblique and transverse abdominal muscles are released, leaving a 0.5- to 1-cm remnant of aponeurosis attached to the iliac crest to enable repair during closure (Fig. 41–2). A Cobb elevator is used to initiate stripping of the iliac muscle from the inner aspect of the ilium. Continued elevation in a medial, inferior, and posterior direction is then accomplished by blunt technique using a sponge-covered elevator or a gloved finger until the prominent thickening, which is the anterior fascial capsule of the sacroiliac joint, is identified. Bone wax is used to control osseous bleeding. By gently retracting the iliac muscle medially, the exact location of the joint may be determined by probing this area with a scalpel blade. The capsular attachments may be incised or elevated as desired, allowing full exposure of the underlying sacroiliac joint as well as the adjacent osseous portions of the sacrum and ilium.

After completing the intended procedure, suction drains are placed within the depths of the wound—one within the sacral hollow, the other deep to the abdominal wall. Meticulous hemostasis is obtained. Closure is accomplished in the layered technique, repairing the aponeuroses of the abdominal muscles to the remnant of soft tissue left attached to the iliac crest during the approach.

TABLE 41–1. MALIGNANT BONE TUMORS INVOLVING THE SACROILIAC JOINT AT MEMORIAL SLOAN-KETTERING CANCER CENTER

	Five-Year Survival NED*
Ewing's sarcoma	60% (6/10)
Chondrosarcoma	67% (6/9)
Osteogenic sarcoma	25% (1/4)

*After wide surgical incision. NED = no evidence of disease.

POSTERIOR APPROACH

With the patient in the prone position, an incision is made along the posterior third of the iliac crest, curving distally at the posterosuperior iliac spine for a distance of 5 to 8 cm (Fig. 41–3). The incision is deepened to expose the iliac crest, from which the attachments of the gluteus maximus muscle and the

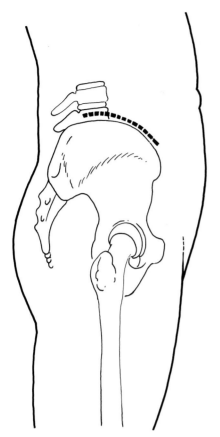

FIGURE 41–1. An incision is made parallel to and 1 cm above the iliac crest from the anterosuperior iliac spine, extending posteriorly for approximately 10 to 12 cm.

otomy of the area shown in Figure 41–6 is made, removing the iliac tuberosity to allow excellent exposure of the posterior aspect of the sacroiliac joint for its full extent.

Closure of the wound is accomplished in standard fashion. Soft tissue hemostasis is obtained using electrocautery, and bone wax is applied to the bleeding margin of the ilium. A suction catheter is placed within the depths of the wound, followed by reapproximation of the cut edges of the gluteus maximus and erector spinae muscles.

COMBINED ANTEROPOSTERIOR APPROACH

This extensive surgical dissection provides access to the posterior pelvic anatomy, allowing resection of tumors in this area (Figs. 41–7 and 41–8). It is recommended that the surgeon review the anterior and posterior approaches described above before proceeding with the study of this surgical exercise.

In any procedure of such magnitude, excellent preparation of both surgeon and patient is critical to success. It is mandatory that the operator possess a thorough familiarity with the involved anatomy. The patient must be fully informed as to the extent of the surgery and the possible complications and must be provided with a clear understanding of the goals of the procedure. A full bowel preparation is recommended. Depending on surgeon preference, the anus may be sewn. Because blood loss is generally significant, adequate amounts of replacement blood

lumbodorsal fascia are incised. The Cobb elevator is used to elevate the gluteus maximus and medius muscles in a subperiosteal fashion from the lateral surface of the ilium. As described by Hoppenfeld, the area of the posterior gluteal line is of concern,[4] and care must be exercised to closely follow the undulating contour of the ilium and to remain in the subperiosteal plane (Fig. 41–4). As the dissection continues posteriorly and inferiorly, a sponge-covered elevator or a gloved finger is used to complete the elevation of the periosteum and soft tissues, thereby affording protection for the superior gluteal vessels lying adjacent to the inferior margin of the ilium, which forms the osseous border of the greater sciatic notch (Fig. 41–5). A Taylor retractor may be used as needed to safely improve exposure. Using a curette, the outer table of the ilium overlying the area of the sacroiliac joint is removed (Fig. 41–6). The inner cortex is next windowed, using an osteotome or a curette to expose the articular cartilage of the joint, confirming correct anatomic location.

An alternative surgical approach may be considered. After exposing the lateral cortex of the iliac tuberosity by elevating the gluteus maximus muscle as described above, the posterior and medial aspects of the superior spine are freed of the attachments of the lumbodorsal fascia, the erector spinae muscles, and the posterior sacroiliac ligament. Next an oste-

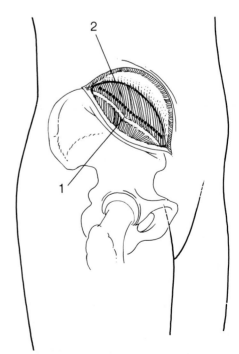

FIGURE 41–2. The inferior margin of the incision is raised to expose the iliac crest (1). The aponeuroses of the abdominal muscles (2) are released leaving a 1-cm remnant attached to the iliac crest to facilitate closure.

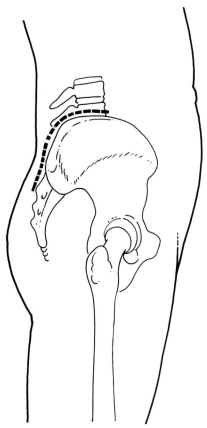

FIGURE 41–3. An incision is made along the posterior third of the iliac crest, curving distally at the posterosuperior iliac spine for a distance of 5 to 8 cm.

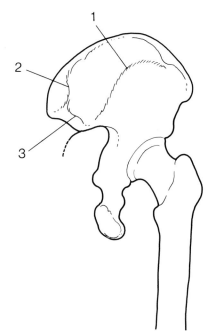

FIGURE 41–4. It is important to closely follow the undulating contour of the iliac bone in the area of the prominence, that is, the posterior gluteal line (2 and 3), to stay in the subperiosteal plane.

should be available and the anesthetist should be warned of potential excessive blood loss. Hypotensive anesthesia may be used to minimize blood loss. Urologic stents should be placed bilaterally to facilitate identification during dissection.

After placement of monitoring lines and induction of general anesthesia, the patient is placed in the lateral decubitus position. As shown in Figure 41–9, an incision is made from the anterosuperior iliac spine coursing posteriorly, remaining parallel and 1 to 1.5 cm above the margin of the iliac crest as described in the anterior approach. It is then extended medially where it is curved distally in the midline along the spinous processes of the lumbar and sacral vertebrae (Fig. 41–9). The incision is then deepened to expose the underlying aponeurosis of the external oblique muscle and the lumbodorsal fascia. The inferior margin of the incision is elevated, revealing the superior aspect of the iliac crest. The aponeurotic attachments of the internal and external oblique and transverse abdominal muscles are released using electrocautery, making certain a 1-cm remnant of aponeurosis is left attached to the crest of the ilium to facilitate closure (see Fig. 41–2). A Cobb elevator is used to strip the iliac muscle from the inner aspect of the iliac wing. Continued elevation in a posterior direction is then accomplished using a sponge-covered elevator, proceeding as far posteriorly as necessary to identify the margin of the tumor

or the prominent thickening that indicates the location of the sacroiliac joint. The greater sciatic notch is located by continued elevation in a slightly more distal direction, using a blunt technique to afford protection of the superior gluteal vessels lying adja-

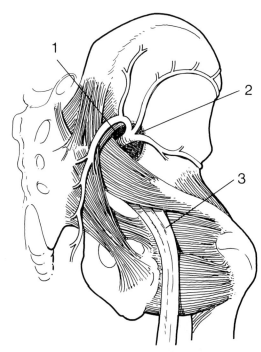

FIGURE 41–5. Caution must be exercised in the area of the greater sciatic notch (2), that area of passage of neurovascular structures exiting the pelvis posteriorly. The superior gluteal artery (1) and the sciatic nerve (3) are shown with their relationship to the piriformis muscle.

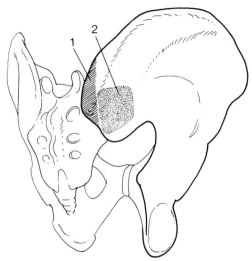

FIGURE 41–6. The sacroiliac joint may be approached laterally through the overlying area of the ilium (2) or posteriorly by osteotomizing the iliac tuberosity (1).

cent to the inferior margin of the ilium, which forms the osseous border of the greater sciatic notch (see Fig. 41–5).

At this point, attention is returned to the area of the iliac crest, from which the attachments of the gluteus maximus and lumbodorsal fascia are incised. The Cobb elevator is used to elevate the gluteus maximus and medius muscles in a subperiosteal fashion from the lateral aspect of the ilium. At the area of the posterior gluteal line, care is exercised to closely follow the undulating contour of the ilium and remain in the subperiosteal plane (see Fig. 41–4). As the dissection continues posteriorly and inferiorly, a sponge-covered elevator is used to complete the soft tissue elevation, thereby protecting the superior gluteal vessels residing within the greater

sciatic notch (see Fig. 41–5). A gloved finger may now be passed through the notch, and the superior gluteal vessels and sciatic nerve may be identified.

The posterior portion of the incision now becomes the center of attention. The sacrospinalis muscles are elevated subperiosteally from the vertebrae or are divided transversely as needed to obtain a margin around the tumor. The underlying posterior aspect of the sacrum is exposed at the site of the intended osteotomy, and hemostasis is obtained. The osteotomy is delayed until the anterior exposure is complete and packed with sponges, providing excellent protection for the anterior structures from an errant osteotome. Additionally, by delaying the osteotomy, stability is maintained until the soft tissue dissection is nearly complete and the important neurovascular structures are identified and secured.

The anterior dissection is completed by retracting the iliac and psoas muscles and the overlying abdominal viscera medially, remaining deep to the iliac muscle in an effort to protect the femoral nerve and iliac vessels. This exposure continues medially to the area of the intended sacral osteotomy. This portion of the dissection is modified as needed to maintain the desired margin around the tumor mass.

Posteriorly, again guided by tumor extent, the lateral and medial portions of the dissection are connected. Electrocautery is used to divide the gluteus maximus muscle, which is raised in continuity with the skin flap to support viability. The sacrospinous and sacrotuberous ligaments and piriformis muscle are similarly transected, with the surgeon ever aware of the sciatic nerve lying nearby (see Fig. 41–5).

The sciatic notch is exposed by retracting the anterior iliopsoas and posterior gluteal muscles in their respective directions. A gloved finger is passed through the sciatic notch, identifying and ensuring adequate mobilization of the superior gluteal vessels.

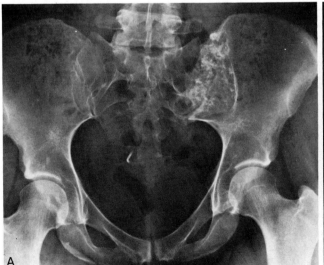
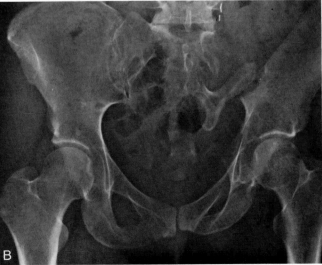

FIGURE 41–7. A, Radiograph of a 33-year-old female with a chondrosarcoma involving the left posterior iliac wing. B, Radiograph of same patient following en bloc resection of the sacroiliac joint, including adjacent portions of the ilium and sacrum.

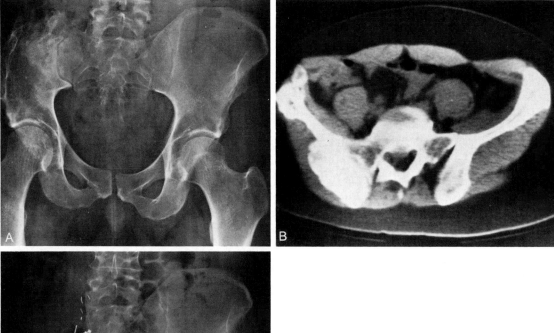

FIGURE 41–8. *A,* Radiograph of a 44-year-old male with an osteogenic sarcoma of the right posterior ilium, sacroiliac joint, and sacral ala. *B,* Computed tomographic scan showing extent of the iliac involvement. *C,* Radiograph following resection of the ilium, sacroiliac joint, and lateral sacrum.

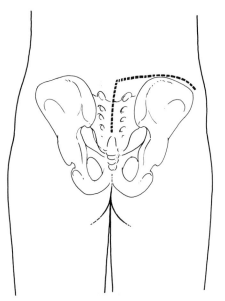

FIGURE 41–9. An incision is made parallel to and 1 cm above the iliac crest from the anterosuperior iliac spine, extending posteriorly to the midline, where it is directed inferiorly.

An Aufranc retractor is carefully placed within the notch to protect these vital structures, after which a Gigli saw is passed and the iliac osteotomy accomplished.

The anterior structures are further retracted medially, sponges are placed for protection, and the sacrum is osteotomized in the posteroanterior direction. The tumor is removed en bloc from the operative field. Osseous bleeding may be significant and is controlled with bone wax. Soft tissue hemostasis is obtained, and the area is examined for evidence of residual tumor. Involved nerve roots are identified, injected with lidocaine, and sharply incised using a scalpel. Following irrigation, drains are placed as needed within the depths of the wound.

Reconstruction is significant following this extensive resection. Posteriorly the gluteus maximus is repaired to the midline fascia if possible or is left in position to form scar tissue. Anteriorly the closure is accomplished in layers, reattaching the aponeuroses of the abdominal muscles to the remnant of the soft tissue left attached to the iliac crest during the exposure. The gluteal fascia is then repaired to the iliac

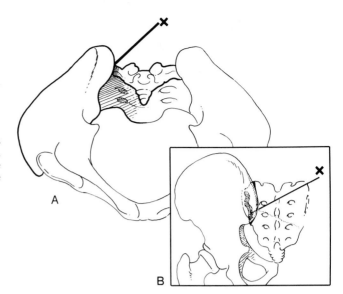

FIGURE 41–10. *A,* Direct vertical entry into the sacroiliac joint is prevented by the overlying medial projection of the iliac tuberosity. Posterior access is possible by passing a needle at a 45-degree lateral angle. *B,* The needle is angled inferiorly approaching the sacroiliac joint 0.5 to 1 cm above its inferior border.

crest in standard fashion. Skin closure is accomplished as desired. A compressive Ace wrap dressing is applied to support the soft tissues and to decrease hematoma formation.

ASPIRATION

Aspiration of the sacroiliac joint from the posterior approach was described by Miskew and colleagues in 1979.[5] The technique is complicated by the medial projection of the posterior ilium (Fig. 41–9), which makes direct vertical entry to the joint impossible. With the patient prone on a radiographic operating table, the area is prepared in sterile fashion, and the midline is anesthetized locally at the level of the midpoint of the sacroiliac joint as confirmed by the image intensifier. An 18-gauge spinal needle is inserted at a 45-degree lateral angle as shown in Figure 41–10A, passing deep to the iliac tuberosity. Using image intensification, the needle is angled inferiorly as needed to approach the joint 0.5 to 1 cm above its inferior border (Fig. 41–10B). Aspiration is then performed, sterile saline is injected, followed by re-aspiration if no specimen is retrieved on the initial attempt.

REFERENCES

1. Avila L Jr: Primary pyogenic infection of the sacro-iliac articulation. A new approach to the joint. Report of seven cases. J Bone Joint Surg 23:922–928, 1941.
2. Crenshaw AH: Surgical approaches. *In* Edmonson AS, Crenshaw AH (eds): Campbell's Operative Orthopaedics. 6th ed. St. Louis, C. V. Mosby, 1980, pp 80–81.
3. Enneking WF: Musculoskeletal Tumor Surgery. New York, Churchill Livingstone, 1983, pp 338–354 and pp 494–501.
4. Hoppenfeld S, de Boer P: Surgical Exposures in Orthopaedics—The Anatomic Approach. Philadelphia, J. B. Lippincott, 1984.
5. Miskew DB, Block RA, Witt PF: Aspiration of infected sacroiliac joints. J Bone Joint Surg 61A:1071–1072, 1979.
6. Simon MA: Biopsy and local resection of the pelvis. *In* Evarts CM (ed): Surgery of the Musculoskeletal System. Vol 2. New York, Churchill Livingstone, 1983, pp 52–53.

TECHNIQUE OF COMPLETE SPONDYLECTOMY IN THE THORACIC AND LUMBAR SPINE

BERTIL STENER

INTRODUCTION

The term complete spondylectomy (or vertebrectomy) is used to describe the removal of all parts of one or more vertebrae. Above the sacrum, the author has performed complete spondylectomy for extirpation of tumors in eight patients; the first operation was carried out in May, 1968. The following description of the technique of complete spondylectomy in three different regions of the spine is based on this experience.

REMOVAL OF MIDDLE THORACIC VERTEBRAE INCLUDING CONSIDERABLE PARTS OF ADJACENT VERTEBRAE

If a malignant tumor, originating in the body of a middle thoracic vertebra, protrudes anteriorly into the mediastinum so that it extends over the adjacent bodies, then it may be suitable to include in the surgical specimen the anteroinferior half of the vertebral body above and the anterosuperior half of the vertebral body below the originally affected vertebra. With such oblique transvertebral osteotomies, it is possible to avoid entering the tumor. A technique will be described for the removal of the whole of T7 and about half of T6 and T8 (Fig. 42–1).

The whole operation can be performed from behind with the patient in the prone position. Using the incision illustrated in Figure 42–1B, a flap is raised bilaterally, consisting of skin, subcutaneous tissue, and the underlying trapezius, rhomboids, and latissimus dorsi muscles. The erector spinae muscles are detached from the spinous processes, the laminae, and the medial part of the transverse processes of T3 to T10 on both sides; they are then severed transversely, level with T7. The dural sac is exposed by removal of the spinous process and the inferior articular processes of T6; by removal of the spinous process, the lamina, the superior and inferior artic-

ular processes, and the transverse processes of T7; and by removal of the superior articular processes of T8 (Fig. 42–1A). Both pleural cavities are then opened by resecting the seventh rib bilaterally from the costotransverse joint to the midaxillary line. To gain adequate exposure within the thorax, the fifth, sixth, and eighth ribs are transected just lateral to the costotransverse joint, with care taken not to damage unnecessarily the intercostal nerves and vessels. After dissecting adjacent mediastinal organs free from the tumor, the intervertebral discs between T5 and T6 and between T8 and T9 are exposed. Then starting at the anterior edge of these discs, oblique osteotomies are done through the bodies of T6 and T8; using a Gigli saw, the osteotomy is directed posteroinferiorly through the body of T6 and posterosuperiorly through the body of T8 (Fig. 42–1A). The last part of the osteotomy is performed with a chisel directed transversely from one side to the other. Thereby the specimen (Fig. 42–1C) becomes loose and can be pushed forward enough to allow one of the pedicles of the vertebra to pass anterior to the spinal cord, while the entire specimen is taken out through one of the thoracotomy openings.

Reconstruction of the spine is performed according to Figure 42–1A. ASIF plates with twelve holes, having been bent to fit the thoracic curve, are fastened, one on each side of the spinous processes, with double 1-mm-thick stainless steel wires to the transverse processes of T3 to T6 and T8 to T10. At the upper and lower ends the plates are secured to each other by wires. Thereafter, one corticocancellous block of bone is taken from the posterior part of each ilium using separate incisions. The blocks are given the form illustrated in Figure 42–1A (bottom right), and they are inserted side by side between T6 and T8. By pressing them posteriorly a good contact is obtained between the obliquely cut ends and the obliquely cut vertebral bodies. A transverse bore-hole is made through the superior and inferior ends of the blocks and through the bodies of T5 and T9. Via

432

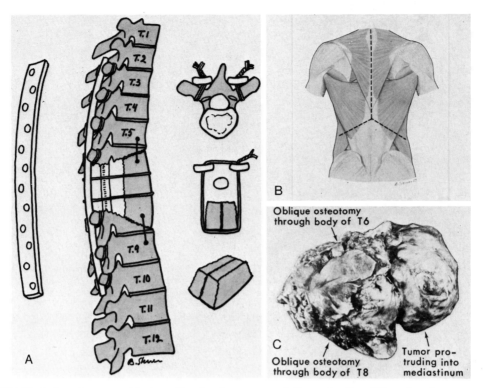

FIGURE 42–1. Complete spondylectomy for chondrosarcoma. *A,* Reconstruction of the spine after removal of the anteroinferior half of the body, the inferior articular processes, and the spinous process of T6, all of T7, and the anterosuperior half of the body and the superior articular processes of T8. Two ASIF plates have been fastened with double steel wires to the transverse processes of T3 to T6 and of T8 to T10. Two iliac bone-blocks with obliquely cut ends have been put together and inserted between the obliquely cut bodies of T6 and T8. The blocks have been fastened to the spine with silk threads passed through holes in the blocks and the vertebrae. Further fixation has been provided by two steel wires fastened to the plates and gripping the bone-blocks. *B,* Interrupted lines indicate incisions by which a flap could be raised on either side, consisting not only of the skin and subcutaneous tissue but also the underlying trapezius, rhomboids, and latissimus dorsi muscles. *C,* Right aspect of the surgical specimen. The tumor protruded from the body of T7 not only anteriorly and to either side but also posteriorly into the spinal canal (not visible here). The patient is still well after 20 years. (*A* from Stener B: Total spondylectomy in chondrosarcoma arising from the seventh thoracic vertebra. J Bone Joint Surg 23B:288–295, 1971.)

these bore-holes the blocks are fastened to the spine with sutures of nonabsorbable material. Further fixation is provided by two steel wires gripping around the anterior cortical surface of the blocks and fastened to the steel plates. The wires are tightened so that the cancellous surfaces meeting at the superior and inferior ends of the blocks are pressed firmly together.

After reconstruction of the spine, two suction tubes are inserted into each pleural cavity, one anteriorly and one posteriorly. The thoracotomy wounds are closed, and the trapezius, rhomboids, and latissimus dorsi muscles are reattached to the spine. After completion of the operation it is advisable to put the patient in a bed allowing convenient changing of position, prone to supine and vice versa (e.g., a Stryker or a Circle-Electric bed).

REMOVAL OF LOW THORACIC VERTEBRAE AND THE FIRST, SECOND, AND THIRD LUMBAR VERTEBRAE

At all these levels the whole operation can be performed from behind in one stage with the patient in the prone position; the author has removed T11, T12, L1, L2, and L3 in six patients. It is important that the patient is positioned to avoid compression of the inferior vena cava.

A suitable incision for removal of L3 is illustrated in Figure 42–2A; a similar incision is used for other levels. The erector spinae muscles are exposed by raising, on each side, a flap consisting of skin, subcutaneous tissue, and the aponeurotic part of the thoracolumbar fascia. The erector spinae muscles are completely detached from the spine so that they can be retracted laterally while working on the posterior elements of the vertebrae (central arrows in Fig. 42–2B), and medially while exposing bilaterally the vertebral bodies, the aorta, and the vena cava (lateral arrows in Figure 42–2B). It is advisable to ligate and divide, at a safe distance from their origin, the segmental arteries and veins at the affected level and the two adjacent levels.

The continued technique is illustrated in Figure 42–3A–G, which shows a complete spondylectomy of L1. The dural sac is exposed by removing those posterior elements of the affected vertebra that are free from tumor (Fig. 42–3C). For better exposure it is usually necessary to also remove parts of the

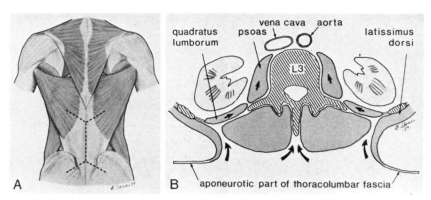

FIGURE 42–2. Posterior approach for complete spondylectomy (L3). *A,* Interrupted lines indicate incisions through the skin, the subcutaneous tissue, and the aponeurotic part of the thoracolumbar fascia. The angles formed between the midline incision and the lateral extensions are 120 degrees. The superior lateral extension divides the latissimus dorsi muscles more or less in their fiber direction. By raising the two flaps the underlying erector spine muscles are exposed as shown in *B. B,* Diagrammatic transection level with L3. Once the erector spinae muscles have been detached from the spine, they can be retracted laterally to expose the posterior elements of the spine (*middle arrows*) and medially to expose the vertebral bodies from both sides, which is done by transecting the quadratus lumborum and psoas muscles (*lateral arrows*). The patient is in the prone position during the whole operation. This approach was used in the case illustrated in Figure 42–5. (From Stener B: Complete removal of vertebrae for extirpation of tumors—a sixteen year experience. Clin Orthop 245:72–82, 1989.)

posterior elements of the adjacent vertebrae (Fig. 42–3*D* and *E*). If the nature of the tumor indicates performing the spondylectomy with wide margins, it is advisable to ligate and divide the spinal nerve roots at the tumor level close to their exit from the dural sac. An osteotomy is then performed through the vertebral bodies above (Fig. 42–3*C*) and below the affected vertebra so that the discs confining the lesion are included in the specimen. Once the two transvertebral osteotomies have been performed, the specimen is gently removed (arrow in Fig. 42–3*C*), with care taken not to damage the contents of the dural sac.

After removal of the specimen, the spine is reconstructed using the method illustrated in Figures 42–3*D* and *E* and 42–4*A*–*C*. Approaching from the right and using a handsaw, a groove is made inferiorly in the vertebral body above the gap and superiorly in the vertebral body below the gap. After diminishing the gap somewhat, three corticocancellous blocks of bone from the posterior ilium, as shown in Figure 42–4*A*, are inserted and fixed with three screws. With the patient in the prone position, the large, match-box-like graft is inserted into the grooves obliquely from the right, and the screws are inserted obliquely from the left (Figs. 42–3*D* and *E* and 42–4*B*). Strips of cancellous bone, omitted in the drawings, are placed outside the reconstructed part of the spine (Fig. 42–3*F* and *G*). Posteriorly, metallic fixation is used above and below the inserted graft. Meurig-Williams plates, fastened to spinous processes as shown in Figures 42–3 and 42–4, have been used successfully in two cases (T11 and L1), but in a third case (L3) we used ASIF plates to obtain good immediate stability. Plates with 12 holes were placed in the sagittal plane, one on each side of several spinous processes above and below the resected part of the spine. The plates were wired to the spinous processes

in such an oblique way that the tightening of the wires resulted in axial compression of the inserted grafts (Fig. 42–5).

The described use of corticocancellous iliac grafts for reconstruction of the spine has consistently resulted in the formation of a block-vertebra, allowing vertical loading after about four months.

REMOVAL OF THE FOURTH LUMBAR VERTEBRA

For complete removal of the fouth lumbar vertebra it is advisable to use both an anterior and a posterior approach. There are two reasons for this: one is the close relation of the lower lumbar spine to the large vessels (aorta, vena cava, common iliac arteries, and veins); the other is the hindrance caused by the iliac wings in exposing the body of L5 from behind.

Figure 42–6 illustrates a technique for complete spondylectomy of L4 which was successful for total removal of a giant cell tumor. The biologic behavior of these tumors allows such intralesional surgery. The operation was performed in two stages: first through an anterior approach and then, four weeks later, through a posterior approach. For the anterior approach a large V-shaped incision (Fig. 42–6*B*) was made through the abdominal wall down to the parietal peritoneum, which was pushed away for exposure of the aorta, the vena cava, and the common iliac arteries and veins. The large myocutaneous flap, with the underlying viscera enclosed in the peritoneal sac, was retracted to the left while working on the right side and to the right while working on the left side. After ligation and division of the third, fourth, and fifth lumbar arteries and veins on both sides, a space was dissected free between the large vessels and the lower lumbar spine. Thus released, the aorta

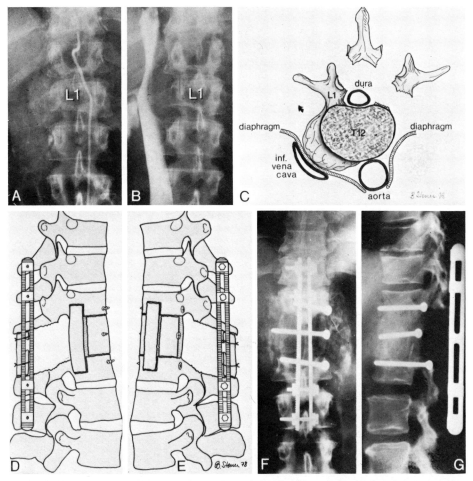

FIGURE 42–3. Complete spondylectomy for metastasis or renal cancer. As revealed by late phase of aortography (*A*), the tumor has expanded outside the affected vertebra (L1) on the right side, making an impression in the inferior vena cava (*B*). The right crus of the diaphragm, located between the tumor and the vena cava (*C*), facilitated removal of the whole of L1, including the adjacent discs and parts of T12 and L2, without damaging the vein. The spinous process, lamina, and left pedicle were free from tumor and could be removed separately to allow extraction of the specimen (*arrow*) without damaging the dural sac with its contents. *D* and *E,* The spine was reconstructed using three corticocancellous blocks of iliac bone. The largest graft, formed as a matchbox, was placed obliquely in grooves made inferiorly in the body of T12 and superiorly in the body of L2; it was inserted posteriorly on the right side (*D*) and came out anteriorly on the left side (*E*). The three grafts were fixed with three screws inserted posteriorly on the left side (*E*). Meurig-Williams plates were used for posterior fixation; pieces of rib were placed between them for creating a bony bridge between the spinous processes of T12 and L2. *F* and *G,* Pieces of cancellous iliac bone were placed outside the inserted grafts as visible on radiographs taken 4 weeks after operation. The reconstruction of the spine resulted in a block-vertebra that permitted ambulation after 4 months. Unfortunately, the patient died from metastases after 15 months. (From Stener B, Henriksson C, Johansson S, et al: Surgical removal of bone and muscle metastases of renal cancer. Acta Orthop Scand 55:491–500, 1984.)

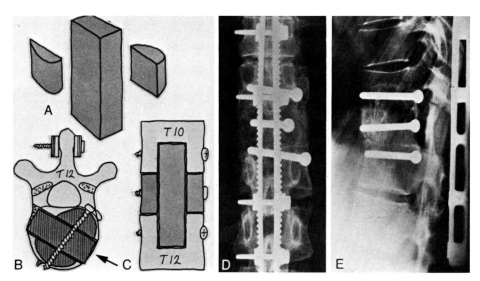

FIGURE 42–4. Complete spondylectomy for giant cell tumor. *A–C,* Reconstruction of the spine after complete removal of T11, including the adjacent discs and parts of T10 and T12. Three corticocancellous blocks of iliac bone (*A*) were inserted between the bodies of T10 and T12 and were fixed by three screws (*B*) and (*C*). In *B* the grafts have been transected level with the screw used to hold them together. The aspect of the vertebral bodies and grafts in *C* is indicated by an arrow. (For the sake of simplicity the posterior parts of the vertebrae have been omitted.) With the patient in the prone position, the large graft was inserted obliquely from the right and the screws obliquely from the left. Meurig-Williams plates were fastened to the spinous processes above and below the resected part of the spine. Strips of cancellous iliac bone (omitted in the figures) were placed outside the inserted grafts, laterally and anteriorly. *D* and *E,* Roentgenograms two years after operation. *D,* Anteroposterior view (see *B*); *E,* lateral view. The bone grafts have formed a block-vertebra with the remaining parts of the bodies of T10 and T12. The patient, who gave birth to a child 3½ years after the operation, remains well after 14 years. (*A–C* from Stener B: Total spondylectomy for removal of a giant cell tumor in the eleventh thoracic vertebra. Spine 2:197–201, 1977. *D* and *E* from Stener B: Complete removal of vertebrae for extirpation of tumors—a 20-year experience. Clin Orthop 245:72–82, 1989.)

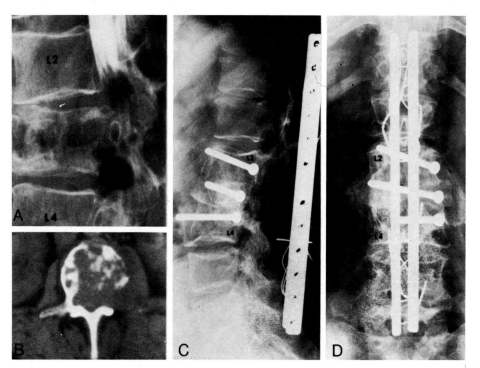

FIGURE 42–5. Complete spondylectomy for chordoma. The tumor has grown outside the body of L3 as revealed by myelography (*A*) and computed tomography (*B*). After removal of the whole of L3 and parts of L2 and L4, the spine was reconstructed by inserting iliac bone grafts anteriorly, using the method illustrated in Figure 42–4*A–C,* and by wiring ASIF plates to spinous processes posteriorly in such an oblique way that the tightening of the wires resulted in axial compression. *C* and *D,* Roentgenograms 15 months after operation. A block-vertebra has been created by the grafts and the remaining parts of L2 and L4. The patient is still free of evidence of tumor after 8 years. (From Stener B: Surgical treatment of giant cell tumors, chondrosarcomas, and chordomas of the spine. *In* Uhtoff H (ed): Current Concepts of Diagnosis and Treatment of Bone and Soft Tissue Tumors. Berlin, Springer-Verlag, 1984, pp 233–242.)

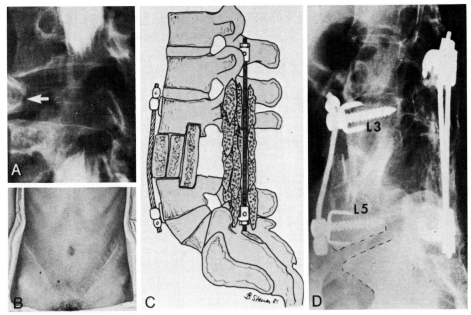

FIGURE 42–6. Complete spondylectomy for giant cell tumor. *A,* The lumen and the dural sac have been obliterated by the tumor, which has destroyed the body of L4 almost completely; a small remaining part *(arrow)* is displaced anteriorly. *B,* Postoperative scar indicates anterior extraperitoneal approach. *C,* After removal of the whole of L4 and parts of L3 and L5, the spine was reconstructed using corticocancellous iliac bone-blocks and a Dwyer tension wire anteriorly, and strips of cancellous iliac bone and a Harrington compression rod on both sides posteriorly. *D,* Roentgenogram two years after operation. Fusion has occurred between the bone grafts and the remaining parts of L3 and L5. The patient, who remains well after 9 years, has borne three children after the operation, and works as a dentist's nurse. (From Stener B: Surgical treatment of giant cell tumors, chondrosarcomas, and chordomas of the spine. *In* Uhtoff H (ed): Current Concepts of Diagnosis and Treatment of Bone and Soft Tissue Tumors. Berlin, Springer-Verlag, 1984, pp 233–242.)

and the vena cava could be retracted to either side as required for suitable exposure. The diseased body of L4 was then removed along with the adjacent intervertebral discs. Corticocancellous blocks of iliac bone, easily available through the anterior approach from the inside of the pelvic wings, were inserted between the bodies of L3 and L5 (Fig. 42–6C). The largest bone block, formed as a matchbox, was inserted in the coronal plane in grooves made inferiorly in the body of L3 and superiorly in the body of L5. For fixation of the blocks, axial compression was achieved using a Dwyer tension wire (Fig. 42–6C). During the posterior approach all remaining parts of L4 and some posterior parts of L3 and L5 were removed along with all residual tumor. Strips of cancellous iliac bone were placed on each side along a Harrington compression rod joining L2 to L5 (Fig. 42–6C). After both the anterior and posterior operations, the patient was placed in a bed allowing convenient turning without jeopardizing the reconstruction of the spine.

We have only used this technique for the removal of a giant cell tumor. If L4 is affected by a tumor, a chordoma for instance, which must be removed without being exposed in any place, let alone being entered, the described technique must be modified as required for achieving a suitable margin. It is advisable in this case to start with the posterior approach for removal of the posterior elements of L4 that are free from tumor, as illustrated in Figure 42–3C.

REFERENCES

1. Stener B: Total spondylectomy in chondrosarcoma arising from the seventh thoracic vertebra. J Bone Joint Surg 23B:288–295, 1971.
2. Stener B: Resección de columna en el tratamiento de los tumores vertebrales. Acta Orthop Latinoam 1:189–199, 1974.
3. Stener B: Total spondylectomy for removal of a giant-cell tumor in the eleventh thoracic vertebra. Spine 2:197–201, 1977.
4. Stener B: Surgical treatment of giant cell tumors, chondrosarcomas, and chordomas of the spine. *In* Uhtoff H (ed): Current Concepts of Diagnosis and Treatment of Bone and Soft Tissue Tumors. Berlin, Springer-Verlag, 1984, pp 233–242.
5. Stener B: Complete removal of vertebrae for extirpation of tumors—a 20-year experience. Clinic Orthop 245:72–82, 1989.
6. Stener B, Henriksson C, Johansson S, et al: Surgical removal of bone and muscle metastases of renal cancer. Acta Orthop Scand 55:491–500, 1984.
7. Stener B, Johnsen OE: Complete removal of three vertebrae for giant-cell tumour. J Bone Joint Surg 53B:278–287, 1971.

43

COMPLETE SPONDYLECTOMY FOR MALIGNANT TUMORS

NARAYAN SUNDARESAN, GEORGE V. DiGIACINTO, GEORGE KROL, and JAMES E. O. HUGHES

INTRODUCTION

Primary osseous tumors are relatively rare and account for less than 0.5 per cent of all cancers. The American Cancer Society estimates that approximately 1000 malignant neoplasms of bone are diagnosed annually each year.[1] The majority of primary malignant bone tumors involve the appendicular skeleton, and less than 10 per cent originate from the axial skeleton (ribs, spine, and pelvis). In addition to primary neoplasms, the spine is a frequent site of metastatic disease. In these patients, a small proportion have no areas of involvement other than the vertebrae.[24, 25] Surgical resection of solitary (or even multiple metastatic tumors) is traditionally advocated in patients for selected anatomic sites such as the lung, liver, and brain,[14] and this has resulted in long-term palliation and occasional cures. However, such an approach for solitary metastases involving the spine has never been considered. This is largely because the goal of total tumor resection is believed to be impossible, and thus surgery has been performed mainly for neural decompression and pain relief.[12, 15]

Over the past two decades, improvements in imaging techniques as well as in combined modality treatments for a variety of malignant bone tumors (such as osteosarcoma) have considerably improved the prognosis for patients with tumors originating in the extremities.[9, 12, 13, 17] As a result, it is standard practice to perform wide local excision or radical compartmental resection of most malignant tumors and to reconstruct large segmental skeletal defects with the use of allografts.[10] In combination with systemic chemotherapy, such strategies have resulted in improved survival and quality of life in most patients with malignant bone tumors. Unfortunately, these improvements have had little impact on the prognosis of patients when the spine is involved.

It is generally accepted that complete surgical removal of all gross disease is the minimal prerequisite for cure[9, 17, 27]; this entails removal of all parts of a single or contiguous vertebra for tumors involving the spine. The term *spondylectomy* is used to indicate complete surgical removal of all parts of one or more vertebrae above the sacrum. The first spondylectomy was performed by Lievre and colleagues[8] in 1966 for a giant cell tumor of the lumbar spine. In the first stage, a laminectomy was performed for neural decompression. Two weeks later, the body of the vertebra was removed. In 1968, Stener and Johnsen removed portions of three vertebrae (T11, T12, and L1) for a giant cell tumor of the spine.[20] Since then, several sporadic reports of the procedure for the treatment of a variety of malignant tumors have been reported in the literature.[6, 19, 21–23, 29] These earlier reports suggest that complete resection of a vertebra is not only technically feasible but also appropriate local treatment for patients with primary malignant neoplasms and for selected cases of metastases. In this chapter, we describe our technique of spondylectomy for malignant tumors involving the true vertebra, which we have successfully carried out in 16 patients.

GENERAL CONSIDERATIONS

The spine consists of four major segments: cervical, thoracic, lumbar, and sacrococcygeal. Although a major principle in tumor surgery is resection of the tumor in one piece without violation of its capsule (using wide local excision or marginal excision), only tumors below S1 can safely be removed using the technique of high sacral amputation. Elsewhere in the true vertebra, the close proximity of the dura and neural elements precludes safe en bloc excision. In the cervical region, an additional technical impediment to en bloc resection is the presence of the vertebral arteries. For these reasons, we recommend that spondylectomy should be carried out in stages. Adequate radiographic evaluation of the local tumor by computed tomography (CT) and magnetic resonance imaging (MRI) scans, as well as appropriate systemic staging by CT scans of the chest and abdomen and radionuclide bone scans, are indicated for high grade tumors. Since the majority of primary spine tumors and some metastatic tumors (such as kidney cancer) are hypervascular, we recommend the use of selective spinal angiography and presurgical embolization to reduce intraoperative blood loss.

Most tumors of the spine involve the anterior elements predominantly, with extension into the soft tissues anteriorly and into the epidural space posteriorly; varying degrees of involvement of the middle column (facets, pedicles) and posterior elements may be seen. Careful anatomic delineation of tumor extent must be sought by evaluation of high quality MRI studies. We believe that the extent of abnormal signal represents actual microscopic tumor involvement. In pretreated patients, the use of gadolinium-enhanced scans is recommended to differentiate tumor from fibrosis or scar.

If a solitary lesion of the spine is the presenting feature of malignancy, the radiologic distinction between a primary and metastatic tumor (or even infection) may be impossible to make. A biopsy may often be required prior to more definitive therapy, and planning of this procedure is required. At present, it is customary to perform CT-guided needle biopsies in most centers as the initial procedure; whereas accurate histologic diagnoses in up to 80 per cent of needle biopsies have been reported, our experience with this procedure is less optimistic. If open biopsy is decided upon, the approach should be carefully planned and careful attention should be paid to asepsis, skin-handling, hemostasis, and wound closure.[11] The skin incision should be placed so as not to compromise subsequent surgery; in this regard, we strongly urge that decompressive laminectomy *not* be performed, since this makes subsequent reconstruction more difficult. An anterior approach should be used for resection in the first stage, since most tumors predominantly involve the anterior elements. A unilateral approach to the spine (except in the cervical segments) does not allow complete resection of the vertebral body because the dura does not permit complete access to the opposite posterolateral corner. Thus a subtotal resection of the body is performed initially, leaving behind a thin shell of cortex and cancellous bone that is beyond reach from a unilateral approach (Fig. 43–1). Tumor resection is performed by intralesional curettage using a variety of specially designed spinal curettes and rongeurs as well as a high speed drill. This technique results in violation of the tumor pseudocapsule, since resection is carried out piecemeal. During the initial Stage 1 spondylectomy, it is important to resect enough of the vertebral body so that the second or posterior stage can be used to complete the resection. Following resection, stabilization is carried out, and the tumor is histologically analyzed. If a low grade aggressive tumor, such as giant cell tumor, is found, the second stage may be carried out within two weeks depending on patient recovery from the initial operation. With the advent of effective systemic chemotherapy for high grade malignant tumors, we believe that the second stage of spondylectomy should be delayed until several cycles of chemotherapy are completed to minimize the risk of tumor dissemination. This strategy—using chemotherapy prior to definitive surgery—is termed neoadjuvant chemotherapy and has proved to be an extremely important strategy in the management of bone sarcomas.

Stage 1 Spondylectomy: Anterior Phase

In the thoracic and lumbar regions, the initial surgical procedure and approach should be planned on the basis of CT scans and MRI. In the thoracic segments, a posterolateral thoracotomy with resection of the involved rib is used; in the lumbar regions, a retroperitoneal flank approach is used. After exposure of the anterior spine, the involved vertebral body is carefully isolated from the rest of the soft tissues and vascular structures by lap pads to minimize tumor spillage into the operative site. If the tumor is purely intraosseous, radiologic confirmation of the correct vertebral level should be obtained prior to osteotomy of the vertebral body. In most cases,

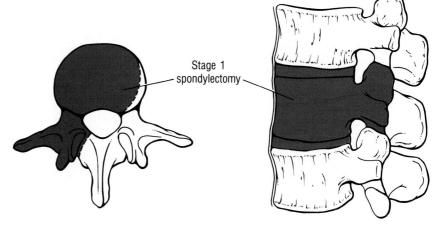

FIGURE 43–1. Line diagram illustrating planned subtotal resection of the vertebral body, pedicle, and facet (*shaded area*) during Stage I spondylectomy.

Stage 1 spondylectomy

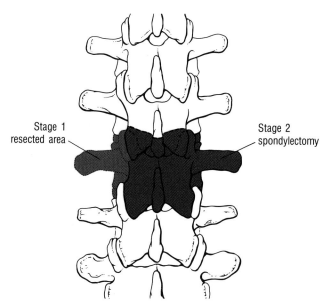

FIGURE 43–2. Line diagram illustrating the proposed resection of posterior elements during the Stage 2 posterior approach.

the tumor can be seen by its soft tissue extension either anterior or anterolateral to the body of the vertebra.

The initial surgical strategy should be to define the superior and inferior limits of normal anatomy, that is, the intervertebral discs. For intraosseous tumors, a small cortical window (1 cm × 1 cm) is then made with osteotomes, and the soft tissue portion of the tumor is removed by intralesional curettage. At all times, suction tips under high pressure are used within the cortical window, and every effort should be made to prevent spillage of gross tumor into the surrounding soft tissues. Frequently, the soft tissue tumor may be multifocal within bone with islands of

harder bony trabeculae. These bony trabeculae should be removed with curettes and rongeurs. Once all soft tissue tumor has been removed, the rest of the vertebral body is removed by a combination of rongeurs and high speed drill. Dissection should carefully proceed toward the dura. Finally, removal of the posterior longitudinal ligament should be carried out to remove tumor adjacent to the dura. This may require sharp dissection with microinstruments as well as the use of small Kerrison punches. More tenacious tumors may require the use of the Cavitron ultrasonic tumor aspirator. *Posteriorly* the resection should include the *pedicle and superior facet* on the side of operation. In the thoracic region, the pedicle is generally hidden by the head of the rib. The most important aspect of this procedure is to remove enough of the vertebral body at the Stage 1 procedure so that the rest of the body can be removed by a subsequent posterior procedure (Fig. 43–2).

Following tumor resection, stabilization is carried out with either polymethyl methacrylate or an iliac strut graft. If the histology of the tumor is clearly known to be benign, autologous bone grafts are preferable. If the use of radiation therapy is required in the postoperative period, we prefer to use methyl methacrylate for the immediate stability that it affords. The methacrylate is allowed to polymerize in situ and is held in place by Steinmann pins straddling the intact segments above and below (Fig. 43–3). A variety of other anterior devices to provide distraction, such as Knodt or Harrington rods, as well as a variety of anterior plates have also been recommended to augment stability, but we have rarely found them necessary. Wound closure is carried out in routine fashion.

Postoperatively, patients should be ambulated early (within 48 hours) and are fitted with a prefabricated brace for comfort. The extent of resection is evaluated by CT scans and MRI.

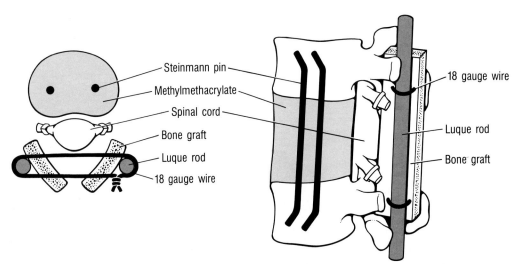

FIGURE 43–3. Line drawings illustrating completed spondylectomy and reconstruction. For malignant tumors, anterior reconstruction is carried out with methyl methacrylate, and posterior stabilization is achieved with bone grafts and Luque rods using segmental fixation. Posterior fixation may be carried out with a variety of stabilization devices including Cotrel-Dubousset instrumentation.

Stage 2 Spondylectomy: Posterior Phase

The second phase of the spondylectomy is performed within weeks if the patient has a benign aggressive tumor or a radioresistant tumor such as kidney cancer or chondrosarcoma. If the patient has a high grade sarcoma, it is preferable to delay the second stage until several cycles of chemotherapy are completed. Accurate staging studies are required to document localized disease before completing the second stage.

For the posterior phase, patients are positioned prone, although a semiprone position may be used. A long midline incision is extended horizontally (Fig. 43–4) across the involved segments. If the patient has received prior radiation therapy, the midline should be avoided, and a paramedian skin incision approximately 3 inches off midline is used and the flaps raised. At least three spinal segments above and below the site of involvement should be dissected subperiosteally. Careful intraoperative radiographic control is used to restrict removal of posterior elements to the pathologically involved lamina and spine. The intraspinous ligaments are carefully bitten off with rongeurs, and the involved lamina and spine are removed piecemeal using rongeurs. Removal of the superior articular facets bilaterally is facilitated by removal of the overhanging portion of the inferior facet of the vertebra above. Once the posterior elements are removed, the paraspinal muscles are transsected or retracted, and the rest of the vertebral body is removed. When the spondylectomy is complete, it should be possible to visualize the dura circumferentially without bony remnants. Using a dental mir-

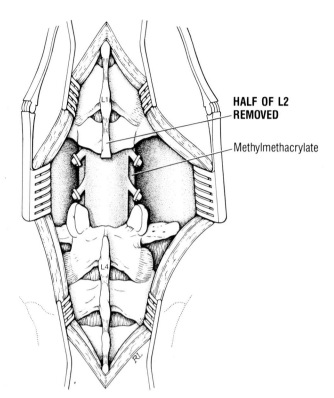

FIGURE 43–5. Completion of posterior resection; note that there is no remaining bone around the dura circumferentially. Nerve roots should be carefully isolated and clipped to prevent cerebrospinal fluid leakage.

ror, care should be taken to ensure that there are no bone or tumor remnants around the dura (Fig. 43–5).

Following tumor resection, the final phase consists of stabilizing the spine with a combination of instrumentation and bone grafts. At present, we prefer to use Luque rods with segmental sublaminar wiring two segments above and below the level of involvement. Heavy double 18-gauge wires or single 16-gauge wires are used for segmental fixation. In addition to the Luque rods, corticocancellous bone is harvested from the iliac crest and laid parallel to either side of the spine to reconstruct the posterior elements. These are wired in place to the Luque rods (Fig. 43–6). Chips of cancellous bone are laid down to also enhance the fusion. Wounds are then closed with suction drains. We generally allow early ambulation in a molded clam-shell jacket. Intraoperative and perioperative broad-spectrum antibiotics are used during surgery. If the dura was inadvertently opened, drainage by the suction drains should continue until the skin flaps seal.

Whereas Luque rods are versatile and generally easy to use, newer forms of instrumentation such as the Cotrel-Dubousset or Universal instrumentation are currently advocated because they allow more stable fixation.[3] Clearly the choice of instrumentation would depend upon the level of fixation, the need for corrective distractive or compressive forces as well as for contouring the implant to maintain physiologic spinal curvatures, and the discretion of the

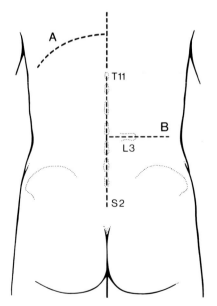

FIGURE 43–4. Skin incisions used for posterior Stage 2 spondylectomy. Lateral exposure is enhanced by extending the midline incisions in a transverse direction, as shown in the dotted lines A and B. At all times, skin incisions should be placed to avoid radiation portals. In preirradiated patients, paramedian skin incisions should be used.

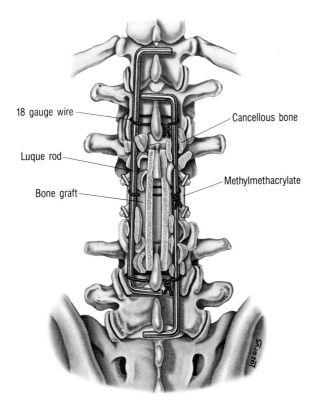

18 gauge wire

Luque rod

Bone graft

Cancellous bone

Methylmethacrylate

FIGURE 43–6. Diagram showing posterior fixation with L-shaped Luque rods and bone graft (sublaminar wiring not shown in the diagram). A combination of corticocancellous struts and cancellous chips is used for posterior reconstruction.

surgeon. Facility with a wide variety of instrumentation systems is required to determine the optimal system for each patient.

DISCUSSION

Our experience suggests that local control and long-term disease-free survival are possible in patients with malignant tumors of the spine if spondylectomy is considered part of the treatment strategy. In the past, spine tumors have been considered unresectable, with surgical efforts limited to intralesional curettage through laminectomy approaches.[2] Therefore, it is not surprising that such procedures have resulted in high rates of local recurrence (exceeding 80 per cent), with the majority of patients dying from complications secondary to paraplegia.[25] Since the histology of the tumors in our series is diverse, it is not possible to compare the length of survival of our patients with a similar group. However, a review of the literature suggests that the median survival time ranges from 6 to 8 months when either primary or metastatic tumors involve the spine. In the two largest series of osteosarcoma arising in the spine, the median survival time was 6 months, but there was an occasional long-term survivor; complete resection of the tumor was not accomplished in any patient.[2, 15] In patients with dedifferentiated chondrosarcoma, the reported median

survival time was 8 months, and the two-year survival rate ranged from 0 to 20 per cent.[5, 7] In patients with adenocarcinoma from an occult primary site, the reported median survival time ranged from 3 to 8 months.[16] Although the prognosis of breast cancer patients with exclusively osseous metastases is favorable, the prognosis is considerably poorer when the spinal cord is involved. In such patients, the median survival time is approximately 6 months, although 10 to 15 per cent live much longer with effective treatment. Similarly, when patients with kidney cancer are treated by palliative radiation therapy or laminectomy, the reported median survival time following the onset of spine metastases is approximately 6 months. With our approach, we have been able to extend the median survival in a diverse group of malignancies to more than 2 years, with 25 per cent of patients living for 5 years. Many patients have required reoperation for tumor recurrences either locally or elsewhere, but all patients have remained ambulatory with satisfactory pain relief. Our experience with spondylectomy corroborates the pioneering work of Stener,[23] who reported eight patients treated with spondylectomy for a variety of bone malignancies, including chordoma, giant cell tumor, and chondrosarcoma. In all of his patients, long-term disease-free survival was achieved.

Our spondylectomy technique differs from that of Stener in several aspects. During the anterior resection, reconstruction of the vertebral body is carried out with methyl methacrylate rather than with bone grafts. A major advantage of methyl methacrylate is that immediate stability is ensured, thus allowing the patient to walk early in the postoperative period. In addition, postoperative radiation therapy can be given safely without weakening the methyl methacrylate construct. If bone grafts are used, radiation therapy would result in nonunion of the graft and a failed fusion. Our experience suggests that the long-term use of methyl methacrylate and instrumentation is not associated with late mechanical failure unless the tumor recurs in the adjacent vertebra. We also prefer a staged procedure rather than the single-stage operation advocated by Stener. Staging the operation minimizes the possibility of neurologic deficit resulting from ischemic damage. Although the spinal cord has an ample collateral supply from the intercostal and lumbar vessels, the thoracic region is a potential watershed zone and is therefore potentially vulnerable if the feeding intercostal vessels are ligated bilaterally. Selective spinal angiography should be performed both to visualize the segmental supply of the spinal cord and to identify hypervascular tumors. The risk of neurologic deficit from spinal angiography in experienced medical centers is less than 2 per cent, and our experience suggests that presurgical embolization is associated with a similar low risk.

Since our technique evolved over several years, the number of patients requiring multiple operations in this series is considerable. We originally assumed that resection of all radiologically visible tumor and the use of postoperative radiation therapy would be sufficient to provide local control. However, local recurrences were noted in the remnants. These observations suggest that spondylectomy is required to achieve adequate local control. Although this is seemingly self evident, there were no data in the literature to support this concept. As a result, our initial spondylectomies were both technically inadequate, and the second stage was frequently deferred until radiographic confirmation of recurrent tumor was obtained.

We recommend that spondylectomy be considered in all patients with primary malignant neoplasms and also in selected patients with solitary metastases to the vertebrae (Figs. 43–7 through 43–9). It is therefore indicated in patients with high grade spindle cell tumors such as osteosarcoma, Paget's sarcoma, malignant fibrous histiocytoma, and dedifferentiated chondrosarcoma. In addition, it is also appropriate therapy for lower grade tumors such as chordomas and giant cell tumors of the spine if radiologic studies indicate involvement of both the anterior and posterior elements. Current data also indicate that patients with solitary metastases to bone from kidney and breast cancer have a favorable prognosis, and thus selected patients with spinal metastases from these sites should also benefit from more aggressive surgery. The interval between the first and second operations should be based on several factors: tumor histology, radiologic extent of tumor, and need for systemic therapy. In patients with low grade aggressive tumors (such as giant cell tumor), the second stage may be performed within two weeks after the first stage. In patients with malignant chemosensitive tumors, the second stage should be delayed for several months to allow several cycles of systemic therapy.

In the management of high grade sarcomas, the traditional surgical procedure is radical resection (removal of the tumor along with the entire anatomic compartment). Staged spondylectomy therefore violates a fundamental surgical principle, since tumor resection is achieved through intralesional curettage. However, with the use of early systemic chemotherapy in combination with radiation therapy, the risk of local seeding can be minimized. Early systemic therapy can also be expected to eradicate presumed systemic micrometastases. This strategy is based on the experience of Rosen and others[12, 13, 18] who advocate the use of neoadjuvant chemotherapy following biopsy. By delaying the second stage until several cycles of chemotherapy are complete, it is possible to determine the histologic response of the tumor. Further modifications can thus be based on the response. If histologically viable tumor is still noted at the second stage, we advocate local radiation therapy to the involved segments after healing of the surgical wound; if bone grafts are used, radiation therapy may need to be delayed for at least 3 months to allow for solid fusion. Although these recommendations are based on our experience with a small series of patients, the oncologic principles on which they are

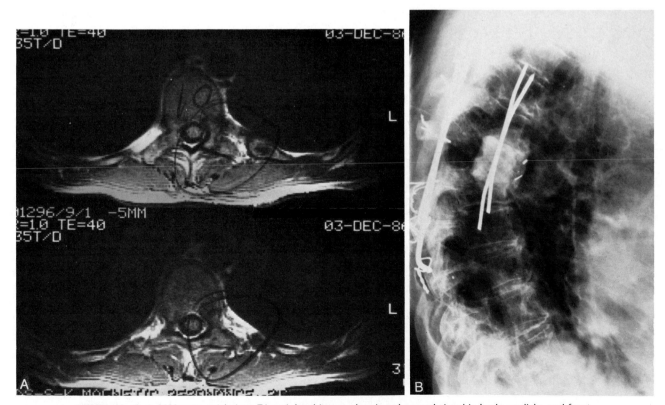

FIGURE 43–7. *A,* MRI scan, axial view, T1-weighted image showing abnormal signal in body, pedicle, and facet with extension into posterior elements. Biopsy revealed malignant fibrous histiocytoma. *B,* Lateral x-ray showing completed spondylectomy, anterior reconstruction with methyl methacrylate and Steinmann pins, and posterior stabilization with Luque rods and bone graft.

FIGURE 43–8. *A*, Axial CT scan showing dedifferentiated chondrosarcoma. *B*, Lateral x-ray showing completed spondylectomy.

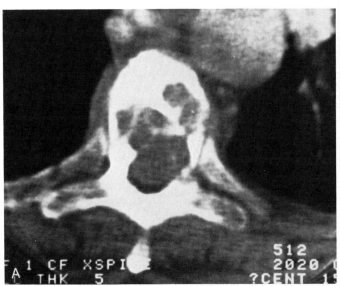

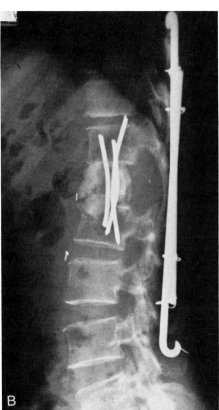

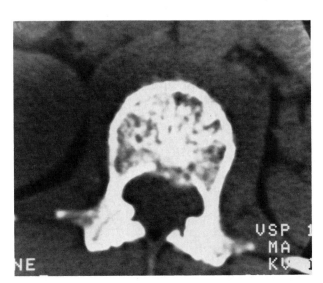

FIGURE 43–9. Solitary metastases to the spine from kidney cancer. All patients with solitary relapse sites in the spine should be considered candidates for spondylectomy if radiologic studies (especially MRI scans) suggest involvement of anterior and posterior elements.

based have proven effective in the treatment of other histologically similar bone tumors.

REFERENCES

1. American Cancer Society: Facts and Figures, 1988.
2. Barwick KW, Huvos AG, Smith J: Primary osteogenic sarcoma of the vertebral column: A clinico-pathologic correlation of 10 patients. Cancer 46:595–604, 1980.
3. Cotrel Y, Dubousset J, Guillamat M: New universal instrumentation in spinal surgery. Clin Orthop 227:10–23, 1988.
4. Enneking WF, Spanier SS, Goodman MA: A system for the surgical staging of musculo-skeletal sarcoma. Clin Orthop 153:106–120, 1980.
5. Frassica FJ, Unni KK, Beabout JW, Sim FH: Dedifferentiated chondrosarcoma—a report of the clinico-pathological features and treatment of twenty eight cases. J Bone Joint Surg 68A:1197–1205, 1986.
6. Hamdi FA: Prosthesis for an excised lumbar vertebra: A preliminary report. Can Med Assoc J 100:576–581, 1969.
7. Johnson S, Tetu B, Ayala AG, Chawla SP: Chondrosarcoma with additional mesenchymal component (dedifferentiated chondrosarcoma). Cancer 58:278–286, 1986.
8. Lievre JA, Darcy M, Pradat P, et al: Tumeur à cellules geantes du rachis lombaire, spondylectomie totale en deux temps. Rev Rhum 35:125–130, 1968.
9. Malawer MM, Abelson HT, Suit HD: Sarcomas of bone. In DeVita VT, Hellman S, Rosenberg SA (eds): Cancer: Principles and Practice of Oncology. 2nd ed, Vol 2. Philadelphia, J. B. Lippincott, 1985, pp 1293–1342.
10. Mankin HJ, Fogelson FS, Thrasher A, et al: Massive resection and allograft transplantation in the treatment of malignant bone tumors. N Engl J Med 294:1242–1255, 1976.
11. Mankin HJ, Lange TA, Spanier SS: The hazards of biopsy in patients with malignant primary bone and soft-tissue tumors. J Bone Joint Surg 64A:1121–1127, 1982.
12. Rosen G, Caparros B, Huvos AG, et al: Preoperative chemotherapy for osteogenic sarcoma: Selection of post-operative adjuvant chemotherapy based upon the response of the primary tumor to preoperative chemotherapy. Cancer 49:1221–1250, 1982.
13. Rosen G, Marcove RC, Caparros B, et al: Primary osteogenic sarcoma: The rationale for preoperative chemotherapy and delayed surgery. Cancer 43:2163–2177, 1979.
14. Rosenberg SA: Surgical Treatment of Metastatic Cancer. Philadelphia, J. B. Lippincott, 1987.
15. Shives TC, Dahlin DC, Sim FH, Pritchard D: Osteosarcoma of the spine. J Bone Joint Surg 68A:660–668, 1986.
16. Sherman ML, Garnick MB: Adenocarcinoma of unknown anatomic origin: Evaluation and therapy. In Fer MF, Greco FA, Oldham RK (eds): Poorly Differentiated Neoplasms and Tumors of Unknown Origin. Orlando, Grune & Stratton, 1986, pp 121–152.
17. Sim FH (ed): Diagnosis and Treatment of Bone Tumors: A Team Approach (Mayo Clinic Monograph). Thorofare, NJ, Charles B. Slack, 1983.
18. Simon MA, Nachman J: The clinical utility of preoperative therapy for sarcomas. J Bone Joint Surg 68A:1458–1463, 1986.
19. Stener B: Total spondylectomy in chondrosarcoma arising from the seventh thoracic vertebra. J Bone Joint Surg 53B:288–295, 1971.
20. Stener B, Johnsen OE: Complete removal of three vertebrae for giant-cell tumour. J Bone Joint Surg 53B:278–287, 1971.
21. Stener B: Total spondylectomy for removal of a giant cell tumor in the eleventh thoracic vertebra. Spine 2:197–201, 1977.
22. Stener B, Henricksson C, Johansson S, et al: Surgical removal of bone and muscle metastases of renal cancer. Acta Orthop Scand 55:491–500, 1984.
23. Stener B: Surgical treatment of giant cell tumors, chondrosarcomas and chordomas of the spine. In Unthoff HK (ed): Current Concepts in Diagnosis and Treatment of Bone and Soft Tissue Tumors. Berlin, Springer-Verlag, 1984, pp 233–242.
24. Sundaresan N, Galicich JH, Lane JM, et al: The treatment of neoplastic epidural cord compression by vertebral body resection. J Neurosurg 63:676–684, 1985.
25. Sundaresan N, DiGiacinto GV, Hughes JEO: Surgical treatment of spinal metastases. Clin Neurosurg 33:503–522, 1986.
26. Sundaresan N, DiGiacinto GVD, Hughes JEO, Krol G: Spondylectomy for malignant tumors of the spine. J Clin Oncol 7:1485–1491, 1989.
27. Sundaresan N, DiGiacinto GV, Hughes JEO: Surgical approaches to primary and metastatic tumors of the spine. In Schmidek HH, Sweet WH (eds): Operative Neurosurgical Techniques: Indications, Methods, Results. Vol 2. Orlando, Grune & Stratton, 1988, pp 1525–1537.
28. Sundaresan N, Galicich JH, Lane JM, Scher H: Stabilization of the spine involved by cancer. In Dunsker SB, Schmidek HH, Frymoyer J, Kahn III (eds): The Unstable Spine. Orlando, Grune & Stratton, 1986, pp 249–274.
29. Szara I, Ciugudean C, Kallo T: Evaluari asupra criteriilar si technicii de eradicase a neoplasmelor colanei prior exerza corporeala si verebrectomie totala. Chirurgia (Bucun) 23:603–630, 1974.

44

OSSEOUS FUSION OF THE CERVICAL, THORACIC, AND LUMBAR SPINE WITH PRIMARY AND METASTATIC SPINE TUMORS

ROBERT C. CANTU

HISTORICAL PERSPECTIVE

While an assortment of wire, silk, rods, screws, and, more recently, plastics have been employed individually and in combination to stabilize the vertebral column, spinal fusion refers to a surgical procedure performed on adjacent vertebrae which leads to an immobilized bony continuity. Using this definition, Russell A. Hibbs and Fred H. Albee ushered in the history of spinal fusion in New York in 1911.[5] For Hibbs, intervertebral fusion was the natural end result of his interest in techniques of arthrodesis which commenced some 29 years earlier in 1882 with Albert in Vienna. Among the earliest to popularize arthrodesis in the United States, Hibbs carried out the first recorded operation of fusion of the spine at the New York Orthopedic Hospital on January 9, 1911.[6] The fusion was achieved by overlapping locally derived osseous elements. Eventually this included spinous processes, laminae, and intervertebral articulations (facet joints). The procedure was reported on May 28, 1911 in the *New York State Journal of Medicine*,[21] and it became known throughout the orthopedic world as the Hibbs fusion operation. With only minor modifications, it has remained the standard for over a half century.

Fred H. Albee, also of New York City, was primarily interested in improving bone graft operations. After exposing the spinous processes and laminae, he split the former in the sagittal plane and inserted a tibial cortical graft into the cleft thus formed. He first performed such a fusion in 1909 and reported his work before the American Orthopedic Association in 1911.[5] His paper was subsequently published in the *Journal of the American Medical Association*.[1] Albee's fusion technique had considerable acceptance during his lifetime because of his worldwide travels, but it eventually lost popularity to the Hibbs procedure.

Other major contributions to spinal fusion include a report by MacKenzie-Forbes of Montreal in 1920 of a technique that denudes the cortical surfaces of the spinous processes and laminae, leaving the cortical slivers overlapping adjacent counterparts.[35] In 1922, Samuel Kleinberg first reported the use of beef-bone grafts and continued to use beef bone until his death in 1957.[34]

Ralph Ghormley of the Mayo Clinic in 1933 recognized the easily accessible abundant supply of autogenous bone from the iliac crest.[17] His report led to a flood of reports regarding the relative merits of cancellous bone versus the stiffer bracing factor offered by the rigid cortical bone. A third minor voice advocated specially prepared beef bone, but cancellous bone from the ilium won the most adherents.

The first two anterior approaches to the lumbar spine both appeared in British journals in 1936. Walter Mercer of Edinburgh described using bone from the iliac crest as an anterior bone graft between the fifth lumbar vertebra and the sacrum.[37] J. A. Jenkins reported in the *British Journal of Surgery* on the abdominal approach for exposing the fifth lumbar vertebra and the sacrum. A bone drill was passed from L5 into S1, and a cortical tibial graft was inserted into the hole.[30] Both of these reports were on cases of spondylolisthesis.

Interfacet screws—metal screws placed across denuded articular facets—were suggested in an effort to improve the efficiency of spinal fusion by James W. Toumey of the Lahey Clinic in Boston in 1943[52] and by Don King of San Francisco in 1944.[33]

Posterior interbody fusion through a laminectomy exposure following disc excision was first reported in *Surgery, Gynecology, and Obstetrics* in 1946 by Irwin A. Jaslow, an orthopedic surgeon in New Bedford, Massachusetts.[29] Ralph B. Cloward of Honolulu in 1952 reported the first large series of his variation of this procedure.[13]

Anterior cervical spine fusion was reported by Robinson and Smith in 1955[45] and by Cloward in 1958.[12]

After the sketch of the salient milestones in the history of spine fusion, a personal and practical approach to the indications and recommended types of spinal fusion for primary and metastatic tumors of the cervical, thoracic, and lumbar regions is given.

ANATOMIC AND PHYSIOLOGIC RATIONALE

Primary tumors of the spine—for example, neurofibroma, meningioma, ependymoma, giant cell tumor, lymphoma, plasmacytoma, aneurysmal bone cyst, chordoma, rhabdomyosarcoma—are less common than metastatic lesions. The spine is the most frequent site of bone metastases,[41] and according to Black,[7] neurologic deficit may occur in 5 per cent of all cancer patients owing to vertebral metastasis. Sarcomas and malignant tumors of the breast, lung, prostate, and reticuloendothelial system most frequently metastasize to the spine.[2-4, 20] Most spinal tumors involve the anterior structures, less commonly the spinous process, lamina, or pedicle posteriorly, and occasionally both the anterior and posterior structures.[4]

Treatment of primary and metastatic tumors of the spine has been a controversial subject frequently appearing in the literature.[3, 4, 8, 9, 15, 18, 23, 25, 27, 28, 31, 40, 42] Nonsurgical treatment of radiation therapy alone or in combination with high dose corticosteroid therapy has been reported to relieve pain and reverse neurologic deficit in both primary and metastatic tumors of the spine.[14, 16, 19, 32, 36, 38, 39, 43, 44, 46–48, 50, 53] Surgical therapy, with or without radiation therapy or chemotherapy, has achieved similar results.[9-11, 22, 24-26, 31, 36, 49, 54, 55] With both surgical and nonsurgical proponents, it is agreed that the worse the neurologic deficit, or if there is a vertebral body collapse of 50 per cent or more, the worse the prognosis for neurologic recovery.

In the past five years the indications for surgery versus radiation therapy appear to have been clarified. So too has the question of the type of surgery: anterior, posterior, or combined anterior and posterior. Symptomatic benign or low grade malignant tumors of the spine are surgically resected as totally as possible, and fusion is carried out if spine instability exists.

Malignant tumors of the spine cause pain, spinal deformity, instability, and neurologic deficit. Neurologic complications may result from (1) direct tumor compression or infiltration, (2) osseous compression by spinal instability or deformity, or (3) vascular compression by tumor. Whereas factors such as tumor behavior, location and extent of tumor, radiosensitivity, and life expectancy affect the decision-making process, initial medical therapy would seem preferable in situations in which neurologic complications are a result of direct tumor compression or infiltration. Surgery would be initially preferable

TABLE 44–1. INDICATIONS FOR SURGICAL THERAPY OF METASTATIC SPINE TUMORS

1. Spinal instability or deformity causing osseous compression of neural tissue.
2. Intractable pain not relieved by medical therapy.
3. Worsening neurologic deficit with medical therapy.
4. Impending spinal deformity.

when bony compression owing to instability or deformity is causing the neurologic deficit. Such surgery must correct the instability and deformity. Therefore, anterior lesions must be approached and stabilized anteriorly, posterior lesions must be approached and stabilized posteriorly, and extensive anterior and posterior lesions must be approached by a combined one-stage anteroposterior resection and stabilization.

Other surgical indications include (1) pain not relieved by medical therapy, (2) worsening neurologic deficit with medical therapy, and (3) impending spinal deformity.

FUSION FOR TUMORS OF THE CERVICAL SPINE

Tumors involving the anterior structures of the cervical spine do not as commonly produce kyphotic deformity as those in the thoracic and lumbar regions. This is because there is no anterior arm lever with the gravity line and because the articular facets usually can support the weight of the skull. However, in those common cases with anterior vertebral body collapse and osseous compression of spinal tissue, the perferred surgical approach is anterior. The involved vertebral body(s) is removed entirely as well as the adjacent discs. I then prefer to notch two iliac crest corticocancellous grafts into the vertebral bodies above and below. A metal plate is screwed anteriorly over the bone grafts into one or more vertebral bodies above and below. This provides immediate stabilization and prevents dislodging of the bone strut.

For posterior lesions after the laminectomy has been completed and the dura denuded of tumor, I prefer stabilization by the following technique. The last exposed facet joint at the cranial end is slightly opened with an osteotome, and either a suction tip or a No. 4 Penfield dissector is then inserted and the osteotome removed. Using a Hall air drill, a hole is drilled through the inferior facet into the joint space

TABLE 44–2. SURGICAL PRINCIPLES FOR SPINE TUMORS

1. Anterior tumors should be approached and stabilized when needed from an anterior approach.
2. Tumors of the pedicles, laminae, or spinous processes (posterior structure) should be approached and stabilized (when needed) from a posterior approach.
3. Extensive tumors involving both anterior and posterior structures should be approached and stabilized (when necessary) from a one-stage combined anteroposterior approach.

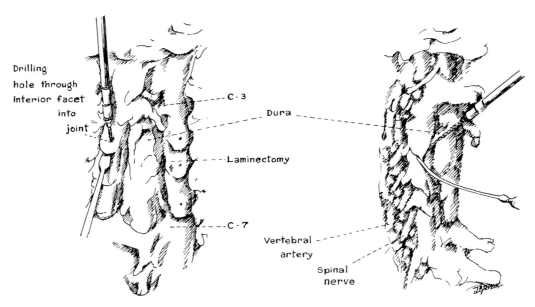

FIGURE 44–1. Cervical vertebrae. *A,* Posterior view; *B,* left lateral view. (From Cantu RC: Techniques of fusion in the cervical, thoracic, and lumbar spine. *In* Schmidek HH, Sweet WH (eds): Operative Neurosurgical Techniques: Indications, Methods, and Results. 2nd ed. Orlando, Grune & Stratton, 1988, p 1472.)

(Fig. 44–1). A No. 20 wire is passed through the hole. Bilaterally, this is carried out from the exposed facet most cranial to the level below the first intact spinous process. A corticocancellous graft 2 cm wide by whatever length is required is taken from the outer table of the posterior iliac crest. Cancellous side down, the graft is securely wired to the facets (Fig. 44–2). Additional cancellous bone may be tucked laterally. Careful wiring of the graft at each

facet ensures the most rapid and secure union. In those rare cases with extensive anterior and posterior tumor involvement meeting the surgical criteria in Table 44–1, I prefer a one-stage combined anteroposterior approach as just discussed.

Comments. I would like to express certain personal biases regarding cervical spine fusion gleaned from more than 25 years of practice and reflection. It has been said that in posterior cervical fusion all that has

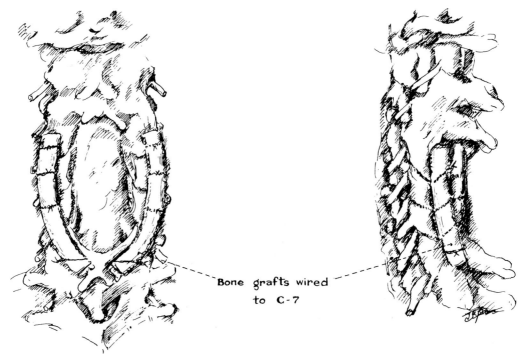

FIGURE 44–2. Bone grafts wired to C7. (From Cantu RC: Techniques of fusion in the cervical, thoracic, and lumbar spine. *In* Schmidek HH, Sweet WH (eds): Operative Neurosurgical Techniques: Indications, Methods, and Results. 2nd ed. Orlando, Grune & Stratton, 1988, p 1472.)

to be done is clean the lamina and lay on the bone. In my experience, I have found that roughening the bed (that is, the laminae, facets, and spinous processes) with a Hall burr, using wire fixation, employing corticocancellous grafts from the posterior iliac crest with the cancellous side down, and using many additional slivers of cancellous bone obtained with gouges maximally ensures the rapidity and solidity of the fusion.

FUSION FOR TUMORS OF THE THORACIC AND LUMBAR SPINE

Extensive tumor involvement of the anterior thoracic or upper lumbar spine is especially prone to produce anterior collapse with osseous compression of neural structures. Adequate surgical treatment requires a lateral extrapleural (thoracic spine) or extraperitoneal (lumbar spine) approach. This approach affords stabilization, correction of deformity, and removal of lesions that cannot safely be reached by laminectomy or costotransversectomy and has a lower morbidity and complication rate than thoracotomy or laparotomy.

Lateral Thoracic Extrapleural Fusion

The patient is placed in the prone position, and a midline incision is made from well above to well below the lesion, curving laterally inferiorly for about 10 cm. The back muscles are stripped from the ribs. The number of vertebral levels to be approached determines the number of ribs to be removed, but it is usually desirable to remove at least two ribs. The rib is transected 8 cm lateral to the costotransverse joint and is removed with rongeurs (Fig. 44–3). The pleura is very carefully stripped from the endothoracic fascia with blunt finger dissection, the neurovascular bundle is located, and the intercostal nerve is separated from the vessels. The costovertebral articulation and transverse processes are removed (Fig. 44–3). The intercostal nerve is traced to its foramen, and it along with the segmental artery and vein are doubly clipped and divided. The pedicle is removed with a rongeur. When the anatomy is particularly distorted, it is often advantageous to first remove the pedicle above and below the lesion. At this point, turning the operating table on a 30- to 45-degree tilt laterally aids in viewing the spinal canal. The annulus is now incised below the level of the posterior longitudinal ligament, and the entire disc and adjacent cartilaginous plates are removed with curettes. The curette stroke is always downward and lateral into the cavity. Epidural bleeding can be controlled with cotton packing. An angled dental mirror may aid in assessing the completeness of the disc excision. I prefer a Smith-Robinson type bone graft from the iliac crest that, with the aid of Cloward spreaders, is tapped into place with a mallet and tamper. The wound is now closed in layers. If a bronchopleural fistula has occurred, a chest tube connected to a closed drainage system is required.

Lateral Lumbar Extraperitoneal Fusion

A skin incision similar to that used for lateral thoracic extrapleural fusion is employed. The lumbodorsal fascia is incised laterally, and the latissimus and erector spinae muscles are split. At least two transverse processes are identified (an x-ray film may be required), and their superior and inferior surfaces are cleared of erector spinae and quadratus lumborum muscles, respectively. Then the transverse processes and associated intertransversarii muscles are removed (Fig. 44–4). The lumbar plexus is identified, and the spinal nerve, which has just exited from the level above, is noted. Complete removal of the transverse process affords exposure of the nerve at the level of the lesion. It may be necessary to remove the pedicles above and below to afford good exposure of the spinal canal.

Division of connecting rami to the sympathetic chain permits sufficient mobility of the spinal nerves to allow good exposure for removal of the disc and adjacent cartilaginous plates. The technique of disc excision and lateral interbody fusion using a Smith-Robinson bone graft is the same as that described for the thoracic spine (Fig. 44–4).

Posterior Thoracic or Thoracolumbar Fusion

For posterior lesions of the thoracic or thoracolumbar spine with instability or with a one-step combined approach for extensive anteroposterior neoplastic involvement, I favor a wide laminectomy with Harrington rod stabilization and deformity correction in combination with a posterior lateral iliac crest corticocancellous fusion as described above. Other excellent fixation measures include Hall distraction rods, Dwyer screws, and segmental spine plates with pedicle screw fixation.[51]

The laminectomy should be at least one level above and below tumor involvement and/or pathologic fracture, and the pedicles should be preserved when free of tumor. I favor intraoperative x-ray films to confirm realignment with the Harrington apparatus. Figure 44–5 shows the deformity in a combined anteroposterior lesion. Figure 44–6 shows the anteroposterior, and Figure 44–7 the lateral view, of the high grade but incomplete myelographic block. Harrington hooks are notched into the facet joints several levels above and below the laminectomy. The outrigger is installed and extended to correct the dislocation and to realign the spine (Figs. 44–8 through 44–10). With the outrigger in place, twin distraction rods are inserted until snug. X-ray films are then taken to assess alignment (Figs. 44–9 and 44–10).

Text continued on page 455

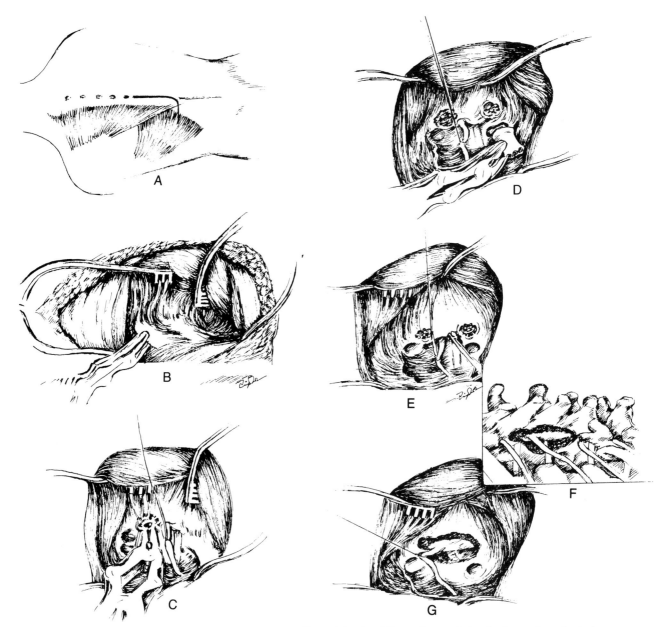

FIGURE 44–3. Lateral retropleural approach. *A,* Skin incision in midline and curved laterally; *B,* muscles retracted to expose ribs; *C,* rib resected; *D,* rib, including costovertebral articulation removed; *E,* annulus incised and disc removed; *F* and *G,* contiguous portions of bone removed from dorsal portions of vertebral bodies. (From Cantu RC: Techniques of fusion in the cervical, thoracic, and lumbar spine. *In* Schmidek HH, Sweet WH (eds): Operative Neurosurgical Techniques: Indications, Methods, and Results. 2nd ed. Orlando, Grune & Stratton, 1988, p 1476.)

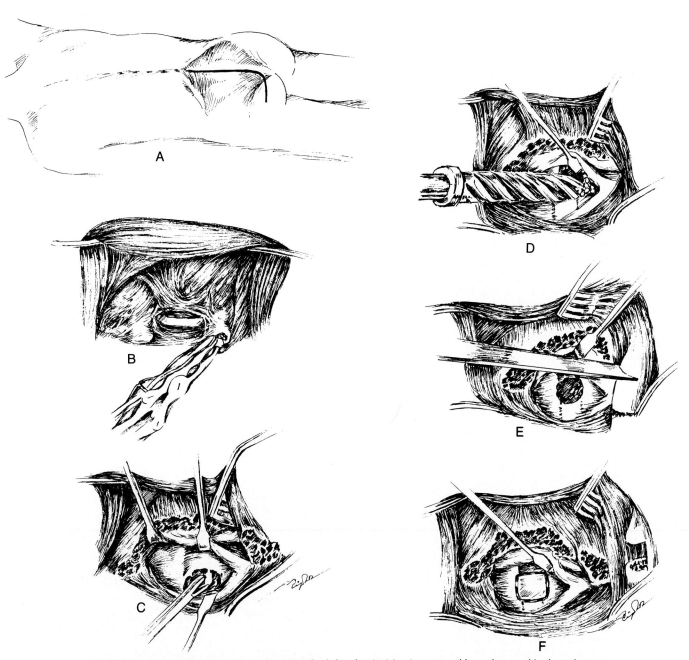

FIGURE 44—4. Lateral retroperitoneal approach. *A,* Lumbar incision is comparable to that used in thoracic area; *B,* lumbar fascia is incised, transverse processes and intertransversarii muscles resected; *C,* disc is removed; *D–F,* bone is removed from vertebral body and fusion is achieved with iliac bone graft. (From Cantu RC: Techniques of fusion in the cervical, thoracic, and lumbar spine. *In* Schmidek HH, Sweet WH (eds): Operative Neurosurgical Techniques: Indications, Methods, and Results. 2nd ed. Orlando, Grune & Stratton, 1988, p 1477.)

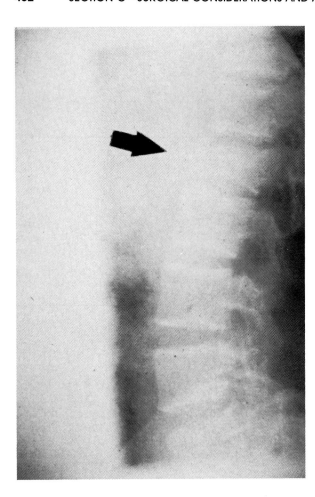

FIGURE 44–5. (From Cantu RC: Techniques of fusion in the cervical, thoracic, and lumbar spine. *In* Schmidek HH, Sweet WH (eds): Operative Neurosurgical Techniques: Indications, Methods, and Results. 2nd ed. Orlando, Grune & Stratton, 1988, p 1478.)

FIGURE 44–6. (From Cantu RC: Techniques of fusion in the cervical, thoracic, and lumbar spine. *In* Schmidek HH, Sweet WH (eds): Operative Neurosurgical Techniques: Indications, Methods, and Results. 2nd ed. Orlando, Grune & Stratton, 1988, p 1478.)

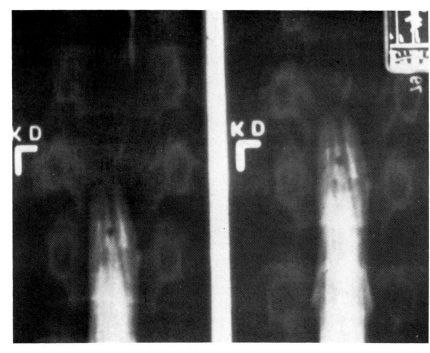

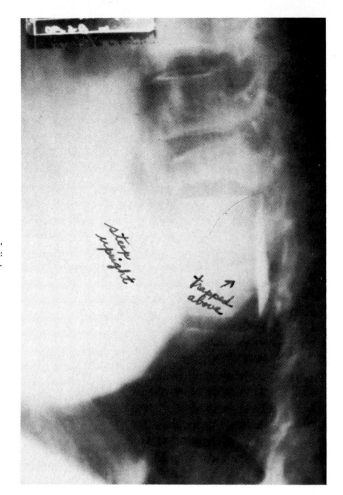

FIGURE 44—7. (From Cantu RC: Techniques of fusion in the cervical, thoracic, and lumbar spine. *In* Schmidek HH, Sweet WH (eds): Operative Neurosurgical Techniques: Indications, Methods, and Results. 2nd ed. Orlando, Grune & Stratton, 1988, p 1479.)

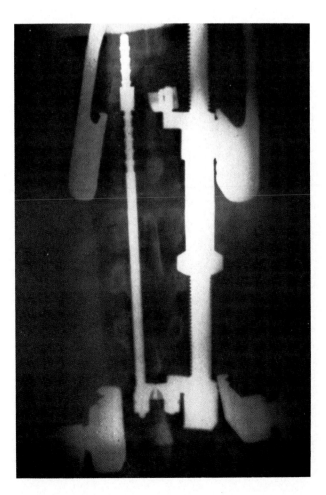

FIGURE 44—8. (From Cantu RC: Techniques of fusion in the cervical, thoracic, and lumbar spine. *In* Schmidek HH, Sweet WH (eds): Operative Neurosurgical Techniques: Indications, Methods, and Results. 2nd ed. Orlando, Grune & Stratton, 1988, p 1479.)

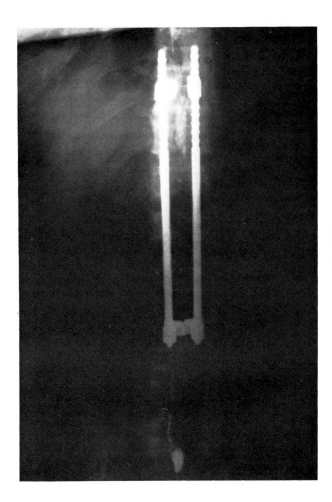

FIGURE 44–9. (From Cantu RC: Techniques of fusion in the cervical, thoracic, and lumbar spine. *In* Schmidek HH, Sweet WH (eds): Operative Neurosurgical Techniques: Indications, Methods, and Results. 2nd ed. Orlando, Grune & Stratton, 1988, p 1479.)

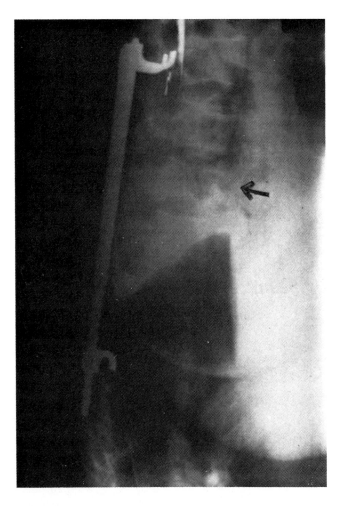

FIGURE 44–10. (From Cantu RC: Techniques of fusion in the cervical, thoracic, and lumbar spine. *In* Schmidek HH, Sweet WH (eds): Operative Neurosurgical Techniques: Indications, Methods, and Results. 2nd ed. Orlando, Grune & Stratton, 1988, p 1480.)

REFLECTIONS ON GRAFT CHOICE AND SITE

Methyl methacrylate is usually employed in fusions where life expectancy is 3 to 6 months. Bone is indicated as the graft material in benign and neoplastic lesions with a life expectancy in excess of 6 months. Today the surgeon has available not only autologous bone but also cadaver bone. Common sites for autologous bone include the iliac crest, the fibula, and the rib.

I prefer to use iliac crest bone primarily because this is strong corticocancellous bone and abundant fresh cancellous bone. By widely exposing the iliac crest posteriorly with a separate incision made right over the crest, and with careful use of straight and curved ½-inch and 1-inch osteotomes, I have been able to remove a large corticocancellous graft of sufficient length to open up to four vertebrae. The initial corticocancellous graft is usually cut with osteotomes into two struts of the desired length. Any additional corticocancellous bone is slivered. Using gouges, copious quantities of cancellous bone are removed from the exposed cancellous bone. If there is any doubt as to whether an adequate amount of bone has been obtained, and in virtually all instances in which a combined procedure is being done, the graft(s) must be harvested from both iliac crests.

REFERENCES

1. Albee FH: Transplantation of portions of the tibia into the spine for Pott's disease. JAMA 57:885, 1911.
2. Alexander E Jr, Davis CH Jr, Field CH: Metastatic lesions of the vertebral column causing cord compression. Neurology 6:103–107, 1956.
3. Barron KD, Hirano A, Araki S, Terry RD: Experiences with metastatic neoplasms involving the spinal cord. Neurology 9:91–106, 1959.
4. Bhalla SK: Metastatic disease of the spine. Clin Orthop 73:52–60, 1970.
5. Bick EM: An essay on the history of spine fusion operations. Clin Orthop 35:9, 1964.
6. Bick EM: Source Book of Orthopedic Surgery. 2nd ed. Baltimore, Williams & Wilkins, 1948.
7. Black P: Spinal metastasis: Current status and recommended guidelines for management. Neurosurgery 5:726–746, 1979.
8. Boland PJ, Lane JM, Sundaresan N: Metastatic disease of the spine. Clin Orthop 169:95–102, 1982.
9. Botterrell EH, Fitzgerald GW: Spinal cord compression produced by extradural malignant tumors: Early recognition, treatment, and results. Can Med J 80:791–796, 1959.
10. Brice J, McKissock W: Surgical treatment of malignant extradural spinal tumors. Br Med J 1:1341–1344, 1965.
11. Bucy PC: The treatment of malignant tumors of the spine: A review. Neurology 13:938–944, 1963.
12. Cloward RB: The anterior approach for removal of ruptured cervical discs. J Neurosurg 15:602, 1958.
13. Cloward RB: Changes in vertebra caused by ruptured intervertebral discs. Observations on their formation and treatment. Am J Surg 84:151, 1952.
14. Cobb CA, Milam EL, Eckles N: Indications for nonoperative treatment of spinal cord compression due to breast cancer. J Neurosurg 47:653–658, 1977.
15. Cusick JF, Larson SJ, Walsh PR, Steiner RE: Distraction rod stabilization in the treatment of metastatic carcinoma. J Neurosurg 59:861–866, 1983.
16. DiLorenzo N, Spallone A, Nolletti A, Nardi P: Giant cell tumors of the spine: A clinical study of six cases with emphasis on the radiologic features, treatment and follow-up. Neurosurgery 6:29–34, 1980.
17. Ghormley RK: Low back pain. With special reference to the articular facets with presentation of an operative procedure. JAMA 101:1773, 1933.
18. Giannotta SL, Kindt GW: Metastatic spinal cord tumors. Clin Neurosurg 25:495–503, 1978.
19. Gilbert H, Apuzzo M, Marshall L, et al: Neoplastic epidural spinal cord compression: A current perspective. JAMA 240:2771–2773, 1978.
20. Gilbert RW, Kim J, Posner JB: Epidural spinal cord compression from metastatic tumor: Diagnosis and treatment. Ann Neurol 3:40–51, 1978.
21. Goodwin GM: Russell A. Hibbs. New York, Columbia University Press, 1935.
22. Gorter K: Results of laminectomy in spinal cord compression due to tumors. Acta Neurochir 42:177–187, 1978.
23. Greenberg HS, Kim J, Posner JB: Epidural spinal cord compression from metastatic tumor: Results with a new treatment protocol. Ann Neurol 8:361–366, 1980.
24. Haerer AF, Smith RR: Neoplasms involving the spinal cord: An analysis of 85 consecutive cases. South Med J 61:801–807, 1986.
25. Hall AJ, MacKay NNS: The results of laminectomy for compression of the cord of cauda equina by extradural malignant tumor. J Bone Joint Surg 55B:497–505, 1973.
26. Harries B: Spinal cord compression. Br Med J 1:611–614, 1970.
27. Harrington KD: The use of methylmethacrylate for vertebral body replacement and anterior stabilization of pathologic fracture-dislocations of the spine due to metastatic disease. J Bone Joint Surg 63A:36–46, 1981.
28. Hermodsson S, Unander-Scharin L: Palliative surgery in epidural malignant tumour. Acta Orthop 54:768–771, 1983.
29. Jaslow IA: Intercorporal bone graft in spinal fusion after disc removal. Surg Gynecol Obstet 82:215, 1946.
30. Jenkins JA: Spondylolisthesis. Br J Surg 24:80–85, 1936.
31. Kennady JC, Stern WE: Metastatic neoplasms of the vertebral column producing compression of the spinal cord. Am J Surg 104:155–168, 1962.
32. Khan FR, Glicksman AS, Chu CH, Nickson JJ: Treatment by radiotherapy of spinal cord compression due to extradural metastases. Radiology 89:495–500, 1967.
33. King D: Internal fixation for lumbosacral fusion. Am J Surg 66:357, 1944.
34. Kleinberg S: Operative treatment for scoliosis. Arch Surg 5:631, 1922.
35. MacKenzie-Forbes A: Technique of an operation for spinal fusion as practiced in Montreal. J Orthop Surg 2:509, 1920.
36. Marshall LF, Langfitt TW: Combined therapy for metastatic extradural tumors of the spine. Cancer 40:2067–2070, 1977.
37. Mercer W: Spondylolisthesis. Edinb Med J 43:545, 1936.
38. Millburn L, Hibbs GG, Hendrickson FR: Treatment of spinal cord compression from metastatic carcinoma: Review of the literature and presentation of a new method of treatment. Cancer 21:447–452, 1968.
39. Mones RJ, Dozier D, Berrett A: Analysis of medical treatment of malignant extradural spinal cord tumors. Cancer 19:1842–1853, 1966.
40. Nather A, Bose K: The results of decompression of cord or cauda equina compression from metastatic extradural tumors. Clin Orthop 169:103–108, 1982.
41. Ominus M, Schraub S, Bertin D, et al: Surgical treatment of vertebral metastases. Spine 11:883–891, 1986.
42. Perese DM: Treatment of metastatic extradural spinal cord tumors: A series of 30 cases. Cancer 11:214–221, 1958.
43. Posner JB: Neurological complications of systemic cancer. Med Clin North Am 55:625–646, 1971.
44. Raichle ME, Posner JB: The treatment of extradural spinal cord compression. Neurology 20:391, 1970.

45. Robinson RA, Smith GW: Anterolateral cervical disc removal and interbody fusion for cervical disc syndrome. Bull Johns Hopkins Hosp 96:223, 1955.

46. Rubin P: Extradural spinal cord compression by tumor. I. Experimental production and treatment trials. Radiology 93:1243–1248, 1969.

47. Rubin P, Mayer E, Poulter C: Extradural spinal cord compression by tumor. II. High daily dose experience without laminectomy. Radiology 93:1248–1260, 1969.

48. Silverberg IJ, Jacobs EM: Treatment of spinal cord compression in Hodgkin's disease. Cancer 27:308–313, 1971.

49. Smith R: An evaluation of surgical treatment for spinal cord compression due to metastatic carcinoma. J Neurol Neurosurg Psychiatry 28:152–158, 1965.

50. Solisio EO, Akbiyik N, Alexander LL: Spinal cord compression from metastatic breast carcinoma: Treatment by radiation therapy alone. J Natl Med Assoc 71:229–230, 1979.

51. Steffee AD, Biscup RS, Sitkowski DJ: Segmental spine plates with pedicle screw fixations. Clin Orthop 203:45–53, 1986.

52. Toumey JW: Internal fixation in fusion of the lumbosacral joints. Lahey Clin Bull 3:188–191, 1943.

53. Ushio Y, Posner R, Kim J, et al: Treatment of experimental spinal cord compression caused by extradural neoplasms. J Neurosurg 47:380–390, 1977.

54. Vieth RG, Odom GL: Extradural spinal metastases and their neurosurgical treatment. J Neurosurg 23:501–508, 1965.

55. White WA, Patterson RH, Bergland RM: Role of surgery in the treatment of spinal cord compression by metastatic neoplasm. Cancer 27:558–561, 1971.

POSTERIOR STABILIZATION USING HARRINGTON ROD INSTRUMENTATION

GEORGE W. SYPERT

INTRODUCTION

The role of surgical therapy in the management of spinal neoplasms, both primary and secondary (metastatic), has evolved such that its goals of maximizing neurologic function, stabilizing the spine, and preventing chronic pain and progressive myelopathies and radiculopathies are now generally accepted. One of the most important surgical advances has been the development of stabilizing spinal implants for the thoracic and lumbar spinal regions. The first truly successful spinal implant adopted and modified for the surgical management of spinal instability and deformity was the Harrington rod system.[7, 8, 9, 12, 15] Subsequently, a variety of new posterior and anterior stabilizing spinal implants have been successfully applied in the surgical management of thoracic and lumbar spine disorders including neoplastic processes. Concurrently, improved anterolateral and posterolateral surgical approaches to the diseased thoracic and lumbar spine have been developed which permit decompression of the neural elements with reconstruction of the compromised spinal canal[2, 6, 11, 13, 14, 16, 17, 24, 26, 28–30, 33, 36, 38, 39, 41–47] Another important advance is the development of radiographic imaging techniques such as polytomography and, more recently, computed tomography (CT) scans. With the development of precise imaging techniques, particularly CT-myelography[23, 34] and magnetic resonance imaging (MRI), in conjunction with advances in the biomechanical understanding of the normal and pathologic spine,[7, 8, 48] application of the appropriate spinal neoplasm resection technique and of the appropriate spinal stabilizing instrumentation is now possible. Knowledge of the benefits, biomechanical limitations, and complications of available posterior spinal instrumentation is requisite for successful surgical management of neoplastic diseases affecting the spine. This chapter discusses the application of posterior distraction and compression spinal instrumentation, excluding the segmental wiring technique, which will be described in another chapter of this text.

GENERAL CONSIDERATIONS

The goals of surgical management of neoplastic diseases affecting the thoracic and lumbar spine which produce neural compression and/or spinal instability (including progressive deformity) include decompression of the neural elements by returning the configuration of the spinal canal to its normal shape and restoration of the normal biomechanical characteristics. These goals are dependent on knowledge of the individual neoplastic process affecting the spine, the level of spinal involvement (thoracic/T1-T10, thoracolumbar/T11-L1, lumbar/L2-S1), the location of any neural compression, and the biomechanical nature of the inherent instability of the spinal column. Conventional anteroposterior lateral spinal radiography, high-resolution CT scanning with sagittal reconstruction, and CT-myelography in combination with a detailed history, general physical, and neurologic examination are generally sufficient to gain this knowledge. MRI may also be helpful in special circumstances.

The spinal surgeon can then select an appropriate surgical procedure to excise the neoplasm, decompress the neural elements, and reconstruct the spine. The type of spinal instrumentation selected will depend upon the methods used to achieve excision of the neoplasm and decompression of the neural elements and upon the nature of the neoplastic process destroying the spinal integrity. Generally, the spinal implant should produce optimal correction of any spinal deformity and give rigid internal fixation, as this offers the greatest probability of a successful outcome. Each of the available spinal implants has advantages and disadvantages. It must further be kept in mind that when used improperly all of the spinal instrumentation systems can result in significant complications. Finally the spinal implant should be considered a temporary device. Given time and stress, all of the implants will fail if solid osseous union across the instrumented area is not ultimately achieved. Therefore, with the exception of incurable high grade malignancies with short life expectancies, strict attention to bony fusion must be made simultaneously with the application of the spinal instrumentation.

POSTERIOR SPINAL INSTRUMENTATION

Excluding the techniques for vertebral body resection and replacement with a fast-setting acrylic compound such as methyl methacrylate, posterior spinal instrumentation has received the greatest application in the correction and stabilization of the diseased thoracic and lumbar spine. In many cases, proper use of such instrumentation reduces the spinal deformity and fixates the unstable spine and may occasionally improve neurologic function by restoring vertebral alignment and reconstructing the spinal canal. Although recovery of neurologic function occurs infrequently if direct surgical decompression of the neural elements is not performed, evidence indicates that realignment and internal fixation decreases the risk of progressive spinal deformity and subsequent pain.[6, 11, 13, 14, 37, 44] Surgical stabilization also permits earlier rehabilitation and decreases the incidence of complications related to prolonged bedrest and immobilization.

A wide variety of devices have been developed for posterior spinal element stabilization. Some of these implants, including various plates and screws, have not withstood with test of time. In contrast, Harrington distraction and compression systems and Luque intersegmental rods have been utilized with excellent results by various clinicians treating neoplastic diseases of the spine. A recently developed system, the Universal instrumentation of Cotrel-Dubousset (CD rods), has undergone extensive clinical trials and now plays a substantial role in the surgical management of certain thoracic and lumbar spine neoplasms, largely surpassing the aforementioned systems.

Each posterior spinal implant has both advantages and disadvantages that must be considered carefully in determining the appropriate instrumentation for an individual patient. In general, compression systems are used for isolated posterior ligamentous injuries where the anterior bony column is largely intact or the vertebral body has been replaced by a rigid construct of either bone or cement which will bear compressive forces without vertical collapse. Distraction systems are generally used for isolated anterior vertebral column diseases that produce vertebral body collapse and kyphotic deformity. Disease that produces combined injuries in which the posterior osseous-ligamentous complex as well as the anterior vertebral column have been significantly injured cannot be satisfactorily stabilized with distraction instrumentation alone. Luque segmental instrumentation fails to support the vertical compressive load and may be associated with collapse of the vertebral body when weakening by neoplastic disease due to sliding of the wires down the rod. Hence, a variety of surgical strategies have been proposed to address these complex spinal processes.

In addition to an understanding of the biomechanics of the vertebral disease and its requirements for reduction and stabilization, consideration must be given to the experience of the surgical team, the ease of application of the spinal implant, patient factors, and the potential for complications related to the stabilizing spinal instrumentation. If posterior instrumentation is to be used, the surgical procedures may be accomplished in a single stage via a posterior or posterolateral excision of the neoplasm and decompression of the neural elements with appropriate vertebral body reconstruction and application of the posterior instrumentation all via a posterior approach. The surgery may also be accomplished in two stages with anterolateral excision of the neoplasm and decompression of the neural elements via an anterolateral approach with secondary application of appropriate posterior instrumentation via a posterior approach. The latter could be accomplished simultaneously using two operating teams.

The Harrington distraction rod system is used most often in the treatment of traumatic thoracolumbar spine fractures. The distraction rods apply axial forces through two sublaminar hooks attached to the rods by means of a hub on one end and a ratchet-locking mechanism at the other end. Two different mechanisms are provided by the distraction rod–hook complex to correct and fixate a spinal deformity: (1) a pure distraction force, and (2) three-point bending (Fig. 45–1A). The combination of the lon-

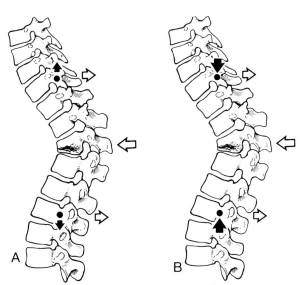

FIGURE 45–1. *A,* The forces applied to the spine by a posterior distraction instrumentation system. *B,* The forces applied to the spine by a posterior compression rod system. The black arrows represent axial bending of the spine as the rod is inserted between the two hooks attached to the laminae.

gitudinal spinal distraction and the application of sagittal bending movements corrects the spinal malalignment and deformity.[12] The Harrington compression system consists of thinner threaded rods, hooks, and small nuts. Compression and three-point bending forces (Fig. 45–1B) are generated by tightening the nuts threaded onto the rod above each hook. As this system acts in a sagittal plane, the three-point bending tends to correct a kyphotic deformity, whereas the compression increases the angulation of the deformity.[48] The bending movements created by the distraction system are more efficient in the correction of a kyphotic spinal deformity, whereas the compression system provides more stability by means of impaction, particularly for severely disrupted spines.[40, 48] In situations where the anterior portion of the spine has been adequately decompressed (e.g., vertebrectomy for neoplasia) and the spinal deformity has been reduced and reconstructed by bone grafts or cement, such that the anterior column can handle a compressive load, a compression system, which can be used effectively over fewer motion segments, would yield more inherent stability than a distraction system. In situations where substantial instability exists, especially with disruption of the anterior longitudinal ligament, and strong correctional forces are required, combined compression and distraction rods have been recommended.[35, 48]

Harrington Rod Instrumentation

The ligaments of either the anterior or posterior column, particularly the anterior longitudinal ligament, are exceedingly important for maintaining the structural integrity of the spine when using distraction systems.[1, 35, 48] Combined destruction of the anterior, middle, and posterior columns[7, 8] presents a major problem for the application of a distraction system. While resisting bending of the spine and restoring vertebral body height, distraction instrumentation requires some intact structure to provide the necessary counterforce in order to hold the laminar hooks and prevent overdistraction. Therefore, Harrington distraction instrumentation should be used with great caution whenever there is destruction of the anterior longitudinal ligament. It should always be kept in mind that this spinal implant can produce disastrous overdistraction and neural injury. In most clinical situations, the Harrington distraction rods should be used primarily to produce bending movements to correct the deformity and then serve as internal splints. The distraction force is primarily employed to lock the rods in place via the sublaminar hooks. Another consequence of excessive force applied to the sublaminal hooks is fracture of the lamina and dislodgement of the hooks.

Generally, Harrington distraction instrumentation is applied via a posterior midline longitudinal incision. This requires that the patient be carefully turned onto a four-poster frame, permitting the spine to go into some extension without compression of the abdominal cavity. In cases of severe spinal instability, awake positioning of the patient may be helpful to ensure that the positioning does not compromise the neural elements. An intraoperative radiograph should be obtained to be absolutely sure that the correct levels are exposed and that spinal alignment has not been adversely affected by the patient's position. Once the correct levels are identified, a careful subperiosteal exposure of the spine is performed, which permits the erector spinae muscles to be retracted laterally. Further dissection is carried out to the tips of the transverse processes of the exposed vertebrae if a posterolateral fusion is to be accomplished.

In general, the spinal exposure should extend in the rostral direction sufficiently to allow placement of the superior ratcheted hook (#1262) under the lamina of the second or third intact vertebra below the diseased level(s). A small laminotomy is often necessary to achieve optimal placement and orientation of the hooks. Since the Harrington distraction system is used primarily as an antibending device, the rods must be carefully *contoured* to achieve a normal curvature that maintains appropriate thoracic kyphosis and lumbar lordosis. In addition, the rod should be contoured in such a manner that the maximal bending force is applied to intact laminae rostral and caudal to the diseased segment(s) to preclude posterior laminar intrusion into the spinal canal with a resultant neurologic catastrophe. Maintaining the plane of the rod curvature in the sagittal plane of the spine necessitates some form of fixation of the rods to the hooks which will mitigate rotation of the rods. This may be accomplished by using the Moe modification of the Harrington distraction rods, which have square-ended rods and square holes in the caudal hooks. The latter system does require very precise determination of the final position of the hooks prior to contouring the rods. Another modification of the Harrington distraction system which appears to overcome many of the limitations of the original system is the locking-hook spinal distraction rod system developed by Jacobs and colleagues.[20, 21] The Jacobs rod system features special hooks that permit rotational adjustments and lock around the rostral lamina to reduce dislodgement of the rostral fixation. An even more versatile system is the Universal system of Cotrel-Dubousset (see below).

When applying a distraction system the author has found it useful to perform a partial or complete laminectomy at the involved level(s), with removal of a pedicle and facet complex on the side of maximal neural compression. A well-machined drill with a cutting burr is very useful in safely accomplishing this exposure and decompression. This exposure allows direct visual inspection and intraoperative real time ultrasound evaluation of adequacy of the reconstruction of the spinal canal and, if necessary, decompression of the spinal canal via a posterolateral transpedicular approach (Fig. 45–2). In fact, a complete vertebrectomy can be accomplished posteriorly using a radical bilateral posterolateral transversope-

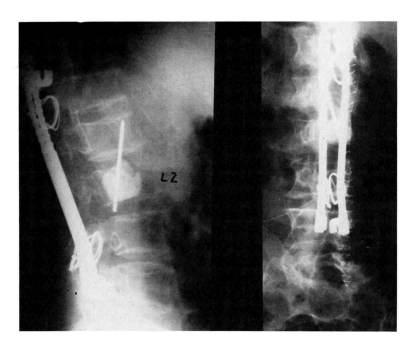

FIGURE 45–2. Combined posterolateral decompression of the spinal canal, including corpectomy of L2 with methyl methacrylate reconstruction and posterior Harrington distraction rod–sublaminar wire reconstruction and fixation of the vertebral column. The patient was a 71-year-old male with a progressive cauda equina syndrome and intractable pain secondary to neural compression from progressive collapse and deformity of the L2 vertebral body from metastatic carcinoma of the lung. Postoperatively, the patient completely recovered all neurologic function and was relieved from spinal pain until his death 13 months later.

diculofacetectomy approach to the vertebral body and discs. The decompression can be accomplished before or after application of a contralateral distraction rod. Optimal reduction and fixation must be confirmed with an intraoperative radiograph. Upon achieving decompression of the neural elements and reconstruction of the spinal canal, verified by either palpation or intraoperative ultrasound, the second ipsilateral distraction rod is applied and a radiograph obtained to verify the reduction. If the reduction and fixation are satisfactory, then the C washers are applied. A posterolateral fusion may then be performed using iliac autograft matchstick grafts obtained with an AO gauge, and the wound is closed over a Hemovac drain. The patient may then be mobilized in a polyform clam-shell prosthesis on or about the third postoperative day.

Despite rather extensive literature on the use of Harrington distraction rods in trauma, its role in neoplastic spinal instability has been infrequently reported.[6, 37, 44] Similarly, although an extensive effort has been made to develop criteria for the definition of instability in traumatic spinal disorders,[7, 8, 48] such criteria have not been rigorously defined for neoplastic spinal disorders. In 1983, Cusick and colleagues[6] reported their results of surgical stabilization in seven patients suffering metastatic carcinoma of the thoracic and upper lumbar spine using Harrington distraction rods supplemented by posterior acrylic fusion. Their indications for this procedure included (1) intractable mechanical pain, (2) absent or minimal evidence of neurologic deficit, (3) clinical and neurodiagnostic imaging verification that the predominant neoplastic involvement localized anteriorly to the vertebral body and adjoining structures, and (4) poor general medical condition. After stabilization, pain relief was reported to be almost total and sustained, and the patients' neurologic status remained largely unchanged from preopera-

tive status. These investigators suggest that this form of spinal stabilization may offer substantial relief of incapacitating pain, may lessen the risk of neoplastic fracture-dislocation, and may reduce the local compressive effects of the spinal cord related to the ventrally located neoplasm.

More recently, Sundaresan and coworkers[44] reported their experience with 19 patients who had neoplasms involving the thoracolumbar spine that were managed with Harrington distraction rod stabilization following decompressive laminectomy. They found that this approach may be useful in providing postoperative stability and restoring spinal alignment following laminectomy for spinal neoplastic disease, but it carries an increased risk of wound breakdown if used in a previously irradiated region. They suggest that this procedure may be indicated in the following situations: (1) progressive vertebral body collapse on serial radiographs, (2) following extensive bilateral resection of facets to provide nerve root decompression or access ventral to the spinal cord, and (3) pathologic fracture-dislocations with marked instability to reinforce anterior decompression and arthrodesis. The ultimate role of this approach in the management of instability related to tumors of the thoracic and lumbar spine will have to await further clinical trials.

Harrington Compression System

Instability owing to posterior spinal destructive processes, in which the anterior columns of the thoracic or lumbar vertebrae are sufficiently intact for supporting anterior compressive loads, is ideal for the application of posterior compression systems, such as the Harrington compression system, the Knodt rods used in a compression configuration, or the Kempf's instrumentation. With respect to neoplastic processes in which both the anterior and posterior elements of the spine are not infrequently destroyed, reconstruction of the vertebral body with cement or bone may not yield adequate stability. The latter circumstance would also represent an ideal situation for the application of a compression system. Clinical experience indicates that the application of hooks to the intact laminae immediately above and below the involved segment(s) to bilateral compression rods, with a posterior fusion across the levels of instrumentation, is generally effective in providing a rigid, stable internal fixation. The results of biomechanical testing are also consistent with the clinical experience.[22] Direct inspection of the spinal canal via either careful palpation or intraoperative ultrasound is essential to be sure that fragments of the diseased vertebra or intervertebral disc are not displaced into the spinal canal by the internal reduction. In addition, when the rostral hooks are applied to the superior margins of the lamina, particularly in the thoracic region with its small spinal canal, great care must be exercised to ensure that the hooks do not compromise the spinal canal and produce an injury of the neural elements.

When Harrington compression rods are used to span multiple vertebral levels of the thoracic and lumbar spine, the rostral compression rod hooks are generally attached to the thoracic vertebral transverse processes. These rostral hooks should rest easily under the transverse processes at the junction of the process and the lamina. Often two or three hooks above or below the level of maximal kyphotic deformity are applied to each compression rod. Below T11, the transverse processes are not suitable for application of the compression rod hooks. At these levels, the hooks must be placed under the upper margin of the lamina as close as possible to the facet joints. Harrington compression rods are supplied in two sizes (⅛ inch and 5/16 inch). The smaller rods are more flexible and easier to use for posterior internal reduction and fixation. After the hook sites are prepared, the threaded compression rods with the hooks and locking nuts attached are inserted. The compression rod assembly is tightened using rod and hook holders and spreaders similar in principle to the distraction system. The hooks are tightened and fixed in position with locking nuts. An intraoperative radiograph is necessary to verify adequacy of reduction and fixation. After final adjustment of the nuts, it is recommended that the threads adjacent to the nuts be crushed to prevent the nuts from loosening, with a subsequent loss of reduction and fixation.

An innovative approach to the application of compression instrumentation in the surgical management of metastatic lesions of the thoracic and lumbar spine has been proposed by Lozes and associates.[30] They have recommended a single-stage posterior approach to these lesions which includes aggressive excision of the neoplasm, reconstruction of the vertebral body with a methyl methacrylate prosthesis, and stabilization with Kempf's compression instrumentation (resembles Harrington distraction rods with the ratchets reversed). The surgery is carried out in the prone position with a midline longitudinal incision that extends one level above and below the involved segment(s). A decompressive laminectomy and *bilateral* transversopediculofacetectomy using a rotatory burr are performed with piecemeal gross total excision of all neoplasms, including retropleural or retroperitoneal tumor. Total or subtotal vertebrectomy is also performed, reconstructed with an acrylic prosthesis incorporating Steinmann or Kirschner pins placed under radiographic control. The compression instrumentation is then applied to the first intact lamina rostral and caudal to the level(s) of involvement. Patients are permitted to ambulate within 2

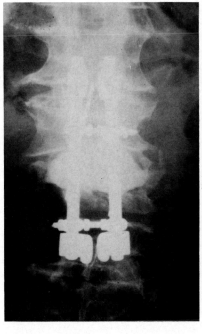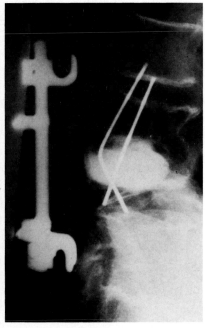

FIGURE 45–3. Combined bilateral posterolateral transversopediculofacetectomy, including corpectomy of L3 with vertebral body reconstruction using methyl methacrylate and posterior Universal (CD) distraction rod reconstruction and fixation of the vertebral column. The patient was a 69-year-old male who developed a progressive cauda equina syndrome and intractable pain secondary to extradural compression at L3. He underwent a decompressive laminectomy and was found to have metastatic prostatic carcinoma. During the postoperative recovery, he developed progressive collapse of L3, with retropulsion of the vertebral body into the spinal canal and worsening of his cauda equina syndrome and pain. The patient was then transferred to the University of Florida Health Center, where he underwent posterior vertebrectomy and reconstruction. Postoperatively, his neurologic function recovered and his pain was relieved. He was doing well at last follow-up 3 months after hospital discharge.

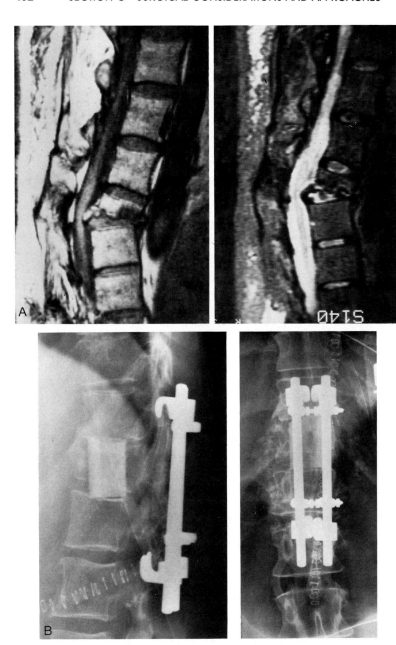

FIGURE 45–4. Combined anterolateral retroperitoneal T12 corpectomy with femur allograft vertebral body reconstruction and posterior Universal (CD) compression rod fixation of the vertebral column. The patient was a 48-year-old female with a progressive loss of neurologic function secondary to a pathologic fracture of T12 with kyphotic deformity. The patient's paraparesis was so severe that she could not bear weight without two assistants and had urinary incontinence. Magnetic resonance imaging revealed severe anterior neural compression from retropulsed bone (*A*). During the same anesthesia, a two-stage surgical procedure was performed (*B*). Postoperatively, an excellent reconstruction of the spinal canal was achieved with return of neurologic function. When last seen 6 months later, the patient had maintained neurologic recovery and demonstrated stable fusion of the allograft to T11 and L1.

days of the surgery without an external orthosis. Using this technique, the authors have achieved excellent results in 15 patients.

Universal Instrumentation

The most recent development of posterior spinal instrumentation designed to correct and stabilize spinal deformities is the Universal instrumentation system, or Cotrel-Dubousset (CD) system. This system permits the three-dimensional correction of complicated spinal deformities. The Universal rods may be used in either a distraction or compression mode (Figs. 45–3 and 45–4), or both, and may accomplish three-point bending and derotation. The Universal system is potentially so versatile that it can be used to manage a wide range of thoracic and lumbar spine

disorders, including spinal neoplastic diseases. The instrumentation consists of two types of rods (the Cotrel rod and a DTT or transverse loading rod) and three types of hooks (thoracic sublaminar hooks, lumbar sublaminar hooks, and pedicle hooks). There are also a large number of special-purpose hooks and sacral staples for unique circumstances. Like the Harrington distraction rods, a number of specially designed instruments are required for insertion of the rods, even for relatively simple spinal deformities.

Although the author's experience with this system is limited to date, he is very impressed with his initial clinical applications of this elegant instrumentation. In fact, this instrumentation has come to replace all prior posterior spinal instrumentation including Harrington rods, Knodt rods, and the Luque systems. Major advantages of this system are that multiple distraction and/or compression sublaminar hooks can be attached to each Cotrel rod, consequently reducing the stress on an individual lamina, and that sublaminar hooks surround a lamina, locking the rod rigidly to one or more laminae. Further clinical experience with this innovative spinal instrumentation will be required in order to determine the advantages and limitations of Universal instrumentation.[10, 27, 46]

CONCLUSION

As with the recent evolution of surgical approaches to decompression and stabilization of spinal neoplastic diseases, understanding of the ultimate role of posterior spinal instrumentation in the surgical management of neoplastic diseases of the thoracic and lumbar spine will have to await further clinical applications. The author predicts that posterior compression systems will have a major role in the surgical management of spinal neoplastic diseases, whereas distraction systems will have limited clinical application. Combined distraction-compression systems may prove to have a substantial role, particularly when one can use the hooks to lock about a lamina, preventing the problem of biologic creep (elasticity over time with hook dislodgement). New concepts concerning the biomechanics of spinal instability, new technology for spinal imaging, further evolution of the role of neurologic decompression, and the development of improved systems and techniques for achieving anatomic reconstruction and fixation of the spine will continue to improve the care of patients suffering from neoplastic diseases of the spine. This field of medicine is in rapid evolution. An understanding of all of these developments as well as their limitations and potential complications is necessary if we are to optimize the quality of life of patients suffering from tumors of the spine.

REFERENCES

1. Anden U, Lake A, Nordwall A: The role of the anterior longitudinal ligament in Harrington rod fixation of unstable thoracolumbar spinal fractures. Spine 5:23, 1980.
2. Bailey RW, Badgley CE: Stabilization of the cervical spine by anterior fusion. J Bone Joint Surg 42A:565–594, 1960.
3. Benzel EC, Larson SJ: Functional recovery after decompressive operation for thoracic and lumbar spine with paralysis. Neurosurgery 19:772–778, 1986.
4. Bohlman HH, Freehafer A, Dejac J: The results of treatment of acute injuries of the upper thoracic spine with paralysis. J Bone Joint Surg 67A:360–369, 1985.
5. Bradford DS, Akbarnia BA, Winter RB, Seljeskog EL: Surgical stabilization of fractures and fracture-dislocations of the thoracic spine. Spine 2:185–196, 1977.
6. Cusick JF, Larson SJ, Walsh PR, Steiner RF: Distraction rod stabilization in the treatment of metastatic carcinoma. J Neurosurg 59:861–866, 1983.
7. Denis F: The three column spine and its significance in the classification of acute thoracolumbar spinal injuries. Spine 8:817–831, 1983.
8. Denis F: Spinal instability as defined by the three-column spine concept in acute spinal trauma. Clin Orthop 189:65–88, 1984.
9. Dickson JH, Harrington PR, Erwin WD: Results of reduction and stabilization of the severely fractured thoracic and lumbar spine. J Bone Joint Surg 60A:799–805, 1970.
10. Dubousset J, Graf H, Miladi L, Cotrel Y: Spinal and thoracic derotation with CD instrumentation. Scoliosis Res Soc Abstr 20:142, 1985.
11. Flatley TJ, Anderson MH, Anast GT: Spinal instability due to malignant disease. Treatment by segmental spinal stabilization. J Bone Joint Surg 66A:47–52, 1984.
12. Flesh JR, Leider LL, Erickson DL, et al: Harrington instrumentation and spine fusion for unstable fractures and fracture-dislocations of the thoracic and lumbar spine. J Bone Joint Surg 59A:143–152, 1977.
13. Harrington KD: Anterior cord decompression and spinal stabilization for patients with metastatic lesions of the spine. J Neurosurg 61:107–117, 1984.
14. Harrington KD: The use of methylmethacrylate for vertebral body replacement and anterior stabilization of pathological fracture-dislocations of the spine due to metastatic malignant disease. J Bone Joint Surg 63A:36–46, 1981.
15. Harrington PR: Instrumentation in spine stabilization other than scoliosis. S Afr J Surg 5:7–12, 1967.
16. Harrington PR, Dickson JH: An eleven year clinical investigation of Harrington instrumentation. Clin Orthop 93:113–117, 1973.
17. Harrington PR, Johnston JO, Turner RH: The use of methylmethacrylate as an adjunct in the internal fixation of malignant neoplastic fractures. J Bone Joint Surg 54A:1665–1676, 1972.
18. Herring JA, Wenger DR: Segmental spinal instrumentation: A preliminary report of 40 consecutive cases. Spine 7:285–298, 1982.
19. Hodgson AR, Stock FE, Fang HSY, et al: Anterior spinal fusion. The operative approach and pathological findings in 412 patients with Pott's disease of the spine. Br J Surg 48:172–178, 1960.
20. Jacobs RR, Asher MA, Snider RK: Thoracolumbar spine injuries: A comparative study of recumbant and operative treatment of 100 patients. Spine 5:463–477, 1980.
21. Jacobs RR, Casey MP: Surgical management of thoracolumbar spinal injuries. Clin Orthop 189:22–35, 1984.
22. Jacobs RR, Nordwall A, Nachemson A: Reduction, stability, and strength provided by internal fixation systems for thoracolumbar spinal injuries. Clin Orthop 171:300–308, 1982.
23. Jelsma RK, Dirsch PT, Rice JF, Jelsma LF: The radiographic description of thoracolumbar fractures. Surg Neurol 18:79–92, 1982.
24. Johnson JR, Leatherman KD, Holt RT: Anterior decompression of the spinal cord for neurological deficit. Spine 8:396–405, 1983.
25. Laborde JM, Bahniuk E, Bohlman HH, Samson B: Comparison of fixation of spinal fractures. Clin Orthop 152:303–310, 1980.
26. Larson SJ, Holst RA, Hemmy DC, Sances A Jr: Lateral extracavitary approach to traumatic lesions of the thoracic and lumbar spine. J Neurosurg 45:628–637, 1976.
27. Lesion F, Kabbaj K, Debout J, et al: The use of Harrington's rods in metastatic tumors with spinal cord compression. Acta Neurochir 65:175–181, 1982.
28. Lesion F, Mathevon H, Villette L, et al: Use of universal instrumentation in the dorso-lumbar spine pathology. AANS/CNS Joint Section on Spinal Disorders Abstr 2:13, 1986.
29. Livingston KE, Perrin RG: The neurosurgical management of spinal metastases causing cord and cauda equina compression. J Neurosurg 49:839–843, 1978.
30. Lozes G, Fawaz A, Jomin M, et al: Use of methylmethacrylate for vertebral body replacement and interest of Kempf's rods in thoraco-lumbar metastases with spinal cord compresssion (1986 unpublished data).
31. Maiman DJ, Sances A Jr, Larson SJ, et al: Comparison of the failure biomechanics of spinal fixation devices. Neurosurgery 17:574–580, 1985.
32. Mascolm BW, Bradford DS, Winter RB, Chou SN: Post-traumatic kyphosis: A review of forty-eight surgically treated patients. J Bone Joint Surg 63A:891–899, 1981.

33. McAfee PC, Bohlman HH: Complications of Harrington instrumentation for fractures of the thoracolumbar spine. A ten-year experience. J Bone Joint Surg 65A:672–686, 1985.

34. McAfee PC, Yuan HA, Fredrickson BE, Lubicky JP: The value of computed tomography in thoracolumbar fractures. An analysis of one hundred consecutive cases and a new classification. J Bone Joint Surg 65A:461–473, 1983.

35. Murphey MJ, Southwick WO, Ogden JA: Treatment of the unstable thoracolumbar spine with combination Harrington distraction and compression rods. Orthop Trans 6:9, 1982.

36. Paul RL, Michael RH, Dunn JE, Williams JP: Anterior transthoracic surgical decompression of acute spinal cord injuries. J Neurosurg 43:299–307, 1975.

37. Perrin RG, Livingston KE: Neurosurgical treatment of pathological fracture-dislocation of the spine. J Neurosurg 52:330–334, 1980.

38. Siegal T, Siegal T, Robin G, et al: Anterior decompression of spine for metastatic epidural cord compression: A promising avenue of therapy? Ann Neurol 11:28–34, 1982.

39. Siegal T, Siegal T: Surgical decompression of anterior and posterior malignant epidural tumors compressing the spinal cord: A prospective study. Neurosurgery 17:424–432, 1985.

40. Stauffer ES, Neil JL: Biomechanical analysis of structural stability of internal fixation in fractures of the thoracolumbar spine. Clin Orthop 112:159–164, 1975.

41. Sundaresan N, Bains MS, McCormack P: Surgical treatment of spinal cord compression in lung cancer. Neurosurgery 16:350–356, 1985.

42. Sundaresan N, Galicich JH: Treatment of spinal metastases by vertebral body resection. Cancer Invest 2:383–397, 1984.

43. Sundaresan N, Galicich JH, Bains MS, et al: Vertebral body resection in the treatment of cancer involving the spine. Cancer 53:1393–1396, 1984.

44. Sundaresan N, Galicich JH, Lane JM: Harrington rod stabilization for pathological fractures of the spine. J Neurosurg 54:187–192, 1984.

45. Sundaresan N, Galicich JH, Lane JM, et al: Treatment of neoplastic epidural cord compression by vertebral body resection and stabilization. J Neurosurg 63:676–684, 1984.

46. Sypert GW: Stabilization procedures for thoracic and lumbar fractures. Clin Neurosurg 34:340–377, 1987.

47. Watkins RG: Surgical Approaches to the Spine. Berlin, Springer Verlag, 1983.

48. White AA III, Punjabe MM: Clinical Biomechanics of the Spine. Philadelphia, JB Lippincott, 1978.

49. Yosipovitch Z, Robin CC, Mankin M: Open reduction of unstable thoracolumbar spinal injuries and fixation with Harrington rods. J Bone Joint Surg 59A:1003–1015, 1977.

46

SEGMENTAL FIXATION OF THE SPINE WITH THE LUQUE ROD SYSTEM

SANFORD J. LARSON and WADE MUELLER

INTRODUCTION

Segmental fixation can be defined as the attachment of a metallic device at each level of the vertebral column to be immobilized rather than only at the extremities of the system, as with the conventional use of Harrington rods. Segmental fixation has the advantages of distributing the load across the extent of the system and of providing resistance to flexion, extension, and rotation at each vertebral level.

The modified Weiss spring is a relatively simple form of segmental fixation in which the rodded portion of the spring is fixed to the spinous processes by Parham bands. Modified Weiss springs have the advantage of easy, rapid, and safe application and, when necessary, rapid and easy removal. However, in the case of vertebral tumor, the spring (or any compression device) should be used only in conjunction with vertebrectomy and interbody fusion (Fig. 46–1). Modified Weiss springs should not be used in patients with flexion deformity who have had a laminectomy and are not practical in the case of severe angulation that extends over many vertebral levels (Fig. 46–2). Also because of the lumbar lordosis the springs should not be used in lesions below the second lumbar vertebra.

Cotrel-Dubousset rods can also be used for segmental fixation. With this system, rods are passed through opposing hooks placed on the pedicles and transverse processes at each thoracic level to be fixed and through opposing laminar hooks for the lumbar vertebrae. This avoids sublaminar instrumentation, but application can be difficult and tedious. More recently, pedicle fixation has been employed for lumbar fixation, but long-term results in cases of metastatic tumor are not available.

TECHNIQUE

Segmental fixation is usually achieved by sublaminar wiring. This method is time consuming, and the incidence of neurologic complication is greater than with other forms of posterior instrumentation. Either Harrington or Luque rods can be used. Because application of Harrington rods is considered in Chapter 45, this discussion is limited to sublaminar fixation of Luque rods. These rods are available in $\frac{3}{16}$ and $\frac{1}{4}$ inch diameters. The $\frac{3}{16}$-inch rods are much easier to bend and cut and are sufficiently strong for use in cases of vertebral body tumor. They are supplied in various lengths, either as a straight rod, a prebent rod, or a closed rectangular loop. Regardless of the size or type employed, fixation to bone is necessary. Wiring to the spinous processes is an alternate, but less frequently used, technique. The safety of sublaminar wiring depends upon (1) an adequate space between the spinal cord and the undersurface of the lamina (Fig. 46–3), and (2) maintenance of contact between the wire and the undersurface of the lamina from introduction of the wire into the sublaminar space until the last turn of the wire has been completed. Adequacy of the space between the cord and lamina is best assessed by contrast-enhanced computed tomography (CT) scanning. Magnetic resonance imaging (MRI) is less reliable because the space available is not as precisely shown on a single film. Gas myelography with polytomography is superior to both CT scanning and MRI because direct measurements can be made, but this imaging technique is not available at most institutions. It is also more time consuming and uncomfortable.

Maintenance of contact between the wire and lamina depends upon proper preparation of the lamina. Exposure of the laminar edges can be achieved by resection of the spinous process, although this entails loss of the supraspinous and interspinous ligaments. To spare these structures, a few turns of a conical burr, such as the D'Errico, on either side of the spinous process will remove the trailing edge of the superior lamina (Fig. 46–4). The ligamentum flavum can then be removed with the use of small curved curettes and Kerrison punches with a thin foot plate.

465

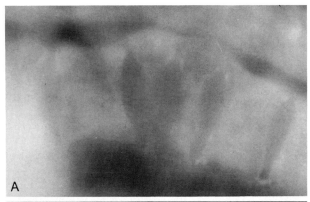

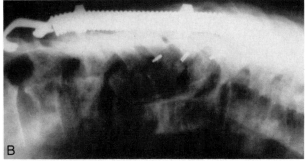

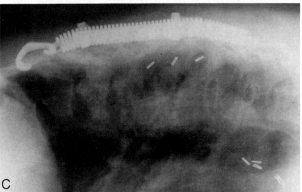

FIGURE 46–1. *A,* Gas myelogram performed in a patient with metastatic breast cancer and progressive myelopathy secondary to deformity of the spinal cord at T6. Chemotherapy had been suspended because of leukopenia. There is translational displacement of T5 on T7, suggesting instability. *B,* Film taken two weeks following a lateral approach for resection of T6, interbody fusion from T5 to T7, and posterior fixation with modified Weiss springs. Neurologic function returned to normal. *C,* Film from the same patient one year later. Neurologic function remained normal during the postoperative survival of more than 3 years.

The ligamentum flavum must be completely removed from the area beneath which the wire will be passed. If this is not done, residual ligament could direct the tip of the wire toward the spinal cord. A small notch should be made at the leading edge of the lamina to facilitate identification of the wire as it emerges from beneath the lamina and to prevent deflection of the wire toward the cord (Fig. 46–4). This curve of the wire should approximate one quarter of a circle to conform to the lamina (see Fig. 46–3). Only fingertip grasp is used, and contact is continuously maintained between the wire and the undersurface of the lamina. If any resistance is encountered, the wire is withdrawn and the situation reassessed. The emerging wire tip can be grasped in a curved needle holder, which is then used to pull the wire beneath the lamina. Upward tension is maintained on both ends until they are of approximately equal length. With continued traction on the wires, they are bent down over the outer surface of the lamina to prevent migration of the sublaminar portion of the wire toward the spinal cord (Fig. 46–5). For purposes of

orientation, the beaded portion of either the single or the prebent double wires can be bent laterally. This facilitates subsequent application of the rods, since with multilevel fixation, a bristling hedge of wires can be a source of confusion.

The rods are bent to the desired configuration for the vertebral column. A template made from a relatively stiff, but malleable, length of wire substantially decreases the length of time required for this part of the procedure. The rods can then be placed between the lateral and medial ends of the wires. The wires are twisted down sequentially to achieve gradual correction of deformity. The end point for twisting occurs when bending the end of the wires backward and forward does not produce any motion of the wire on the rod.

The prebent rods are very suitable for correction of deformity in patients with multilevel disease and severe angulation. The straight end should be placed over the bent end to prevent rotation (Fig. 46–6). Telescoping of at least some extent can be anticipated with prebent rods. This is not a disadvantage and

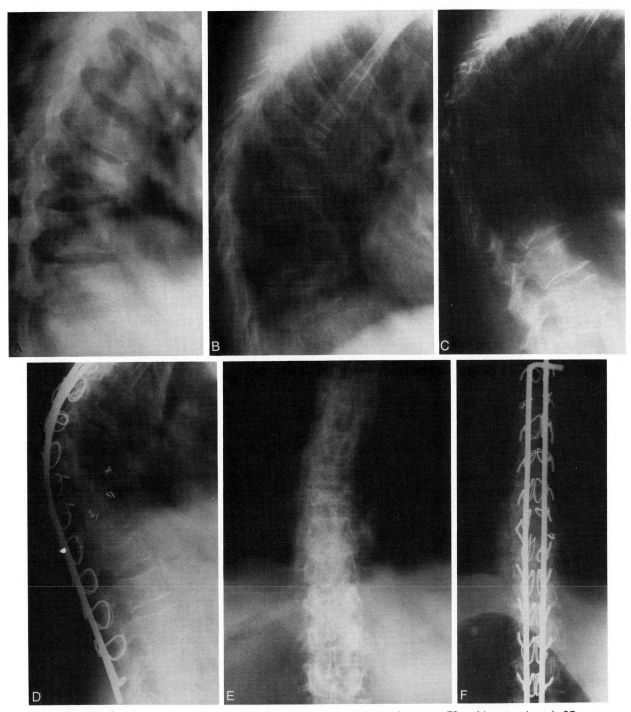

FIGURE 46–2. *A,* The major angulation in this patient with multiple myeloma is at T9 and is approximately 27 degrees. *B,* One year later, the flexion deformity has increased to nearly 50 degrees. *C,* Six weeks after the film in *B,* angulation has increased to 90 degrees. Magnetic resonance imaging demonstrated deformity of the spinal cord produced by a posteriorly displaced portion of T9. *D,* A single stage resection of the posterior portion of T9, interbody fusion of T9-T11, and application of Luque rods were done. Following operation, deformity has decreased to approximately 60 degrees. It was necessary to extend segmental fixation as high as T4 and as low as L2, so that at least two vertebral bodies of relatively normal appearance could be included at either end of the construct. *E,* Preoperative anteroposterior view of the same patient. *F,* Postoperative film demonstrates partial correction of the scoliosis. During application, wires cut through the lamina of T5 and were replaced by wires passed through holes in the pedicles.

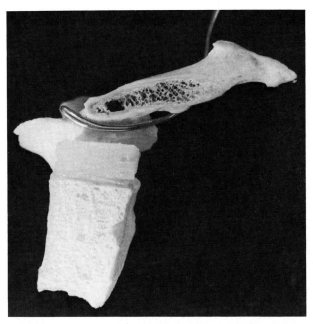

FIGURE 46–3. Photograph of a midsagittal section through the seventh thoracic vertebra. The silastic representation of the spinal cord has an anteroposterior diameter of 8 mm. The sublaminar portion of the wire has been bent to a one-quarter-circle curve.

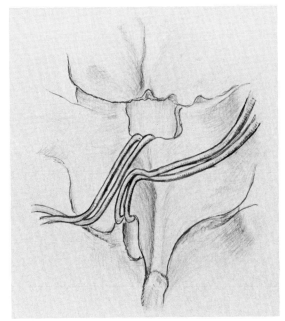

FIGURE 46–5. The wires are crimped down on the lamina to prevent migration of the sublaminar portion toward the spinal cord. The right side of the inferior lamina is shown intact for purposes of comparison.

may even be an advantage if vertebrectomy and interbody fusion have been performed; however, it may cause problems in patients who have had only posterior instrumentation.

Rod migration can be prevented by using a system

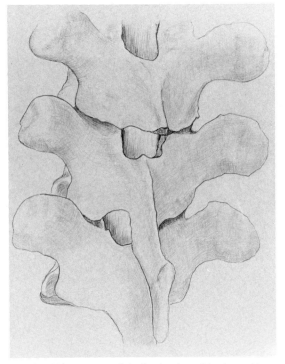

FIGURE 46–4. Preparation of the lamina for sublaminar wiring can be accomplished by spinous process resection (upper) or limited laminotomy lateral to the spinous process (lower). This is done bilaterally.

consisting of a rod, each end of which is bent at a right angle in the same direction and combined with a straight rod. This configuration, however, may permit some rotation.

The closed rectangular loop provides strong vertical support without telescoping and minimizes rotation. The closed loop lacks flexibility since it can be bent only in one plane, and a large inventory of many lengths is required. The best application for the closed loop is in the lumbar area with disease confined to the vertebral body, where fusion and instrumentation should be coextensive to minimize the number of segments immobilized (Fig. 46–7). They are particularly useful for lumbosacral fixation where the usual lordosis does not permit application of Harrington rods or modified Weiss springs.

A single rod bent into a U shape with one of the free ends bent at a right angle also provides vertical support, resists rotation, and permits bending in more than one plane. The end with the right angle can be passed either between spinous processes or through a hole in the base of a spinous process.

Pelvic fixation with intraosseous iliac rodding provides excellent immobilization,[1] but it requires extensive exposure of the iliac bone and has the undesirable feature of fixation across unfused sacroiliac joints. In most instances the closed Luque loop serves very well for lumbosacral fixation. The loop can be fixed to the sacrum by passing wires beneath the sacral lamina, either from burr holes or from the first dorsal sacral foramina if CT scanning demonstrates the sublaminar space to be adequate. If not, a wire can be passed through a drill hole made obliquely downward from medial to lateral in the sacral facet. However, a long pelvic lever arm is

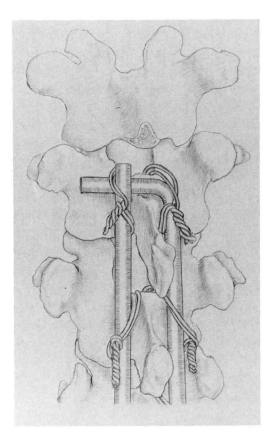

FIGURE 46–6. The wires have been twisted down. The straight end is over the bent end to inhibit rotation, and the wires run diagonally across the rod junction. The relationship at the lower end is similar but opposite.

required to resist very strong stresses at the lumbosacral junction, such as those encountered in scoliosis surgery, where the long lever formed by fixed thoracic and lumbar vertebrae cannot be satisfactorily opposed by a short sacral lever. This situation may be encountered occasionally in tumor surgery. For example, the patient whose x-ray films are shown in Figure 46–8 had several previous operations for chordoma involving L5 and the sacrum with extension into the paravertebral muscles. He was paraplegic and, while comfortable when recumbent, developed severe back pain shortly after sitting up. The tumor had also extended into the abdomen and the pelvis with early encroachment on the iliac vessels and ureters. Since the laminae of L3-L5 had been removed and the tumor involved the sacrum, neither sublaminar wiring nor pedicle fixation were practical. The patient was treated in two stages. The Luque rods were placed at the first operation, and at the second operation a transabdominal approach was used for subtotal resection of the tumor and placement of fibular grafts from L4 into the intact portion of the sacrum. The patient experienced excellent relief of symptoms and is able to sit in a wheelchair.

For pelvic fixation, the erector spinae muscles are separated from the lumbar spinous processes and laminae, from the upper sacrum, and from the medial portion of the iliac crest down to the posterosuperior iliac spine. At this point, rather than work around the muscle, it is more convenient to transect it, reflecting the cut ends superiorly and inferiorly. The gluteal muscles are separated from the outer

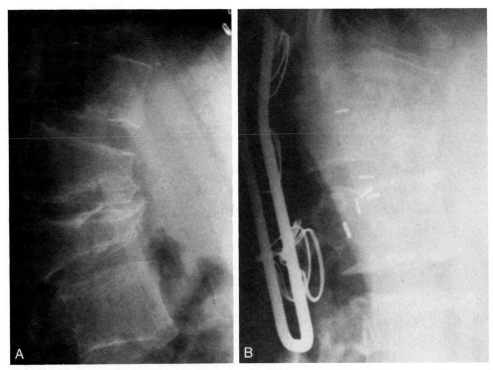

FIGURE 46–7. *A,* This patient with carcinoma of the lung presented with radicular pain and progressive paraparesis. *B,* Film from the same patient after a lateral approach for vertebrectomy and interbody fusion with closed Luque loop fixation from L1 to L3. Postoperative CT scans demonstrated a satisfactory resection of the bone that had been deforming the conus medullaris. A shorter rod might have been more suitable.

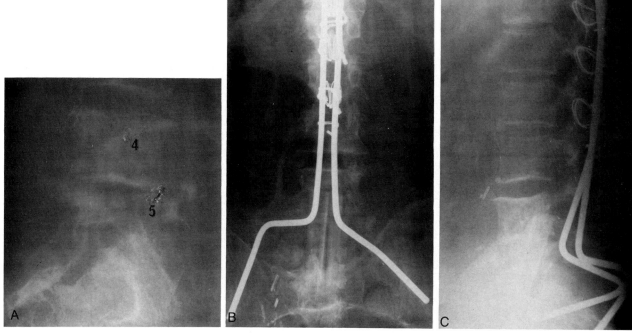

FIGURE 46–8. *A,* Preoperative lateral view of the patient with a cordoma involving L5 and the sacrum. *B,* Anteroposterior view of the same patient following application of Luque rods and anterior approach for placement of fibular graft from L4 to the sacrum. *C,* Postoperative lateral view of the same patient.

table of the ilium until the sciatic notch is identified. The iliac crest is perforated with a drill 2 cm rostral to the posteroinferior iliac spine, and a guide pin of the same diameter as the rod to be used for fixation is driven toward the sciatic notch parallel to but beneath the posterior gluteal line for a distance of 6 or 7 cm. The pin is withdrawn and is replaced by a heavy but malleable wire which will form a template. The material sometimes used to stiffen endotracheal tubes during intubation serves this purpose very well. The wire is bent down onto the sacrum and then superiorly, conforming to the lumbar lordosis. At the desired rostral end of fixation the wire is bent medially at a right angle. Using bending sleeves, a bending press, and a rod holder or two vise grips (the rod is held by one, which in turn is grasped by the other for leverage), a 3/16-inch Luque rod is bent to conform to the template. A similar procedure is followed on the opposite side. The lumbar laminae are prepared for sublaminar wiring, the iliac ends are put in place, and the rods are wired down as previously described.

If it becomes necessary to remove the rods, the sublaminar portion of the wires should be left in place, because withdrawal of the wires may lacerate the dura or injure the neural elements. Instead, the wires should be cut as close to the lamina as possible. Once the rods have been removed, any residual protruding portion of the wire can be bent down onto bone.

INDICATIONS

Although many patients with vertebral body metastases with intact posterior elements can be effec-

tively treated by vertebrectomy and replacement with bone graft[3] or by methyl methacrylate in conjunction with pins or distraction rods and hooks,[2, 4, 6] posterior segmental fixation is indicated in several situations. For example, an interbody construction will not effectively oppose translational deformity (see Fig. 46–1A) or flexion deformity in the presence of osteopenia (see Fig. 46–7A). A strictly anterior approach is also difficult in the lumbosacral region because of the relationship of the iliac vessels and lumbosacral plexus to the vertebral bodies. Although in these situations posterior devices can be used alone, segmental fixation provides additional support in cases where failure of the system can be disastrous. Posterior segmental fixation is also desirable when the deformity is extensive and complex, particularly when the bone is of suboptimal quality (see Fig. 46–2).

Posterior segmental fixation in conjunction with interbody fusion has been employed in 36 patients treated at the Medical College of Wisconsin Affiliated Hospitals between 1977 and 1987. Modified Weiss springs with Parham bands were used in 9 patients, Harrington distraction rods with sublaminar wiring in 13, and Luque rods in 14. Of this group, 13 patients were doing well as far as spinal stabilization was concerned when lost to follow-up 5 months to 2 years after operation. Fourteen patients died 2 months to 28 months postoperatively, with a mean postoperative survival of 7 months. Of the seven patients who died within 6 months of operation, four had carcinoma of the lung and three had undifferentiated adenocarcinoma of unknown origin. Nine patients are living 8 months to 52 months after surgery, with a mean of 25 months.

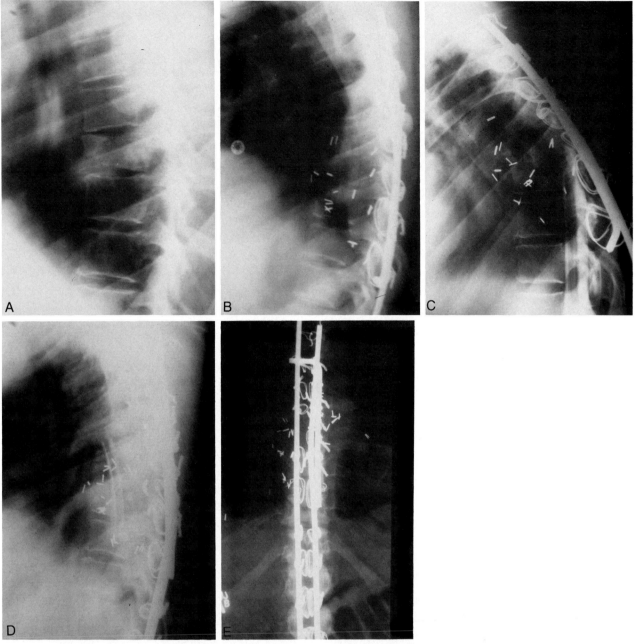

FIGURE 46–9. *A,* Lateral view of patient with metastatic breast tumor to the body of T8. *B,* Lateral film following resection of the body of T8 with rib graft from T7-T9 and application of Luque rods with sublaminar wiring from T5 to T10. *C,* Lateral film taken one year later. The tumor had invaded the seventh vertebral body, causing failure of the anterior fusion and subsequent failure of the wires at T10 followed by substantial flexion deformity. The patient remained neurologically normal. *D,* Lateral film following resection of the bodies of T7-T8, placement of rib graft from T6 into T9, and replacement of the Luque rods. *E,* Postoperative anteroposterior view. The original rod on the right side has been removed with a longer rod inserted through the original wire loops and then fixed with additional sublaminar wires from T2 through L2. On the left side, the distal portion of the original rod was removed, and a second rod was fixed by wiring the remaining portion of the original rod and by sublaminar fixation from T11 to L2.

Failure of fixation occurred in one patient, whose x-ray films are shown in Figure 46–9. This patient had carcinoma of the breast and had received radiation therapy for a metastasis to T8. The presenting symptom was bilateral radicular pain, and the neurologic examination was normal. Using the lateral approach,[5] vertebrectomy of T8 with interbody fusion from T7 to T9 was done. Posterior segmental fixation was used to support what appeare to be demineralized vertebral bodies. The patient was free of pain and fully active (except for symptoms related to a C7 metastasis which failed to respond to radiation and which was successfully treated by fusion) until a year later when the original symptoms recurred. Radiologic examination demonstrated invasion of T7 destroying the fusion with subsequent failure of the wires at T10, allowing substantial flexion deformity. Spinal cord function was unimpaired, but it is possible that, without additional support supplied by the rods, neurologic deficit might have been associated with failure of the fusion. With the lateral approach, tumor was resected and interbody fusion done from T6-T9, and segmental fixation was extended superiorly and inferiorly. The patient is alive and without pain from this lesion 14 months later, although surgical treatment has been necessary for metastases to L2, L3, and L5.

Posterior fixation with sublaminar wiring is tedious and potentially hazardous. However, it is useful in the management of metastatic disease of the vertebral column when lower lumbar and lumbosacral stabilization is necessary, when the posterior elements of the involved vertebrae have been disrupted, and when vertebral deformity is extensive and complex, particularly where bone is of suboptimal quality.

REFERENCES

1. Allen BL, Ferguson RL: Basic considerations in pelvic fixation cases. *In* Luque ER (ed): Segmental Spinal Instrumentation. Thorofare, NJ, Charles B. Slack, Inc., 1984, pp 185–220.
2. Harrington KD: Anterior cord decompression and stabilization for patients with metastatic lesions of the spine. J Neurosurg 61:107–117, 1984.
3. Harrington KD: Metastatic disease of the spine. J Bone Joint Surg 68A:1110–1115, 1986.
4. Siegal T: Surgical decompression of anterior and posterior malignant epidural tumors compressing the spinal cord: A prospective study. Neurosurgery 17:424–432, 1985.
5. Larson SJ: The thoracolumbar junction. *In* Dunsker SB, Kahn A, Schmidek H, Frymoyer J (eds): Orlando, Grune & Stratton, 1986, pp 127–152.
6. Sundaresan N, Bains M, McCormack P: Surgical treatment of spinal cord compression in patients with lung cancer. Neurosurgery 16:350–356, 1985.

TREATMENT OF MALIGNANT TUMORS OF THE SPINE WITH POSTERIOR INSTRUMENTATION

R. ROY-CAMILLE, Ch. MAZEL, G. SAILLANT,
and Ph. LAPRESLE

INTRODUCTION

In cases of malignant extradural tumors of the spine, surgery has two main objectives. The less ambitious one is decompression of the cord and stabilization of the spine without attempts at major tumor removal. This is palliative and improves the quality of the patient's life, which is important, but does not change the ultimate prognosis. A second, more ambitious, objective is to perform a curative resection with complete removal of tumor by spondylectomy. In both cases, a reliable fixation system is necessary. Since 1963, we have been using posterior plates, which have proved both reliable and highly effective. To date, we have treated more than 150 patients with spinal metastases and more than 50 patients with primary spinal tumors with this system.

The clinical presentation of both primary spinal tumors and metastases is similar, with back pain being the most frequently encountered symptom. Radicular involvement and compression of the cord may also inaugurate the evolution of the neoplastic process. In the majority, the plain roentgenographic appearance will demonstrate a lytic lesion with vertebral body collapse. Correct histologic diagnosis is essential, for treatment will depend on it. Metastases are the most frequent vertebral tumors, and the diagnosis is easily confirmed by knowledge of an existing primary site. In such instances, the diagnosis of a bony metastasis demonstrates a new stage in the evolution of the tumor biology, and the prognosis must be considered in the treatment plan. When no primary tumor is evident, it is essential to establish correct diagnosis by biopsy. Different techniques may be used depending on the level and location of the tumor on the vertebrae.

The simplest way is a direct, open biopsy using an appropriate approach: an anterolateral approach for vertebral body tumors, a posterior approach for posterior arch locations. Such a biopsy requires a complete surgical procedure with its potential discomfort and morbidity. For this reason, we favor the use of either needle biopsy or transpedicular biopsy.

At the cervical level, the complex surroundings of the spine may present obstacles, and it is necessary to use thin needles. Results may often be inadequate, and in comparison an anterolateral open biopsy represents a simple alternative. It is in this site that we usually advocate open biopsy. At the thoracic and lumbar levels, a needle biopsy can be performed with a large trocar 3 to 5 mm in diameter. The body is located through a posterolateral puncture 5 to 7 cm lateral to the midline. The computed tomography (CT) scan is useful in directing the biopsy. This is relatively easily accomplished at the lumbar level but may be more difficult in the thoracic region. In such cases, we use a transpedicular biopsy approach (Fig. 47–1). This is performed through a small posterior incision, which can be done from C7 to S1. It is possible to go far anteriorly within the vertebral body itself. The biopsy is done with a curette after transpedicular drilling and a small hemilaminotomy. In our experience with a consecutive series of 47 transpedicular biopsies, histologic diagnosis was established in 46. A major advantage of this technique is the ability to excise the wound tract if a resection is subsequently decided upon.

Tumor Evaluation

In all cases, radiologic evaluation should determine the extent of tumor and involvement of surrounding elements. Plain tomography is a simple and easy way to assess the mechanical consequences of the tumor as well as the bony extension into adjacent vertebrae. The CT scan is currently the most complete and efficient diagnostic investigation. Both bony exten-

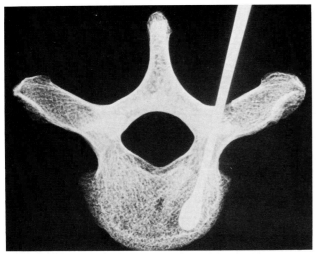

FIGURE 47–1. Transpedicular biopsy through a small posterior approach can give a simple histologic diagnosis.

sion and soft tissue components are well demonstrated. It is thus possible to analyze the tumor and its extensions into the canal and muscle as well as to assess vascular compression or invasion. The visualization of epidural extension may sometimes be difficult with a CT scan. Myelography still represents an important aspect of final tumor investigation. It provides visualization of the spinal dura and the cord in the sagittal as well as the coronal plane. Its major advantage is demonstrating epidural extension as well as the location of compression, that is, anterior or posterior to the cord. One should be careful with the type of contrast material used. We avoid the use of iodine-containing compounds if thyroid cancer is suspected, preferring air myelography instead. It

provides the same results and allows the use of radioactive iodine treatment and iodine body scans in the future.

Magnetic resonance imaging (MRI) will certainly become more important in the evaluation of spinal tumors. Soft tissues, muscles, and vessels, as well as the cord, epidural fat, and cerebrospinal fluid (CSF) are perfectly visualized. The horizontal, sagittal, and coronal representations allow a thorough analysis.

Arteriography is necessary in most cases in which an aggressive treatment is planned. It can include arteriography of the tumor with possible embolization as well as selective angiography of the spinal cord. The type of vascularization may in some instances provide an orientation to the tumor origin. For example, thyroid and kidney metastases are well known to be hypervascular tumors. A second aspect is to perform preoperative embolization, which will considerably decrease bleeding during surgery, in known hypervascular tumors (Fig. 47–2). Arteriography may frequently be used prior to a posterolateral approach to both decrease blood supply and prevent injury to the blood supply of the cord.

General Extent-of-Disease Evaluation

Before treatment, it is important to assess the general extension of the tumor. This is valid for both primary as well as metastatic tumors. The three other major locations to evaluate include the lungs (with plain x-rays and CT scans), the liver (with CT scans and ultrasonic imaging), and bone (with MDP technetium bone scans). These extent-of-disease evaluations will enable a definitive treatment plan to be developed.

Two major groups will be identified with opposing

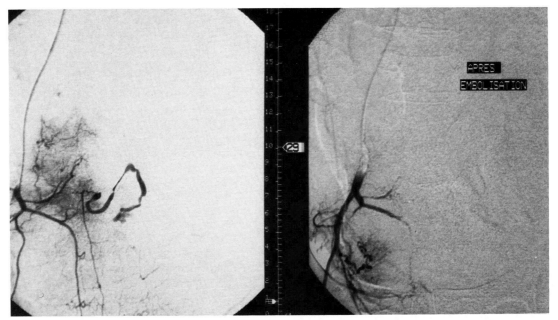

FIGURE 47–2. Preoperative embolization of a hypervascularized tumor can be extremely helpful and can decrease bleeding during surgery.

goals. In the first are isolated tumors without any other sites of involvement. In this group, we also include isolated metastases for which a primary site has not been established. This group will account for treatment approaches with curative intent; the largest possible tumor resection and best antineoplastic treatment should be offered in all possible cases. In the second group are all other tumors. Primary spinal tumors with metastatic foci or metastatic tumors with known primary origin will account for a large subgroup for palliative treatment associated with decompression fixation, but without the goal of cancer resection. One exception in this group are patients with thyroid cancer. In such patients, more extensive resections have to be done because of the better efficiency of tumor control through iodine treatment.

SURGICAL CONSIDERATIONS

Spinal tumor surgery relies on two major fixation techniques, which we will describe first. The indications will then be based on the level of the tumor and the surgical goal.

Lower Cervical Spine Fixation with Plates and Screws

This technique is based on the use of special plates with screws implanted into the cervical articular masses. It is simple, safe, and efficacious and can be used by itself or in conjunction with an anterior approach. Through a posterior approach to the cervical spine, it is necessary to visualize the position of the spinal cord, the vertebral arteries, and the cervical roots. This is accomplished by the knowledge of some specific landmarks of the posterior arch of the vertebra. On each site, the lamina goes down from the spinous process to a small groove located between the lamina and the bulging articular mass laterally. This groove runs all along both sides of the cervical spine, resembling a valley at the bottom of the articular masses, which represent the hills. The vertebral artery runs anterior just in front of the valley, the cord is in front of the spinous process and lamina, and the roots are located above and below the hills in the foramina in front of the facet joints. To be safe, the surgeon must implant the screws at the top of the hills, precisely in the middle (Fig. 47–3). The screws should be driven straight anteriorly or, even better, with a 10-degree oblique lateral and outward direction to the vertebral artery in between the nerve roots. We have designed special plates for this type of excision. They are premolded to fit the normal cervical spine lordosis. They are 2 mm thick and 1 cm broad. They have two to five holes to enable two to five vertebrae fixation; the holes are positioned every 13 mm. These plates are made of chrome-cobalt alloy or stainless steel. The screws are self-tapped and 3.5 mm in diameter. They are short,

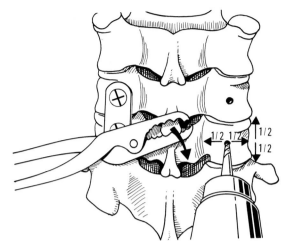

FIGURE 47–3. Cervical spine—implantation of screws is done on top and in the middle of the articular mass. Two bone cortices must be drilled to have a correct fixation.

measuring 16 or 19 mm, depending on the patient morphology.

Experimental studies performed with the help of Rollin Johnson, M.D., at the Veterans' Adminstration Hospital in New Haven, Connecticut, have evaluated the osteosynthetic mechanical properties in flexion and extension. Two cervical vertebrae from a fresh cadaver were fixed posteriorly together with a symmetrical pair of two-hole plates after removal of all ligaments and interbody disc material. The lower vertebra was firmly fixed, and a stress was applied to the upper vertebra. Displacements were analyzed with gauges during the stress. The entire experiment was performed in a large glass box to keep a constant hydrometric level and to simulate as closely as possible the in vivo situation.

Displacements were measured and radiographed as well. All results were computerized. The average breaking load from extension stress was found to be 2.5 kilograms (515 newton). This represents 60 per cent of the load necessary to dislocate two normal cervical vertebrae. These results were then compared with the other methods of posterior cervical fixation. For extension stresses, a posterior wiring of the spinous processes or in the articular masses was insufficient to stabilize the spine. The posterior fixation technique gave an increase of 60 per cent to the normal stability of the spine. A methyl methacrylate fixation of the spinous process gave a 99 per cent increase in stability. For flexion stresses, the posterior wiring between the spinous processes gave a 33 per cent increase in stability; posterior wiring with bone grafts gave a 55 per cent increase in stability. This was increased to 88 per cent when the wiring went through the articular masses. Our plate fixation technique gave a 92 per cent increase in stability.

Surgical Procedure

The surgery is performed through a midline posterior incision. The patient is positioned prone with a head holder enabling flexion-extension ranges of motion. A traction device, if necessary, can be used and fixed to the operating table. Local xylocaine and epinephrine infiltration helps to minimize bleeding and allows a division of the muscles in the midline. The posterior approach is achieved with electrocautery going down to the lateral side of the articular masses in order to locate the reference landmarks. The exact position where a drill should be used for implantation with screws is located at the top of the articular masses exactly at its midpoint. Drilling is performed with a 2.8-mm drill bit when using a 3.5-mm screw. A special drill with depth gauge at 19 mm limits forward motion. A slow motor drill is necessary. The direction of the drilling should be perpendicular to the vertebral plane or, even better, at a 10-degree lateral inclination, but never in the medial direction. Lateral obliquity increases safety and helps avoid the vertebral artery, which is medial, right in front of the valley. With the surgery performed with such care, we have not noted any complications. The only major contraindication to this plate technique is extensive osteoporosis.

COMPLEMENTARY PROCEDURES

The posterior approach and the use of plates and screws implanted in the articular masses allow different associated procedures. A laminectomy is easily performed when necessary, because the plates are lateral to the laminae and are situated on the masses. A Hibbs fusion centered on the laminae can always be performed if desired. If tumor extension is excessive, an extensive fixation using plates of three, four, or five holes may be necessary. An anterior complementary surgical approach is often necessary for removal of the vertebral body and for grafting. For osteosynthesis, we use original staples that have four fish teeth–like feet. They are implanted on the midline in front of the vertebral bodies, and their size is selected to bridge the graft and find support for the base in the adjacent uninvolved body. To prepare the implant, a flat model to assess the size is used, with a hole in each corner corresponding to the feet in the staple. Through these holes, drilling is performed. The staples are then positioned on a holder and are implanted by hammering.

Upper Cervical Spine Fixation with Plates and Screws

Plates and screws can also be used for the treatment of upper cervical spine instability. Tumor involvement of the C2 vertebral body is the best indication for the technique of occipitocervical fixation using our posterior cervical plates. They restore the upper cervical spine stability and a normal curvature of the spine. The normal occipitocervical angulation is 105 degrees, giving a normal horizontal direction to the patient's eyes. Any osteosynthesis using plates must preserve this important angulation. The longitudinal posterior sinus is in the midline of the occipital bone. Lateral to this sinus, the occipital bone is about 10 to 12 mm thick, with two strong cortical surfaces. It

therefore allows only a short screw implantation, but the cortex gives it strength.

To stabilize the occipitocervical junction, we use special premolded plates (Fig. 47–4). Their shape is designed to restore the normal curvature of the occipitocervical junction with a 105-degree angulation. They are reinforced in the middle at the apex of the curve. The occipital part of the plate is flat to prevent skin necrosis at this level. Fixation to the occiput is achieved laterally with 13-mm-length screws. Drilling is performed with a depth gauge of 12 mm. At the cervical level, fixation is achieved with screws implanted into the articular masses as described previously. Some plates are short, going down to C4, while others go down to C5. Between the two plates, there is a large place for corticocancellous bone grafting. The graft is fixed with a 9-mm screw into the external occipital cortex at its upper end and with a wire on the C4 or C5 spinous process at the lower end.

Transpedicular C2 Fixation

It is difficult to implant a screw into the pedicle of C2. Prevention of injury depends on knowledge of

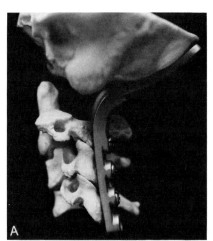

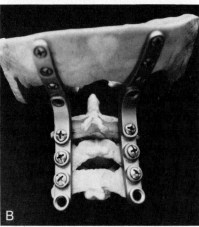

FIGURE 47–4. Occipitocervical fixation and fusion rely on special plates. Correct head position is given by a 110-degree angle of the plate.

precise anatomic landmarks. The C1 ring is normally divided into three equal surfaces: one is the odontoid process, one is the cord, and one is free. At the C2 level, the ring is still large and has no intimate contact between the cord and the pedicles. The vertebral artery is included in the C2 articular mass, making a loop as a horizontal **S**. The posterior aspect of the articular mass, which is discovered through the posterior approach, can be divided into four quarters. The vertebral artery occupies the two inferior quarters and the upper lateral quarter. The upper medial quarter is where a screw can be implanted. The C2 pedicle is at an oblique angle, 10 to 15 degrees upward and inward. An implanted screw must have the same direction.

Surgical Procedure

After clearing the superior border of C2, a slightly curved spatula is introduced into the vertebral canal (which is large) along the medial aspect of the pedicle. On the posterior aspect of the articular mass, the upper medial quarter is located, and the point of penetration of the drill is prepared with a sharp point. This point is as high and medial as possible on the articular mass. From this point, aided by the spatula in the vertebral canal, the drilling is performed obliquely upward and inward 10 to 15 degrees. The drill is as close as possible to the medial and the upper cortex of the pedicle. Drilling extends to a depth of 35 mm. The vertebral artery is lateral and inferior to the drill. A 35-mm-length screw can then be inserted through the cervical plate.

Thoracic, Thoracolumbar, and Lumbar Fixation with Transpedicular Plates and Screws

For this technique, an adequate knowledge of the anatomy of the vertebral pedicles is required.

Pedicle Anatomy. The pedicle is the strongest part of the vertebra. It is mainly a cylinder of cortical bone, with some cancellous bone in its center. From 35 cadaveric dissections, we have determined the characteristics of the pedicles at thoracic and lumbar levels. The study of the horizontal and vertical diameters of the pedicles confirms that there is no problem implanting one or even two screws into a pedicle. The vertical diameter from T1 to L5 increases steadily from 0.7 to 1.5 cm. The horizontal diameter decreases from T1 to T5 (0.7 cm to 0.5 cm); from T5 to L5, it increases from 0.5 to 1.6 cm. The pedicle direction from T1 to T3 is somewhat medially oblique; from T4 to L4, the orientation is almost sagittal. The obliquity never exceeds 10 degrees. At the L4 level, the pedicle is broad and easy to drill straight on. It is the same for L5, where the pedicles are 15 degrees medially oblique. Implantation of 3.5- or 4-mm screws is therefore possible.

Pedicle Relationships. Medially, the cord is close (from 2 to 3 mm); in between are the dura and the CSF. Below L1, the medial aspect of the pedicle is close to the cauda equina and the vertical segment

of the roots. Just below the pedicle lies the root. The inferior portion of the pedicle is thus the most dangerous place in which to drill. The lumbar roots occupy one third of the intervertebral foramen in its anterior and upper part. The pedicle areas located laterally and superiorly are less dangerous, so it is safer to implant a screw too high than too low.

Mechanical Properties. Mechanical properties have been studied at the biomechanical laboratory of L'Ecole Nationale Supérieures des Arts et Métiers (ENSAM) in Paris. They confirm the quality of pedicle fixation. During this experiment, 108 screws have been tested. The pull-out strength is fairly high, with an average of 76 deca newton for a 3.5-mm Phillips screw and of 80 deca newton for a 4-mm Muller screw. This study also demonstrated that pedicle fixation with a cortical bone screw is similar to that with a cancellous bone screw. The average useful implantation length is 3 cm from the posterior aspect of the pedicle. A longer screw does not give a better grip into the cancellous bone of the vertebral body. The length of the screws must be calculated to include the thickness of the plate and will change with the level of the spine. It is not necessary to try to grip the anterior cortex of the vertebral body; on the contrary, it is dangerous.

Instrumentation

The design of the posterior plates follows spinal anatomy. The average distance between two adjacent pedicles is 2.6 cm. The plates are created with holes every 1.3 cm. It is therefore possible to fix two adjacent vertebrae with a transpedicular screw every two holes. The screws used at the thoracic level are 3.1 cm long; at the thoracolumbar junction they are 3.8 cm long; and at the lumbar level they are 4.5 cm long. Between the pedicular screws are holes for optional short articular screws that may complete the

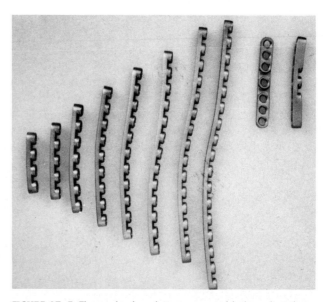

FIGURE 47–5. Thoracolumbar plates are premolded to adapt themselves to normal thoracolumbar curvature. They can be bent before implantation with reinforced pliers and can be used on both sides.

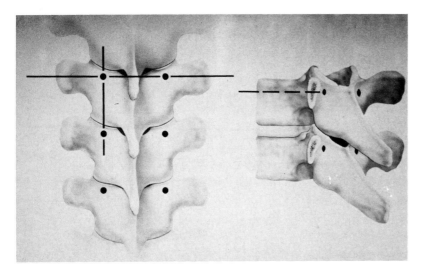

FIGURE 47–6. Thoracic spine—pedicle entrance point is located at the crossing of two lines, at the middle of the inferior articular facet 1 mm below.

fixation. These are 1.9 cm long and thus are fixed into the articular facets.

The plates are premolded into the normal curvature of the spine at the thoracolumbar junction, which is the most common site of fractures. The holes are reinforced on one side by a collar, giving a homogeneous resistance all along the plates. They are made of cobalt-chromium alloy or of stainless steel. Both types of plates can be bent if necessary. Different lengths, ranging from 49 to 190 mm with 5 to 15 holes, have been designed. Special plates also exist for lumbosacral fixation and fusion.

Surgical Procedure

Because it is almost never seen, the pedicle is a dangerous, unknown area of the spine for orthopedic surgeons. To implant a screw into a pedicle correctly without ever seeing it, one must be absolutely sure about its entrance point and direction. The patient lies prone, and the approach is posterior. The vertebral grooves have to be perfectly cleaned on each

side. Only then is it possible to begin looking for the pedicle landmarks. In both the lumbar and thoracic levels, the posterior entrance point for the pedicle is located at the crossing of two lines.

In the thoracic spine (Fig. 47–6), the entrance point of the drill is marked by the crossing of a vertical line, passing through the middle of the inferior articular facets, and a horizontal line, passing through the middle of the insertion of the transverse process. This point is situated 1 mm below the middle of the facet joint.

In the lumbar spine (Fig. 47–7), the landmarks are quite similar: the horizontal line passes through the middle of the insertion of the transverse process, but these are deeper than in the thoracic spine. The vertical line is given by the joint itself, which at this level is sagittal and vertical. The entrance point is thus situated 1 mm below the facet joint on a typical vertical bony crest. This crest is hidden by soft tissues and needs to be cleaned during the approach.

Direction of the Drilling. A bone awl helps to start

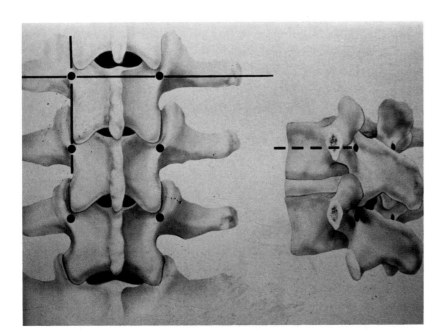

FIGURE 47–7. Lumbar spine—pedicle entrance point is located at the crossing of two lines. Here is a typical bony crest 1 mm below the facet joint.

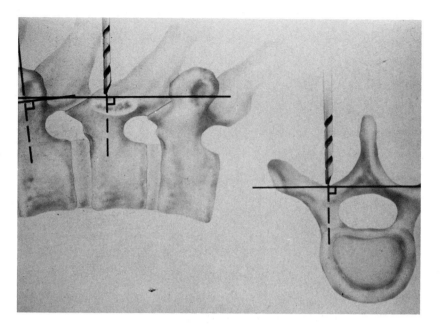

FIGURE 47–8. A 3.2-mm low speed motor drill should be used to drill into the pedicle. It should be perpendicular to the posterior plane of the vertebra.

the drilling, which is done with a low speed drill (Fig. 47–8). The drill is 3.2 mm in diameter. The drill has to be perpendicular to the tangential plane of the posterior aspect of the vertebra and straightforward. It must not go either medially or laterally.

A lateral radiograph taken at the beginning of the surgical procedure placed on the operating room viewer gives the pedicle direction in relation to the ground. This is the direction to follow, preventing drilling too caudally or too cranially. Throughout the drilling for 3 cm, one should feel a continuous, firm bony resistance. To check the position, a new lateral x-ray is taken with metallic pins in the different holes. Afterward, the plates are positioned on the spine with the pins through the holes. They will be replaced by screws. This step is very important because the implantation of the pedicular screws will achieve the full reduction. Indeed, when the plates are applied on the vertebral grooves, the adaptation to the spine is rarely perfect; such factors as a persistent kyphosis, a small lateral translation, or a rotational displacement are often present. The plates are positioned on the spine guided by the pins into the pedicular holes. This is easy because the pins are flexible. The implantation of screws starts from the central portion of the plates and proceeds toward the ends. When the screws are tightened, the spine returns progressively back toward the plates, recovering its normal curvature.

Usually the fixation is very firm with just the pedicular screws, but if necessary the short intermediate articular screws may aid stability. It is better not to implant screws into the pedicles of the tumoral vertebrae because one may not obtain a good quality fixation. At the thoracic level, the normal spine curvature is a lordosis, so the plates are best placed with their concavity and reinforcement collars on the vertebral grooves. Complementary procedures include laminectomy and bone graft.

Thoracic One-Stage Total Vertebrectomy

Thoracic one-stage total vertebrectomy is performed through a simple posterior approach. This way one can perform a bilateral rib resection to extend laterally and then frontally on the vertebral body. The major difficulty is to separate the anterior vertebral plane from the posterior mediastinum with the heart, big vessels, aorta, and vena cava.

Surgical Procedure

The patient is prone on an ordinary operating table, using a head holder if the resection may go above T6. The incision is medial (Figs. 47–9 and 47–10). The spine is cleaned from muscles and fibrous tissues. Dissection is extended laterally in the ribs. The upper and lower ribs adjacent to the tumoral vertebra are dissected 5 to 6 cm from the midline. Periosteum is carefully removed from the ribs, avoiding opening the pleura. Laminectomy is then performed at the level of the tumoral vertebra, typically extending one level in either direction as well. The approach is extended laterally by removing the transverse processes, the articular processes, and the pedicles. Ribs are also resected after dislocation of the rib joint. At that time, the cord is in the middle of the wound unprotected, the roots emerging laterally on both sides lying on the lungs and the pleura (Fig. 47–11).

The major step is the freeing of the anterior vertebral body plane from the posterior mediastinal elements. The dissection is, in fact, fairly easy and nontraumatic. It is a finger dissection (Fig. 47–12). The pleura will be pushed aside from the lateral aspect of the bodies. There is a nonvascular plane, so the vertebral body is freed from the surrounding soft tissues by a slow and progressive posteroanterior dissection. In some cases, it is necessary to ligate one

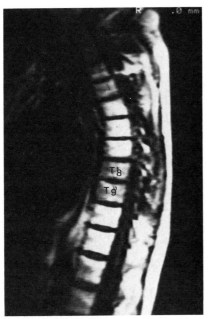

FIGURE 47–9. Thoracic posterior total vertebrectomy. Thyroid metastases of the body of T8 and T9. Radioiodine treatment is no longer effective, so complete carcinologic resection is performed.

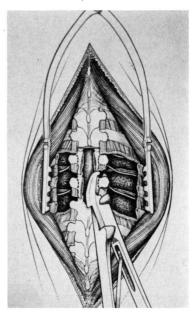

FIGURE 47–11. Rib resection is performed on both sides at the level of the resection and at the adjacent upper and lower levels. Roots are preserved but can be ligated. A complete resection of the laminae and the posterior arch is done.

or two roots. It is the posterolateral extension of the approach that explains the necessity to investigate cord vascularization before surgery. The existence of a main cord artery at the level of the tumoral vertebra or immediately adjacent to it is a contraindication to surgery. Lungs and posterior mediastinum are kept aside with mealleable retractors. It is then possible to go around the entire body without problems. The discs adjacent to the resection are carefully identified and marked with intravenous needles on both sides.

At this point an en bloc spondylectomy is performed. Spinal fixation is mandatory and is performed with a unilateral posterior transpedicular plate taking two or three vertebrae on both sides of the resection.

The spondylectomy is performed with two Gigli saws (Fig. 47–13). Sawing is done from front to back at the level of the adjacent vertebral ends. At the cord, the immediately proximal bone is cut with a cold chisel posterior-to-anterior (Fig. 47–14). The vertebral body is now almost completely free. The posterior longitudinal ligament is cut with a knife carefully anterior to the cord. The vertebral body is

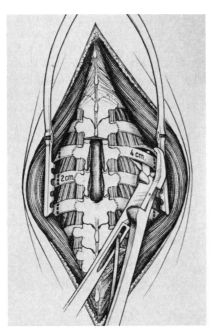

FIGURE 47–10. The first step is a posterior approach extending laterally on the ribs.

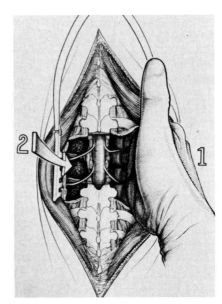

FIGURE 47–12. Posterior mediastinum is carefully pushed forward with a hand dissection. The total vertebral body is thus included.

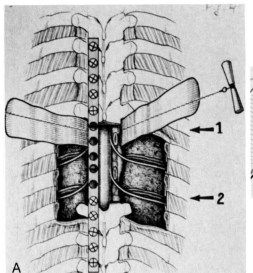

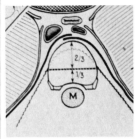

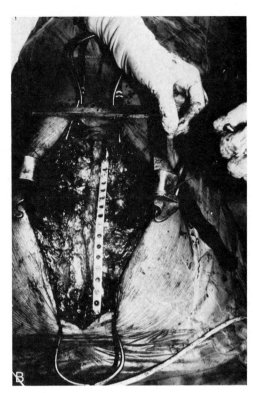

FIGURE 47–13. Stabilization of the spine is mandatory before spondylectomy. Gigli saws are best for cutting both adjacent vertebral end plates.

then pushed aside and removed en bloc (Figs. 47–15 and 47–16).

The cord and spine are then stabilized bilaterally with the plate (Fig. 47–17A). The cord has sustained no trauma, and reconstruction can begin. The best possible body reconstruction is an allograft of femur head and neck bank bone. A 5- to 6-cm-long resection can easily be filled, and the ensuing reconstruction is reliable. In cases with longer resections (two bodies), a fibula reconstruction is indicated. The second posterior transpedicular plate is implanted symmetrically. A complementary tibia graft can be placed lateral to the plates and screwed into the adjacent transverse processes (Fig. 47–15B). The posterior wound is easily closed. A plastic jacket is indicated in all cases. Early walking depends on the quality of the reconstruction.

Two-Stage Lumbar Total Spondylectomy

At the lumbar level, psoas and iliac muscle insertions on the vertebral body, as well as the vascular lumbar pedicles, make the posterior single approach impossible. A two-stage operation is required (Fig. 47–18).

Surgical Procedure

The first step is a posterior approach. The resection includes all the posterior elements, laminae, facet joints, transverse processes, and pedicles. At the time of the pedicle resection, the surgeon should go as far forward as possible in order to ease the anterior resection. The spine is then stabilized with two pos-

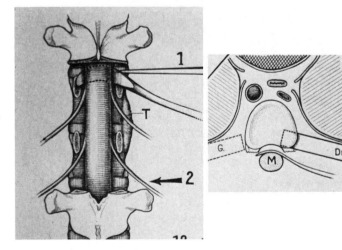

FIGURE 47–14. The posterior part of the body is cut with a bone chisel under careful visual control.

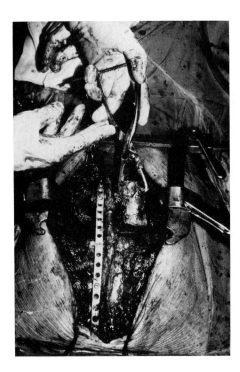

FIGURE 47–15. The tumoral bodies are then completely free and are pushed aside from the cord.

FIGURE 47–16. Roentgenographic study of the anatomic piece demonstrates the en bloc resection.

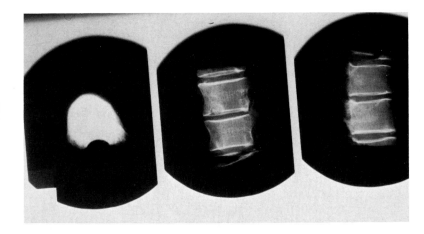

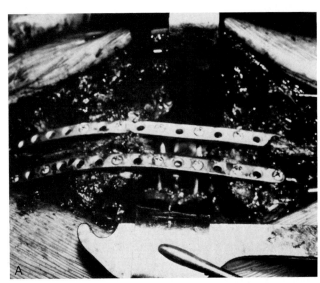

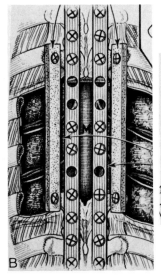

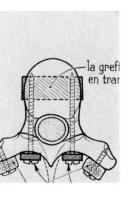

FIGURE 47–17. A second posterior plate is implanted. Reconstruction is performed with tibial bone grafts and fibular or femur head and neck bank bone.

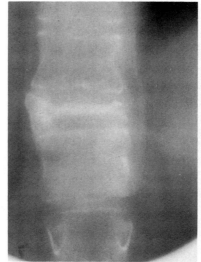
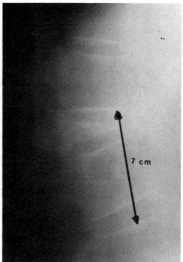

FIGURE 47–18. Lumbar two-stage total vertebrectomy. Two-level primary histiocytofibrosarcoma in a 30-year-old patient. Total vertebrectomy is performed after chemotherapy and radiotherapy.

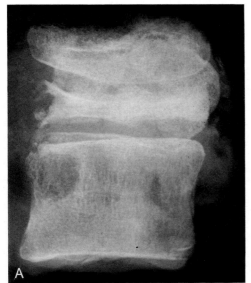
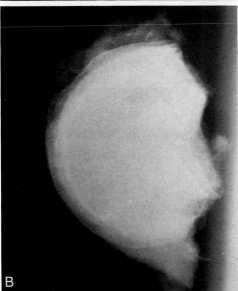

FIGURE 47–19. En bloc resection is achieved.

terior transpedicular plates. A complementary bone graft can be added on both sides.

The second step is performed the same day or a few days later using a retroperitoneal approach. The vertebral body is resected. The level of the posterior wall is easily found if pedicle resection has been deep enough. The entire body of the vertebra is then freed from the surrounding muscles, vessels, and soft tissues. Adjacent discs are resected, but resection can be done in the adjacent vertebral plateaux. The en bloc spondylectomy can then be performed (Fig. 47–19).

Reconstruction is performed with an allograft or with iliac crest (Fig. 47–20). Early walking is possible in all cases with a plastic jacket.

Cervical Spondylectomy

At the cervical level, two major problems—the vertebral artery and the roots—are encountered in total spondylectomies. Vascular surgical techniques enable vertebral artery ligation as well as bilateral vascular bypass, allowing resection of both vertebral arteries at tumor level. Root preservation is much more difficult, and in some cases roots will have to be sacrificed. Cervical spondylectomy is rare, and this surgical procedure requires a high degree of skill.

INDICATIONS

Metastasis Palliation

The goal of metastasis palliation is to give a comfortable survival. Radiotherapy and chemotherapy are usually offered for the treatment of vertebral metastases when the spine is stable. In two instances, however, surgery is indicated: (1) When mechanical complications arise owing to the vertebral brittleness of an osteolytic lesion. Trabecular microfractures are painful and lead to collapse of the vertebral body.

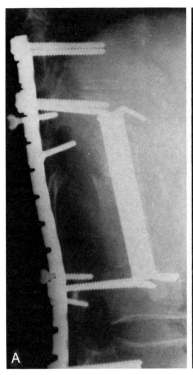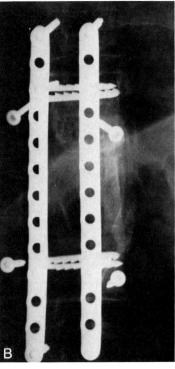

FIGURE 47–20. The first step is posterior resection of the entire posterior arch and plate stabilization. Through a second anterolateral approach, the two-level spondylectomy is performed. Reconstruction is achieved with iliac bone graft, tibial graft, and femur head and neck bank bone.

Stabilization of the spine is then necessary to treat the pain and to prevent deformity. (2) When neurologic complications occur owing to many somewhat related pathologic problems. An epidural tumor occurs most frequently, typically responsible for medullar or radicular involvement, with somewhat rapid-paced compression. Bone metastases extending into the canal are less frequent, but the deformity induced by vertebral collapse and protrusion into the canal can cause neurologic deficit. These complications require decompression of the cord and roots. A laminectomy must be performed, with exploration of the canal to remove any epidural metastases. Cord ischemia is rare but can be suspected when there is a sudden neurologic deficit without associated deformity or epidural tumor. Surgery is ineffective in these cases.

General Considerations

Decompression of the cord and stabilization of the spine are often necessary on an emergency basis, in cases of sudden tetraplegia or paraplegia.

In our experience, a posterior approach is more efficient than an anterior approach. The surgery is quick and less aggressive than thoracotomy or an abdominal procedure. The vertebral canal exploration so permitted, on multiple vertebral levels, is much larger and allows an easier removal of epiduritis than with an anterior approach. After decompression, stabilization is achieved by posterior pedicular screw plating, which is known to be quite strong.

When the cord is involved, laminectomy and decompression are done first. The laminectomy must be wide and should be guided by a preoperative myelogram, indicating the superior and inferior levels of compression. If the posterior arch is tumoral, one must begin on a safe nontumoral level where the dura mater is easily located. Epidural tumor has to be separated and removed from the dura. Most of the time there is a cleavage plane between them. The tumor is removed with a curette or with disc forceps. Its consistency is smooth or firm. Posterior decompression may thus be treated with classic laminectomy, but for lateral or anterior compression an enlarged posterior approach may be required. This would include resection of the pedicle and the transverse process with the head rib at the thoracic level. Such an approach allows encircling the cord without ever contacting or injuring it.

Reducing the vertebral deformity is the second step. At the cervical level, a head holder on the operating table, which causes cervical lordosis, reduces the deformity. At the thoracic level, reduction is given by fixation on the premolded plates. The screws, tightening on the plates, pull back the vertebrae, and the spine recovers its normal curvature. At the thoracolumbar or lumbar level, the deformity is corrected on the orthopedic operation table with the patient in the supine position. If necessary, the lordosis can be improved by lifting the lower limbs upward. If reduction is not complete, the plate fixation will achieve it. The spine fixation is the third step. However, this step alone may be indicated in cases of painful metastases with brittle vertebrae.

Surgical Techniques

The actual level of the metastasis will determine the specific action to be taken.

Upper Cervical Spine (C1-C3). The risk of possible occipitocervical dislocation is greater than that of

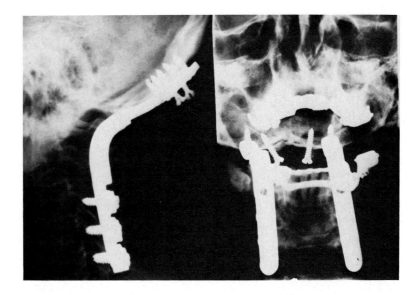

FIGURE 47–21. Fixation is performed on the cervical spine in the articular masses and into the occiput. It is mostly indicated to avoid catastrophic upper cervical dislocations.

cord compression. Treatment is thus limited to occipitocervical fusion as already described (Fig. 47–21). An associated graft between the plates depends on the patient's life expectancy. An iliac unicortical graft is fixed over the occiput with a direct screw, and its lower part is tied on the spinous process of C4. The patient should wear a complementary Minerva corset until fusion, which occurs at the third month.

Lower Cervical Spine (C4-C7). The narrowness of the canal at this level accounts for the rapid onset of medullar compression. Instability increases the neurologic risk. In most cases, a double posterior and anterior approach is necessary (Fig. 47–22). The posterior approach is performed first for laminectomy and fixation of the cervical spine. The length of the fixation is usually greater than for emergency treatment of vertebral injuries. Indeed, the poor quality of the bone often requires a fixation including two levels above and two levels below the tumoral vertebrae.

An anterior complementary tumor resection is often done in the same surgical procedure or a few days later. The anterolateral approach is easy to perform and is not very aggressive. The reconstruction with iliac bone gives a very strong fixation. A postoperative Minerva corset is worn for 3 months after the surgery.

Thoracic and Lumbar Spine. The ribs give a certain degree of stability to the thoracic spine; the problem is more one of possible neural compression than instability. At the lumbar level, root compression is often incomplete. Vertebral collapse gives immediate, significant spinal instability. A posterior procedure can meet all these goals, enabling an extended exploration of the vertebral canal through a more or less long laminectomy. The pedicular screw plating has biomechanically and clinically demonstrated its fixation qualities. Most of the patients have an osteoporosis; the best stabilization, as for the cervical spine, is given by a long instrumentation. This would extend three levels on each side of the tumoral vertebra at the thoracic level (Fig. 47–23) and usually two on each side at the lumbar level (Fig. 47–24). A posterolateral graft will be added only in cases of long life

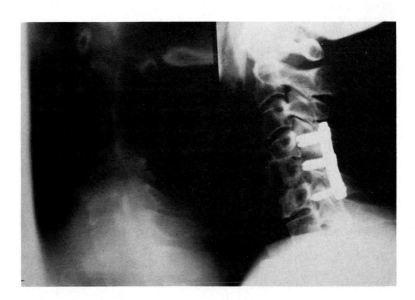

FIGURE 47–22. A C5 lytic tumor (breast) is stabilized by a successive posterior and anterior surgery. The patient remained free from pain and neurologic deficit until death two years later.

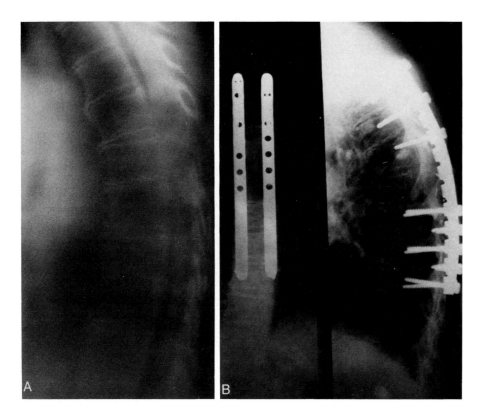

FIGURE 47–23. A thoracic lung metastasis with extended tumor epiduritis is discovered in an acute presenting paraplegia. Air myelography gives the exact extension of the compression.

expectancy. A complementary light plastic Böhler-like corset will be necessary for early ambulation. In cases of major neurologic deficit, no complementary corset is necessary.

Complementary Treatment. Radiotherapy and/or chemotherapy is the last step of the treatment un-

impeded by surgery; this depends on the histologic findings. Radiotherapy should be started only after wound healing (3 weeks). When radiotherapy is given just prior to surgery, one observes wound nonhealing with major skin problems, removing all the palliative benefits of such treatment. The radiation dosage is

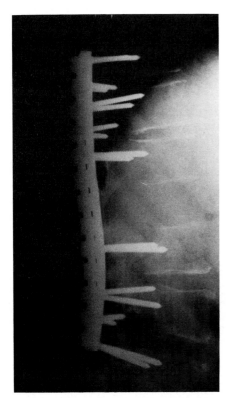

FIGURE 47–24. A lytic kidney lumbar metastasis has been stabilized by a simple posterior procedure. No collapse was observed even immediately before death, 8 months later.

also important to prevent a postradiation myelopathy with secondary paraplegia or tetraplegia. The maximum dosage to the cord is 4500 cGy delivered over a one-month period. In some cases of extended primary vertebral tumors, possibly with metastases, palliative treatment can be justified.

Indications for Curative Surgery (Total Spondylectomies)

Large resections as well as total spondylectomies are indicated for those patients with long life expectancies. We have already emphasized the importance of preoperative biopsy and of localization and determination of extent. Only in isolated tumors are these large resections ever justified. These are rare, but if carefully selected, long-term survival and even healing are observed.

CONCLUSION

The importance of preoperative diagnosis as well as correct patient evaluation has been demonstrated. Only on completion of these can correct treatment be undertaken. Palliative posterior fixation with laminectomy and transpedicular plate fixation has demonstrated its quality and efficiency on pain as well as neurologic improvement. Curative surgery is rarely indicated but can be tremendously important for some lethal tumors.

48

POSTERIOR AND POSTEROLATERAL SURGICAL APPROACHES TO THE SPINE

SETTI S. RENGACHARY

INTRODUCTION

The spinal column may be approached posteriorly, posterolaterally, anteriorly, or anterolaterally. The primary determinant of the choice of surgical approach is the precise location of the pathologic process.[5] If the disease process is extensive, a combination of approaches may be necessary to eradicate the lesion.

Intrinsic neoplasms of the spinal cord are approached exclusively through laminectomy, since this allows extensive craniocaudad intradural exploration. Despite extensive exposure, stability of the spine following these procedures is generally maintained, especially in adults, although postlaminectomy kyphosis and swan-neck deformity may occur if there is weakness of paravertebral muscles. Attempts at replacing the laminae after extensive exploration of the spinal cord have not materially decreased the incidence of postlaminectomy deformities in children as it was once hoped.

Intradural extramedullary neoplasms can frequently be removed through laminectomy. Neurilemomas extending through the intervertebral foramen may require unroofing of the foramen drilling out the zygoapophyseal joint. A "dumbbell" neurinoma, in which the extraspinal tumor is as large as or larger than the intradural component, may require either a concurrent or two-stage intradural and extraspinal exploration. If the surgery is staged, then the intradural component should be removed first to minimize manipulative trauma to the spinal cord.

Epidural neoplasms commonly represent extension into the epidural space of bony neoplasms, the most common being metastatic lesions. The majority of metastatic neoplasms involve the ventral elements of the spine, so that direct access to these lesions requires an anterior exposure of the spine, with posterior approaches to the spine being utilized in unusual instances where the lesion is predominantly in the dorsal or dorsolateral epidural space (Fig. 48–1) or when internal stabilization is necessary. Decom-

pressive laminectomy in patients with ventral epidural lesions seldom offers lasting benefits.

POSTERIOR APPROACHES

The following descriptions apply to the posterior and posterolateral approaches to the spine. Ventral approaches are described elsewhere in this volume. The posterior approaches to the cervical, thoracic, and lumbar spine are the same; however, some regional differences are worth mentioning.

Upper Cervical Spine

To explore the upper cervical spine posteriorly the patient is positioned in either the sitting or the prone position. Complications related to the sitting position

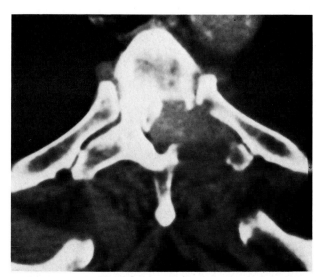

FIGURE 48–1. CT scan showing predominant posterior/posterolateral metastatic epidural tumor amenable for removal through laminectomy.

488

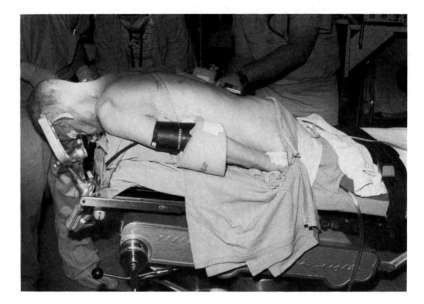

FIGURE 48–2. Optimal position for cervical laminectomy.

(air embolism, hypotension, pneumocephalus, intracranial hematoma) have resulted in its declining use in neurosurgical practice. Alternatively, for surgery in the prone position the patient is placed on chest rolls, and the patient's head is secured in a three-pin Mayfield head rest (Fig. 48–2). This device is preferable to the horseshoe head rest, which carries the risk of injury to the eyes and does not provide secure fixation. Excess neck flexion during positioning can impede the venous drainage and should be avoided.

The incision extends in the midline from the inion to the third or fourth spinous process, prior to which the skin is infiltrated with 1 per cent xylocaine containing 1:100,000 epinephrine, which reduces the skin bleeding. It takes about 7 minutes for the peak vasoconstrictive effect of epinephrine to occur, and therefore the line of the incision is infiltrated prior to draping the region. The skin is incised with the scalpel, and the deeper dissection is carried out with electrocautery. It is often possible to use the coagulation mode alone to complete the dissection if the cautery control mechanism is set sufficiently high. Use of cutting current results in less complete hemostasis and requires one to pause after each layer of dissection to coagulate the bleeders. Self-retaining retractors are inserted, and the wound is held open with some degree of tension, which also helps in hemostasis. Dissection should be maintained along the avascular midline plane until the tips of the spinous processes are reached; however, it is commonly observed that this avascular midline plane does not stay exactly in midline but tends to deviate in a zigzag fashion from side to side.

As the incision is deepened, the self-retaining retractors are moved correspondingly deeper to maintain a steady tension on the tissue planes. The nuchal muscles are best detached from the occipital bone using electrocautery. The cautery dissection is continued over the broad lamina of C2 up to the facet joint while maintaining tension on the muscle with a Cobb elevator. Further dissection laterally is carried out

with a Cobb elevator. The posterior tubercle of the atlas is then identified by palpation. The rectus capitis posterior minor muscle, which arises from the tubercle of the atlas, is divided with electrocautery. This is the only muscle attached to the superior border of the atlas (Fig. 48–3), and, once detached, further lateral dissection is safely carried out with a Cobb elevator and injury to the vertebral artery is avoided. During this dissection direct pressure against the posterior arch of C1 should be avoided, since in some cases the posterior arch may be extremely thin or may even be replaced by a fibrous membrane.

Most lesions that require exposure of high cervical epidural space also require exposure of the caudal posterior fossa. It is best to start with occipital craniectomy first and then proceed with laminectomy of C1 and C2. The occipital craniectomy is customarily

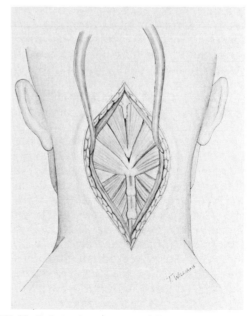

FIGURE 48–3. Operative exposure of the upper cervical region.

done by placing multiple burr holes and excising the intervening bone. The posterior arch of the atlas is then separated from the underlying dura and is removed using a thin-nose Kerrison rongeur. The lamina of C2 is then excised using Kerrison or Leksell rongeurs. The lateral epidural gutter is packed with thrombin-soaked Gelfoam or with Oxycel. After appropriate resection of the tumor, the nuchal muscles are closed in several layers avoiding any dead space. The subcutaneous tissue and the skin are then closed. A suction wound drain is seldom necessary.

Mid and Lower Cervical Region

Patient positioning for surgery in this region is the same as described in the high cervical approach. The length of incision will vary depending upon the extent of pathology, but generally it extends from the spinous process of C2 to the spinous process of C7. These two spinous processes are the most prominent of the cervical spinous processes, and it is often easy to palpate them. When the C2 spinous process is included in the operative field, positive identification of the level of dissection may be made by palpating the spinous processes in the craniocaudad direction. When a more limited exposure is made without access to the spinous process of C2, then x-ray confirmation of the level of the dissection is mandatory.

The skin alone is incised with a knife. The rest of the dissection is carried out using electrocautery at high setting. Initially the dissection should be carried strictly in midline along the ligamentum nuchae until the spinous processes are reached. The spinous processes of C2 through C6 are bifid; that of C7 is not. The spinous processes of C3, C4, and C5 are small and are not always quite lined up in the midline. Cautery dissection is continued around the spinous processes with firm digital pressure and application of tension on the muscles attached to them. The nuchal muscles are arranged in three layers: a superficial layer consisting of the trapezius, a middle layer consisting of the splenius capitis, and a deep layer consisting of the semispinalis capitis, cervicis, multifidi, and rotatores. From a practical point of view these muscles are seldom identified individually. The goal is to carry the dissection in the subperiosteal plane to keep the bleeding at a minimum. Dissection over the laminae is carried out with a large-blade sharp periosteal elevator such as the Cobb elevator (Fig. 48–4). Separation of multifidus and rotator muscles is completed by cautery dissection. Dissection is continued until the lateral margin of the articular capsule of the facet joint is reached.

After separation of the muscles on the side, the paralaminar gutter is packed tightly with dry sponges to provide hemostasis while the other side is worked on. When the muscle dissection on both sides is completed, self-retaining retractors are inserted. The interspinous ligaments are sectioned with a knife, and the spinous processes are rongeured off. The next step is to separate the ligamentum flavum from

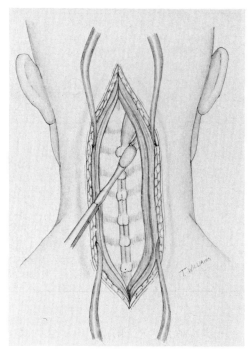

FIGURE 48–4. Separation of the paraspinal muscles from the laminae.

the ventral surface of the cephalad lamina, and this is best started at the lowest limits of the surgical exposure. The laminae are then removed piecemeal using Leksell or Kerrison rongeurs (Fig. 48–5). Alternatively the laminae may be removed en bloc using a high speed drill. The lateral dural gutter is packed with Gelfoam soaked in thrombin. Tumor dissection is completed and hemostasis is achieved with bipolar electrocoagulation and Gelfoam packing. The wound is closed in multiple layers using heavy absorbable sutures. A suction drain is seldom necessary.

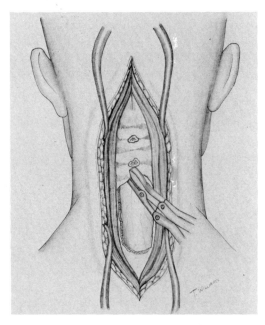

FIGURE 48–5. Laminectomy using Leksell rongeurs.

Thoracic Region

The principles involved in the posterior approach to the thoracic spine are the same as those involved in the exposure of the cervical and lumbar spines and are not discussed separately.

Lumbar Spine

A crucial factor in the successful outcome of lumbar spine surgery is the appropriate positioning of the patient. Every effort should be made to avoid pressure on the anterior abdominal wall. The Wilson frame is satisfactory to achieve this end; however, we prefer the knee-chest position. Various commercially available frames facilitate proper positioning in the knee-chest mode (Fig. 48–6).

The plain roentgenograms of the lumbar spine should be carefully reviewed for the presence of supernumerary lumbar vertebrae or spina bifida occulta. In most patients, the spinous processes are readily palpable. The last interspinous space corresponding to the L5-S1 space is marked with a skin marker. The space above should correspond to the highest point of the iliac crests. In obese patients or in patients with congenital anomalies of the vertebrae, intraoperative radiologic confirmation of the level of the spine is mandatory.

The skin incision is vertical in the midline over the spinous processes. The subcutaneous bleeder is grasped with a fine-toothed Adson pickup and is coagulated with electrocautery. It is not necessary to dissect the subcutaneous fatty layer from the lumbodorsal fascia, except in situations where one plans to utilize fascial grafts. Further dissection is continued with electrocautery around the spinous processes. The spinous processes in the lumbar area are heavy and bulbous. After making cautery cuts in the lumbodorsal fascial muscles attached to the spinous processes, a Cobb elevator is used to strip the paraspinal muscles from the laminae. The multifidus and rotator

muscles are sharply divided with either heavy scissors or electrocautery. When dissection is carried close to the facet joints, branches of segmental arteries bleed and should be coagulated. Modified Hoen-type self-retaining retractors are then inserted. At this point one should define the superior and inferior articular processes. The pedicles lie directly ventral to the base of the superior articular facets. The inferior articular facet is continuous with the lamina above the interspace, and the superior articular process is continuous with the lamina below the interspace. The interspinous ligaments are sharply divided. The ligamentum flavum is separated from the ventral surface of the lamina above using a small, straight, sharp periosteal elevator or a curette. After the spinous processes are rongeured off, the laminae are removed using either rongeur or high speed drill. The dura is protected during drilling if the latter is used. If facet joints had to be removed to facilitate exposure of the pathologic lesion, consideration should be given to internal stabilization at the end of the tumor resection.

COSTOTRANSVERSECTOMY

Costotransversectomy provides access to the lateral and dorsolateral aspects of the vertebral bodies, the intervening discs, and the ventral aspect of the spinal canal.[1] The standard technique entails removal of one or two ribs and their related transverse processes and pedicles. Extended costotransversectomy involves removal of additional bony structures, including the facet joints and in some instances the corresponding hemilaminae.[2] The extended approach gives greater exposure of dural sac and provides better anatomic orientation.

The major advantage of costotransversectomy over laminectomy is the direct access it provides to the ventrolateral spinal canal without the need to retract the spinal cord. This virtually eliminates the morbidity associated with spinal cord retraction. A biopsy of a suspected neoplasm of the vertebral body can usually be accomplished through this approach. A more common indication for costotransversectomy is anterolateral decompression of the spinal cord with resection of primary or metastatic neoplasms involving mostly the anterior elements of the spine. A limited anterior spinal fusion may be accomplished utilizing the rib removed during exposure or a more extensive posterior fusion using Harrington or similar systems at the same sitting.

The fact that the dissection remains extrapleural, with the pleural cavity never intentionally violated, minimizes the postoperative surgical morbidity. Thus costotransversectomy may be preferred over an open thoracotomy in debilitated or elderly individuals, or for a palliative rather than a curative operation.[3] Thoracotomy, however, provides a far more extensive craniocaudal exposure of the spine, which can only be achieved through a costotransversectomy with the removal of too many ribs to be practical.

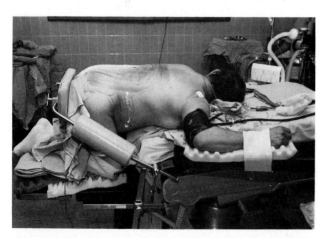

FIGURE 48–6. Knee-chest position utilizing a commercially available frame.

Surgical Technique

The technique of costotransversectomy is virtually the same regardless of the level at which the thoracic spine is exposed. Indeed, access to dorsolateral lumbar vertebral bodies may be obtained through a similar approach.

The operation is performed under general endotracheal anesthesia. The use of a Robert-Shaw double-lumen endobronchial/endotracheal tube is optional. The patient is positioned prone on chest rolls; the side to be operated on is elevated about 30 degrees by tilting the operating table. The tilt may be obtained either at the time of original positioning or after the rib resection is complete and the vertebral exposure is about to begin. It is mandatory to positively identify the vertebral level by radiologic means either before or just at the start of surgery. It is usually done in one of two ways. A sterile needle may be inserted into the spinous process of the appropriate vertebra with radiologic guidance, and this may be left throughout the operative procedure; or the rib to be resected may be positively identified fluoroscopically, and 0.1 ml of sterile methylene blue may be injected into its subperiosteal layer.

The lesion may be approached from either side of midline, but the right side is preferred if the lesion is symmetric because the artery of Adamkiewicz originates almost invariably from the left side from about T8 to L2. If the lesion is off to one side, it may be approached from that side. The incision is arc-shaped with the maximum point of the convexity extending 10 cm from the midline (Fig. 48–7A). The incision should extend for about 12 cm in a craniocaudad direction. The skin along with subcutaneous fat and deep fascia are reflected medially. The trapezius muscle is split and retracted (Figs. 48–8 and 48–9). The rhomboid, if encountered, is divided. The paraspinal muscles either are separated from their deep attachments and retracted medially or are divided transversely and retracted in a craniocaudal direction. Since the paraspinal muscles are innervated segmentally, dividing them horizontally is not likely to result in significant weakness. The rib to be removed is carefully identified and denuded of all

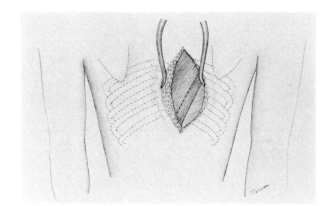

FIGURE 48–8. Exposure of the trapezius muscle.

muscle attachments. Using a Doyen separator the periosteum is separated from the rib. The intercostal nerve and vessels are preserved if possible. The transverse process is rongeured off. The rib is divided about 8 cm away from the midline, lifted up, separating it from the periosteum and endothoracic fascia and disarticulated from the vertebra after dividing the ligaments attaching the head of the rib to the vertebral body. At least two ribs are removed to gain adequate exposure of the vertebral bodies (Fig. 48–10).

Subsequent dissection is done with magnification utilizing either 3.5-power magnifying loupe or an operating microscope. The parietal pleura is dissected away bluntly from the thoracic cage above and below and from the spinal column and is held down with a medium Deaver retractor. The pedicles are removed using micro Kerrison rongeurs or high speed drill. The tumor in the vertebral body is removed using a combination of curettes, rongeurs, or high speed drill depending upon its consistency. The rib(s) that was removed is then trimmed to span the gap left by the removal of the vertebral bodies and is impacted in place. Depending upon the extent of the bony removal and the nature of the tumor, internal stabilization may be accomplished with either intervertebral rib strut graft as described above or posterior instrumentation, or both. Meticulous he-

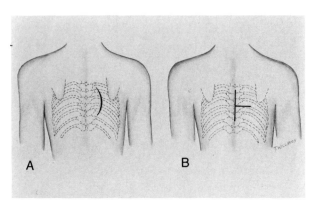

FIGURE 48–7. Incisions used for costotransversectomy (A) and for extended costotransversectomy (B).

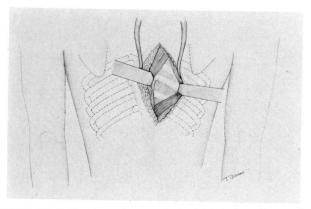

FIGURE 48–9. The trapezius muscle is divided along its muscle fibers.

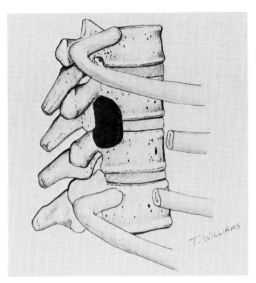

FIGURE 48–10. Costotransversectomy procedure. Two ribs have been resected. The dark area represents the area of the removed vertebral body.

mostasis is obtained with use of bipolar or monopolar cautery. The lung is expanded and the parietal pleura is inspected for any air leaks. Should they exist, placement of a chest tube is essential. The wound is closed by approximating chest wall muscles and subcutaneous tissue with heavy absorbable sutures and the skin with nylon or staples. A suction wound drain is generally not necessary.

TRANSPEDICULAR APPROACH

The transpedicular approach in itself gives very limited access to the vertebral body.[4] It is specifically

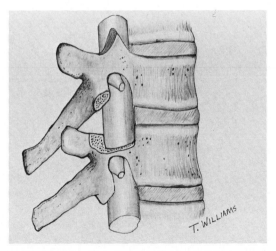

FIGURE 48–11. Illustration depicting the transpedicular approach.

indicated for the biopsy of an unknown vertebral lesion in instances where a Craig needle biopsy has been unsuccessful or contraindicated. Because of limitations of exposure, extensive tumor removal is not possible with this approach.

The patient is placed on chest rolls. A vertical incision is made, and the paravertebral muscles are stripped subperiosteally from the spinous process and the lamina on the side of interest. The muscle reflection should extend laterally well beyond the zygoapophyseal joint. A hemilaminectomy is done, and the facet joints and the corresponding pedicle are drilled away. It is well to remember that the pedicle is situated immediately caudal and ventral to the superior articular facet. Completion of the drilling of the pedicle leads one to the dorsal surface of the vertebral body. Appropriate biopsy of the body is taken, or in cases of small benign lesions, such as an osteoid osteoma, excision of the lesion is accomplished. After meticulous hemostasis, the wound is closed in layers without leaving a drain.

EXTENDED COSTOTRANSVERSECTOMY

Extended costotransversectomy entails the removal of hemilaminae and the zygoapophyseal joint in addition to the removal of usual structures during costotransversectomy. The skin incision is T-shaped with the horizontal limb of the **T** centered on the lesion (see Fig. 48–7*B*). The paraspinal muscles are separated from the spinous processes and laminae and the zygoapophyseal joints, transected horizontally, and retracted in a cephalocaudal direction. After completing the removal of the rib and transverse process, in a manner described in the previous section, the hemilaminae, zygoapophyseal joints, and the pedicles are removed. This gives extended exposure of the dural sac, roots, and epidural space.

REFERENCES

1. Capner N: The evolution of lateral rhachotomy. J Bone Joint Surg (Br) 36:173–179, 1954.
2. Giarrido E: Modified costotransversectomy: A surgical approach to ventrally placed lesions in the thoracic spinal canal. Surg Neurol 13:109–113, 1980.
3. Hoppenfeld S, deBoer P: Surgical Exposures in Orthopedics: The Anatomic Approach. J. B. Lippincott, Philadelphia, 1984, pp 269–273.
4. Patterson RH Jr, Arbit E: A surgical approach through the pedicle to protruded thoracic discs. J Neurosurg 48:768–772, 1978.
5. Perrin RG, McBroom RJ: Anterior versus posterior decompression for symptomatic spinal metastasis. Can J Neurol Sci 14:75–80, 1987.

49

SPINAL ORTHOTICS

GEORGE W. SYPERT

INTRODUCTION

The management of pain of spinal origin and the correction of spinal deformity utilizing external braces or appliances date back to as early as the fifth Egyptian dynasty (2750–2625 BC).[17] The basic principles of many of our present spinal orthoses may be traced to the devices used by Hippocrates and the armorers of the Middle Ages. Currently there are many spinal orthoses available to the spinal surgeon. These devices are often known by eponyms based on the inventor's name, where the device was designed, or its physical description. In spite of the large number of such appliances, sufficient information concerning the biomechanical principles of external spinal orthoses exists, such that rational application of these appliances can be made in each clinical situation.[21] Relatively few external appliances merit application by the majority of spinal surgeons treating spinal disorders, because such surgeons are seldom involved in the use of these devices for the correction of severe developmental spinal deformities that involve large numbers of pathologic motion segments.

CLINICAL RATIONALE

The objective of the clinician in the application of external spinal orthoses is control of the position of the spine by the use of external forces. Control of spinal position may be necessary for protection, immobilization, support, correction of deformity, or diagnostic trial. Of these various reasons, protection of the neural elements (spinal cord and nerve roots) is most important.

The application of external forces to the body alters the preexisting patterns of deformation and kinematics of the spine. When it is necessary to protect the neural elements from spinal instability or deformity related to various diseases (traumatic, neoplastic, and so forth), the orthosis generally performs functions normally achieved by the intrinsic structure of the spine and its axial musculature. If inaccurate clinical assessments or fallacious assumptions are made regarding the biomechanics of either the spinal disorder or the external orthosis, there is danger of

injury to the patient. It may be appropriate to put the spine at rest to limit the range of spinal motion when certain positions or movements are painful to the patient. In the latter circumstance, the orthosis is used largely as a substitute for or as an assistant to the actions of the axial musculature. It may also sometimes function as a psychologic reminder owing to the irritative properties of the orthotic device. Finally, the external orthosis may be used in the therapeutic correction of spinal deformities such as scoliosis and kyphosis.

COMPLICATIONS

The clinical applications of spinal orthoses are associated with some undesirable effects, including skin breakdown and local pain, weakening of the axial musculature, contracture of the soft tissues, psychologic dependence, and aggravation of symptom patterns.[10] Because most spinal orthoses function through the transmission of external forces that act directly on the skin, local pressure pain and cutaneous and underlying soft tissue breakdown are potential complications of these appliances. Certain biologic functions of the skin limit the magnitude and duration of the external forces that can be applied to it. The skin requires cleansing and ventilation; without these, serious decubitus ulcerations may ensue.

Axial muscle weakness and atrophy are caused by a reduced functional demand on these muscles when an orthosis substitutes for their role in maintaining an upright posture. To prevent this complication, the orthosis should be used in conjunction with an appropriate exercise program, especially isometric exercises to the limit of the patient's tolerance.

A goal of therapy should be to discontinue the external appliance as soon as its therapeutic value has been achieved. To prevent fixed soft tissue contractures, a rehabilitation mobilization program should be instituted as quickly as possible after removal of the orthosis. Physical dependence can occur because of weakening of the axial muscles and tightness and contracture of the soft tissues supporting the spine (e.g., frozen neck, frozen back). In addition, psychologic dependence may occur or augment any physical dependence. Psychologic dependence is frequently encountered in patients with substantial emotional problems or if major psychosocial-economic elements play a role in the spinal disorder. In cases of continuing compensation or litigation, there is frequently a tendency on the part of the patient to continue therapy because of secondary and tertiary gains. The clinician should be cognizant of these factors, and if they are recognized as major reasons for the patient's continued use of the orthosis, its termination should be strongly considered.

Finally, orthoses may aggravate the patient's symptoms. By reducing movement of the spinal segments within the confines of the external device, the spinal orthoses may cause increased spinal motion at the ends of the immobilized segments. This complication is particularly relevant to the lumbosacral segments, where increased symptoms may occur when the orthosis does not include a thigh extension.[9, 14] In addition, increased electromyographic activity in the erector spinae musculature during walking has been reported while the patient has been wearing a spinal orthosis.[24] This increase in axial muscular activity is thought to be due to increased demands on the spinal musculature to provide the normal spinal rotations related to walking which are limited by the orthotic device. Another potential source for aggravation of a patient's symptoms by a spinal orthosis is compression or obstruction of venous return, with consequent shunting to Batson's plexus, and increased compression and irritation of the spinal neural elements. Despite these various negative effects of spinal orthoses, their appropriate use provides substantial therapeutic benefits for many patients suffering a wide range of spinal disorders.

BIOMECHANICS

The biomechanical consequences of the application of a spinal orthosis are the result of the forces exerted by the device on the body. The point(s) of application, direction(s), and magnitude(s) of these forces depend on the design of the device, the tightness with which it is worn, the patient's attempts to move against it, and the patient's body shape. The correct use of any spinal orthosis depends on an understanding of these factors. Moreover, an understanding of the pathophysiology and biomechanics of the spinal disorder under treatment and an accurate evaluation of the effects of the orthosis are required. To develop a rational approach to the clinical application of spinal orthotics, full understanding of spinal and orthotic biomechanics is essential.

The spine has been described as a series of semirigid bodies (vertebrae) separated by viscoelastic linkages (discs and ligaments).[25] To complete a biomechanical analysis of the spine, one must remember that its linkages are suspended in the body; viscoelastic structures of various stiffness are attached to the spine. From the standpoint of spinal orthotics, all of these elements have been viewed as sitting inside a cylinder—the body—that varies in size. The goal of spinal orthotics is to transmit forces through this cylinder to the vertebral column.

Force cannot be applied directly to the spine by orthotic devices. The major mechanical factor limiting the application of forces to the spine is the stiffness of the structures through which the forces must be transmitted.[25] Therefore, the fundamental problem of external spinal orthoses is transmitting sufficient forces to the vertebral column through low-stiffness viscoelastic transmitters. This problem is further complicated because these transmitters vary considerably in stiffness. For example, the skull, ribs, and pelvis (although not particularly stiff) may be the stiffest available transmitters. In contrast, the fat, viscera, and muscles of the abdominal cavity are of much lower stiffness. Therefore, it should not be surprising that it is possible to apply more corrective forces to a thoracic scoliosis than to a scoliosis in the lumbar region. In fact, it is well known that spinal orthotics are less effective at holding or correcting lumbar curves than thoracic curves.

An additional problem is encountered in the cervical spine, which lies in a smaller cylinder, the neck, which is filled with many vital structures (e.g., major cerebral vessels, the larynx, and the trachea) that cannot withstand any significant direct pressure or force. Hence, to be effective, an orthosis for the cervical spine must grip structures at each end of the neck, that is, the skull and face and the thoracic cage. Another limiting factor is the sensitivity of the skin and deeper structures, because the effectiveness of an orthotic device is, in part, dependent on the firmness of its attachment to these structures.

To understand the biomechanics of spinal orthoses, consideration must be given to the normal kinematics of the vertebral column. The cervical spine is the most mobile. Greater flexion is permitted than extension. Most of this motion is in the sagittal plane, and motion is greatest in the midpoint, at C5-C6, and at the craniovertebral junction (0-C2). The C1-C2 articulation has the greatest degree of axial rotation. The lower cervical spine allows a generous amount of axial rotation and lateral bending. Although there is significant motion of the thoracic spine, it is considerably less mobile than either adjacent vertebral region. Its flexion is also greater than its extension, whereas axial rotation decreases in a caudal direction. Lateral bending increases in a caudal direction. There is little axial rotation in the lumbar spine. The greatest motion of the lumbar spine is flexion-extension. Some increase in rotation occurs at the lumbosacral junction. Any pelvic motion results in movement of the lumbar spine.

Besides the normal regional kinematics of the spine, the control of the spine by an orthosis may depend on the six principles of freedom of the involved motion segments.[25] The clinician evaluates these factors and the nature of the spinal instability or deformity under treatment to decide which of the movements to restrict or what deformity to correct. Based on this analysis, the most appropriate orthosis for achieving control of the spine can then be selected. For example, if an orthosis is used to compensate for spinal instability, a basic understanding of the clinical instability in the individual patient is essential. In general, loss of structural integrity of the spine owing to destruction of the posterior elements tends to make the spine more unstable in flexion, and destruction of anterior elements makes it more unstable in extension. Certain orthoses protect better against anterior flexion displacement, whereas others protect better against posterior extension displacement. Attention must also be given to how rigid and how firmly attached the orthosis should be. Is it certain that an orthotic appliance can compensate for the spinal instability or correct the spinal deformity under consideration? The clinician should select the orthotic device that is most appropriate for each spinal disorder.

Four positive biomechanical effects of spinal orthoses have been described: (1) motion control, (2) spinal realignment, (3) trunk support (with lumbar orthoses), and (4) weight transfer (with cervical orthoses).[12] These positive physiologic effects result from the application of one or more of the six biomechanical principles used in the design and application of spinal orthoses: (1) the balance of horizontal forces (mechanical three-point pressure system), (2) fluid compression, (3) distraction, (4) the sleeve principle (construction of a cage around the patient), (5) irritative restraint (reminder), and (6) skeletal fixation (e.g., halo fixation, halo-pelvic fixation).[25]

Motion Control

All orthotic devices are designed to reduce gross trunk motion between the two ends of the appliance. Skeletal fixation appears to be the most effective method for reliable control of spinal motion. Two other principal mechanisms for restraining spinal motion include the mechanical three-point pressure system and irritative restraint of gross trunk motion. Quantitative information on the degree of motion control (particularly at the motion segment level) is difficult to obtain in vivo and is necessarily incomplete. It is known that no external appliance, especially those used in the lumbosacral region, can completely immobilize the vertebral column because of the intervening compressible, nonstiff soft tissue. In fact, there is evidence that segmental motion may be increased at the ends of the externally stabilized vertebral column when a patient attempts to move.

Spinal Realignment

Correction of spinal deformities or realignment is generally accomplished by the application of balanced horizontal forces (three-point pressure system) and irritative restraint. Balanced horizontal forces may be used to provide bending moments for ky-

photic (flexion), scoliotic (lateral), and rotational deformities. The bending moments are most efficient when the apex of the curve or deformity is placed at the middle force equidistant from the two opposing end forces. Irritative restraint stimulates corrective muscle action patterns in response to the presence of uncomfortable pressure points.

Trunk Support

Trunk support is used primarily in thoracolumbar and lumbar orthoses. Fluid compression by elevating the intraabdominal pressure through compression of the abdomen and application of balanced horizontal forces are the major biomechanical actions of these devices. Essentially elevation of intraabdominal pressure with compression of the soft abdominal contents converts the abdomen into a semirigid cylinder that can transmit a portion of the vertical load imposed on the trunk, thereby relieving some of the load on the vertebral column.

Weight Transfer

Weight transfer is frequently used in cervical orthotic appliances. Resembling trunk support, weight transfer relieves some of the vertical gravitational load on the spine. Distraction forces are the most efficient in transferring weight; therefore, maximal head support is obtained through skeletal fixation, such as that provided by cranial tongs and the halo-vest orthosis. The other means to achieve weight transfer for cervical spine disorders is with chin and occipital supports incorporated in the orthotic device.

CERVICAL ORTHOSES (0-T3)

As mentioned, the vital soft tissues of the neck cannot withstand compressive forces. Hence, the efficacy of an orthotic appliance designed for the cervical spine depends upon the adequacy of fixation at the ends of the cervical spine, that is, the skull and face and the thorax. Cervical orthoses have been classified into four basic types, which are listed from the least restrictive to the most restrictive in the following order: the cervical collar, the poster-type orthosis, the cervicothoracic orthosis, and the halo orthosis.[26]

Cervical Collars

Collars have long been popular in managing a variety of conditions of the cervical spine. These appliances have the advantage of low cost, ease of fabrication, convenience, and high patient comfort. Unfortunately, they do little to restrict motion or transfer weight. They do provide warmth and psychologic comfort and support. There are three gen-

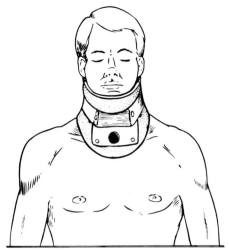
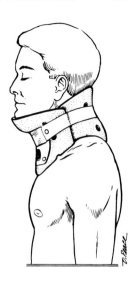

FIGURE 49–1. The Philadelphia collar.

eral types of cervical collars: the soft collar, the hard collar (e.g., the Thomas collar), and the Philadelphia collar. The soft collar does not significantly immobilize the cervical spine, according to studies in which soft-collar wearers were compared with normal controls without collars.[2, 5–8, 15] The hard plastic collar is also not very effective in restricting motion of the cervical spine.[5, 15] Therefore, these devices serve largely as psychologic reminders and have little role in the management of clinical cervical spine instability. Adding an anterior and posterior reinforcement under the chin and occiput, such as in the relatively rigid Philadelphia collar (Fig. 49–1), significantly restricts cervical spine motion, particularly flexion and extension.[5–7, 15] However, the latter device is generally ineffective in controlling rotation and lateral bending. Hence, the Philadelphia collar serves largely to remind patients whose cervical spines are essentially stable that excessive cervical spine motion should be restricted.

Poster-Type Orthoses

A wide variety of poster-type braces are available. Examples include the four-poster brace, the two-poster (e.g., Guilford orthosis), and the sternooccipitomandibular immobilizer (SOMI). The four-poster, like the Philadelphia collar, has chin and occipital fixation. There are anterior and posterior pieces that grip the chest, but not firmly. The four-poster does add more control of cervical spine motion than the Philadelphia collar, especially in restricting flexion in the middle cervical segments. It is not very effective in restricting rotation, lateral bending, and sagittal plane motion in the upper cervical spine. The Guilford orthosis (Fig. 49–2), with its circumferential straps to secure the chest, is significantly more effective than the conventional four-poster brace in controlling cervical spine motion.[5, 6, 26] The Guilford device is the most effective conventional brace, but it also remains poor at controlling flexion at the cranio-

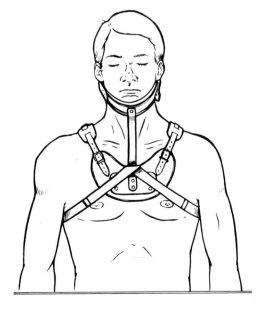
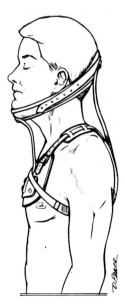

FIGURE 49–2. The Guilford orthosis.

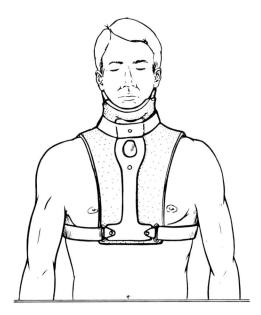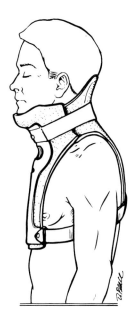

FIGURE 49–3. The cervicothoracic orthosis.

cervical junction as well as rotation and lateral bending. Unfortunately, most patients find this orthosis uncomfortable. The SOMI, in contrast, is reasonably comfortable and is readily applied with the patient lying supine. This device is effective in controlling flexion of the upper cervical spine (C1-C3). However, it is less effective than the other poster-type orthoses in controlling every other motion.[5, 6, 27]

Cervicothoracic Orthoses

The cervicothoracic orthoses (Fig. 49–3) are reasonably comfortable and relatively easy to fabricate by a well-equipped, experienced orthotic laboratory. Moreover, they control motion as well as the Guilford orthosis, providing at least 90 per cent restriction of flexion, extension, and rotation.[5, 6, 28] Lateral bending

is reduced to 50 per cent of the unrestricted movements of normal controls. Upper cervical spine motion is less well controlled than the middle and lower cervical spine. An example of this type of orthosis is the Yale cervical orthosis, which consists of a Philadelphia collar with molded fiberglass extensions riveted to the collar and extending over the chest, front, and back. A circumferential chest strap anchors the orthosis to the trunk.

Halo Orthoses

There are two basic types of halo appliances that are used to control cervical spine motion: halo casts and halo vests (Fig. 49–4). These orthoses provide the most secure control of all cervical spine motions.[5, 6, 26, 27] Of great importance are the findings that halo

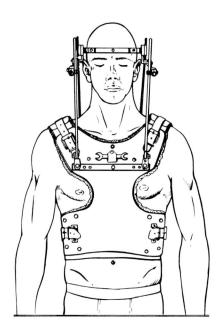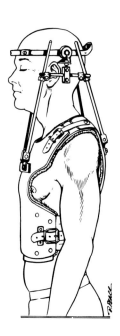

FIGURE 49–4. The halo-vest orthosis.

orthoses control rotation, lateral bending, and flexion-extension motion over the upper cervical spine, planes of motion, and levels, which the other orthoses control poorly. However, even these orthoses do not eliminate all cervical motion.

Control of cervical motion can be improved with the halo systems by increasing the distraction forces across the neck. The amount of distraction that the neck can tolerate is limited, particularly if there is severe instability. Therefore, there are clinical situations in which the cervical spine is so unstable that no external orthosis will adequately control the spinal segments involved. In these cases, internal surgical fixation and fusion may be required, with supplementary external orthotic support.

Although the halo devices are the gold standard for all external cervical orthoses, it must be recognized that there are serious risks associated with the application of halo systems. These complications include penetration of the skull, brain abscess, and cranial nerve palsies.[22] The clinical application of halo orthoses thus requires great care and careful neurologic observation and follow-up.

Recommendations

With the exception of the cervical collars without mandibular and occipital supports, the various cervical orthoses provide similar control of cervical spine motion. Each orthotic device has advantages and limitations that depend on specific mechanical goals: to support (rest, assist), to immobilize (protect), or to correct a deformity. All of the cervical orthoses find it difficult to control rotation between the occiput and C2. In addition, all conventional orthoses poorly control flexion-extension and rotation at 0-C1, as well as rotation and lateral bending over the whole spine. Only the halo system controls these various motions well. In general, increasing the length and rigidity of a cervical orthosis improves its effectiveness. To be effective, a cervical orthosis must fix the head directly (halo) or hold the chin and occiput through adequate molding. Another factor to consider in choosing an orthosis is familiarity with the benefits, limitations, and complications of specific devices by both the clinician and the local orthotist. Because it is not reasonable to stock all of the devices, it is recommended that the clinician become experienced with selected orthoses that correct the various spinal disorders treated by the clinical staff. The cervical orthoses that the author has found useful and recommends for the adult spinal surgeon are listed in Table 49–1.

THORACOLUMBAR ORTHOSES (T3-L3)

External orthotic appliances for the thoracic spine, thoracolumbar junction, and upper lumbar spine (T3-L3) may be divided into two general categories: (1) immobilizing or supportive, and (2) corrective.

TABLE 49–1. CERVICAL ORTHOSES: RECOMMENDATIONS

ORTHOSIS	SPINAL DISORDER
Soft collar Hard collar	None
Philadelphia collar	Stable spine Cervical strain Interbody fusion
Guilford orthosis Cervicothoracic orthosis	Mild instability Stable fractures Postoperative internal fixation
Halo orthosis	Unstable spine (0-T3)

Immobilizing or supportive devices are principally used for traumatic fractures, neoplastic disorders, and infectious disorders and after surgical treatment of spinal instability or deformity. Corrective devices are generally used for the specialized treatment of children suffering progressive scoliosis or kyphosis. Like cervical orthoses, a wide variety of external devices have been designed for the thoracic and lumbar spine. Such orthoses include long thoracic corsets, dorsolumbar braces, hyperextension braces, the Milwaukee brace, and molded polyform or Risser plaster jackets.

Thoracic Corsets

Long thoracic corsets, when well fitted, can offer some restriction of spine motion. They do not, however, immobilize the thoracic and lumbar spine as well as other orthoses. The author has not encountered patients who were deemed appropriate for these devices.

Dorsolumbar Braces

The Taylor brace is the prototypal dorsolumbar brace. This appliance consists of a wide, circumferential, fitted pelvic band with two long posterior vertical bars extending from the pelvic band to the shoulders. The vertical bars are joined by a short transverse bar in the midthoracic region. Straps attached to the vertical bars pass around the shoulders and under the axillae. Finally, a full-length abdominal pad is attached by straps and buckles to the vertical bars. The device functions in part on the sleeve principle as a splint and as a three-point fixation, with force applied in the region of the thoracolumbar junction posteriorly and counterforce applied on the upper chest and the lower abdomen and pubis posteriorly.[12, 24] Although this orthosis offers some resistance to flexion-extension motions, it provides very little resistance to lateral bending or rotational motions. Therefore, it appears to act largely as a reminder not to move excessively in flexion and extension. The role of this type of orthosis in the management of spinal disorders is therefore very limited.

Hyperextension Braces

The hyperextension braces, such as the Jewett or Griswold brace, are designed to use three-point fixation for resistance of motion, primarily flexion.[12, 24] Such appliances generally consist of a rectangular metal frame over the anterior and lateral sides of the trunk, which maintains hyperextension by backward pressure from fixation points at the manubriosternal area and the symphysis pubis, and a transverse strap, which maintains counterpressure in the midthoracolumbar region. These braces offer little resistance to extension, lateral bending, and rotational motions. When such braces can be adjusted to achieve some degree of hyperextension, it appears that they may shift some of the weight-bearing axis of the spine toward the posterior elements. They may decrease the stresses of the vertebral bodies. These braces do not prevent additional vertical collapse in cases of severely comminuted thoracolumbar fracture nor do they prevent vertebral body collapse in case of neoplasia and osteoporosis. Therefore, a well-molded full-body jacket or cast should be applied in hyperextension whenever significant vertebral collapse or deformity is a concern.

Milwaukee Brace

The Milwaukee brace and its modifications are very sophisticated, complex orthotic appliances used in the correction of progressive developmental scoliosis, lordosis, and kyphosis. An adequate description of these dynamic orthoses, which are used to redirect spinal growth by stimulating corrective trunk muscle patterns, is beyond the scope of this chapter.

Molded Body Jackets

Circumferential, well-molded, full-length body jackets extending anteriorly from the manubriosternal region to the symphysis pubis, laterally from the axillae to the pelvis, and posteriorly from the upper thoracic region to the sacropelvic region yield the most effective control of the thoracic, thoracolumbar, and upper lumbar spinal regions (T3-L3). If the upper thoracic spine (T3-T7) is to be immobilized, an extension of the jacket to include mandibular and occipital supports should be incorporated. Moreover, if kyphotic deformity or vertebral body collapse is a clinical consideration, the jacket should be applied in hyperextension, with the posterior fulcrum at the site of potential deformity. When appropriately designed and applied, these orthoses exert control against axial rotation and effectively control flexion-extension and lateral bending motions. They require fabrication by an experienced and well-equipped orthotics laboratory. Molded body jackets may be fabricated from light cast material, plastics, or heat-sensitive polyform. The author prefers the latter. These jackets may be split like a clam-shell with Velcro straps connecting the anterior and posterior

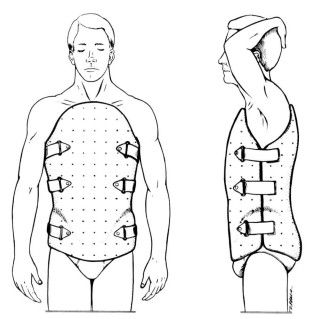

FIGURE 49–5. The polyform clam-shell orthosis.

halves of the shell (Fig. 49–5). The clam-shell permits reliable patients to lie in one half of the shell while removing the other half to bathe and care for the skin.

Recommendations

Although a variety of orthoses have been developed and used for disorders of the thoracic and upper lumbar spine, the author has found that the majority are not useful to the surgeon treating nondevelopmental spinal disorders. None of these devices can completely immobilize this region of the spine because of its viscoelastic properties. Therefore, the author's recommendations are very straightforward. As can be seen in Table 49–2, the molded body jackets are the principal orthoses recommended for the T3-L3 spinal regions.[21, 22]

LUMBOSACRAL ORTHOSES (L3-S1)

Lumbar spine orthoses are most frequently used for the management of low back pain disorders. They are also used for vertebral support or immobilization after lumbosacral fusion, lumbosacral spinal trauma,

TABLE 49–2. THORACOLUMBAR ORTHOSES: RECOMMENDATIONS

Orthosis	Spinal Disorder
Thoracic corset	None
Dorsolumbar brace Hyperextension brace	Stable fractures (<50% compression)

Molded body jacket
  Clam-shell
  Plaster jacket
	Unstable spine (T3-L3)
	Postoperative instrumentation fusion

**TABLE 49–3. LUMBOSACRAL ORTHOSES:
RECOMMENDATIONS**

Orthosis	Spinal Disorder
Lumbosacral corsets	None
Lumbosacral braces/jackets	None
Lumbosacral spica	Instability (L3-S1)

and lumbosacral spine neoplastic and infectious destructive diseases. Application of lumbosacral orthoses in the management of low back pain disorders remains controversial among expert clinicians. Some think that there is little, if any, scientific basis for using such devices. A significant reservation frequently cited is the adverse development of physical (muscle atrophy, contractures) and psychologic dependence. Others think that the temporary application of some form of external support may help manage episodes of acute low back pain or evaluate the effect of immobilization when considering spinal fusion (diagnostic trial). In any event, a long, confusing list of orthotic devices has been developed, consistent with the confusion and complexity inherent in the management of low back pain. Lumbosacral orthoses may be classified from the least to the most effective immobilizers as follows: corsets, braces and jackets, and spicas (Table 49–3).

Lumbosacral Corsets

The lumbosacral corset has been used for at least 400 years.[3] In its present form, the prototypal canvas lumbosacral corset is generally made or fitted individually by an orthotist for the patient suffering a lumbosacral spine disorder.[1, 13] The corset usually extends from around the lower rib cage to over the iliac crests laterally and to just above the symphysis pubis anteriorly and includes the sacrum and upper part of the buttocks posteriorly. The corset is frequently reinforced with two posterior vertical steel bars stitched between the layers of canvas.

Lumbosacral Braces and Jackets

A partial listing of braces and jackets that have been used in the management of lumbosacral spine disorders includes short lumbar spine braces (e.g., Williams) or jackets (e.g., flexion body jacket); intermediate length lumbar spine braces (e.g., Knight, MacAusland, chairback); and long lumbar spine braces (e.g., Taylor, Arnold) or jackets (e.g., plaster, polyform clam-shell).

The flexion body jacket has recently become a relatively popular support for the management of low back pain disorders. It consists of anterior and posterior custom-fitted shells made of lightweight rigid thermosensitive polyform material connected by side straps using buckles or Velcro. The front panel is indented toward the abdomen to provide abdominal compression and increased abdominal pressure. Both the flexion body jacket and the Williams lumbar orthosis provide lumbar support by increasing abdominal pressure and immobilization by three-point fixation that tends to reverse any excessive lumbar lordosis.

The intermediate length lumbar spine braces, although differing in the degree of rigidity, are largely derived from the original concepts underlying the Knight brace. The latter brace consists of a circumferential wide pelvic band and a circumferential band at about T8, joined by two posterior vertical bars and an anterior pad or corset. The points of fixation anteriorly are the lower rib cage and the epigastrium superiorly and the symphysis pubis inferiorly. The posterior force is directed to the midlumbar region.

The long lumbar spine braces and jackets (see thoracolumbar orthoses) shift the anterosuperior fixation point rostrally to the manubriosternal region, with a tendency for the posterior force to rise toward the thoracolumbar junction.

Lumbosacral Spicas

Lumbosacral spica-type orthoses may be fabricated individually using light cast or thermosensitive polyform material. These jackets are usually applied on the standing patient by an experienced orthotist. Generally, these jackets extend from 2 cm below the shoulder blades to the midportion of the sacrum posteriorly, from the xiphisternum to the symphysis pubis anteriorly, and from around the rib cage to 3 cm below the level of the anterosuperior iliac crests laterally. Careful molding about the pelvic structures is required because the device should be tightly fitted. A thigh extension, usually on the most symptomatic side, is extended to 5 cm above the patella. The hip is held in 15 to 20 degrees of flexion to prevent lumbar lordosis, to facilitate sitting, and to permit swing through of the leg in walking. Usually, the patient in physical therapy is instructed in walking with a cane. Most younger patients will eventually find the cane an inconvenience and will stop using it. If the spica is always to be worn while weightbearing, the patient will require a raised toilet seat. As in the polyform clam-shell lumbosacral spica illustrated in Figure 49–6, the appliance may be constructed so that the patient can remove half of the shell for skin care or can completely remove the device when recumbent (nonweightbearing) for sleep. The author has found the latter modification to be an excellent orthosis when treating highly reliable patients.[18]

Although there are only a few biomechanical studies of lumbosacral orthoses, the studies that have been performed are very useful for an understanding of the benefits, limitations, and adverse effects of lumbosacral external immobilizing appliances. Early investigators found that when a subject wore a long lumbosacral spinal brace, paradoxically, increased motion was observed at the lower lumbar motion segments (L4-L5 and L5-S1) compared with that observed when the subject was wearing no external

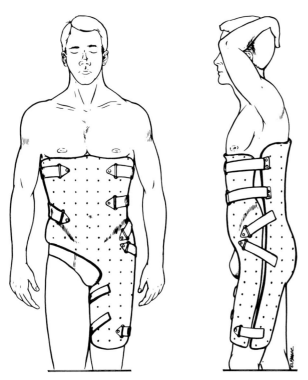

FIGURE 49–6. The polyform clam-shell lumbosacral spica orthosis.

orthosis. This appeared to be a result of the more secure fixation of the appliance to the thoracic and thoracolumbar junction than to the pelvis. This creates a more rigid thoracic and upper lumbar vertebral column, transmitting motion to the relatively free lower portion of the spine. Therefore, it appears that if substantial restriction of movement in the L3-S1 spinal region is desired, secure fixation of the pelvis is a prerequisite. This implies that an effective lumbosacral orthosis must include a thigh extension (lumbosacral spica).

More recently, the efficacy of the canvas corset,[1, 13] the Raney flexion jacket,[16] the long lumbosacral light cast jacket, and the light cast jacket with inclusion of the thigh (spica) on the segmental mobility of the lumbosacral spine in normal volunteers has been investigated.[4] Consistent with the aforementioned conclusions, the light cast spica was found to be the most effective in restricting angular movements below L3, particularly at the L4-L5 and L5-S1 motion segments. Therefore, it is reasonable to conclude that if significant restriction of motion of the lumbosacral spine is a goal of the application of a lumbosacral orthosis, then a carefully molded body cast or polyform jacket with a thigh extension to control pelvic motion is essential.

Based on the observations that the long lumbosacral orthoses may aggravate movements in the lumbosacral spine, it has been assumed that the shorter the orthosis, within reason, the better the restriction of lumbosacral spine motion. The short lumbosacral orthoses do appear to decrease flexion-extension angular movements.[4, 14] However, none of the many lumbosacral orthoses carefully studied effectively im-

mobilized the lumbosacral spine.[14] In fact, walking while wearing a lumbosacral orthosis without a thigh extension may actually increase the rotation of the lumbosacral spine.[9] Electromyographic studies of the intrinsic spinal musculature indicate that paraspinous muscle activity is increased with the application of a lumbosacral orthosis.[24] This may be due to an attempt of the paraspinous musculature to produce normal rotatory motions against the resistance of the appliance. Electromyographic activity of the abdominal muscles, in contrast, was decreased with the application of both the lumbosacral corset and the chairback brace. Intradiscal pressure is also apparently reduced to 15 to 20 per cent in an individual wearing a tight lumbosacral support that produces significant abdominal compression.[11] It appears that the application of a well-fitted, tight lumbosacral orthosis may take over some of the function of the abdominal muscles and relieve some of the load on the lumbosacral spine by compression of the abdomen, converting its contents into a semirigid cylinder.

One of the adverse effects of application of a lumbosacral orthosis in which abdominal compressive forces are important is a decrease in vital capacity (about 10 per cent).[11] An increase in abdominal pressure and, thereby, lower extremity venous pressure also results from the use of these devices. Hence, patients who suffer from poor pulmonary reserve, hemorrhoids, and varicose veins are poor candidates for management of lumbosacral spine disorders with tight lumbosacral orthoses.

In general, the effectiveness of the various lumbosacral orthoses in lumbosacral immobilization (excluding the spica-type devices) is related more to their discomfort than to the actual magnitude of the forces (abdominal compression, three-point fixation) transmitted from the appliance to the body.[25] Thus, the functions of most lumbosacral orthoses are to remind and irritate the patient to restrict movement, to support the abdomen to alleviate some of the load on the lumbosacral spine, to provide some movement restriction of the upper lumbar and thoracolumbar spine by three-point fixation, and to reduce excessive lumbar lordosis to provide a straighter and more comfortable low back.

Recommendations

The clinician should attempt to select an appropriate lumbosacral orthosis based on the goals to be achieved by the orthosis. The role of conventional lumbosacral spine orthoses in the management of low back pain disorders remains controversial. The adverse physiologic and psychologic factors inherent in these devices appear to far outweigh any advantage they may have. This is particularly true for the individual suffering a chronic low back pain disorder, where myofascial contractures play a major role in the continuance of the chronic pain syndrome.[18–20] In contrast, the use of a lumbosacral spica-type orthosis, which is highly effective in immobilizing the lumbosacral spine, is recommended for the management of lumbosacral instability produced by various spinal disorders (Table 49–3).

REFERENCES

1. Ahlgren SA, Hansen T: The use of lumbosacral corsets prescribed for low back pain. Prosthet Orthot Int 2:101–104, 1978.
2. Colachis SC, Strohm BR: Cervical spine motion in normal women: Radiographic study of effect of cervical collars. Arch Phys Med Rehabil 54:161–169, 1973.
3. Evans E: The Palace of Minos at Knossos. Vol 1. London, MacMillan, 1921, p 503.
4. Fidler MW, Plasmans CMT: The effect of four types of support on the segmental mobility of the lumbosacral spine. J Bone Joint Surg 65A:943–947, 1983.
5. Hartman JT, Palumbo F, Hill BJ: Cineradiography of the braced normal cervical spine: A comparative study of five commonly used cervical orthoses. Clin Orthop 109:97–102, 1975.
6. Johnson RM, Hart DL, Simmons EF, et al: Cervical orthoses: A study comparing their effectiveness in restricting cervical motion in normal subjects. J Bone Joint Surg 59A:332–339, 1981.
7. Johnson RM, Owen JR, Hart DL, et al: Cervical orthoses: A guide to their selection and use. Clin Orthop 154:34–45, 1981.
8. Jones MD: Cineradiographic studies of the collar immobilized cervical spine. J Neurosurg 17:633–637, 1960.
9. Lumsden RM, Morris JM: An in vivo study of axial rotation and immobilization at the lumbosacral joint. J Bone Joint Surg 50A:1591–1602, 1968.
10. Lusskin R, Berger N: Prescription principles. In American Academy of Orthopaedic Surgeons (eds): Atlas of Orthotics: Biomechanical Principles and Application. St. Louis, CV Mosby, 1975, pp 364–372.
11. Morris JM: Spinal bracing. In Wilkins RH, Rengachary SS (eds): Neurosurgery. New York, McGraw-Hill, 1985, pp 2300–2305.
12. Morris JM, Lucas DB: Biomechanics of spinal bracing. Ariz Med 21:170–176, 1964.
13. New York University, Post-Graduate Medical School Prosthetics and Orthotics: Measurement, layout and pattern design for lumbosacral F-E and L corsets. In Spinal Orthotics Including Orthotist's Supplement. New York, New York University, 1975, pp 167–196.
14. Norton PL, Brown T: The immobilizing efficiency of back braces: Their effect on the posture and motion of the lumbosacral spine. J Bone Joint Surg 39A:111–139, 1957.
15. Podolsky S, Baraff LJ, Simon RR, et al: Efficacy of cervical spine immobilization methods. J Trauma 23:461–464, 1983.
16. Raney F: Royalite flexion jacket: Report on the Spinal Orthotics Workshop. Sponsored by the Committee on Prosthetics Research and Development of the Division of Engineering of the National Research Council. Washington, DC, National Research Council, 1969, pp 85–91.
17. Smith GE: The most ancient splints. Br Med J 1:732, 1908.
18. Sypert GW: Low back pain disorders: Lumbar fusion? Clin Neurosurg 33:457–483, 1986.
19. Sypert GW: Lumbar disc disease. Part I. Natural history and diagnosis. Neurol Neurosurg Update Ser 7(11):1–8, 1987.
20. Sypert GW: Lumbar disc disease. Part II. Therapy. Neurol Neurosurg Update Ser 7(12):1–8, 1987.
21. Sypert GW: External spinal orthotics. Neurosurgery 20:642–649, 1987.
22. Sypert GW: Stabilization procedures for thoracic and lumbar fractures. Clin Neurosurg 34:340–377, 1988.
23. Victor D, Bresnan M, Keller R: Brain abscess complicating the use of halo traction. J Bone Joint Surg 55A:635–637, 1973.
24. Waters RL, Morris JM: Effect of spinal supports on the electrical activity of muscles in the trunk. J Bone Joint Surg 52A:51–60, 1970.
25. White AA III, Panjabi MM: Clinical Biomechanics of the Spine. Philadelphia, JB Lippincott, 1978.
26. Wolf JW, Johnson RM: Cervical orthoses. In The Cervical Spine Research Society (eds): The Cervical Spine. Philadelphia, JB Lippincott, 1983, pp 54–61.
27. Zeleznik R, Chapin W, Hart DL, et al: Yale cervical orthosis. Phys Ther 58:861–865, 1978.

50

WOUND MANAGEMENT IN SPINAL SURGERY

MAHMOUD B. EL-TAMER and TED CHAGLASSIAN

INTRODUCTION

The management of wounds has varied throughout history and with various cultures. The Navajo tribe chanted to the gods to promote healing, and the Kapelli tribe of Liberia packed wounds with rodent hair and used papaya slices for wound debridement.[69] The management of wounds was also addressed by the ancient Egyptians in the Edwin Smith Papyrus.[5] Management of open wounds with exposed vital structures remains a major problem. The spine represents a vital structure because it protects the spinal cord and plays a primary role in posture. In this chapter, the pathophysiology and management of wound complications in spinal surgery are discussed. Systemic factors that impair wound healing in general as well as decrease host resistance to infection, such as old age, obesity, hypovolemia, malnutrition, diabetes mellitus, chemotherapy, corticosteroids, sepsis, and shock, are not specifically addressed. We limit the discussion to the following issues: anatomy of the cutaneous arteries of the posterior trunk, cutaneous sequelae of radiation, management of cutaneous infections following spinal surgery, safe closure of incisions in the posterior spinal approach, and musculocutaneous flaps for coverage of the spine.

BLOOD SUPPLY

The cutaneous blood supply of the back has been investigated by several different authors. In 1889 Carl Manchot delineated anatomic territories of cutaneous arteries in his book *Die Hautarterien Des Menschlichen-Korpus*[45] (Fig. 50–1). Similarly, in 1936 Michel Salmon outlined the arterial blood supply of the skin in his manuscript *Les Artères de la Peau* (Fig. 50–2). Depending on the anatomic area, the blood supply of the skin may be considered in four zones: neck, thorax, lumbar, and sacral regions (Fig. 50–3).

The neck is defined anatomically by the following boundaries: superiorly, the occipital protuberance; medially, the midline; laterally, the edge of the trapezius muscle; and inferiorly, the spinous process of C7. The blood supply of this region is based on branches of two major arteries (Fig. 50–4): the occipital artery and the transverse cervical artery. The occipital artery originates from the external carotid, with the end segment reaching the skin of the upper part of the posterior neck. It sends branches that perforate the trapezius muscle and supply the upper zone of the neck region. The transverse cervical artery arises commonly from the thyrocervical trunk and separates into two branches—the superficial transverse cervical artery and the deep dorsal scapular artery. These vessels supply the trapezius muscle through vertical perforators and perfuse the skin. The contribution of the deep cervical artery is minimal in the neck.

In the thorax, the skin is supplied by nine pairs of intercostal vessels distributed through the lower nine intercostal spaces. The first and second intercostal spaces are supplied by the supreme intercostal artery, which is a branch of the costocervical trunk that originates from the subclavian artery. The intercostal arteries arise from each side of the aorta and send dorsal branches that run posteriorly. These dorsal branches give origin to the spinal artery, which supplies the spinal cord through the intervertebral foramina, and continues posteriorly to ramify in two segments—the medial and lateral dorsal cutaneous branches—which supply the skin through muscular perforators (Fig. 50–5).

The lumbar zone is vascularized through four lumbar arteries that arise lateral to the first four lumbar vertebral bodies. They send dorsal branches that bifurcate at the medial and lateral segments. The lumbar branch of the iliolumbar artery replaces the fifth pair of lumbar arteries. These arterial branches supply the skin through muscular perforators. The sacral arteries send branches that traverse posteriorly to the sacrum to perfuse the overlying skin. These cutaneous branches supply a limited area surrounding the sacrum (see Fig. 50–3). The major contribution is through musculocutaneous perfora-

therapy may frequently be combined with multimodality therapy, and patients are often referred following failure of such treatment. Radiation initiates changes in the vascular connective tissue of the skin, decreasing its healing capacity and predisposing it to wound complications. To understand these changes, the physiology and changes secondary to radiation are considered.

The integument is an important organ system that protects the body from external factors. Histologically, the skin is composed of three layers: the epidermis, the dermis, and the subcutaneous tissue (Fig. 50–6). The epidermis is a stratified squamous epithelium with variable thickness. It is made of five strata of cells: from within outward, the germinal or basal layer, the spinosum, the granular layer, the clear or lucidum layer, and the horny or corneum layer (Fig. 50–7). The basal cell layer, which is the deepest of

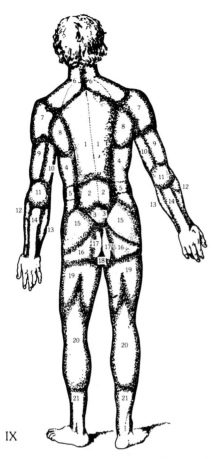

FIGURE 50–1. Review schema of the branching of skin arteries. (From Carl Manchot's book, Die Hautarterien Des Menschlichen Körpers [1889].)

1. Hautgebiet der Rr. dorsales aus den Aa. intercostales
2. Hautgebiet der Rr. dorsales aus den Aa. lumbales
3. Hautgebiet der Rr. dorsales aus den Aa. sacrales
4. Hautgebiet der Rr. perforantes posteriores der Aa. intercostales
5. Hautgebiet der Rr. perforantes posteriores der Aa. lumbales
6. Hautgebiet des Truncus thyrocervicalis
   a. der A. cervicalis superficialis
   b. der A. transversa scapulae
   c. der A. transversa colli
7. Hautgebiet der A. deltoidea subcutanea posterior
8. Hautgebiet der A. circumflexa scapulae superficialis
15. Hautgebiet der A. glutaea
16. Hautgebiet der A. ischiadica
17. Hautgebiet der A. pudenda interna
18. Hautgebiet der A. obturatoria

tors and communicating branches from the superior and inferior gluteal arteries.

Obliteration of the cutaneous blood supply is a major factor in initiating wound complications. It predisposes to infection and poor healing, culminating ultimately in wound dehiscence or necrosis. The cutaneous blood supply should be taken into consideration throughout the operative procedure, starting from the skin incision, exposure of the operative field, retraction, the major surgical procedure, as well as wound closure.

EFFECT OF RADIATION ON THE SKIN

External radiation therapy is frequently used in the treatment of spinal tumors. In addition, radiation

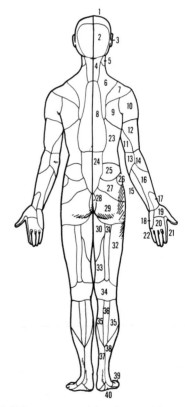

FIGURE 50–2. Schema summarizing the arterial cutaneous areas of the dorsal plane. (From Michel Salmon Plate 71 "Les Artères de la Peau" [1936].)

1. Artère temporale superficielle
2. A. occipitale
3. A. auriculaire postérieure
4. A. cervicale profonde
5. A. sterno-cleido-mastodiennes
6. A. scapulaire postérieure
7. A. sous-scapulaire
8. A. intercostale, branche dorso-spinale
9. A. scapulaire inférieure
10. A. circumflex postérieure
23. A. intercostales (rameaux perforants)
24. A. lombaires (rameaux dorso-spinaux)
25. A. lombaires (rameaux perforants)
26. A. circumflex iliac superficielle
27. A. fessiere
28. A. honteuse internes
29. A. ischiatique

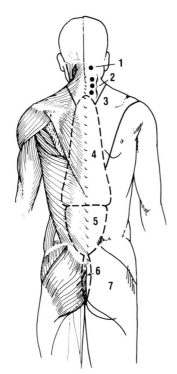

FIGURE 50–3. Arterial supply of the midback.
1. Occipital artery
2. Superficial transverse cervical artery
3. Deep transverse cervical artery
4. Dorsal cutaneous branch of intercostal arteries
5. Lumbar arteries
6. Sacral arteries
7. Superior and inferior gluteal arteries

the germinal stratum, is in continuous active mitosis and thus is responsible for the regeneration of epidermal cells. The last two strata consist of dead cells. Since sensitivity to radiation varies directly with mitotic activity, the basal stratum is the most sensitive. The viability of the basal cell layer depends on tissue fluids that infiltrate through capillaries of the dermis, as the epidermis is a nonvascular structure. A basement membrane separates the dermis from the epi-

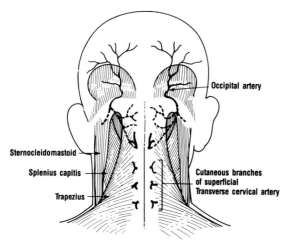

FIGURE 50–4. Cutaneous arterial anatomy of the neck.

dermis. This dermis is composed of connective tissue layered by fibroblasts. The suppleness of skin is determined by the thickness, number, cross-linkages, and elasticity of the collagen and elastic fibers. The dermis contains sweat glands, hair follicles, sebaceous glands, capillaries, and nerve endings. In the ill-defined plane between the dermis and hypodermis runs a network of arteries parallel to the surface. This arterial network sends capillaries to perfuse the dermis. In addition the hypodermis contains loose connective tissue that binds the skin to the underlying structures and allows it to slide over these surfaces.[34]

Radiation effects range from a minor degeneration of the germinal layer of the epidermis to complete necrosis of the skin. The spectrum of the damage is related to multiple factors: dose and type of beam utilized, daily fractionation and duration, as well as intrinsic biologic factors. Although skin complications frequently occur from the use of orthovoltage radiation, 25 per cent of patients treated with megavoltage techniques through parallel opposing ports will have observable skin reactions, but only a small percentage will have erythema or desquamation.[41] Radiation changes may be divided into acute and chronic phases, often separated by a subacute stage; this is illustrated diagrammatically in Figure 50–8. Under standard arbitrary radiation conditions (250 Kv irradiation, HVL 1.0 mm Cu, field size 15 × 15 cm, daily skin dose 200 cGy), the acute reaction entails an erythema in the third week associated with edema and local tenderness. The histologic findings are characterized by an inflammatory exudate, degranulation of mast cells,[87] as well as vascular dilatation with endothelial swelling. This erythema reaches its peak with the onset of desquamation in the fourth week. If the treatment is limited to 3000 cGy over three weeks, the desquamation is generally dry and the clinical picture is characterized by pruritus, scaling, and an increase in melanin production. The skin recovers to nearly normal turgor, except for permanent changes in the vascular or connective tissue.

When larger doses are used (more than 4000 cGy), the reaction may progress to a wet desquamation phase, in which there is collection of fluid above the basal cell layer or under it in more severe reactions. The fluid collection is histologically similar to bullae found in second-degree burns,[1] leading eventually to sloughing of the epidermis. Healing is related to the ability of the germinal cell layer to repopulate the epidermis. Failure to do so will result clinically in acute ulceration[93] for up to two months. Another vital factor in healing is the status of the overlying dermis, the depth of injury, and its capacity to nourish the epidermis.

Superimposed trauma and/or infection on an irradiated area have unfavorable effects on healing, as they can destroy any remnants of the germinal stratum.

The subacute phase extends from 6 to 12 months following treatment. The specialized structures of the dermis may be replaced by a dense, less resilient, fibrous tissue. The vascular changes are more significant,[46, 86] and histologically they are noted as an

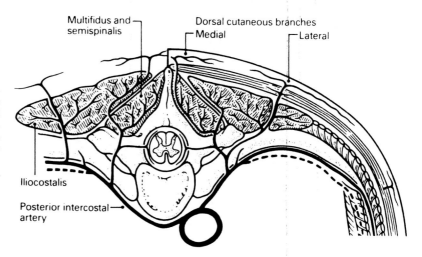

FIGURE 50–5. Schematic oblique transverse section through one half of a lower intercostal space illustrating the branches of a typical intercostal artery. Alternative arrangements of the dorsal cutaneous branches are shown on either side of the spine. (Courtesy of Drs. Cormack and Lamberty and Churchill-Livingstone.)

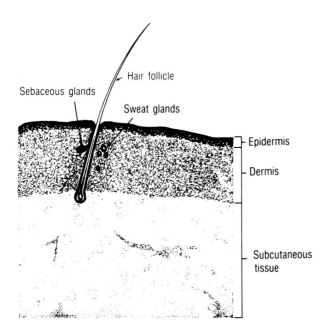

FIGURE 50–6. Schematic depiction of the skin. The blood vessels and nerve endings were omitted.

FIGURE 50–7. Diagrammatic representation of the epidermis.

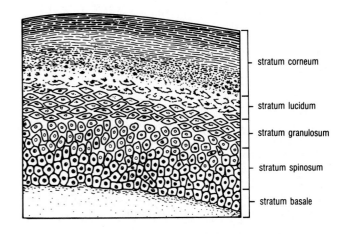

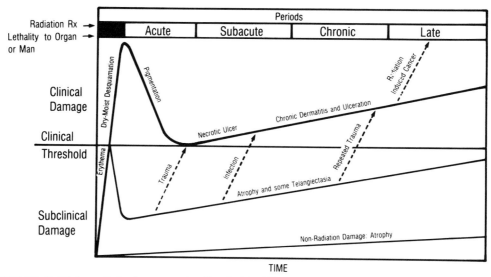

FIGURE 50–8. Clinicopathologic course: irradiated skin. When radiation damage is viewed against a background of a normal aging skin in which atrophy occurs, two possible courses out of many are illustrated. The lower line illustrates the effect of an erythematous dose level with rapid recovery and minimal changes, an effect that rarely reaches clinical significance. Trauma or infection may unmask latent radiation changes, since irradiated skin has less resistance and heals more slowly than normal skin. The top line shows the probable damage from a large dose of radiation in which moist desquamation occurs and in which atrophy and pigmentation are immediately evident. A necrotic ulcer may occur as a result of minimal trauma. Chronic dermatitis, telangectasia, ulceration, and in some instances radiation-induced cancer may follow in time. The most typical course in patients receiving therapeutic radiation lies in the zone between the two heavy lines; with supervoltage radiation the typical course lies closer to the lower line. (Courtesy of Drs. Rubin and Casarett.)

endothelial cell swelling followed by a proliferation, subintimal fibrosis, and narrowing of the capillary lumen.[10] These changes ultimately lead to loss of capillary tone and an obstructive endarteritis in the arteries.

The chronic phase is dictated by the previous reactions and also on whether there has been superimposed trauma or infection. When the acute reaction is substantial, the cutaneous change after one year is that of an atrophic dry and depilated epidermis through which telangiectatic capillaries are seen. The dryness is attributed to loss of cellular activity of the sweat and sebaceous glands. Hair loss is secondary to the destruction of hair follicles. The collagen fibers and subcutaneous fat are replaced by dense fibrous tissue that may produce, in severe cases, a leathery appearance.[21]

With this perspective, several preventive measures have to be emphasized in planning surgery to irradiated tissue.

1. Skin incisions should be planned based on the anatomic description of the cutaneous blood supply. Midline incisions are preferred whenever possible, although for paraspinal tumors the transverse incision parallel to the ribs is advisable, which can be extended vertically over the midline, provided the skin is elevated with the overlying muscle.

2. The exposure of the spine is achieved by dissection and retraction of the paraspinal muscles. The dissection should be in the subperiosteal plane, and extensive retraction should be avoided to spare the blood supply to the erector spinae muscles (Fig. 50–9). In previously irradiated patients, details of the port, dose, duration, as well as the acute radiation reaction and interval since radiation should be known. The condition of the skin overlying the spine is a critical factor in planning the closure of the wound. The possibility of primary rotation flaps should be considered when the condition of the skin is unfavorable.

3. A multiple layered watertight closure is advisable in irradiated wounds. This is especially important when a portion of the dura has to be removed and a dural patch is used.

4. Debridement of irradiated wounds should not be extended to bleeding edges as is generally done in nonirradiated infected or necrotic wounds. It should be extended to soft and resilient tissue that is capable of adequate healing.

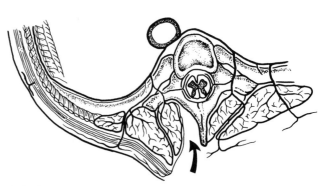

FIGURE 50–9. Subperiosteal plane of spine exposure. Severe retraction may compromise the blood supply of the muscle and predispose the wound to postoperative complication.

WOUND INFECTION

Wound infection following spinal surgery is not infrequent. The reported incidence ranges from 0.6 to 11.6 per cent.[25, 28, 56, 60, 77, 79, 82, 98] In irradiated tissue and in cancer surgery, the incidence may increase to 30 per cent.[85] The use of prophylactic antibiotics is a well-established modality for spinal surgery.[18, 23, 28, 36, 58] Since the organism most frequently responsible for wound infection is *Staphylococcus aureus*,[19, 23, 35, 42, 60, 63, 64, 97] a penicillinase-resistant prophylactic antibiotic is suggested for patients undergoing spinal surgery but is especially mandatory in cancer patients who have undergone prior radiation. Oxacillin, 1 to 2 gm, is started preoperatively and is continued postoperatively until removal of drains; the dosage is 1 gm every 6 hours over a minimum of 72 hours if drains are not inserted. In patients with allergy to penicillin, we recommend the use of vancomycin.

The clinical features of wound infection following surgery have been well outlined by Crock,[16] but the diagnosis of discitis or deep-seated wound infection may sometimes be very difficult. Healing of the skin edges and fascia is compromised in irradiated fields and also when a deep-seated infection is present. Patients present with erythema, back and incisional pain, wound discharge, systemic signs of sepsis or meningitis, and occasionally signs of nerve or spinal cord compression.

Management of wound infection following spinal surgery depends on whether prior radiation has been used (Fig. 50–10). Early and adequate surgical debridement is indicated in all patients. In nonirradiated infected wounds, primary closure can be performed following debridement if suction-irrigation systems are used,[34, 59] or alternatively a delayed primary closure may be performed following frequent dressing changes.[60] The timing of delayed primary closure is based on the appearance of a healthy granulating wound and a quantitative bacterial count of less than 10^5 per gram of tissue.[17, 38–40, 43, 65–68]

When the spinal surgery is associated with the use of foreign material such as Harrington rods or methyl methacrylate for spinal stabilization procedures, primary closure of irradiated tissue following an infection is hazardous. We prefer to use a triple antibiotic regimen initially and recommend intravenous oxacillin, aminoglycoside, and metronidazole. This is followed by debridement, frequent change of local dressings using sodium hypochloride solution (Dakin's) or antibiotic solution (bacitracin 50,000 units/liter in normal saline), and a healthy tissue transfer in the form of a myocutaneous flap. All foreign material should be removed or replaced whenever possible prior to closure of the treated infected wound. When such removal of stabilizing devices is not feasible, wound closure is preferred with the use of antibiotic beads.[11, 12, 37, 100] The use of prophylactic impregnated polymethyl methacrylate (PMMA) cement in irradiated patients is advocated. Early reports suggest that the use of such impregnated cement may decrease the incidence of postoperative deep-seated infections[7, 20, 32, 70, 88, 89, 92] by delivering a higher local antibiotic concentration than through systemic routes.[26] The use of this cement has not been associated with complications.[29, 47, 78, 90, 91] The primary closure of infected wounds with foreign material is generally associated with high failure rates, and therefore a musculocutaneous flap should be used in such patients.

METHODS OF CLOSURE OF BACK WOUNDS

When operating on previously irradiated areas, especially when a portion of the dura has to be removed and reconstructed with a fascial graft, a watertight closure is advised to decrease the possibility of cerebrospinal fluid (CSF) leak. The fundamental basic principle is that of multiple-layer closure with mobilization of the muscular and fascial layers to allow approximation without tension. An understanding of the muscular anatomy of the back (Fig. 50–11) is essential and is highlighted later in this chapter. The back can be divided into four regions based on the muscular anatomy as shown in Figure 50–12.

Cervical Zone

The musculofascial coverage of this region is composed of three layers: the trapezius muscle superficially, the semispinalis capitis and splenius capitis muscles in the middle zone, and the erector spinae muscle deeply. The semispinalis capitis is the largest muscle mass of the back, originating from the superior and inferior nuchal line. It also originates from the transverse processes of C7 through T6 and inserts

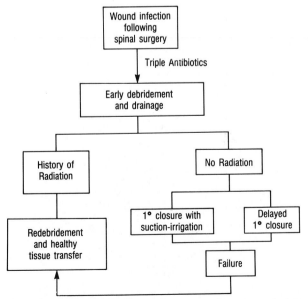

FIGURE 50–10. Management of wound infection following spinal surgery. The suggested triple antibiotic therapy is penicillin, aminoglycoside, and metronidazole.

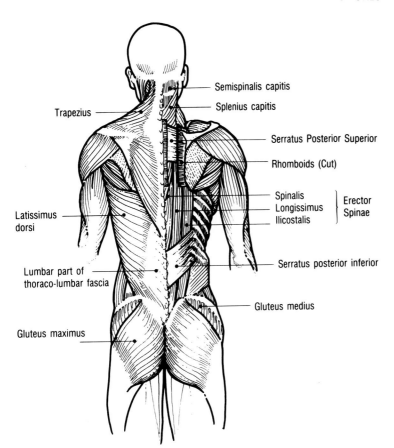

FIGURE 50–11. Muscular anatomy of the posterior trunk.

into the occipital bone. The splenius capitis takes origin from the spinous processes of the 7th cervical to the 6th thoracic vertebrae and the ligamentum nuchae. It inserts onto the lateral third of the superior nuchal line and the mastoid process and partially covers the inferior part of the semispinalis capitis.[21]

The erector spinae is made of small and thin muscle fibers that are not suitable for closure in the cervical region. Since the trapezius is also thin at this level, a one-layer closure is advised consisting of the trapezius, semispinalis, and splenius. If the tumor involves the vertebrooccipital junction, the trapezius and semispinalis muscles should be detached bilaterally and rotated medially for coverage (Fig. 50–13). The

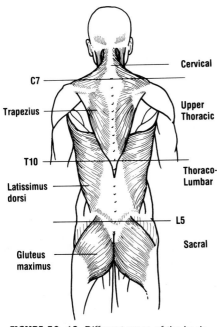

FIGURE 50–12. Different areas of the back.

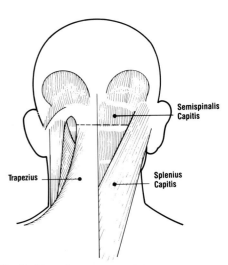

FIGURE 50–13. Muscular anatomy of the neck. Note: the dotted line delineates the level at which the semispinalis capitis and trapezius muscles are transected and rotated medially to cover the vertebrooccipital bony defects.

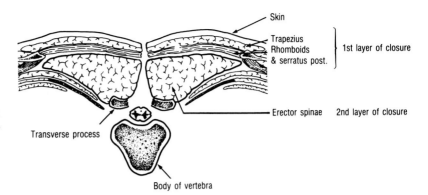

FIGURE 50–14. Notice the absence of the dorsal spinous process for exposure. Burring down the lateral processes at the edge of the incision would allow a safer closure. We suggest burring down the dorsal processes if unresected, to a level that permits adequate approximation of the trapezius and rhomboids layer.

occipital artery should be spared since it provides an important cutaneous blood supply. It emerges between the lateral edge of the semispinalis and the medial edge of the splenius capitis. The rotated muscles should be anchored to the periosteum or other available tissue. We suggest sparing a 1-cm edge of the superior nuchal fascia to allow attachment of the rotated muscles. If this edge of tissue is unavailable, drill holes are performed in the bone and used for approximation.[99]

Upper Thoracic Zone

Anatomically, this area extends from the first to the 10th thoracic vertebrae and consists of a superficial and deep layer. The muscles are of uniform thickness, and the erector spinae is composed of three groups: iliocostalis, longissimus, and spinalis (see Fig. 50–11). Each group is made of three segments. The thoracis and cervicis segments are common to all three groups. The lumborum segment is part of the iliocostalis, and the capitis segment is part of the longissimus and spinalis groups.[55] For all practical purposes, the erector spinae should be elevated bilaterally from the spinous processes of the vertebrae in the subperiosteal plane and should be approximated at the time of closure. The superficial layer, composed of the trapezius and a variety of other muscles at different levels, forms the primary defense barrier against CSF leakage. Other muscles in this region include the rhomboids, serratus posterior superior, and latissimus dorsi. The separation of the superficial and deep layers should be performed by blunt dissection after identifying the areolar tissue plane between these two layers. After elevating both sides, the muscular layers should be approximated to each other (Fig. 50–14). The lower thoracic and upper thoracic zones are most commonly associated with wound dehiscence because of the tension produced by movement of the scapula over the wound edges. We therefore recommend the use of a figure-of-eight dressing over the shoulder such as that used in clavicular fractures. This dressing will decrease the mobility of the shoulders and keep them in extension at rest, as shown in Figure 50–15, and should be worn for a period of four to five weeks.

Lower Thoracic and Lumbar Spine

This zone extends between T10 and L5 and consists of two layers. The superficial layer is mostly fascial and is composed of the thoracolumbar fascia, the latissimus dorsi, and serratus posterior inferior. The deep layer is the continuation of the erector spinae. These layers may be separated by a transverse incision in the edge of the wound. A two-layer closure should be achieved by approximating each layer by its counterpart, similar to the upper thoracic spine.

Sacral Region

The tissue covering the bony sacrum is mostly fascia, being composed of extensions of the erector

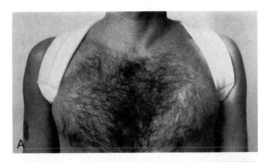

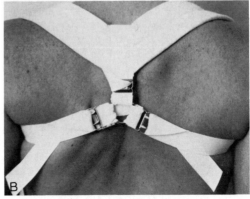

FIGURE 50–15. Figure-of-eight garment. Note the release of tension over the midback skin in *B*. Ready-made garments have a buckle that might apply pressure over the wound; it is preferable to pad the underlying incision. When ready-made garments are unavailable, a 4-inch stockinette filled with sheath wadding and secured with safety pins would be satisfactory.

spinae and the thoracolumbar fascia. The difficulties in closure of this region depend on the amount of fascia excised during tumor resection. Whenever possible, this fascia should be elevated from the bone and spared, since it may be the sole layer available for closure. If resection of tumor by total sacrectomy includes this layer, closure depends on approximation of both gluteus maximus muscles. These muscles should be elevated from their attachment to the edges of the sacrum and iliac crest and sutured to each other as a muscular layer.

WOUND CLOSURE

In general, surgical closure should be performed with delicate instruments following adequate debridement of necrotic and fibrotic tissues. The approximated edges as well as the skin should be healthy and have a good blood supply. Copious irrigation and adequate hemostasis should be secured. A nonabsorbable suture material is preferred, or otherwise absorbable sutures with very long half-lives, such as Vicryl or Dexon, should be used. We recommend the use of a 0 or 00 suture size. The sutures should be evenly spaced and applied in a figure-of-eight fashion. When using nonabsorbable suture material, it is important to invert the knots in the previously irradiated patient to prevent erosion of the suture through the skin. The closure should be tested for watertightness by injecting saline in the underlying layer. All leaking spots should be sealed with simple 00 absorbable sutures. Relaxing incisions in the fascia of the muscle may be required for a tension-free approximation of the musculofascial layer. This is achieved by elevating the skin from the underlying fascia for a distance of 3 to 5 cm. However, relaxing incisions should be avoided at the thoracolumbar fascial level.[99] Skin approximation should be performed in two layers, using absorbable sutures for subcutaneous tissue and nonabsorbable sutures such as nylon or polypropylene in a subcuticular manner for the dermis. Skin sutures may be left in and removed one month following surgery. If a CSF leak is anticipated, suction drains are mandatory. These drains have to be exteriorized through a separate incision that is located in a healthy nonirradiated field by tunneling in the subcutaneous tissues for a distance of 10 cm. It has been recommended that the exit site should be handled like that of a chest tube drain[99] by applying a purse-string suture that will be closed after removal of the drain. In addition, one or two transcutaneous sutures encircling the drain tract will prevent a potential CSF leak through the drain site. Drains should be removed after clearing of the drainage in 48 to 76 hours. To decrease the chances of CSF leakage, it may be advisable to keep patients with dural tears on complete bed rest for a short period.

MANAGEMENT OF WOUND DEHISCENCE

Wound dehiscence is a common complication that results frequently from wound infection. The presence of foreign material in the wound increases the possibility of this complication, especially if prior radiation has been used. An incidence of 30 per cent wound dehiscence may be encountered following instrumentation in spinal surgery.[74] When this complication arises in healthy tissue, mobilization and coverage of the defect are required. Skin grafts alone applied to an irradiated bed are futile, as they are associated with a failure rate of 100 per cent.[73] Musculocutaneous flap transfers are therefore required, and their timing depends on the status of the recipient bed and the precipitating factors. It is important to differentiate between the two major causes of dehiscence: radiation and infection. When associated infection is present, the wound should be rendered clean with healthy granulation tissue and a bacterial count of less than 10^5 prior to primary closure. In an irradiated bed, healthy granulation tissue is rarely evident in a short time, so that its appearance is not a prerequisite if colonization of the wound is absent. Our experience parallels that of others,[44] in that debridement of the radiated wound should be carried beyond the bleeding edges and all fibrotic soft tissue should be excised, following which rotation flaps can be performed. In the usual setting, both infection and radiation are causative factors, and the first priority should be clearing the infection with frequent debridements and dressing changes, followed by tissue coverage. The choice of flap depends on the site and can be conveniently divided into three separate zones—cervical, thoracolumbar, and sacral. In the next few sections, both the pertinent anatomy and the most common and applicable myocutaneous flaps are discussed. We strongly advise a review of the suggested references for further details.

Cervical Zone

The most frequently used flap to cover the posterior aspect of the neck and skull base is the trapezius myocutaneous flap.[51, 76] A conventional latissimus dorsi or an extended upper trapezius[15] based on the occipital artery may also be used, but the arc of rotation will cover only the lower cervical or upper thoracic vertebrae.

The trapezius is a fan-shaped muscle originating from the spinous processes and supraspinous ligament of the cervical and the thoracic vertebrae as well as the medial third of the superior nuchal line. The muscle has three different directions, with the superior fibers running downward and inserting into the lateral third of the clavicle, the middle fibers proceeding horizontally and inserting into the medial margin of the acromion, and the inferior fibers running superiorly and inserting onto the spine of the scapula (see Fig. 50–11). This muscle is innervated by the accessory nerve and has multiple actions in coordination with other muscles to stabilize the scapula and shoulder girdle during upper limb movement. With the levator scapulae, the upper fibers elevate the scapula; acting with the serratus anterior, it rotates the scapula forward so that the arm can be raised over the head; in conjunction with the rhomboids, it retracts the scapula, thereby bracing the shoulder girdle.

The trapezius is a type II muscle and has a dominant vascular pedicle composed of the transverse cervical artery, which bifurcates into a superficial branch and deep branches that supply the middle and lower segments. In addition, minor vascular pedicles, the most prominent of which are branches of the occipital artery, perfuse the superior segment of the muscle. The deep transverse cervical artery has a variable origin, arising from the subclavian artery in 66 per cent of patients and from one of its branches in the remainder.[15] It courses medially to the vertebral border of the scapula underneath the rhomboids and gives muscular branches to the trapezius at the level of the scapular spine (Fig. 50–16).

The cutaneous paddle is designed either as an island or a pedicled flap (Fig. 50–17). For extra length, the pedicle design is preferred. While planning the flap, the skin should overlap the edge of the muscle, but it is preferable to limit the distal end

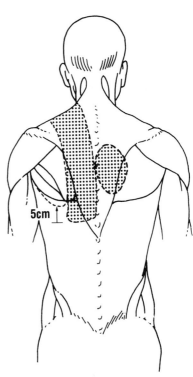

FIGURE 50–17. Cutaneous paddle of the trapezius flap. Pedicled flap on the left has a longer arc of rotation. Avoid extending the skin beyond 5 cm distal to the lower edge of the scapula. On the right is a cutaneous island paddle.

of the flap to 5 cm below the lower pole of the scapula. Patients may be positioned prone or with the ipsilateral donor site up. After skin incisions are performed, the muscle should be approached inferolaterally and elevated from the latissimus by sharp and blunt dissection. The muscle is then detached from its origin over the spinous processes and reflected superiorly. The muscular branch of the dorsal scapular artery and its associated veins are identified on the undersurface of the muscle and are dissected free. This may require division of the upper fibers of the rhomboid minor. The flap is then rotated or tunneled to cover the defect, with the donor site being closed primarily or with a split-thickness skin graft.

Thoracolumbar Zone

The muscle of choice for this region is the latissimus dorsi, and coverage is achieved by either a conventional or a reverse latissimus dorsi flap. The lower thoracic and upper lumbar regions are best covered with a reverse latissimus dorsi muscle flap[4, 48, 53, 84] (Fig. 50–18).

The latissimus dorsi originates from the spinous processes of the lower six thoracic vertebrae, the thoracolumbar fascia, and the posterior iliac crest. It also originates by muscular fibers from the posterior aspect of the outer lip of the iliac crest (see Fig. 50–11) and three or four ribs, interdigitating with the

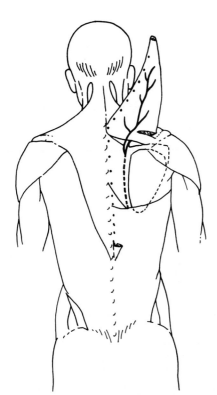

FIGURE 50–16. Trapezius flap elevated. The muscular branch of the dorsal scapular artery may arise under the rhomboid minor. Transecting the lateral edge of the muscle, under direct visualization of the vessels, would increase the mobility of the flap.

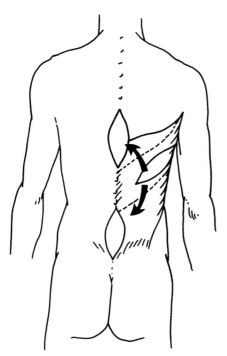

FIGURE 50–18. Reverse latissimus dorsi. The pivot point is the origin of the lateral dorsal cutaneous branches.

external oblique muscle laterally. The fibers run superiorly and obliquely and insert on the intertubercular sulcus of the humerus. The latissimus dorsi is an expendable muscle. It is active in adduction, extension, and medial rotation of the humerus, and when the arm is swung back. It is classified as a type V muscle[48] with one major pedicle—the thoracodorsal artery—and multiple segmental minor pedicles—the dorsocutaneous branches of the intercostal and lumbar arteries (Fig. 50–19). These dorsal branches have a medial and lateral element. The medial dorsocutaneous segments are branches of the lower five intercostal, subcostal, and lumbar arteries.

They are small and lack the ability to carry the flap. Three of the lateral dorsal branches are of a significant size capable of sustaining the flap. These are branches of the 9th, 10th, and 11th intercostal arteries and veins.[84] Accompanied by cutaneous nerves, these vessels pass through the erector spinae (see Fig. 50–5). They perforate the origin of the latissimus dorsi at 4 to 8 cm from the midline and give branches that run through the muscle and perforate it through its skin. The terminal branches communicate with those of the thoracodorsal artery. These communications are poorly developed over the distal third of the muscle and therefore render the placement of a skin paddle over that area hazardous. The muscle is innervated by the thoracodorsal nerve.

Since dissection of a conventional latissimus dorsi is well known, we limit our discussion to the reverse latissimi dorsi. The skin incision is based on the defect size and site and can be used as an island or a pedicled flap. Perforating branches of the 9th, 10th, and 11th intercostal vessels enter the ventral surface of the latissimus dorsi at an intersection of an imaginary line 5 cm lateral and parallel to the midline and at the lower borders of the 10th, 11th, and 12th ribs (Fig. 50–20). Patients are generally positioned prone, and after completing the skin incision the muscle is exposed and elevated from the chest wall, starting laterally and proceeding medially. After detaching its insertion from the humerus and transecting the dominant thoracodorsal vessels, the lateral dorsal branches of the intercostals are encountered at 5 to 8 cm from the midline and should be dissected. By releasing the superior origin of the muscle from the spinous processes of T6-T9, additional flexibility of the flap can be obtained. This detachment can be performed after direct visualization of the lateral dorsal arteries. Mobility of the flap is also increased by incising the lumbar fascia over the erector spinae muscle and dissecting the perforators as they travel cephalad toward the origin. The flap can rotate cephalad or caudad to cover superior or inferior

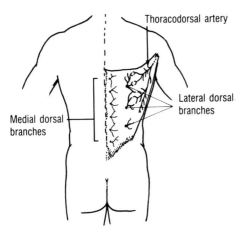

FIGURE 50–19. Latissimus dorsi blood supply. Notice the lack of communication between the lowest lateral thoracic dorsal and thoracodorsal arteries. This anatomy renders the planning of a skin paddle solely over the distal third of a latissimus dorsi, based on the thoracodorsal artery, hazardous.

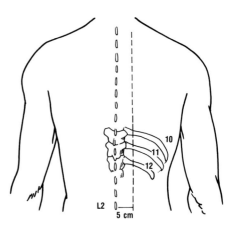

FIGURE 50–20. Cutaneous location of the dorsal perforating branches. The 9th, 10th, and 11th dorsal lateral intercostal branches travel caudally through the erector spinae muscles and perforate the latissimus dorsi muscle at the intersection of an imaginary line, 5 cm lateral and parallel to the midline and the lower edge of the 10th, 11th, and 12th rib.

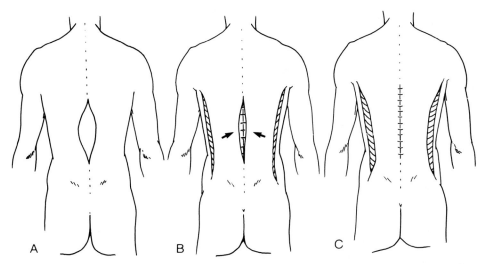

FIGURE 50–21. *A,* Midthoracic large defect. *B,* Bilateral myocutaneous latissimus dorsi advancement flaps. The muscles are approximated as a separate layer. *C,* Wound is closed in two layers. Split thickness skin graft is applied over relaxing incisions.

defects (see Fig. 50–18). The skin paddle can slide medially to cover a midthoracic defect.[48]

Large defects of the midthoracic zone involving more than six vertebrae are difficult to cover with a reverse latissimus dorsi flap. A bilateral musculocutaneous conventional latissimus dorsi flap offers a safer choice. Skin incisions are made over the lateral edges of the muscle bilaterally, and the muscle and overlying skin are elevated from the chest wall. Occasionally, the insertion of the muscle over the humerus has to be released. These flaps are based on the thoracodorsal artery. The segmental dorsal blood supply of the latissimus dorsi is dissected and spared if possible. Both flaps are advanced medially, and a two-layer closure is performed. Skin grafts are used

over the lateral relaxing incisions to achieve a tension-free closure (Fig. 50–21).

Sacral Region

Coverage of sacral defects has evolved over time from large, random flaps[9] to musculocutaneous flaps. Local random cutaneous transfers are frequently unsuccessful, as radiation effects frequently extend beyond the port of treatment. A myocutaneous flap is thus more reliable, since it has an independent blood supply and the potential to improve perfusion of the underlying bed. The gluteus maximus is used in a variety of techniques: turnover flap[49] with a skin graft, musculocutaneous rotation flap,[52] superior or inferior myocutaneous flap (Fig. 50–22), unilateral sliding flap, bilateral V-Y advancement flaps (Fig. 50–23), or thigh or posterior thigh flap.[30]

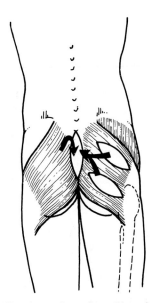

FIGURE 50–22. Gluteus maximus flaps. Muscular turnover on the left is based on the inferior gluteal artery (IGA) or the superior gluteal artery (SGA), with an overlying split thickness skin graft (STSG). Myocutaneous flaps on the right may be rotated, based on either or both vessels (IGA, SGA).

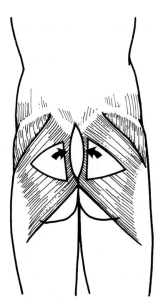

FIGURE 50–23. Gluteus maximus unilateral or bilateral advancement flaps.

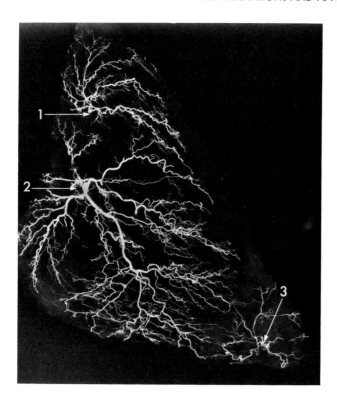

FIGURE 50–24. Gluteus maximus blood supply: (1) Superior gluteal artery; (2) inferior gluteal artery; (3) first perforator of deep femoral artery.

The gluteus maximus originates from the posterior iliac crest and inferiorly from the sacrospinalis fascia, the coccyx, the posterior iliosacral ligament, and the posterior surface of the sacrotuberous ligament. It inserts into the iliotibial tract, the ascending tendon, and the femur. This muscle has a type III vasculature, with two dominant arteries—the superior and inferior gluteal arteries—and a third blood supply as shown by our injection studies from the first perforator of the deep femoral artery (Fig. 50–24). Its innervation is solely by the inferior gluteal nerve (L5-S1, S2), which accompanies the inferior gluteal artery. Contraction of the superior portion of the muscle abducts the thigh, allows one-legged support, and assists in running and climbing stairs. Its inferior portion is associated with thigh extension. Blood vessels enter the muscle from its ventral aspect as they branch from the internal iliac artery. The gluteus flap is very versatile, and many designs can be planned based on the defect and vessel use. The flap can be perfused by either pedicle separately or by using all three vascular supplies. In large defects, both glutei should be used. In our experience, the most valuable and physiologic flap in ambulatory patients is a bilateral sliding V-Y advancement flap. After completion of debridement, a cutaneous triangle is drawn over each gluteus maximus, with the base at the edge of the defect. The skin incision is formed, and the surrounding skin is elevated. The origin of the muscle is detached from the sacrotuberous ligament.

Attention should be directed toward sparing the inferior gluteal artery (IGA), which is 1 cm from the superior edge of the sacrotuberous ligament and 3 to 4 cm lateral to the sacral edge. The superior gluteal artery is only 3 cm cephalad to the IGA. After identification of both vessels, the origin is completely detached. All four sacral and the iliolumbar branches should be ligated (if still present). Next the superior border is freed from the gluteus medius. Both musculocutaneous flaps are advanced medially and sutured to each other (Fig. 50–25). Patients are given two weeks of bed rest on a Clinitron bed. Ambulation is gradual, with sitting and pelvic flexion allowed after one month. The success of the reconstruction depends on adequate debridement of the wound and drainage.

Free tissue transfer has not been included in this

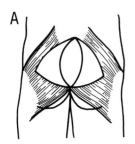
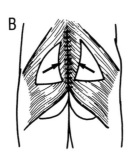
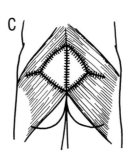

FIGURE 50–25. Gluteus maximus V-Y advancement flap. *A,* Large midsacral defect. Skin triangles are drawn with their bases as the edge of the debrided wound. *B,* Muscles are elevated after debridement and are approximated as a separate layer. *C,* Skin is approximated as a second layer by suturing the bases of the triangles to each other.

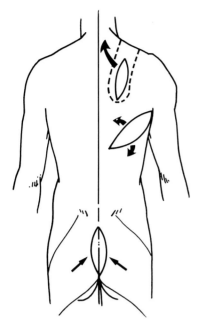

FIGURE 50–26. Musculocutaneous flaps used for midposterior trunk closures.

chapter. It is important to keep in mind the availability of the recipient vessels. An inferiorly based transverse rectus abdominis, positioned vertically over the defect and anastomosed to the occipital or the external carotid artery and the external jugular vein, is suggested in the cervical and upper thoracic zones. In the thoracolumbar areas, although difficult to use, the intercostal vessels are the most accessible. Over the sacral zone the inferior or superior gluteal vessels are candidates. A long saphenous vein and femoral artery delayed fistula could be tunneled to the gluteal area and used as recipient vessels.[75]

In summary, the three most commonly used flaps in reconstruction of defects of the midback are: the myocutaneous rotation or advancement trapezius, the latissimus dorsi, and the gluteus maximus flaps (Fig. 50–26). An adequate understanding of the anatomy and familiarity with the basic principles of wound care are crucial for successful repair.

REFERENCES

1. Ackerman AB: Histologic Diagnosis of Inflammatory Skin Diseases. Philadelphia, Lea & Febiger, 1978, pp 201–202, 765–767.
2. Anson BJ: Morris' Human Anatomy. 12th ed. New York, McGraw-Hill, 1966.
3. Becker H: The distally based gluteus maximus muscle flap. Plast Reconstr Surg 63:653–656, 1979.
4. Bostwick J III, Scheflan M, Nahai F, et al: The reverse latissimus dorsi muscle and musculocutaneous flap: Anatomic and clinical considerations. Plast Reconstr Surg 65:395–399, 1980.
5. Breasted JH: The Edwin Smith Papyrus in Facsimile and Hieroglyphic Transliteration with Translation and Commentary. Chicago, University of Chicago Press, 1930.
6. Buchanan DL, Agris J: Gluteal plication closure of sacral pressure ulcers. Plast Reconstr Surg 72:49, 1983.
7. Buchholtz HW, Elson RA, Engelbrecht E, et al: Management of deep infection of total hip replacement. J Bone Joint Surg 63(B):342, 1981.
8. Campbell J, Pennefather CM: An investigation into the blood supply of muscle with special reference to war surgery. Lancet 1:294, 1919.
9. Campbell RM, Delgado JP: The pressure sore. In Converse JM (ed): Plastic and Reconstructive Surgery. Philadelphia, WB Saunders, 1977.
10. Casarett GW: Radiation Histopathology. Boca Raton, CRC Press, 1980, p 41.
11. Cierny G III: Soft tissue reconstruction of the lower leg (expert commentary). Perspec Plast Surg 1:24–31, 1987.
12. Cierny G III, Mader JT, Couch L: Adjunctive local antibiotics in the management of contaminated orthopedic wounds. Orthop Trans 10:465, 1986.
13. Clemente CD: Anatomy. Baltimore, Urban & Scharzenberg, 1981, Fig. 456.
14. Copenhaver W, Kelly D, Wood R: Bailey's Textbook of Histology. 7th ed. Baltimore, Williams and Wilkins, 1978, pp 423–446.
15. Cormack GC, Lamberty BGH: The Arterial Anatomy of Skin Flaps. Edinburgh, Churchill Livingstone, 1986.
16. Crock HV: Practice of Spinal Surgery. New York, Springer Verlag, 1983, pp 238–241.
17. Duke WF, Robson MC, Krizek TJ: Civilian wounds, their bacterial flora and rate of infection. Surg Forum 23:513, 1972.
18. Ecker J, Erschbaumer H: Antibiotic prophylaxis in orthopedics with special reference to spinal surgery. Z Orthop 121(6):738–740, 1983.
19. El-Gindi S, Aref S, Salama M, et al: Infection of intervertebral discs after operation. J Bone Joint Surg (Br) 58:114–116, 1976.
20. Elson RA: Prophylaktiche verwendung von gentamycin Palacos im Northern General Hospital, Sheffield, England. Aktuel Probl Chir Orthop 12:206, 1979.
21. Fajardo LF: Pathology of Radiation Injury. New York, Masson Publishing, 1982, pp 186–200.
22. Fisher J, Arnold PG, Waldorf J, Woods JE: The gluteus maximus musculocutaneous V-Y advancement flap for large sacral defects. Ann Plast Surg 11:517, 1983.
23. Fogelberg EV, Zitzmann EK, Stinchfield FE: Prophylactic penicillin in orthopedic surgery. J Bone Joint Surg (Am) 52:95–98, 1970.
24. Garrido E, Rosenwasser RH: Experience with the suction-irrigation technique in the management of spinal epidural infection. Neurosurgery 12:678–679, 1983.
25. Gurdjian ES, Ostrowski AZ, Hardy WG, et al: Results of operative treatment of protruded and ruptured lumbar discs. Based on 1176 cases with 82 percent follow up of 3 to 13 years. J Neurosurg 18:783–791, 1961.
26. Hoff SF, Fitzgerald RH, Kelly PJ: The depot administration of penicillin G and gentamycin in acrylic bone cement. J Bone Joint Surg (Am) 63:798, 1981.
27. Hollingshead WH: Textbook of Anatomy. Hagerstown, Md, Harper & Row, 1974.
28. Horwitz NH, Curtin JA: Prophylactic antibiotic and wound infection following laminectomy for lumbar disc herniation. J Neurosurg 43:727–731, 1975.
29. Hughes S, Field CA, Kennedy MRK, et al: Cephalosporin in bone content. J Bone Joint Surg (Br) 61:96, 1979.
30. Hurwitz DJ, Swartz WM, Mathes SJ: The gluteal thigh flap: A reliable, sensate flap for closure of buttock and perineal wounds. Plast Reconstr Surg 68:521, 1981.
31. Jolles B, Harrison RG: Enzymic processes and vascular changes in the skin radiation reaction. Br J Radiol 39:12–18, 1966.
32. Josefsson G, Lindberg L, Wiklander B: Systemic antibiotic and gentamycin containing bone cement in prophylaxis of postoperative infection in total hip arthroplasty. Clin Orthop 159:194, 1981.
33. Joseph J, Williams PL: Electromyography of certain hip muscles. J Anat 91:286, 1957.
34. Junqueira LC, Carneiro J: Basic Histology. 4th ed. Los Altos, Lange Medical Publications, 1983, pp 383–396.
35. Keller RB, Pappas AM: Infection after spinal fusion using

internal fixation instrumentation. Orthop Clin North Am 3(1):99–111, 1972.

36. Ketcham AS, Bloch JH, Crawford DT, et al: The role of prophylactic antibiotic therapy in control of staphylococcal infections following cancer surgery. Surg Gynec Obstet 114:345–352, 1962.

37. Knoringer P: PMMA in the area of the skull and spine experiences with cement containing antibiotics and anti-biotic-free cements. Aktuel Probl Chir Orthop 31:308–313, 1987.

38. Krizeck TJ, Robson MC, Kho E: Bacterial growth and skin graft survival. Surg Forum 18:518, 1967.

39. Lawrence JC, Lilly HA: A quantitative method for investigating the bacteriology of skin: Its application to burns. Br J Exp Pathol 53:550, 1972.

40. Levine NS, Lindberg RB, Mason AD, et al: The quantitative swab culture and smear: A quick, simple method for determining the number of viable aerobic bacteria on open wounds. J Trauma 16:89, 1976.

41. Liegner LM, Michaud NJ: Skin and subcutaneous reactions induced by supervoltage irradiation. Am J Roentgenol Radiat Ther Nucl Med 85:533–549, 1961.

42. Lindholm TS, Pylkkanen P: Discitis following removal of intervertebral disc. Spine 7:618–622, 1982.

43. Loebl EC, Marvin JA, Heck EL, et al: The use of quantitative biopsy culture in bacteriologic monitoring of burn patients. J Surg Res 16:1, 1974.

44. Luce EA: The irradiated wound. Surg Clin North Am 64(4):821–829, 1984.

45. Manchot C: Die Hautarterien des Menschlichen Körpers. Leipzig, FCW Vogel, 1889.

46. Marino H: Biologic excision: its value in the treatment of radionecrotic lesions. Plast Reconstr Surg 40:180, 1967.

47. Marks KE, Nelson CL, Lautenschlager EP: Antibiotic impregnated acrylic bone cement. J Bone Joint Surg (Am) 58:358, 1976.

48. Mathes SJ, Nahai F: Clinical Applications for Muscle and Musculocutaneous Flaps. St. Louis, CV Mosby, 1982, pp 12–13, 28–29, 46–49, 106–107, 118–119, 352–357, 470–471, 646.

49. Mathes SJ, Nahai F: Clinical Atlas of Muscle and Musculocutaneous Flaps. St. Louis, CV Mosby, 1979.

50. Mathes SJ, Nahai F: Classification of the vascular anatomy of muscles: Experimental and clinical correlation. Plast Reconstr Surg 67:177, 1981.

51. Mathes SJ, Vasconez LO: Head, neck and truncal reconstruction with musculocutaneous flap: Anatomic and clinical considerations. Transactions of the VII International Congress of Plastic and Reconstructive Surgery. Sao Paulo, Brazil, 1980, pp 178–182.

52. Minami RT, Milles R, Pardoe R: Gluteus maximus musculocutaneous flaps for repair of pressure sores. Plast Reconstr Surg 60:242, 1977.

53. Muldowney JB, Magi E, Hein K, Birdsell D: The reverse latissimus dorsi myocutaneous flap with functional preservation—Report of a case. Ann Plast Surg 7:150, 1981.

54. Napier J: The antiquity of human walking. Sci Am 216:56, 1967.

55. Netter FH (ed): The Ciba Collection of Medical Illustration. Volume 8: Musculoskeletal System. Part I. Ciba-Geigy Corporation, 1987, pp 2–8.

56. Odom GL, Hart D, Johnson P, et al: Neurosurgical operation infections. A seventeen year survey of the use of ultraviolet radiation. Presented at the 23rd Meeting of the American Academy of Neurological Surgeons, New Orleans, November, 1962.

57. Parry SW, Mathes SJ: Bilateral gluteus maximus myocutaneous advancement flaps: Sacral coverage for ambulatory patients. Ann Plast Surg 8:443, 1982.

58. Pavel A, Smith RL, Ballard A, et al: Prophylactic antibiotic in clean orthopedic surgery. J Bone Joint Surg (Am) 56:777–782, 1974.

59. Probst C, Costabile G, Rafaisz A: Treatment of local infections, cranial and spinal, with suction-irrigation drainage. Experience in 60 patients. Neurochirurgia (Stuttg) 30:139–142, 1987.

60. Prosser AJ, Waddell G: Wound infections in lumbar spinal surgery: Clinical features and management. J R Coll Surg Edinb 31(5):296–299, 1986.

61. Ramirez OM, Hurwitz DJ, Futrell WJ: The expansive gluteus maximus flap. Plast Reconstr Surg 74:757, 1984.

62. Ramirez OM, Orlando JC, Hurwitz DJ: The sliding gluteus maximus myocutaneous flap: Its relevance in ambulatory patients. Plast Reconstr Surg 74:68, 1984.

63. Ravicovitch NA, Spallone A: Spinal epidural abscess. Surgical and parasurgical management. Eur Neurol 21(5):347–357, 1982.

64. Rawlings CE III, Wilkins RH, Gallis HA, et al: Postoperative intervertebral disc space infection. Neurosurgery 13:371–376, 1983.

65. Robson MC, Heggers JP: Bacterial quantification on open wounds. Milit Med 134:19, 1969.

66. Robson MC, Krizeck TJ: Predicting skin graft survival. J Trauma 13:213, 1973.

67. Robson MC, Lea CE, Dalton JB, Heggers JP: Quantitative bacteriology and delayed wound closure. Surg Forum 19:501, 1968.

68. Robson MC, Shaw RC, Heggers JP: The reclosure of post-operative incisonal abscess based on bacterial quantification of the wound. Ann Surg 171:279, 1970.

69. Romm S: Symposium on wound management. Surg Clin North Am 64:623, 1984.

70. Rottger J, Buchholz HW, Engelbrecht E, et al: Gentamycin-PMMA in der gelenkprothetic: Indikation und Technik unter verwendung von Refobaci-Palacos in der gelenk-prothetic. Aktuel Probl Chir Orthop 12:197, 1979.

71. Rubin P, Casarett G: Clinical Radiation Pathology. Philadelphia, W.B. Saunders, 1968, pp 38–119.

72. Rudolph R: Complication of surgery for radiotherapy skin damage. Plast Reconstr Surg 70:179, 1982.

73. Salmon M: Les Artères De La Peau. Paris, Masson, 1936.

74. Scheflan M, Nahai F, Bostwick J III: Gluteus maximus island musculocutaneous flap for closure of sacral and ischial ulcers. Plast Reconstr Surg 68:533, 1981.

75. Serafin D: Delayed arterio-venous fistula as recipient vessels. Symposium on Refinements in Free Flap Surgery. New York, 1988.

76. Seyfer AE, Joseph AS: Use of trapezius muscle for closure of complicated upper spinal defects. Neurosurgery 14:341–345, 1984.

77. Shinners BM, Hamby WB: The results of surgical removal of protruded lumbar intervertebral discs. J Neurosurg 1:117–122, 1944.

78. Soto-Hall R, Saenz L, Tavernetti R, et al: Tobramycin in bone cement. Clin Orthop 175:60, 1983.

79. Spangfort EV: The lumbar disc herniation. A computer aided analysis of 2,504 operations. Acta Orthop Scand (Suppl) 142:1–95, 1972.

80. Stern JT: Anatomical and functional specializations of the human gluteus maximus. Am J Phys Anthropol 36:315, 1972.

81. Stern JT, Susman RL: Electromyography of the gluteal muscle in Hylobates, Pongo and pan: Implication for the evolution of hominid bipedality. Am J Phys Anthropol 55:153, 1981.

82. Stevens DB: Postoperative orthopedic infections. A study of etiological mechanisms. J Bone Joint Surg (Am) 46:96–102, 1964.

83. Stevenson TR, Pollock RA, Rohrick RJ, VanderKolk CA: The gluteus maximus musculocutaneous island flap: Refinement in design and application. Plast Reconstr Surg 79:761, 1987.

84. Stevenson TR, Rohrick RJ, Pollock RA, et al: More experience with the "reverse" latissimus dorsi musculocutaneous flap: Precise location of blood supply. Plast Reconstr Surg 74:237–243, 1984.

85. Sundaresan N, Huvos AG, Krol G, et al: Surgical treatment of spinal chordomas. Arch Surg 122:1479–1482, 1987.

86. Telok HA, Mason ML, Wheelock MD: Histopathologic study of radiation injuries of the skin. Surg Gynecol Obstet 90:335, 1950.

87. Tessmer CF: Radiation effects in skin. In Berdjis CC (ed):

Pathology of Irradiation. Baltimore, Williams and Wilkins, 1971, pp 146–170.

88. Thierse L: Erfahrungen mit Refobacin-Palacos im hinblick auf die tiefen spatinfektionen nach huftendoprothesenoperationen. Z Orthop 116:847, 1978.

89. Torholm C, Lidgren L, Lindberg L, et al: Total hip joint arthroplasty with gentamycin impregnated cement. Clin Orthop 181:99, 1981.

90. Wahlig H, Dingeldein E, Bergmann R, et al: The release of gentamycin from polymethylmethacrylate beads. J Bone Joint Surg (Br) 60:270, 1978.

91. Wahlig H, Dingeldein E, Buchholz HW, et al: Pharmacokinetic study of gentamycin loaded cement in total hip replacements. J Bone Joint Surg (Br) 66:175, 1984.

92. Wannske M, Tscherne H: Ergenbnisse prophylakticher anwendung von Refobacin-Palacos bei der implatation von endoprosthesen des huftgelenkes in Hanover. Aktuel Probl Chir Orthop 12:201, 1979.

93. Warren S: Effects of radiation on normal tissues. XII. Effect on skin. Arch Pathol 35:340–348, 1943.

94. Washburn SL: The analysis of primate evolution with particular reference to the origin of man. Cold Spring Harbor Symp Quant Biol 15:67, 1951.

95. Wheatley MD, Jahnke WD: Electromyographic study of the superficial thigh and hip muscles in normal individuals. Arch Phys Med 32:508, 1951.

96. William PL, Warwick R (eds): Gray's Anatomy. 36th ed. Philadelphia, F.A. Davis, 1980, pp 564–566.

97. Woo JH, Ryu JK: Cefoperazone in the treatment of postsurgical wound infection, sepsis, and abscess of spinal cord and brain. Clin Ther 6:839–843, 1984.

98. Wright RL: Septic Complications of Neurological Spinal Procedures. Springfield, Ill, Charles C Thomas, 1970.

99. Zide BM, Wisoff JH, Epstein FJ: Closure of extensive and complicated laminectomy wounds. J Neurosurg 67:59–64, 1987.

100. Zumkeller M, Gaab MR: Local treatment of infections in neurosurgery with gentamycin PMMA chains (Septopal). Neurochirurgia (Stuttg) 30(5):143–148, 1987.

51

USE OF THE INTERNAL FIXATOR IN SPINE TUMOR SURGERY

MAX AEBI and WALTER DICK

INTRODUCTION

The internal fixator is a posterior spinal instrumentation system that is fixed to the spine by pedicle screws and allows fixation as well as correction of a deformed spinal segment. This instrumentation was developed by Dick in 1982[4, 5] in conjunction with the AO/ASIF group in Switzerland and was intended for use in spinal fracture treatment by overcoming the limitations of the classic Harrington rod system and its modifications. Later it became obvious that this instrumentation was also useful in other spinal disorders.[2, 4]

The internal fixator is an extension of the pioneering work with spinal fixators by Magerl,[14] who initially introduced the external spinal skeletal fixator. Simultaneously, other internal fixator systems were also developed,[9, 20] but these have not had a significant impact on the technical improvements in spinal surgery that the Dick internal fixator has had in Europe. Basically, this system is based on the classic observation, known for more than 15 years, that the pedicle is the strongest and hence most important structure in the vertebra to anchor spinal instrumentation.[18] Pedicle screws together with plates were first used by French orthopedic surgeons.[18] A major disadvantage of the plate-screw construct is the unstable angle between the screw and the plate within the screw hole. Thus, a two-point fixation with screws above and below the spine lesion is necessary. This requires that at least two vertebrae above and below a lesion must be included in the fixation.[1, 2, 4, 5, 14, 22] With the internal fixator, it is possible to achieve stable fixation utilizing only one vertebra above and below the involved segment. Therefore, healthy spinal segments may be spared, while fixation and spinal mobility are maximized.

The initial goals of orthopedic surgery in the treatment of spinal tumors are to stabilize pathologic fracture, to avoid impending fractures by stabilization, and therefore to prevent neurologic deficit, painful deformity, and instability of the diseased segment. Secondly, direct tumor debulking is needed either to prevent or to treat neurologic deficit and to ameliorate pain that may be due to local tissue pressure resulting from extension of the tumor mass into the adjacent tissue. Adequate tumor debulking therefore produces additional instability of a spinal segment invaded by a tumor. Consequently, tumor resection in the spine is only rarely indicated without additional stabilization if life expectancy is reasonable or to avoid an iatrogenic unstable spine.[6, 8, 12, 16, 17, 19, 23, 24]

More than 8 out of 9 tumors involving the spine are metastases; the most frequent primary sites are the breast, lung, prostate, and hematopoietic system.[25] Most metastases involve the vertebral body alone or in combination with the posterior elements; selective involvement of the posterior elements is less common.[3, 6, 8, 12, 16, 19]

A posterior approach to the spine is therefore not a logical approach to metastatic tumors in most instances. Furthermore it is well known that laminectomy alone or in combination with postoperative radiation is not significantly better than radiation alone[19, 21, 24] from the standpoint of preventing neurologic deficit, and that laminectomy may produce an iatrogenic unstable spine.[6–8, 10, 15, 19, 24]

A consideration in using the internal spinal skeletal fixation (ISSF) system is that it is a posterior fixation device and thus requires an additional surgical procedure when the tumor is resected directly from an anterior procedure. In such cases, use of the internal fixator requires a combined anterior and posterior approach. However, it is possible to resect tumor involving the anterior column and both posterior columns using a *single* posterior approach with resection of the body or with a modified eggshell procedure[13] or, alternatively, by a combined posterior and posterolateral approach.[19] In the following presentation we will separately discuss (1) the technique for insertion of the ISSF system, and (2) approaches and technical aspects of tumor surgery in connection with the use of the ISSF, with special reference to metastatic tumors of the spine.

PRINCIPLES AND SURGICAL TECHNIQUE

The ISSF is a bilateral device consisting of hinged coupling clamps that attach the transpedicular Schanz screws to square-ended, threaded spanning rods. The spanning rods connect ipsilateral Schanz screws together (Fig. 51–1). The threads of the spanning rods allow a "locked-nut system" to provide either distraction or compressive forces throughout the entire anteroposterior diameter of the instrumented vertebra through the transpedicular screws (Fig. 51–2). The hinged coupling clamps allow full rotation of the Schanz screws about an axis of 90 degrees to the long axis of the spanning rods. This rotation, along with the long lever arm, allows efficient reduction of the spinal column in the sagittal plane, that is, restoration of lordosis and kyphosis (Fig. 51–3). Once tightened, the angle between the Schanz screws and the rod is completely stable, unlike a hook-rod or plate-screw combination. The hinged coupling clamps are also able to rotate about the long axis of the spanning rods (Fig. 51–3B). This facilitates the rotation or realignment of lateral displacement in a spinal deformity if necessary. The final position of the ISSF is "locked into place" by collared lock nuts that are crimped to the square-ended spanning rods (Fig. 51–4), after having adjusted the height and shape of the diseased vertebra and the distance between the two vertebrae above and below the involved segment.

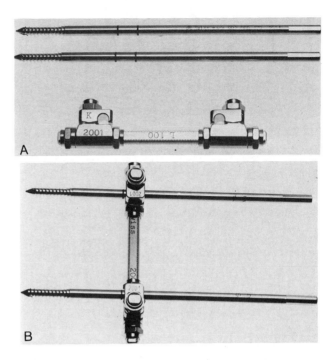

FIGURE 51–1. The internal fixator. *A,* The implant disassembled with two Schanz screws and one threaded rod with mounted proximal and distal hinged clamps. *B,* The implant mounted. Observe the long lever arm of the Schanz screws extending beyond the clamps.

Unlike fracture management, the need for manipulation of the injured vertebra is minimal and consists of restoring the lordotic shape (contouring) of the lumbar spine and reestablishing normal vertebral height through distraction along the threaded rods by approximating the ends of the Schanz screws (Fig. 51–5A and B). An anterior graft—bone or artificial

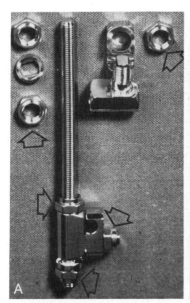
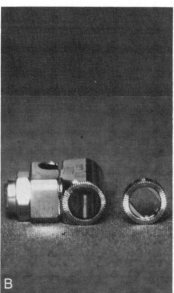
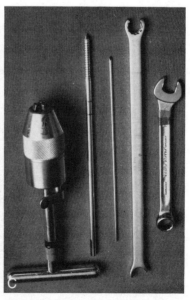

FIGURE 51–2. The internal fixator. *A,* Square-ended threaded rod with a mounted hinge and clamp at the bottom and a hinged clamp disassembled with its serrated lock washers and collard nuts shown at the top. *B,* Isolated clamp with its serrated end and the serrated lock washer as counterpart. *C,* Basic instruments: chuck for Schanz screws, Schanz screw K-wires, speed wrench for preliminary tightening of collard nuts, and standard 10-mm box wrench for final nut tightening.

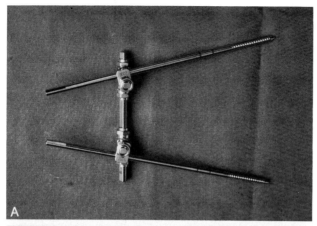

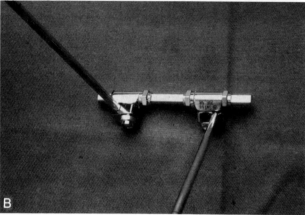

FIGURE 51–3. The internal fixator. *A,* In a lordotic position, given by the fixed angle in the hinged clamp. *B,* Rotation of the hinged clamps around the spanning rod is possible in 6-degree intervals. This is secured by the serrated lock washers and collard nuts.

spacer (cement, biodegradable material, vertebral prosthesis)—can be put under compression through dorsal compression along the threaded rods (Fig. 51–5*C*). In case of a total vertebrectomy, attention should be paid to reestablishing the normal intervertebral distance between the upper and lower vertebral bodies, although a decrease in disc and vertebral body height may not be harmful as long as the roots are visible and are not under compression.[13] This is accomplished by measuring the height of the intact vertebra above or below and adding the height of the intact upper and lower disc spaces on preoperative x-rays (Fig. 51–5*D* and *E*).

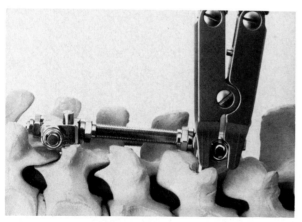

FIGURE 51–4. The collard nuts and washers are crimped to the cut edges of the spanning rods and clamps with a special "crimper."

If both anterior and posterior elements are removed, thereby creating a highly unstable spine, the two parallel rods may be bridged by one or two transverse bars to increase the stability by a closed-frame effect and to protect the instrumentation from parallelogram-like lateral forces (Fig. 51–6). The same effect can also be achieved by twisting two diagonally crossed cerclage wires around the ends of the fixator. The Schanz screws are secured to the clamp by tightening the lateral nuts as well as the nuts and counternuts at the threaded rod above and below every clamp, in order to avoid rotation of the Schanz screws around the rods.

The ISSF allows fixation and fusion to be limited only to the vertebral segments immediately adjacent to those involved in tumor, owing to the stable angle between Schanz screws and threaded rod. In contrast to the traditional Harrington system and its modifications, healthy vertebral segments do not need to be instrumented or fused. Biomechanical studies by Dick and Wörsdorfer[4] have shown the ISSF to be nearly as rigid as plate fixation. Instrumentation using the ISSF is technically demanding and should therefore only be attempted after training and practice with cadavers. As with all transpedicular fixation, the risk of vascular injury or neurologic damage during insertion of the screws is always present, if anatomic landmarks and direction of the screws are not carefully observed.

Following subperiosteal preparation of the arches, the facet joints are identified (Fig. 51–7). With a drill,

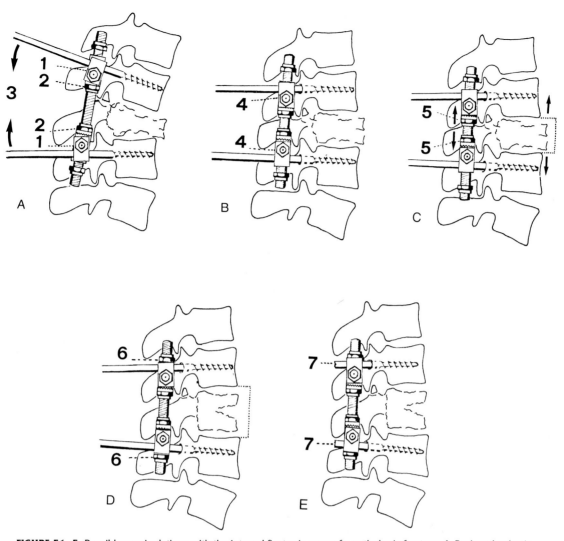

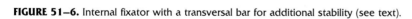

FIGURE 51–5. Possible manipulations with the internal fixator in case of a pathologic fracture. *A,* Reduce kyphotic deformity by squeezing together the dorsal ends of the Schanz screws (3); the lateral nuts (1) are loose; the distraction nuts (2) may be positioned near to the clamps to protect the posterior wall from further compression. *B,* Tighten the lateral nuts (4), thus lordosis is fixed. *C,* Restore vertebral height by the distraction nuts (5). Lordosis will not be altered, since the angle of the Schanz screw with the threaded rod is already fixed. *D,* Tighten the counternuts (6), thus rotation is controlled. *E,* Cut the overstanding ends of Schanz screws (7).

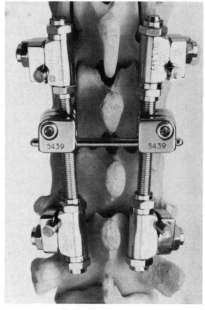

FIGURE 51–6. Internal fixator with a transversal bar for additional stability (see text).

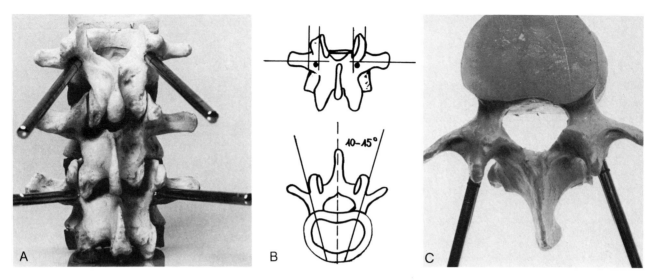

FIGURE 51–7. The surgical landmarks to find the lumbar pedicles. *A,* Schanz screws in situ seen from a posterior aspect. *B,* Schematic drawings of the landmarks. *C,* Schanz screws in situ seen from the top.

2.0-mm Kirschner wires are placed through the pedicle into the vertebral body without perforation of the anterior cortex. *The dorsal entry point of the K-wires corresponds to that described for the transpedicular screw fixation of plates.*[1, 2, 19] The entry points are demonstrated in Figure 51–7. In the lumbar spine the entry point is located at the crossing of a horizontal line, which corresponds to the midline of the transverse processes, and a vertical line, which is perpendicular to the latter one and is tangential to the upper facet joint of the vertebra of interest. From this entry point, the Schanz screw can be inserted with an inclination of 10 to 15 degrees toward the midline of the spine. If the entry point is chosen 2 to 3 mm medially of the mentioned typical localization, the pedicle can be reached securely too, although with lesser inclination.

In the thoracic spine the entry point for the Schanz screw is located 1 to 2 mm below the margin of the lower facet of the upper adjacent vertebra and approximately 3 mm lateral to a line that connects the midpoint of the vertebral joint. At this point the transverse process starts but lies already in a plane slightly more dorsal than the joint itself. Therefore the entry point has to be prepared flat by a Luer.

The K-wires should converge 10 to 15 degrees with respect to the midline (Fig. 51–7). The position of the K-wires is then checked by an image intensifier, and if the wires are correctly placed, they are exchanged with 5-mm Schanz screws. The entry point through the dorsal cortex is drilled with a 3.5-mm drill bit extending only about 5 to 10 mm deep. The Schanz screw is used as a self-tapping screw within the cancellous bone and is driven with the hand chuck to a depth of about 40 mm. There are marks on the Schanz screws at 50 and 60 mm (Fig. 51–8). Usually the Schanz screw is kept within the pedicle by its circumferential cortex. After inserting all Schanz screws, an additional fluoroscopic image is obtained. The screws are then driven further in until

they approach the ventral cortex of the vertebral bodies. Since there is great variety in the size of the vertebrae, the nuts themselves are secured by tightening the lugs of the nuts onto the surface of the rod with pliers, retaining firmly the Schanz screw.

The dorsal projecting Schanz screw ends are then removed with a special bolt cutter (Fig. 51–9). There remains a protruding end of the screw, approximately 5 mm in length, which does not usually prove bothersome to the patient and can be left alone (Fig. 51–10).

The instrumentation area depends on the number of vertebrae involved by tumor. If only one vertebra is involved, the fixation device includes the intact vertebra above and below the lesion. If more than one vertebra is involved, the instrumentation should

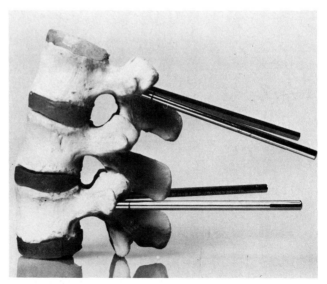

FIGURE 51–8. The position of the Schanz screws seen from a lateral aspect. Note the ends of the Schanz screws, which may be squeezed together, creating a lordosis through a powerful lever arm.

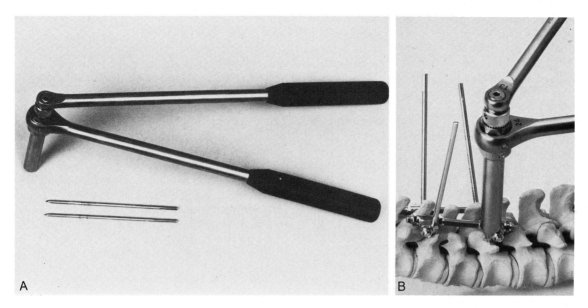

FIGURE 51–9. A, Special bolt cutter with the Schanz screw in a 1:1 proportion. B, The bolt cutter in situ.

extend to reach from proximal to distal intact vertebrae. Postoperative treatment usually includes antibiotic prophylaxis, which is started intraoperatively before performing the skin incision and continues for 48 hours postoperatively. The patient is mobilized postoperatively as soon as possible depending on general condition and neurologic deficit. With or without minor neurologic deficit, the patient usually gets up within the first postoperative week. As an external support, a soft brace or a lightweight three-point corset is often utilized, depending on the construct that was performed. If there is sufficient support of the anterior column by the use of a methyl methacrylate–metal construct, no external support is necessary for mobilization. If the stabilization in benign spinal tumors is combined with a bone fusion, the external support is maintained for 12 weeks postoperatively.

INDICATIONS AND CLINICAL APPLICATIONS

The ISSF system is mostly used at the lumbar spine. Its use can be extended up to the 8th thoracic vertebra and, in some rare cases, even higher. The thoracic spine in elderly patients does not necessarily need to be fixed with a short spinal instrumentation owing to the physiologic immobility of the spinal area with increasing age.

Posterior Fixation Alone

Posterior fixation alone is indicated in combination with posterior decompression following extensive laminectomy and facet joint resection in the face of a largely posterior and posterolateral neural com-

FIGURE 51–10. Lateral (A) and posteroanterior (B) views of the internal fixator in situ after having cut the Schanz screws and tightened all the nuts.

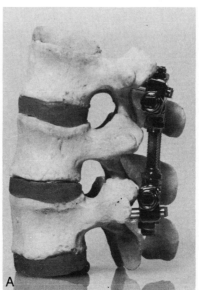
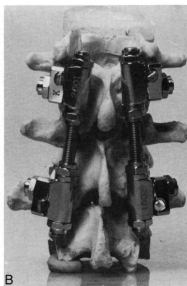

pression.[13] This indication mostly applies to patients with metastatic spinal tumors, in whom the goal of surgery is mainly palliative. The goal is to achieve immediate decompression of a tumor that circumferentially narrows the canal, to prevent progressive neurologic deficit, to ameliorate pain, and to gain time for radiation therapy to work. Such measures are advocated in patients with multiple metastatic sites, in whom poor general condition does not allow extensive two-stage procedures (Fig. 51–11). In benign neural tumors, posterior fixation alone may occasionally be indicated, for example, in a 52-year-old female patient with an egg-sized type I neurofibroma of the L3 root. In this case the neurosurgeon had to remove the L2-L3 and, partially, the L3-L4 joints on one side with an almost complete resection of the L3 pedicle to remove the tumor from the foramen and canal and preserve the root along its length. Posterior fixation was necessary from L2 to L4, which was enforced by posterolateral fusion with autogenous bone graft. The patient is disease free two years postoperatively, with only minor sensory disturbance of the L3 root and no evidence of recurrency to date. In rare conditions, a metastatic tumor may predominantly involve the posterior elements, as in a 74-year-old male patient with metastatic spread of a prostate carcinoma. The spinal tumor was almost exclusively confined to the pedicle, facet joint, and posterior arch. A posterior resection alone was performed, and the defect was bridged by our ISSF system.

Combined Anterior and Posterior Fixation

Most vertebral metastatic tumors involve the vertebral body and contribute significantly to spinal compression either by kyphotic deformity secondary to pathologic fractures or by direct compression of the tumor. Therefore, complete or at least partial body resection is the logical procedure. A single anterior approach combined with anterior fixation would be the procedure of choice.[6, 10, 23, 24] Stable anterior fixation, especially in elderly people with poor bone quality, is generally not possible or can only be accomplished with a cement-metal construct as proposed by Turner and colleagues.[23, 24] However, in benign or malignant tumors that can be controlled by radiation or chemotherapy, complete tumor resection may be advisable, often requiring a combined procedure.[19]

In some cases, it is possible to resect the anterior portion of the tumor in vertebral body through a posterior approach using a modified eggshell procedure or similar technique.[13] This procedure combines the benefits of a combined approach without requiring two incisions. In most of our patients with clear tumor involvement of the anterior column, in whom complete anteroposterior resection is intended, a double approach is performed. The surgery is almost always performed in one stage.

In the initial step, the posterior approach is performed. The implant is inserted on the intact anatomic landmarks, and the posterior decompression or resection is achieved if necessary. This surgical step may be accomplished with the patient supine or in a right lateral position. In the latter position, it is not necessary to interrupt surgery by having to turn the patient for the anterior procedure.

When a deformity is present from tumor destruction or pathologic fracture (compression and/or kyphosis), the ISSF is generally rigid enough to realign the spine by gentle distraction and manipulation into lordosis (see Fig. 51–5). However, if the dural sac is under significant compression according to the computed tomography (CT) or magnetic resonance imaging (MRI) scan, the ISSF is inserted without attempting any correction. The anterolateral approach is performed with the patient in a lateral position with the wound still open. Anterior decompression is then carried out. Only after the dural sac has been decompressed is posterior manipulation to align the

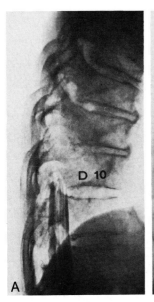
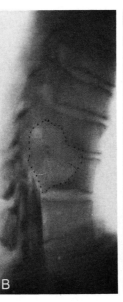
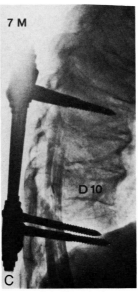

FIGURE 51–11. A 58-year-old male patient with a metastasis of a bronchus carcinoma to the 10th and 11th thoracic vertebrae. Conventional lateral myelographic x-ray (A) and tomography (B) show the destroyed area within D10 and D11. C, Seven months after posterolateral decompression, allogenic bone grafting and stabilization from D9 to D12 with an intact myelogram. The patient survived 10 months.

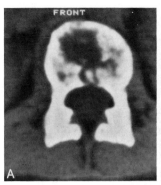
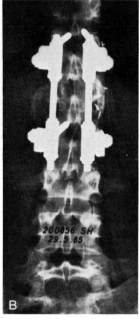
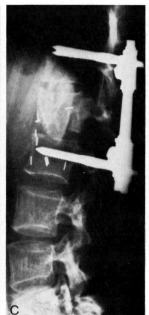
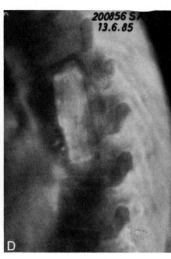

FIGURE 51–12. A 28-year-old female patient with malignant fibrous histiocytoma, first presenting at the 5th–7th thoracic vertebrae, where the tumor was removed and an anterior bony support was achieved by three rib grafts (*D*). Several weeks later a very painful metastasis was discovered at L1 (*A*). Tumor resection, curettage, and bone grafting by an anterolateral approach were carried out after having first installed the internal fixator by a posterior approach (*B* and *C*). Significant pain reduction was noted and the patient was discharged.

spine performed under direct visualization. Bone grafts, calcium apatite or cement, or a vertebral prosthesis can be used for anterior reconstruction. The indication whether a biologic bone graft or an artificial implant is used depends on the type of tumor. Anterior defects after resection of a benign tumor are always reconstructed whenever possible by autogenous bone. However, we also used bone as a substitute in a patient with a tumor, which turned out to be malignant postoperatively (Fig. 51–12).

Resected malignant tumors, which are supposed to have some chance for long-term survival after combined treatment of surgery, radiation, and occasionally chemotherapy, are replaced by calcium apatite (Ceros). This offers a long-term biologic interlocked interface between the bone bed and the substitute (Fig. 51–13). In malignant tumors, however, especially in metastatic tumors, the defect after resection is mostly filled with cement, since it is quick and mechanically sufficiently supportive. The anchorage may even be enhanced by including K-wires within the cement and the adjacent vertebra. Alternatively a vertebral prosthesis like the Polster device may be used as was done in one of our cases (Fig. 51–15). This special vertebral prosthesis offers the possibility to distract and correct a kyphotic deformity caused by the tumor involvement of the anterior column. With the use of the ISSF system, however, especially when inserted in a combined procedure, a vertebral body prosthesis is not necessary, since correction can usually be sufficiently reached by the powerful posterior implant. The Polster implant was used in this series in only one case just to enhance stability and better anchorage in porotic bone by creating a metal-cement compound (Fig. 51–15).

Finally, the anterior space is brought under compression through the adjustment of the ISSF. When using an anterior cement block, we reinforce its fixation to the adjacent vertebral bodies by inserting K-wires bridging the healthy vertebral bodies above and below into the cement.

RESULTS

Our combined experience at the orthopedic departments of the Universities of Basel and Berne totals more than 170 surgically treated cases of spinal tumors; of these, the ISSF system was used in 18 patients seen before 1988. Fifteen patients had spinal metastasis, and three patients had primary tumors. There were 13 male and 5 female patients, with a mean age of 56 years at operation. The metastatic tumors included breast carcinoma (2), malignant histiocytoma (2), hypernephroma (2), bronchial carcinoma (3), prostate carcinoma (2), adenocarcinoma of unknown origin (3), and multiple myeloma (1). The primary tumors included a neurinoma, an enchondroma, and a solitary plasmacytoma. In nine cases the tumor involved more than one vertebra of the lumbar and/or thoracic spine—D11, D12, L1, and L4 (one case each) and L3 (five cases). In six patients intractable back pain alone, and in 11 patients a combination of back pain and neurologic deficit, represented indications for surgery. One patient with a solitary plasmacytoma of L3 was previously operated through an anterior approach. A vertebrectomy was carried out, and the vertebra was replaced by a calcium phosphate spacer (Ceros). This calcium phosphate showed internal fracture lines shortly after

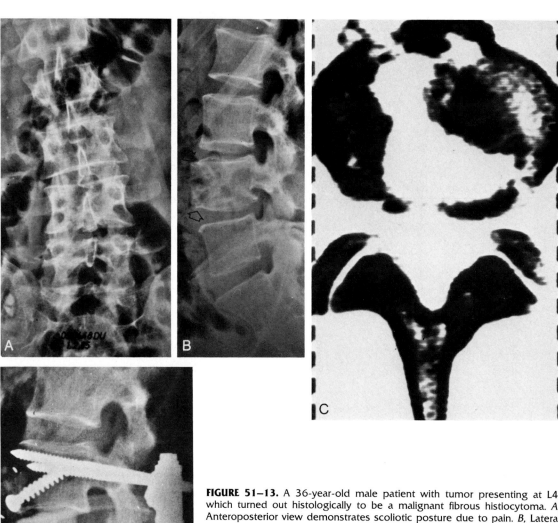

FIGURE 51–13. A 36-year-old male patient with tumor presenting at L4, which turned out histologically to be a malignant fibrous histiocytoma. *A,* Anteroposterior view demonstrates scoliotic posture due to pain. *B,* Lateral view with visible destructive changes at L4 (*arrows*). *C,* Axial CT scan with exclusive involvement of the anterior columns. *D,* Following combined anteroposterior approach and replacement of the anterior column by a calcium phosphate (Ceros) block. In front of the bioprosthesis a corticocancellous bone graft was fixed with a screw in the vertebrae above and below as a ventral "bone bridge."

surgery, and two years later a comminuted fracture with a consecutive localized spinal deformity developed. To reduce the deformity and stabilize the spine, a dorsal instrumentation with the ISSF was performed.

All three patients with a primary spinal tumor are still alive, while the average survival time of patients with metastases was 6.2 months (1 week to 16 months). In six patients the neurologic symptoms improved, in four patients they remained unchanged, and one patient became worse. Sixteen patients reported significant relief of pain, one patient remained unchanged, and one patient experienced more pain after surgery. Thirteen patients were discharged home, and five patients stayed at the hospital for the rest of their lives. Eight patients were supported by a three-point brace, three other patients by a soft corset, and seven patients were mobilized without an external support. Most patients in this series received postoperative radiation therapy.

Different surgical techniques were used. All patients were stabilized posteriorly with the internal fixator. In 10 cases there were only two segments bridged, and in eight cases more than two segments were bridged by the fixation device. In eight patients the posterior fixation was used alone; however, in 10 cases it was used in combination with an anterior procedure. In four cases the anterior tumor resection and the reconstruction of the defect was performed by a posterolateral approach (Fig. 51–11). In six cases the anterior surgery was done through an additional anterior or anterolateral approach, mostly in a one-stage procedure. As anterior implants either bone (4 cases) (Fig. 51–12), calcium phosphate (2 cases) (Fig. 51–13), cement alone (2 cases) (Fig. 51–14), a com-

bination of plate/cement (1 case), or a Polster device (1 case) (Fig. 51–15) was used. In 12 cases the procedure was supplemented by laminectomy.

Technical complications were rare and without consequence for the patients. One Schanz screw was placed in the L5-S1 disc space instead of the L5 vertebral body, one Schanz screw showed a late fatigue fracture, and one Ceros block demonstrated internal fracture lines but with a good incorporation at the bone–calcium apatite interface.

A 72-year-old patient died one week postoperatively during mobilization from a massive pulmonary embolism. In two patients profuse intraoperative bleeding prevented the surgeon from performing the complete vertebrectomy, therefore macroscopic tumor mass was left behind.

CONCLUSION

The ISSF is suitable for a wide range of applications in spinal tumor surgery when posterior fixation is indicated. The decision to perform posterior fixation and decompression alone or in combination with an anterior procedure depends on several factors. With the upcoming development of better anterior fixation devices,[6, 7, 10, 24] with which the goals of stable fixation may be attained allowing immediate mobilization of the patient with minimal external support, indications for the ISSF may become less common. This device was not originally designed for spinal tumor surgery and offers more possibilities for stabilization and correction of deformities than are needed in tumor surgery. Most pedicle plate systems can provide sufficient stabilization as long as correction is not needed. With newer plate development,[20] a stable junction between plate and screws can often

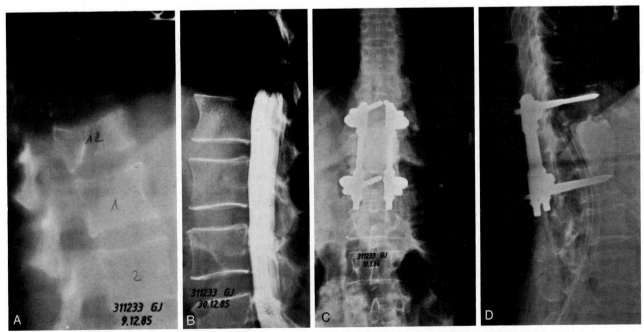

FIGURE 51–14. A 52-year-old male patient with metastatic involvement of D12 by an adenocarcinoma of unknown origin, resulting in a pathologic fracture (A) and complete block on myelogram (B). Combined posteroanterior approach with an anterior support by methyl methacrylate (C and D).

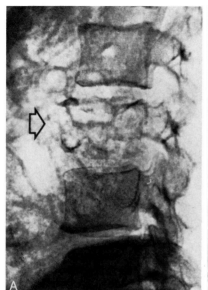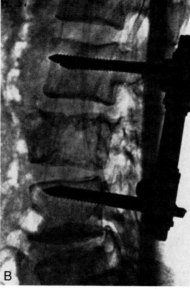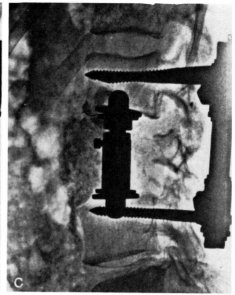

FIGURE 51–15. A 74-year-old male patient with L3 metastatic involvement by a hypernephroma (*A*). Laminectomy and internal fixator in a first stage (*B*). A few days later anterior decompression and tumor resection. Replacement and anterior support by a vertebral prosthesis according to Polster combined with bone cement. The patient survived 11 months and was fully mobile at home.

be achieved. However, in an attempt to simplify stabilization techniques for the spine and to reduce the number of different spinal devices, a well-designed, versatile, "universal" implant system may be a worthwhile goal for future development. The ISSF has proved in applications extending beyond fracture treatment to be a simple and effective device with virtually no significant complications related to the instrumentation. It may be especially useful in the treatment of patients with metastatic disease, allowing them to overcome a difficult and painful period of tumor progression while allowing immediate mobilization and greater independence during hospitalization and at home.

REFERENCES

1. Aebi M, Etter Ch, Kehl Th, Talgott J: Stabilization of the lower thoracic and lumbar spine with the internal spinal skeletal fixation system. Spine 12:544–551, 1987.
2. Aebi M, Etter Ch, Kehl Th, Thalgott J: The internal skeletal fixation system: A new treatment of thoracolumbar fractures and other spinal disorders. Clin Orthop 227:30–43, 1988.
3. Boland PJ, Lane JM, Sundaresan N: Metastatic disease of the spine. Clin Orthop 169:95–102, 1982.
4. Dick W: Innere Fixation von Brust- und Lendenwirbelbrüchen. 2nd ed. Bern, Hans Huber, 1987.
5. Dick W: The "fixateur interne" as a versatile implant for spine surgery. Spine 12:882–900, 1987.
6. Fidler MW: Anterior decompression and stabilization of metastatic spinal fractures. J Bone Joint Surg 68B:83–90, 1986.
7. Fidler MW: Anterior and posterior stabilization of the spine following vertebral body resection. Spine 11:362–366, 1986.
8. Harrington KD: The use of methylmethacrylate for vertebral body replacement and anterior stabilization of pathologic fracture-dislocations of the spine due to metastatic malignant disease. J Bone Joint Surg 63A:36–46, 1981.
9. Kluger P, Gerner HJ: Das mechanische Prinzip des Fixateur externe zur dorsalen Stabilisierung der Brust- und Lendenwirbelsäule. Unfallchir 12:68–79, 1986.
10. Kostuik JP, Errico TJ, Gleason TF, Errico CCh: Spinal stabilization of vertebral column tumors. Spine 13:250–256, 1988.
11. Krag MH, Beynnon BD, Pope MH, et al: An internal fixator for posterior application to short segments of the thoracic, lumbar and lumbosacral spine. Design and testing. Clin Orthop 203:75–98, 1986.
12. Lee CK, Rosa R, Fernand R: Surgical treatment of tumors of the spine. Spine 11:201–208, 1986.
13. Magerl F, Coscia MF: Total posterior vertebrectomy of the thoracic or lumbar spine. Clin Orthop 232:62–69, 1988.
14. Magerl FP: Stabilization of the lower thoracic and lumbar spine with external skeletal fixation. Clin Orthop 189:125–149, 1984.
15. Nather A, Bose K: The results of decompression of cord or cauda equina compression from metastatic extradural tumors. Clin Orthop 169:103–108, 1982.
16. Onimus M, Bertin D: Stabilization chirurgicale des fractures métastatiques du rachis. Rev Chir Orthop 68:369–378, 1982.
17. Onimus M, Schraub S, Bertin D, et al: Surgical treatment of vertebral metastasis. Spine 11:883–891, 1986.
18. Roy-Camille R, Saillant G, Berteaux D, Salgado K: Osteosynthesis of thoracolumbar spine fractures with metal plates screwed through the vertebral pedicles. Reconstr Surg Traumatol 15:2–16, 1976.
19. Roy-Camille R: Les Tumeurs du Rachis. 3-émes Journées d'Orthopédie de la Pitié. Paris, Masson, 1983, pp 3–87.
20. Steffee AD, Biscup RJ, Sitakowski DJ: Segmental spine plates with pedicle screw fixation. A new internal fixation device for disorders of the lumbar and thoracolumbar spine. Clin Orthop 203:45–53, 1986.
21. Sundaresan N, Galicich JH, Lane JM, Scher H: Stabilization of the spine involved by cancer. *In* Dunsker StB, et al (eds): The Unstable Spine. Orlando, Grune and Stratton, 1986, pp 249–274.
22. Thalgott JS, La Rocca H, Aebi M, et al: Reconstruction of the lumbar spine using AO-DCP plate internal fixation. Spine 14:91–95, 1989.
23. Turner PL, Webb JK, Sokal MPJW: Surgery for spinal tumors. J Bone Joint Surg 68B:670–671, 1986.
24. Turner PL, Prince HG, Webb JK, Sokal MPJW: Surgery for malignant extradural tumors of the spine. J Bone Joint Surg 70B:451–456, 1988.
25. Weinstein JN, McLain RF: Primary tumors of the spine. Spine 12:843–851, 1987.

COTREL-DUBOUSSET INSTRUMENTATION:

Indications and Techniques

REGIS W. HAID, JR., and RICHARD L. CARTER

INTRODUCTION

Recent advances in neurodiagnostic imaging, operative exposures, instrumentation, and stabilization techniques have led to a resurgence in the operative treatment of spinal neoplasms. With a better understanding of the tumor's anatomic location afforded by computed tomography (CT) and magnetic resonance imaging (MRI), tumor resection may be undertaken with more precision. Concomitant with these developments, the goals of spinal surgery are evolving to encompass not only neural element decompression but also long-term spinal deformity correction or prevention and fatigue-resistant stabilization. In this way, the optimal environment for pain relief and preservation of neurologic function is provided.[10]

In order to determine the best treatment option for a particular patient, many prognostic factors are considered, including the patient's age, overall medical status, tumor histology, and neurologic status. Sundaresan notes four groups of patients deserving strong consideration for surgical intervention. These include those with (1) pathologic compression fractures, (2) solitary relapse site with a controlled or unknown primary site, (3) neural element compression secondary to direct tumor extension, and (4) spinal metastases with other sites of involvement and a life expectancy greater than six months.[33] Treatment is palliative in terms of pain relief, preservation of neurologic function, and quality of life. However, with a multidisciplinary approach, attempts at "cure" may soon be feasible, especially in those patients with primary bone neoplasms.

The preoperative radiologic evaluation is discussed elsewhere in this text. Needless to say, as thorough a work-up as possible is necessary to determine the best treatment alternative. Plain roentgenographic evaluation is mandatory as the initial diagnostic test. Radionuclide bone scans are used to detect other osseous lesions for staging purposes. Myelography and postmyelography-CT are useful in detecting epidural involvement and bony pathology. MRI is gaining widespread acceptance owing to its sensitivity to pathology, multiplanar views, and contrast resolution.

OPERATIVE APPROACHES

The choice of operative approach and the need for instrumentation must be individualized. Variables include tumor location, vascularity, histology, life expectancy, and the specific goal of intervention.[35]

Anterolateral Approach

The anterolateral approach is generally considered in those patients with (1) anterior osseous destruction or tumor mass, (2) severe kyphotic deformity secondary to an isolated vertebral body collapse, or (3) benign tumor. If the spine is in normal alignment preoperatively and the decompression is at a level of low mobility (e.g., midthoracic vertebrae), stabilization may be obtained by placement of autograft or allograft bone in a "lock and keyed-in" position or by methyl methacrylate covering additional instrumentation. Additional instrumentation should be considered if realignment is needed, if the decompression is at a level of high mobility and less inherent stability (e.g., the thoracolumbar junction), or if there is significant posterior destruction.[2, 3, 23, 26, 30]

Posterior or Posterolateral Approach

These approaches include laminectomy, transpedicular approach, costotransversectomy, and extracavitary. General indications include (1) posterior element disease, (2) multilevel tumor involvement, and (3) instances of spinal instability or deformity that necessitate the need for posterior instrumentation.[21, 28]

ANTERIOR INSTRUMENTATION

Anterior instrumentation implants include the Kaneda device, the Harrington-Kostuik system, or the Zielke system.[14–16] These implants act as a strut and react poorly to torsional loading and lateral bending forces. They often require additional posterior instrumentation or significant external support. They cannot be relied upon for prolonged stabilization without adequate bony fusion.

POSTERIOR INSTRUMENTATION

The goals of internal fixation include (1) correction of a spinal deformity and reconstruction of the normal anatomy, (2) provision for spinal stability to allow early patient mobilization, and (3) establishment of the ideal biomechanical milieu for bony arthrodesis and thus prevention of a progressive deformity.[10]

The durability of methyl methacrylate fusions is not clearly defined.[5, 27] Thus, with the exception of patients with life expectancies of less than 12 to 18 months, bony fusion might be preferred. The concept that long-term treatment of spinal instability requires solid arthrodesis has remained axiomatic since the initial reports of Albee and Hibbs. Harrington rods, Luque rods with segmental wiring, and the combination of these have been utilized with excellent results and have been shown to be important adjuncts to spinal arthrodesis.[13, 34]

Posterior instrumentation has been the mainstay for obtaining alignment and stability in the thoracic, lumbar, and sacral spine. Several types of spinal implants have been developed to treat spinal deformities. Although initially intended for scoliotic deformities, posterior instrumentation is gaining widespread popularity for the treatment of degenerative, traumatic, and neoplastic diseases.

In the United States, the Steffee plate system initiated the use of pedicular fixation,[32] although Roy-Camille in Europe has enjoyed success using pedicular fixation for several years.[29] The Cotrel-Dubousset (CD) or Universal instrumentation system is a recently developed posterior spinal implant. It is a highly versatile system for the treatment of spinal instability or deformity owing to trauma, infection, neoplasm, or congenital anomaly.[6–9, 19, 31]

Each of the available instrumentation systems has inherent advantages and limitations; thus the spinal surgeon should have reasonable knowledge of all of the systems. Whereas this chapter is primarily oriented toward the use of the CD system, a brief review of other systems is also warranted for a broader understanding of instrumentation principles.

Harrington Rods

This system consists of either distraction or compression rods. The distraction rods provide resistance to axial compression via sublaminar hooks on the rostral and caudal end segments. The square distraction Moe rod provides better sagittal plane reconstruction.

There are many reported complications from using Harrington rods. If there is circumferential disruption or loss of the anterior longitudinal ligament, this system may overdistract and cause neural injury.[1] Likewise, caution must be used in distracting over a fixed kyphotic deformity, as this may lead to ventral cord compression. In addition, two-point distraction has also been reported to produce loss of lumbar lordosis with the resultant painful "flat-back syndrome."[15]

Since the majority of the force is located on the upper laminar hook, hook disengagement or "autolaminectomy" (laminar disruption from hook forces) can occur. Rod breakage at the rod-rachet interface is also reported. Since laminar fixation is required, it is not an optimal system to use in conjunction with posterior decompressive procedures. In addition, sacral fixation is often difficult, as the sacral hooks can easily cause sacral root impingement.[22]

To adequately support a one-level instability, the instrumentation needs to span two levels above and two or three levels below the unstable segment, thus immobilizing a longer spinal segment. Rigid fixation is not obtained, thus necessitating a rigid external orthosis.

Compression rods are useful in correcting kyphosis. They may be used in conjunction with a distraction rod to augment rigidity and prevent overdistraction. Compression rods may also be employed after anterior corpectomy and reconstruction to aid in maintaining alignment.[25, 36] Care must be used in middle column pathology to avoid further retropulsion of ventral material into the canal.

Harrington rods may also be used with sublaminar wiring to aid axial and transverse fixation. Advantages include a more evenly distributed biomechanical force and increased rigidity allowing for earlier mobilization.[4, 11, 22, 24] Problems cited include wire breakage, rod fracture at the rod-ratchet junction as a result of a stress riser, and rotation of hooks into the spinal canal.

Luque Segmental Spinal Instrumentation

Segmental spinal instrumentation was first advocated by Luque in the early 1970s and initially consisted of sublaminar wires attached to a Harrington distraction rod. Owing to system complications, a smooth rod system was developed. Advantages include versatility; rigid segmental fixation, thus enhancing arthrodesis; promotion of early mobilization; and dispersement of the biomechanical forces over several segments. By "coupling" the rods into a rectangular configuration, torsional stability is enhanced. The hook-bone interface problem is avoided, although it does not resist axial loading in the coronal plane as well as do Harrington rods.[20] The incidence of neurologic complications is greater with sublaminar wire placement; thus Drummond modified the system by advocating interspinous process wiring. As with the Harrington system, fixation should include two to three levels above and below the level of instability.[18]

Cotrel-Dubousset System

From 1982 to 1984, the concepts of CD instrument design and technical employment were introduced in Paris by Cotrel and Dubousset for treating scoliotic deformities in children. Since the introduction of their system to the United States in 1984, it has gained widespread acceptance among orthopedic surgeons for correcting idiopathic, neuromuscular, and paralytic scoliosis in every age range.

Owing to its versatility, its usage has expanded to manage a wide spectrum of thoracic, lumbar, and sacral disorders. Experience is now being gained in instrumenting spinal pathologies requiring shorter segment posterior instrumentation. Gurr and McAfee reported that in spinal pathology secondary to neoplasm, trauma, and spondylolisthesis, CD instrumentation appeared to offer significant advantages over conventional methods, with an average of 1.6 motion segments preserved per case.[12] In their tumor group, the CD system decreased the number of vertebral levels required for fixation by two segments per patient as compared with Harrington or Luque instrumentation.

A shorter fusion is preferred since unnecessary disruption of normal tissue is avoided and fewer spinal segments are immobilized, which is more biomechanically sound. There is avoidance of the "rod long, fuse short" technique that may require a second operation or induce facet arthropathy.[17]

White and Panjabi have described the loads that are applied to the functional spinal unit and have noted that spinal movements are not pure and that some degree of mechanical coupling occurs with every motion.[37] Kahn states that the implant that provides the greatest amount of stability to the spine in all planes of motion is the one theoretically preferred.[14] The CD system was designed to act in the frontal, sagittal, and axial planes to produce a three-dimensional balanced spine, thus improving spinal deformity correction.

The CD system provides a posterior implant that incorporates the advantages of many systems. Multiple fixation points and rod-coupling increase rigidity. This enhances arthrodesis and permits earlier patient mobilization.[3, 31] Although postoperative orthotics are not used in the majority of idiopathic scoliotic cases, the author usually employs a custom-fit clam-shell orthosis for 6 to 24 weeks in spinal neoplasm cases.

CD Instruments

The availability of certain CD hooks and screws is undergoing considerable change. The basic system includes the following components.

RODS

The rods are produced from 316L stainless steel to enhance rigidity and avoid brittleness. The surface is knurled with diamond-shaped asperities, allowing screw or hook placement at any point on the rod and rotation of the rod in any plane. This allows spinal fixation at multiple points and multiplanar correction. The stress risers generated from knurling the ductile material affect only the surface of the rod, thereby minimizing the reduction in fatigue life. This avoids the stress riser problem inherent in the Harrington rod-ratchet interface. The Harrington rod is also more brittle as a result of cold-working the raw material, which results in residual stresses. The CD rods may be used in a distraction, compression, or neutral mode. Except in scoliosis, the same clinical indications for distraction and compression are employed as with the other posterior instrumentation systems.

HOOKS

The hooks resemble Harrington hooks. Pedicle hooks with a notched, bifid blade are used in the thoracic spine. Laminar hooks are available in many designs for specific anatomic laminar configurations. These include standard and narrow blades, 45-degree slant blades, and standard and long-bodied blades. Laminar hooks are employed in both the thoracic and lumbar levels, although care must be taken in the thoracic region to avoid neurologic injury. Transverse process hooks are also available, although fixation is less secure.

The pedicle and laminar hooks have either an open- or closed-body design. The rod passes through a hole in the closed-body type and is coupled to the open-body type by means of a bushing called a "blocker." The blocker is attached to the rod and is firmly seated into the open hook. Closed hooks are used at the ends of instrumentation, and open hooks are used in the middle.

SCREWS

Screws are used for pedicular fixation. Although only the sacral screw is available in the United States, the sizes allow safe usage in the low thoracic and lumbosacral regions in most adults. The screws currently available are 6 or 7 mm in diameter and come in lengths of 30, 35, or 40 mm. They are available in either a high-profile or low-profile design to adjust for severe spinal curvatures.

SET SCREWS

All hooks and pedicular screws are secured to the rod by means of set screws. Hooks and pedicular screws may be used in combination on the same rod since the coupling mechanism is the same. The rod can be held in position temporarily by slightly tightening the set screws until contact prevents rod migration. Once permanent positioning is obtained after correction of the deformity by rod rotation, compression, or distraction, the set screws are further tightened until the heads of the screws break off.

Once a set screw breaks off, the only recourse for repositioning is drilling or cutting the screw or rod.

DEVICE FOR TRANSVERSE TRACTION (DTT)

The ⅛-inch-diameter transverse loader is a threaded rod that connects the larger rods in a transverse fashion at both the rostral and caudal ends. Preferably, a minimum of two are used, although placement of a second transverse loader is often difficult at the lumbosacral junction. DTTs couple the larger rods into a rectangle and increase torsional stability. Thus, it is possible to obtain the compression or distraction of the Harrington system as well as the torsional stability and rigidity of the Luque system. Additionally, the DTT may "prestress" the screws, which may enhance screw purchase and rigidity.

C-RING

C-shaped rings lock the blockers on the intermediate hooks prior to tightening the set screws. They fixate the hook position during rotation of the large rod. Although mandatory in scoliosis, they are usually not needed in reconstruction for spinal neoplasms.

CD Instrument Selection

It is not within the scope of this chapter to discuss the treatment of scoliotic deformities, which is exceedingly complex with respect to proper placement and rod rotation.

In general, instrumentation used in the treatment of spinal neoplasms is relatively straightforward. The decision to distract or compress is essentially the same as with the Harrington system. However, because pedicle and laminar hook fixation allows bilateral "clawing" of the spine at both the rostral and caudal

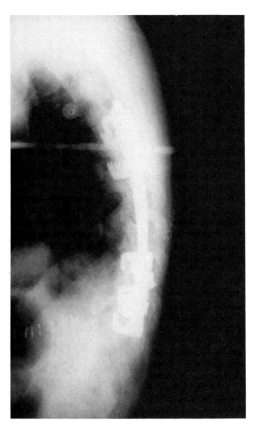

FIGURE 52–2. An example of a midthoracic laminar and pedicle hook system. This patient had a previously staged vertebrectomy for anterior lateral decompression and installation of an allograft strut.

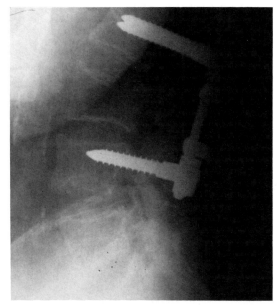

FIGURE 52–1. This illustrates a patient who had lymphoma with posterior element and epidural extension. A laminectomy was done for tissue diagnosis and decompression. A short segment fixation was accomplished utilizing transpedicular fixation from L2-L4.

levels, semisegmental or segmental fixation is obtained which enhances rigidity.

Transpedicular rod instrumentation offers other advantages particularly applicable to the lumbosacral spine. First, it can conform to the contour of lumbar lordosis, and it may also be used in conjunction with decompressive procedures such as laminectomies. Hook systems cannot be used as effectively in this situation (Fig. 52–1).[12, 17]

Other advantages of a transpedicular fixation system include the lack of spinal canal encroachment as is present with sublaminar wires or laminar hooks. The pedicle also seems to be the strongest site from which to obtain a three-dimensional fixation of the vertebrae.[17, 32]

The CD pedicular screw system is a rod system, which has several advantages over a plate system such as the Steffee plate system. A rod system allows gradual deformity reduction and variable screw positioning. Pedicle rod systems allow multiplanar correction and do not impinge on the facet above the level of the fusion. If bone grafting is to be done, the graft site is available for donor bone, as it is not covered up by a plate.[17]

Disadvantages of transpedicular fixation include technical difficulty, a steep surgical learning curve, and the possibility of nerve root impingement. It is the author's opinion that the best application of this type of fixation is at the lumbosacral junction.

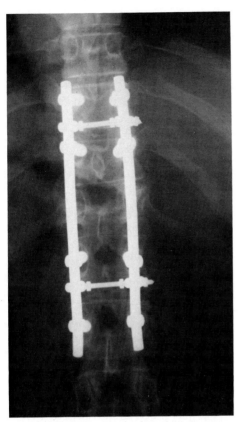

FIGURE 52–3. An example of a patient who had a pathologic thoracolumbar burst fracture. He underwent thoracolumbar transpedicular instrumentation with an excellent clinical response.

The number of segments to be instrumented is individualized. If the instability is at the thoracolumbar junction, or if severe instability is suspected, then instrumentation is often used two segments above and below the pathologic site. If less instability is encountered, then instrumentation is carried out one level above and below the unstable segment. Other determinants include number of levels of neoplastic involvement, quality of the bone (e.g., osteopenia), and the specific surgical goal. The use of pedicular fixation, which provides excellent rigidity, has proved particularly advantageous for short-segment fixation.[12, 17]

In general, for thoracic instrumentation the pedicle and laminar hook system is used (Fig. 52–2). Transpedicular screw fixation is sometimes used at the thoracolumbar junction (Fig. 52–3), although the author prefers hooks except in the setting of T12-L1-L2 vertebral body neoplasms. In this situation, good success has been obtained with an anterolateral decompressive corpectomy with allograft (or autograft) strut placement in combination with posterior transpedicular screw instrumentation spanning one segment above and below the lesion (Fig. 52–4). In this situation, the system is in a slightly compressed or neutral mode. After anterior decompression, these levels are chosen for posterior instrumentation owing to their inherent mobility. At levels above and below the thoracolumbar junction, posterior instrumenta-tion is often not needed after anterior decompression if the posterior elements are intact.

OPERATIVE TECHNIQUES FOR CD INSTRUMENTATION

The patient is placed in a prone position, making sure that all bony prominences are well padded. Free excursion of the abdomen is also ensured to decrease intraoperative blood loss. If transpedicular fixation is to be used, the patient is placed on a pacemaker table with a radiolucent frame to enable anteroposterior and lateral fluoroscopic verification of pedicular anatomy.

A standard midline incision is utilized after infiltration with 0.5 per cent xylocaine with 1:200,000 epinephrine to minimize bleeding. The paraspinous muscles are reflected in a subperiosteal fashion laterally until the facets are readily visualized. All soft tissue is removed to encourage a vigorous osteoblastic fusion response. The transverse processes are isolated and decorticated with a high speed drill. If fusion is to be carried to the sacrum, the alae are identified and are decorticated.

After exposure of the surgical area is complete, the vertebral levels are confirmed and the hook sites are carefully prepared. The thoracic pedicle hooks are placed within the facet joint after the inferior edge of the facet is removed with an osteotome, while

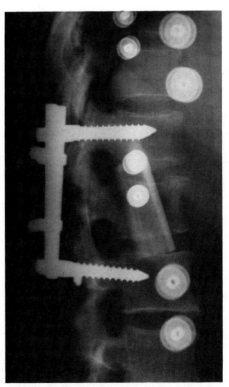

FIGURE 52–4. Lateral radiograph of a patient who underwent a retroperitoneal L1 decompression with placement of a tibial allograft. Transpedicular instrumentation was then carried out from T12-L2. A clam-shell orthosis will be worn for approximately 8 weeks. The radiodense circular areas on the radiograph represent snaps on the clam shell.

leaving the superior portion of the facet intact. Ligamentum flavum is visible at the medial edge of the facet. The pedicle finder is inserted into the facet joint until it is well seated to ensure proper fit of the hook. The pedicular hook is then seated using the hook holder and is inserted until the pedicle is engaged.

Laminar hook placement is essentially the same procedure as with Harrington hooks. The upper or lower edge of the lamina is meticulously cleaned with curettes, and the ligamentum flavum is removed. For hooks placed on the rostral edge of the lamina, it is often necessary to remove a small amount of bone with a Kerrison rongeur to facilitate placement of the hook. The choice between standard or long-bladed laminar hooks depends on the inclination of the lamina. It must be kept in mind that in the thoracic spine the smaller blade is employed.

Fixation of a single or double spine segment on both the rostral and caudal aspect is termed "clawing." A lamina is able to be clawed by placing a rod clamp a short distance from the hook. The spreader is introduced between the rod clamp and the hook, and opening the spreader forces the hook against the pedicle or lamina. As this is done, the set screws are tightened for temporary fixation. This is done sequentially working from a caudal to a rostral direction. It is usually not possible to clamp adjacent laminae between transverse processes and pedicle hooks owing to the limitation of space.

At the thoracic level, pedicular hook fixation is used at the level below the clawed rostral lamina. If the T9 lamina were clawed superiorly with laminar hooks and inferiorly with pedicle hooks, it would be impossible to claw the superior aspect of T10 with laminar hooks. Therefore, the T10 lamina would be stabilized with pedicular hooks caudally. In the lumbar area, the superior (caudally directed) laminar hook is usually applied one lamina rostral to the clawed lamina. For example, if the L4 lamina is clawed at its rostral and caudal edges, it would be difficult to place another laminar hook at the L3 caudal edge. Therefore, a laminar hook would be placed at the rostral margin of the L3 lamina.

Both distraction and compression can be utilized in this system by applying a rod clamp adjacent to a hook and using the distractor or compressor to move the hooks appropriately. After all hook sites have been prepared, the rod is bent into the appropriate curvature and is passed through the various hooks. The rod may be temporarily fixed to the hooks by moderately tightening the set screws. By rotating the prebent rod, multiplanar correction is achievable. Hook selection and rod contour vary with the deformity. For example, in the sagittal plane a rod initially bent in a thoracic lordosis may create a thoracic kyphosis when rotated. Once the proper rod configuration is achieved, the DTTs are applied near the ends of the rods. After this is done, all set screws are tightened until they are broken off. Protruding ends

of the rods or DTTs are cut away to avoid soft tissue damage.

If transpedicular fixation is to be used, then anteroposterior and lateral fluoroscopy is indicated to ensure correct anatomic positioning.[29] It should be noted that it is possible to use both hooks and pedicle screws on the same rod and thus to span several segments (Fig. 52–5).

Identification of the pedicle is of paramount importance. The dorsal portion of the pedicle is located at the junction of the transverse process and the superior articular process of the involved vertebrae. After identifying this intersection, a rongeur or high speed drill is used to remove the superficial aspect of the cortical bone until the cancellous bone of the pedicle is encountered. This may be further delineated by using a short awl. A $5/32$-diameter smooth Steinmann pin is placed into the center of the pedicle under fluoroscopic control. It is mandatory that the image intensifier be used in the anteroposterior and lateral projections to obtain good three-dimensional verification. The Steinmann pins are subsequently removed, and the CD screws are directed along the path created by the Steinmann pin into the pedicle. Continuous fluoroscopic guidance is also used, such

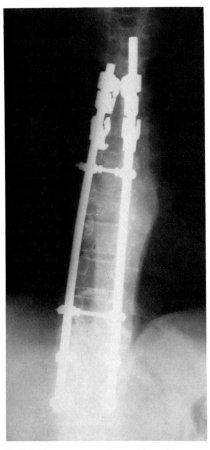

FIGURE 52–5. This illustrates a patient with multisegment midthoracic collapse secondary to metastatic lung carcinoma. Note the versatility of the CD system as the rostral attachments are of the laminar and pedicle hooks, and caudal fixation is achieved via transpedicular screw placement.

that the screw is inserted to a depth of approximately 80 per cent of the vertebral body. Data have shown that an 80 per cent depth of penetration produces an approximate 30 per cent stronger grip on the pedicle compared with a 50 per cent depth of penetration. The most commonly used screw length is 40 mm, but the length of the screw varies with the size of the vertebral body. Placement of the screw deeper than 80 per cent penetration does not offer significant biomechanical advantage.[17]

Choice of pedicle screw diameter varies with the level. Vertebral morphometric studies have shown pedicle diameters are almost constant from T9-L1, with a mean at each level of approximately 7 mm. A very gradual increase in diameter occurs from L1-L5, with almost 100 per cent of the pedicles at L5 being 8 mm in diameter or larger.

The pedicle axis angle relative to the sagittal plane is an important consideration and must be taken into account when the screws are placed. At T12 the pedicle angle is approximately 0 degrees. The angles are approximately 10 to 15 degrees at L1, L2, and L3; 20 degrees at L4; and 25 degrees at L5. An approximation of the pedicle angle may be estimated from a preoperative CT scan.[17]

After all of the screws are placed under fluoroscopic control, the prebent rod is inserted through the openings. Owing to large lumbosacral angles, the passage of a 7-mm rod is often difficult. Experience has been gained using the more flexible 5-mm rod in lumbosacral fusions. A flexible rod is coupled to the screw by means of an adapted blocker. The flexible rod is less technically difficult to place and is more comfortable, which allows for greater freedom in reconstructing the lumbar lordosis. In the author's series of greater than 40 lumbosacral reconstructions using either 7-mm or 5-mm rods, there have been no differences in obtaining initial stability or maintaining long-term alignment. It is important to remember to use the blockers under proper direction in conjunction with the intermediate open screws. The blockers are firmly seated against the intermediate hooks by sequentially tightening them with the rod clamp and spreader.

The decortication of the bony area to be fused is usually best accomplished before rod placement, although this opinion varies among surgeons. Autogenous bone graft is on-laid over the decorticated area. This may be supplemented with allograft bone. Copious irrigation is used, and a Hemovac drain is placed for 24 hours.

The patients are usually mobilized on the second or third postoperative day. Although several surgeons do not use an external orthosis with CD instrumentation, the author prefers a custom polypropylene clam-shell orthosis for a period of 6 to 12 weeks.

Operative Results

In the authors' experience, a total of 29 patients with spinal neoplasms have been instrumented with the CD system. Nineteen had associated decompressive procedures, and 10 were instrumented for pain or instability (Table 52–1). There have been no 30-day operative mortalities. Five patients have died of metastatic disease. There has been one late instrument failure (Fig. 52–6) in a patient who underwent a posterolateral decompression for metastatic breast disease. Postoperative radiation was given. There was rostral laminar claw pull-out with a subsequent open pedicular hook-rod disengagement. This was probably attributable to tumor-infested bone coupled with high biomechanical stress at the rostral lamina.

Another patient with lymphoma had posterior transpedicular instrumentation for pain relief. Radiation therapy had been previously completed. Follow-up radiographs (Fig. 52–7) revealed bending of

TABLE 52–1. CD INSTRUMENT CASE SUMMARY

Anterior decompression and posterior intrumentation	
—thoracic	5
—lumbar	8
Posterolateral decompression and posterior instrumentation	6
Posterior instrumentation without decompression	10
Total	29

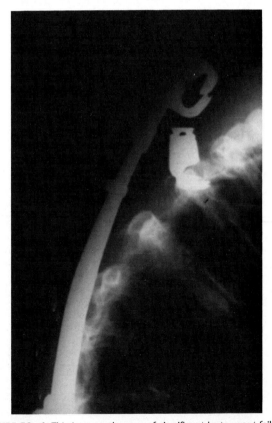

FIGURE 52–6. This is our only case of significant instrument failure. After undergoing a posterolateral decompression for metastatic breast disease, the rostral hooks pulled through the lamina. This resulted in secondary disengagement of the rod from the lower pedicle hook. When instrumenting over a kyphosis, the majority of the biomechanical force is located at the upper lamina. This increased mechanical force coupled with weakened bone resulted in a bone-metal failure.

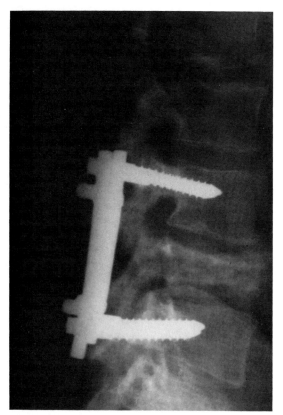

FIGURE 52–7. This illustrates a patient who underwent transpedicular fixation for pain relief. The patient had completed a course of radiation therapy for lymphoma. Note the slight bending of the caudal pedicular screw. Despite this, solid arthrodesis was obtained and a good clinical result was achieved.

the caudal screws, although the clinical response was excellent and arthrodesis was obtained. Possibly an anterior reconstruction may have been beneficial. It was also apparent that the screws did not penetrate to the full 80 per cent depth, thus lessening rigidity. No other complications were encountered.

Neurologic improvement was noted in 20 of 29 patients. Significant pain relief was obtained in 22 of 27 patients. Of the 24 long-term survivors, 17 are ambulatory without assistance and 3 are ambulatory with assistance. Two patients who underwent initial posterior stabilization later required anterior decompression.

Although this series is not large and long-term follow-up is not yet available, CD instrumentation appears to be an effective system for treating spinal neoplasms. The versatility of the system is readily apparent, as is its complexity. Advantages include the ability to obtain fixation at multiple points, increased torsional stability, the applications of distraction and compression within the same rod, and the option of combining this with transpedicular fixation. Disadvantages include the initial mastering of a technically challenging instrument system and the possibility of stress-shielding encountered with excessive rigidity. More experience is needed to fully evaluate the effectiveness of the CD system in treating neo-

plastic spinal disorders. The results of this series suggest that it offers great promise in spinal reconstruction.

REFERENCES

1. Anden U, Lake A, Nordwall A: The role of the anterior longitudinal ligament in Harrington rod fixation of unstable thoracolumbar spinal fractures. Spine 5:23, 1980.
2. Boland PJ, Lane JM, Sundaresan N: Metastatic disease of the spine. Clin Orthop 169:95, 1982.
3. Bridewell K, Jenny A, Saul T, et al: Posterior segmental spinal instrumentation (PSSI) with posterolateral decompression and debulking for metastatic thoracic and lumbar spine disease. Spine 13:1383–1384, 1988.
4. Bryant CE, Sullivan JA: Management of thoracic and lumbar spine fractures with Harrington distraction rods supplemented with segmental wiring. Spine 8:532–537, 1983.
5. Clark CR, Keggi KJ, Panjabi MM: Methyl methacrylate stabilization of the cervical spine. J Bone Joint Surg 66A:40, 1984.
6. Cotrel Y, Dubousset J: New segmental posterior instrumentation of the spine. Orthop Trans 9:118, 1985.
7. Cotrel Y, Dubousset J, Guillaumat M: New universal instrumentation in spinal surgery. Clin Orthop 227:10, 1988.
8. Cotrel Y, Dubousset J, Miladi L, et al: L'instrumentation Universelle (CD) pour l'arthodese postérieure du rachis dans la scoliose idiopathique. In Michel CR, Dubousset J (eds): Cahier d'Euseignment du SOFCOT. Vol 1. Paris, Expansion Scientifique Française, 1986.
9. Dubousset J, Graf H, Miladi L, et al: Spinal and thoracic derotation with CD instrumentation. Scoliosis Res Soc Abstr 20:142, 1985.
10. Flatley J, Anderson M, Anast G, et al: Spinal instability due to malignant disease. J Bone Joint Surg 66A:47–52, 1984.
11. Gaines RW, Breedlove RF, Munson G: Stabilization of thoracic thoracolumbar fracture-dislocations with Harrington rods and sublaminar wires. Clin Orthop 189:195–203, 1984.
12. Gurr K, McAfee P: Cotrel-Dubousset instrumentation in adults. Spine 13:510–520, 1988.
13. Jacobs RR, Nordwall A, Nachemson A: Reduction, stability, and strength provided by internal fixation systems for thoracolumbar spinal injuries. Clin Orthop 171:300–308, 1982.
14. Kahn A: Current concepts of internal fixation. In Dunsker SB, Schmidek HH, Frymoyer J, Kahn A III (eds): The Unstable Spine. Orlando, Grune & Stratton, 1986, pp 45–83.
15. Kaneda K, Abumi K, Fujiya M: Burst fractures of the thoracolumbar and lumbar spine with neurologic involvement—Anterior decompression and fusion with instrumentation. Orthop Trans 7:16, 1983.
16. Kostuik JP: Anterior fixation for fractures of the thoracic and lumbar spine with and without neurologic involvement. Clin Orthop 189:103–115, 1984.
17. Krag M, Beynnon B, Pope M, et al: An internal fixator for posterior application to short segments of the thoracic, lumbar, or lumbosacral spine. Clin Orthop 203:75–98, 1986.
18. Larson SJ: Unstable thoracic fractures: Treatment alternatives and the role of the neurosurgeons. Clin Neurosurg 27:624–640, 1980.
19. Lesion F, Mathevon H, Villete L, et al: Use of universal instrumentation in the dorso-lumbar spine pathology. AANS/CNS Joint Section on Spinal Disorders Abstract, 2:13, 1986.
20. Luque ER: The anatomic basis and development of segmental spinal instrumentation. Spine 7:256–259, 1986.
21. Macedo N, Sundaresan N, Galicich JH: Decompressive laminectomy for metastatic cancer: What are the current indications? Proc Am Soc Am Oncol 4:278, 1985.
22. McAfee PC, Bohlman HH: Complications of Harrington

instrumentation for fractures of the thoracolumbar spine. A ten-year experience. J Bone Joint Surg 67A:672–686, 1985.

23. McAfee PC, Bohlman HH, Yuan HA: Anterior decompression of traumatic thoracolumbar fractures with incomplete neurological deficit using a retroperitoneal approach. J Bone Joint Surg 67A:89–104, 1985.

24. Munson G, Satterlee C, Hammond S, et al: Experimental evaluation of Harrington rod fixation supplemented with sublaminar wires in stabilizing thoracolumbar fracture-dislocations. Clin Orthop 189:97–102, 1984.

25. Murphey MJ, Southwick WO, Ogden JA: Treatment of the unstable thoracolumbar spine with combination Harrington distraction and compression rods. Orthop Trans 6:9, 1982.

26. Overby MC, Rothman AS: Anterolateral decompression for metastatic epidural spinal cord tumors. J Neurosurg 62:344, 1985.

27. Panjabi M, Hopper W, White A, et al: Posterior stabilization with methylmethacrylate. Spine 2:241–244, 1977.

28. Perrin R, Livingston K: Neurosurgical treatment of pathologic fracture-dislocation of the spine. J Neurosurg 52:330–334, 1980.

29. Roy-Camille R, Saillant G, Mazel C: Plating of thoracic, thoracolumbar, and lumbar injuries with pedicle screw plates. Orthop Clin North Am 17:147–159, 1986.

30. Siegel T, Tikva P, Siegel T: Vertebral body resection for epidural compression by malignant tumors. J Bone Joint Surg 67A:375, 1985.

31. Shufflebarger H, Clark C: Cotrel-Dubousset instrumentation. Orthopaedics 11:1435–1440, 1988.

32. Steffee A, Biscup R, Sitkowski D: Segmental spine plates with pedicle screw fixation. Clin Orthop 203:45–53, 1986.

33. Sundaresan N, DiGiancinto GB, Hughes JEO: Surgical treatment of spinal metastases. Clin Neurosurg 33:503, 1986.

34. Sundaresan N, Galicich J, Lane J: Harrington rod stabilization for pathological fractures of the spine. J Neurosurg 60:282–286, 1984.

35. Sundaresan N, Galicich JH, Lane JM, et al: Treatment of neoplastic epidural cord compression by vertebral body resection and stabilization. J Neurosurg 63:676, 1985.

36. Walters CL, Schmidek HH, Krag MH, et al: The management of thoracolumbar fractures. In Dunsker SB, Schmidek H, Frymoyer J, Kahn A III (eds): The Unstable Spine. Orlando, Grune & Stratton, 1986, pp 221–248.

37. White A III, Panjabi MM: Clinical Biomechanics of the Spine. Philadelphia, JB Lippincott, 1978.

INDEX

Note: Page numbers in *italics* refer to illustrations; page numbers followed by (t) refer to tables.